Clinical Dentistry

Clinical Dentistry

Edited by **Kaley Ann**

hayle medical

New York

Published by Hayle Medical,
30 West, 37th Street, Suite 612,
New York, NY 10018, USA
www.haylemedical.com

Clinical Dentistry
Edited by Kaley Ann

International Standard Book Number: 978-1-63241-401-4 (Hardback)

The publisher's policy is to use permanent paper from mills that operate a sustainable forestry policy. Furthermore, the publisher ensures that the text paper and cover boards used have met acceptable environmental accreditation standards.

Trademark Notice: Registered trademark of products or corporate names are used only for explanation and identification without intent to infringe.

Printed in the United States of America.

Contents

Preface

I am honored to present to you this unique book which encompasses the most up-to-date data in the field. I was extremely pleased to get this opportunity of editing the work of experts from across the globe. I have also written papers in this field and researched the various aspects revolving around the progress of the discipline. I have tried to unify my knowledge along with that of stalwarts from every corner of the world, to produce a text which not only benefits the readers but also facilitates the growth of the field.

Many people suffer dental problems these days, this is where clinical dentistry comes into play. It deals with the prevention, diagnosis and treatment of oral problems. It has progressed with the help of specialized alloys and biomaterials. There are different specialties available in this field such as endodontics, forensic odontology, geriatric dentistry, oral medicine periodontology, etc. This book elucidates new techniques and their applications in the area of clinical dentistry. The topics included in this book are of utmost importance and bound to provide incredible insights to readers. It will serve as a valuable source of reference for graduates, postgraduates as well as professionals.

Finally, I would like to thank all the contributing authors for their valuable time and contributions. This book would not have been possible without their efforts. I would also like to thank my friends and family for their constant support.

Editor

Oral Lesions Induced by Chronic Khat Use Consist Essentially of Thickened Hyperkeratinized Epithelium

Ochiba Mohammed Lukandu,[1] **Lionel Sang Koech,**[1] **and Paul Ngugi Kiarie**[2]

[1]*Department of Maxillofacial Surgery, Oral Medicine, Pathology and Radiology, School of Dentistry, Moi University, P.O. Box 4606, Eldoret 30100, Kenya*
[2]*Department of Oral Biology, Anatomy, Physiology and Biochemistry, School of Dentistry, Moi University, P.O. Box 4606, Eldoret 30100, Kenya*

Correspondence should be addressed to Ochiba Mohammed Lukandu; ochiba.lukandu@gmail.com

Academic Editor: Adriano Loyola

Objectives. The habit of khat chewing is prevalent in many Middle Eastern and African cultures and has been associated with various adverse conditions in humans. This study aimed to describe histological changes induced by chronic khat chewing on the buccal mucosa. *Methods.* Biopsies of the buccal mucosa from 14 chronic khat chewers, 20 chronic khat chewers who also smoked tobacco, and 8 nonchewers were compared for epithelial thickness, degree and type of keratinization, and connective tissue changes. *Results.* Tissues from khat chewers depicted abnormal keratinization of the superficial cell layer and showed increased epithelial thickness affecting all layers. Epithelial thickness in control samples was $205 \pm 26\,\mu$m whereas thickness in khat chewers and khat chewers who smoked tobacco was significantly higher measuring $330 \pm 35\,\mu$m and $335 \pm 19\,\mu$m, respectively. Tissues from khat chewers also showed increased intracellular edema, increased melanin pigment deposits, and increased number of rete pegs most of which were thin and deep. *Conclusions.* These results show that oral lesions induced by chronic chewing of khat in the buccal mucosa present with white and brown discoloration due to increased epithelial thickness, increased keratinization, and melanin deposition.

1. Introduction

Khat is an evergreen plant grown in the regions around the horn of Africa and the Southern Arabian Peninsula. Fresh leaves and shoots of the khat plant contain an alkaloid chemical known as cathinone which has psychoactive effects comparable to amphetamine. Since the 13th century [1], populations in these regions have engaged in the habit of chewing khat leaves and shoots as a mood altering drug. In countries such as Yemen, up to 90% of adult males and more than half of adult females are estimated to chew khat for between three and four hours daily [1, 2]. Currently, the habit is spreading to other parts of the world where users are predominantly immigrants from countries where khat use is widespread [2].

The habit of chewing khat is associated with adverse effects in various body systems [3]. It has been reported through evidence from animal studies that khat decreases the systemic capacity of the body to handle reactive oxygen species [4] and therefore has potential to cause damage to cells and tissues. During chewing sessions, large amounts of khat leaves, shoots, and barks are placed in the oral cavity and chewed while being kept in the vestibule in close contact with the buccal mucosa [5]. The khat bolus is chewed gradually and continuously for 2 to 10 hours. On average, 100–500 g of khat is chewed by chronic users per day [6]. Over 90 percent of the alkaloid content of khat is extracted into saliva during chewing and most of it is absorbed through the oral mucosa [7]. Therefore, oral tissues, especially the oral mucosa, are exposed to high doses of khat constituents during khat chewing rendering them susceptible to its potentially toxic effects.

Previous studies have reported various detrimental effects of khat on oral tissues [8]. These effects include various forms

TABLE 1: Standardized criteria used to identify and to take biopsy of khat induced oral lesions.

Parameter	Criteria
Site of lesion	Normally limited to buccal mucosa where khat bolus is placed during chewing, around and especially below (inferior to) the *linea alba*. Most adjacent areas of buccal mucosa remain relatively normal and clearly distinguishable from oral white lesion. Could involve the lateral border of tongue and the gum. Usually does not involve the palate.
Texture	Lesion could be smooth, wrinkled, rough, or plaque-like.
Colour	Mostly white, but could be grey, black, or brown. A mixture of any of these colours could occur. Though rare, it could have red areas within it.
Side of the lesion	On the side identified as the chewing side.
Biopsy taking	Only from buccal mucosa. Biopsy an oval tissue of not more than 1 cm long and not less than 0.3 mm width. Preferably below the *linea alba*, or choose the centre of the lesion on buccal mucosa.

of periodontal disease, mucosal pigmentation, dental caries, tooth wear, and dental staining [9]. Khat is genotoxic to cells of the oral mucosa [10] and has been associated with oral keratotic white lesions which occur in the same region within the vestibule or buccal mucosa where the khat bolus is placed while chewing [11–13]. Some of these lesions have been reported to show histopathological changes like acanthosis, hyperkeratosis, and mild dysplasia [11]. According to some previous studies, the risk for developing these lesions is especially high among khat chewers who also use tobacco products [14]. In another study, khat chewing was found to be a risk factor for developing cellular atypia, in addition to hyperkeratosis and subepithelial infiltration by chronic inflammatory cells [15].

Even though some studies have found a higher incidence of head and neck cancer in khat chewers compared to nonchewers [16, 17], lesions induced by khat have not been considered potentially malignant [18, 19]. Due to the relatively small number of studies on khat [20] and the methodological weaknesses of studies already carried out [19, 21], there is currently no consensus as to whether khat chewing is a potential risk factor for development of oral cancer [21]. A useful point to start in understanding this potential risk would be to have a detailed clinical and microscopic analysis of oral white lesions induced by chronic khat use. This study therefore sought to describe histopathological features induced by khat when used alone and when used alongside tobacco within the oral mucosa of the chronic khat chewers.

2. Materials and Methods

2.1. Study Subjects. The use of human subjects in this study was reviewed and approved by the regional Institutional Research and Ethics Committee (IREC) (approval number 000985). A public call by study assistants for volunteers to participate in the study was made in Eldoret and Meru towns of Kenya, and those willing to participate were requested to visit specified dental clinics for screening. The study was conducted on 42 volunteers who met the inclusion criteria for the study and for biopsy procedures. All participants were

informed of the purpose of the study and were requested to sign consent forms.

Those included in the study as cases were khat chewers who had used khat for more than 5 years (chronic chewers) and who also had clinically detectable pathological oral white lesions based on common protocol/criteria (Table 1). All participants who eventually participated in the study were male, even though this was not a requirement. The study subjects were divided into three groups: (1) a group of 8 volunteers who were neither tobacco smokers nor khat chewers, (2) a study group of 14 volunteers who were chronic khat chewers but nonsmokers, and (3) a second study group of 20 volunteers who were both chronic khat chewers and tobacco smokers. The first group was the control group and consisted of clinically healthy adult male volunteers undergoing surgical removal of wisdom teeth.

2.2. Clinical Procedures. All participants were first subjected to a short interviewer administered questionnaire designed to collect biographic data and information related to khat use, tobacco use, and alcohol drinking. The participants were then subjected to a clinical oral examination on a dental chair with adequate lighting with specific focus on the appearance of their oral mucosa. Clinical images of the buccal mucosa showing the oral lesions were taken prior to biopsy procedures. Control patients were requested to participate in the study by allowing a small piece of buccal mucosal tissue to be biopsied from the incision line during surgical removal of impacted wisdom teeth. For khat chewers, the biopsies were taken from the buccal mucosa at specifically selected sites that were deemed most affected by the habit of khat chewing. The predesigned criteria (Table 1) for oral lesions induced by chronic khat use were used to ensure consistency in the choice of the most affected sites for the purpose of biopsy.

Local anesthesia was achieved through a long buccal nerve block on the side identified for the biopsy. Care was taken to administer the injection away from the site of the biopsy to avoid damage to the tissue. Tissue at the biopsy site was secured and gently retracted using a suture with only one loose knot. An ovoid tissue specimen of about 4 by

8 mm was then excised using a surgical blade. All biopsy specimens were immediately placed in adequate amounts of 4% buffered formalin (pH 7.2) and forwarded to the laboratory for histopathological assessment. Bleeding was controlled by applying pressure and the same suture was then used to stitch and close the wound at the site of the biopsy.

2.3. Tissue Preparation, Staining, and Histopathological Assessment. The tissues were fixed for 48 h at room temperature in 4% buffered formalin. Biopsy specimens were grossed and taken through routine procedures for formalin fixed paraffin embedded preparations. Briefly, the formalin fixed tissues were washed in more formalin solution to remove any loose debris and then dehydrated through a series of graded alcohol solutions (70%, 90%, 100%, 100%, and 100% ethanol 1 h each) and then through three changes of xylene for 1 h each. The tissues were then incubated overnight at 65°C in Paraplast Plus paraffin (Thermo Fisher Scientific) before embedding. The blocks were stored at room temperature for four weeks prior to sectioning.

The tissue blocks were sectioned at 5 μm thickness and placed on glass slides. The slides were dewaxed by placing them in a slide holder and taking them through xylene for 20 min with gentle agitation. The slides were then rehydrated by placing them in graded alcohol (100%, 100%, 90%, and 70% ethanol for 3 min each) and then gently in running tap water. The tissues were stained by placing them in Harris haematoxylin (Sigma Aldrich, Darmstadt, Germany) for 10 minutes. They were then washed slowly in running water and gently distained (using 1% HCl in 95% ethanol), rinsed again in running tap water for 5 min, then placed in Scott's tap water (bluing solution) (Leica Biosystems GmbH, Wetzlar, Germany) for 3 min, and then stained in eosin (Sigma Aldrich, Darmstadt, Germany) for 2 min. The tissues were then dehydrated in graded alcohol (70%, 90%, 100%, 100%, and 100% ethanol 5 h each) and then cleared in three changes of xylene for 5 min each and mounted using Permount mounting medium (Fisher Scientific, Fair Lawn, NJ, USA). Upon drying, the hematoxylin-eosin stained slides were examined under light microscopy.

Histological comparisons between samples from the three groups were made for structural tissue changes such as differentiation patterns, degree and type of keratinization, morphology and number of rete pegs, and connective tissue changes. Histological images were captured using the LASEZ Leica Application Suite EZ software under the Leica DM 750 microscope (Leica Microsystems GmbH, Wetzlar, Germany). Histomorphometric analysis of tissue sections was by computer based digital image analysis software (DinoCapture 2.0) using the DinoEye AM4023 digital eyepiece camera (AnMo Electronics Corporation, Taipei, Taiwan) connected to a computer via USB. Analysis of all tissue sections was done at similar settings at 200-fold magnification under an Olympus CX31 light microscope (Olympus Corporation, Tokyo, Japan).

For comparative histomorphometry, the epithelium was divided into four main components: rete pegs, basal cell layer, spinous cell layer, and superficial cell layer (Figure 1). The superficial cell layer was further subdivided into keratinized

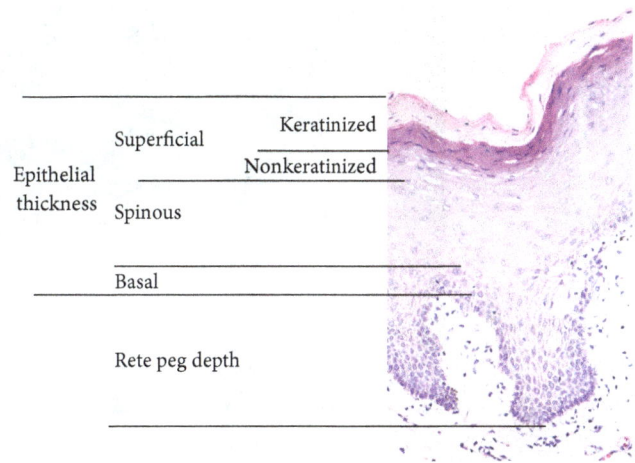

FIGURE 1: Histological preparation of one of the study samples at 200-fold magnification under light microscopy showing how the epithelium was divided into four main components for histomorphometric analysis. Thickness of the various sections was determined by drawing arbitrary lines running vertically and reading off the length/depth as was indicated by the software.

and nonkeratinized components. Thickness of the various sections was determined by drawing arbitrary lines running vertically and reading off the length/depth as was indicated by the software. The layers were assessed for their thickness and compared with each other and with the total thickness of the epithelium.

2.4. Statistical Analysis. Data analysis and generation of figures were done using Sigma Plot software version 12.5 (Systat Software, Inc., San Jose, CA, USA). Data sets from the three groups were first subjected to Shapiro-Wilk normality test and then compared using one-way analysis of variance (ANOVA) or Kruskal Wallis Test. This was followed by multiple comparisons using either the Holm-Sidak or Dunn's methods as appropriate to determine the levels of significance between specific groups. p values less than 0.05 were considered significant. Data were presented as means $\pm$ standard error of the means.

3. Results

3.1. Characteristics of the Study Subjects. The control group of 8 volunteers had a mean age of 28.9 years (range 25 to 37). The first study group of 14 volunteers had a mean age of 33.6 years (range 21 to 52) whereas the second study group of 20 volunteers had a mean age of 39.8 years (range 25 to 55). All selected participants were chronic khat chewers who had used khat for more than 5 years. The only method of tobacco use reported was smoking. Seven (35%) of the smokers had smoked tobacco for less than ten years and the remainder (65%) had smoked for less than 10 years. Four (20%) of the smokers reported that they used 1 cigarette per day, 8 (40%) of them used between 1 and 10 cigarettes per day, 3 (15%) of them used between 1 and 10 cigarettes per day, and the rest (25%) of the smokers used over 20 cigarettes per day.

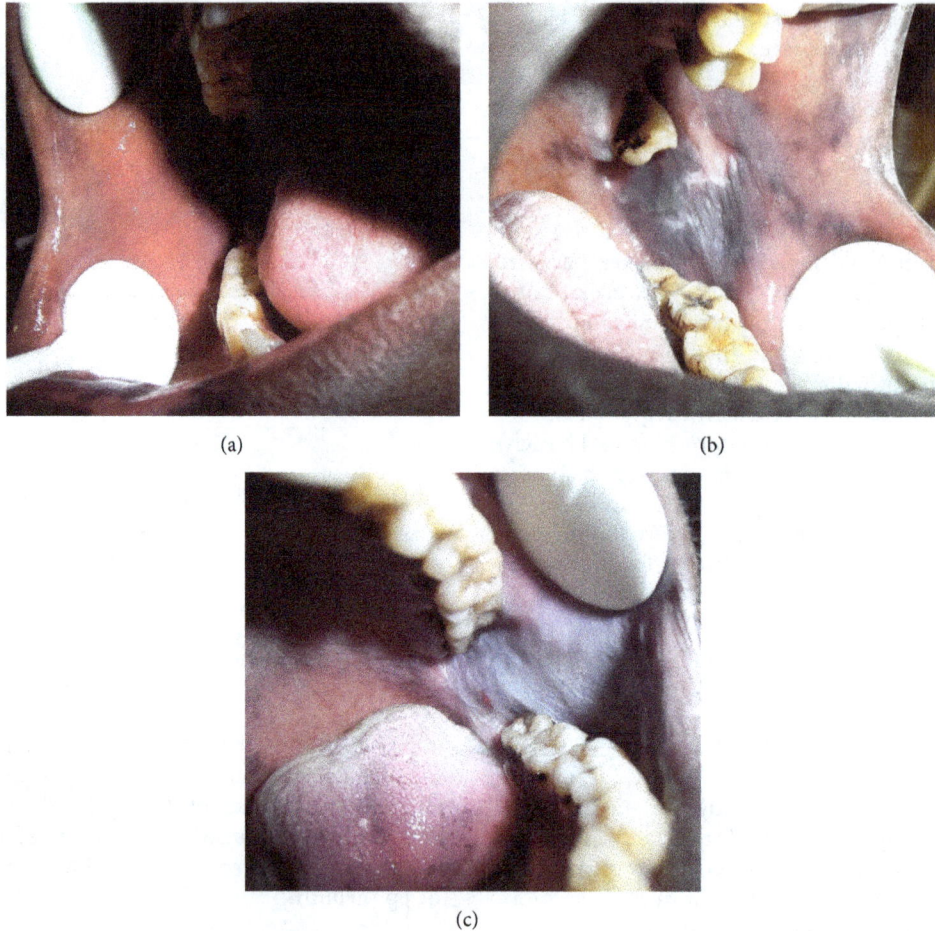

(a)

(b)

(c)

FIGURE 2: Clinical photographs of the buccal mucosa of some of the study participants. (a) Nonchewer (control), (b) a chronic khat chewer, and (c) a chronic khat chewer who was also a heavy smoker.

In the analysis of age differences between the study groups, there was a statistically significant difference in the ages of the control group and the second study group composed of khat chewers who also smoked tobacco. Other than the two habits and the difference in the ages of the control group and the second study group, there were no other differences in health or behavioral characteristics in these groups.

3.2. Tissues from Khat Chewers Showed Abnormal Intracellular Edema and Keratinization. Clinically, khat induced lesions showed varied degrees of white and brown discoloration (Figure 2). Microscopic evaluation of the samples revealed marked acanthosis and an increase in cells showing intracellular edema in the spinous cell layer of tissue samples from khat chewers (Figures 3(b) and 3(c)) when compared to those from nonchewers (Figure 3(a)). Among khat chewers, 75% of those who smoked tobacco showed abnormal intracellular edema compared to only 14% in nonsmokers and 13% in controls (Table 2). Histopathological evaluation showed that superficial layers in samples from chronic khat chewers were keratinized while control samples were nonkeratinized. Only two of the eight samples (26%) from nonchewers showed a keratinized superficial cell layer compared to 71% of samples

from khat chewers and 75% of samples from khat chewers who smoked tobacco (Table 2). The type of keratinization varied from parakeratinization (Figure 3(e)) in most samples to orthokeratinization in a few samples (Figure 3(f)). In some orthokeratinized samples, cells of the deeper section of the superficial cell layer contained keratohyalin granules and resembled the granular cell layer of skin tissue. Both types of keratinization were seen in chronic khat chewers as well as in chronic khat chewers who smoked tobacco with no differences noted in this regard between the two groups. Epithelial dysplasia was not seen in any of the biopsies studied.

3.3. Tissues from Khat Chewers Showed Increased Epithelial Thickness. Total epithelial thickness and thickness of various epithelial layers in samples from khat chewers were markedly increased when compared to samples from nonchewers (Figure 4). Epithelial thickness in control samples was found to be $205 \pm 26\,\mu$m whereas thickness in khat chewers and khat chewers who smoked tobacco was significantly higher measuring $330 \pm 35\,\mu$m and $335 \pm 19\,\mu$m, respectively ($p < 0.05$). The basal cell layer in control samples measured $16 \pm 2\,\mu$m whereas its thickness in khat chewers and khat chewers who smoked tobacco was significantly higher measuring

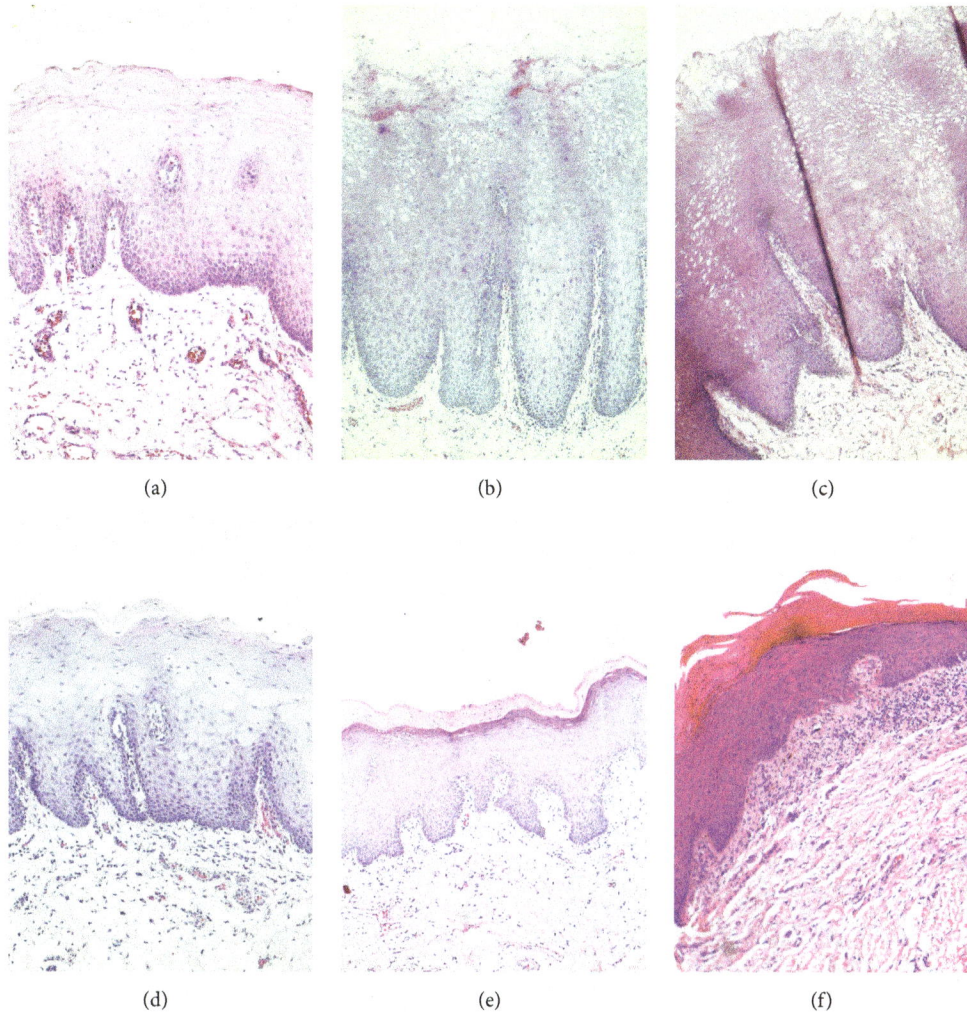

FIGURE 3: Histological preparations of biopsies from a nonchewer (a) and khat chewers. Acanthosis and intracellular edema are seen both in a smoker (b) and a nonsmoker (c). Varying degrees of keratinization are seen in samples from a mild khat chewer (d), a heavy khat chewer (e), and a heavy khat chewer who also smoked tobacco (magnification ×200). There were no histological differences between smokers and nonsmokers.

$26 \pm 3\,\mu$m and $32 \pm 3\,\mu$m, respectively. The thickness of the spinous cell layer in nonchewers, khat chewers, and khat chewers who smoked tobacco was $113 \pm 23\,\mu$m, $195 \pm 28\,\mu$m, and $169 \pm 11\,\mu$m, respectively ($p < 0.05$). For the superficial cell layer, the thickness was $50\pm5\,\mu$m, $81\pm8\,\mu$m, and $79\pm7\,\mu$m in nonchewers, khat chewers, and khat chewers who smoked tobacco, respectively ($p < 0.05$). Even though the overall epithelial thickness and the thickness of constituent layers showed marked increase in tissues from khat chewers, the proportion of each layer relative to total epithelial thickness remained unchanged in all the groups measuring about 10%, 63%, and 27% for the basal, spinous, and superficial layers, respectively (Table 2).

The keratinized component of the superficial cell layer in nonchewers, khat chewers, and khat chewers who smoked tobacco was $1\pm0.5\,\mu$m, $34\pm7\,\mu$m, and $31\pm6\,\mu$m, respectively ($p < 0.01$) (Figure 4(e)). Whereas less than 1% of the superficial cell layer in control samples was keratinized, the proportion of superficial cell layer that was keratinized in khat chewers and khat chewers who smoked tobacco was 36.8% and 33.6%, respectively ($p < 0.01$). There was an increase in number of rete pegs per $100\,\mu$m horizontally from 6.1 ± 0.4 in controls to 9.5 ± 0.8 and 7.8 ± 0.5 in khat chewers and khat chewers who smoked tobacco, respectively ($p < 0.01$). The rete pegs in khat chewers also appeared thinner and longer particularly among khat chewers who smoked tobacco. The differences noted between the groups with regard to number of abnormally shaped rete pegs were not significant (Table 2).

3.4. Abnormal Connective Tissue Changes in Tissues from Khat Chewers. Within the submucosa, an increase in the amount of collagen fibres (fibrosis) was noted in one control sample (13%), in four samples from khat chewers (29%), and in 7 samples among khat chewers who smoked tobacco (35%) (Table 1). Vessels within the submucosa of khat chewers were noted to be increased in number and were also more tortuous. There were deposits of melanin pigment and aggregates of melanophages scattered within the subepithelial

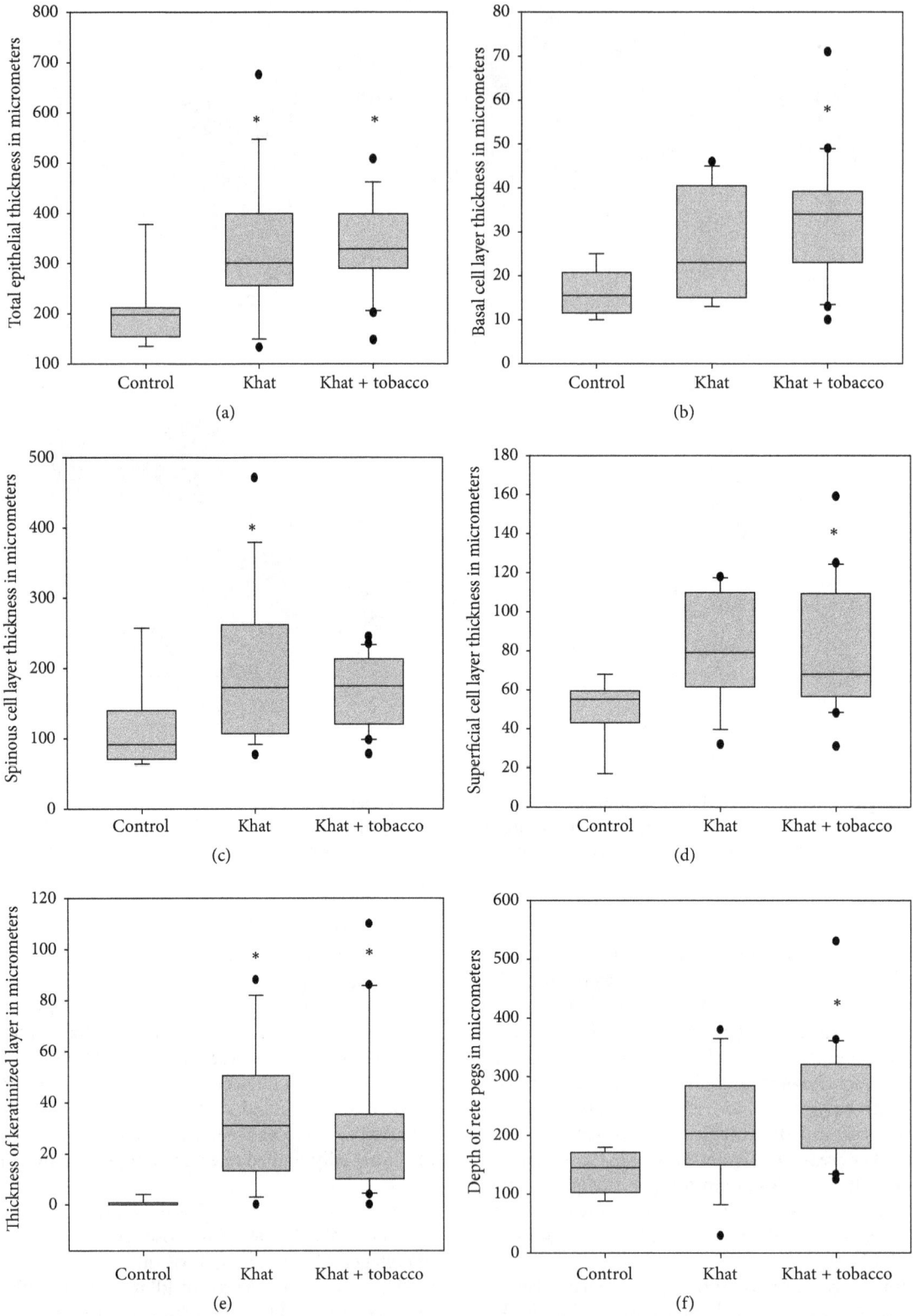

FIGURE 4: Analysis of the thickness of the buccal epithelium in controls and in study groups. Asterisk ($*$) shows statistically significant differences ($p < 0.05$) between study groups when compared to the control after multiple comparisons.

TABLE 2: Analysis of histological changes in the buccal mucosa.

| | Nonchewers ($n = 8$) | Khat chewers ($n = 34$) | | p value |
		Nonsmokers ($n = 14$)	Smokers ($n = 20$)	
Samples with fibrosis (%)	13	29	35	—
Samples with intracellular edema (%)	13	14	75	—
Samples with keratinization (%)	26	71	95	—
Percentage of superficial layer keratinized	0.7 ± 0.3	36.8 ± 8.8	33.6 ± 6.2	$p < 0.01$
Number of rete pegs/100 μm	6.1 ± 0.4	9.5 ± 0.8	7.8 ± 0.5	$p < 0.01$
Abnormally shaped rete pegs (%)	8.1 ± 2.8	9.8 ± 0.4	14.2 ± 2.4	$p > 0.05$
Rete peg depth as % of whole thickness	38.3 ± 3.0	34.8 ± 3.7	42.6 ± 2.7	$p < 0.01$
Proportion of basal cell layer (%)	8.9 ± 0.2	8.6 ± 0.5	11.4 ± 0.4	$p > 0.05$
Proportion of spinous cell layer (%)	61.3 ± 4.4	64.6 ± 4.6	60.4 ± 5.5	$p > 0.05$
Proportion of superficial cell layer (%)	27.9 ± 3.4	26.8 ± 6.3	28.2 ± 3.4	$p > 0.05$

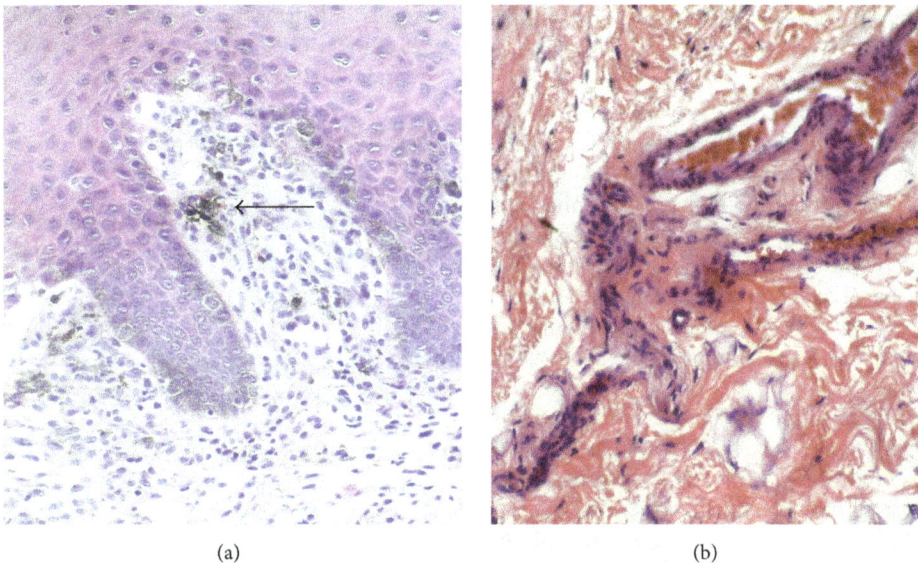

(a)   (b)

FIGURE 5: Connective tissue features in khat induced oral lesions. (a) Melanin pigment (arrow). (b) Fibrosis and tortuous blood vessels in the submucosa of chronic khat chewers.

area (Figure 5) and melanin was also seen within basal keratinocytes. A few samples from khat chewers also showed abnormal subepithelial infiltration of chronic inflammatory cells (Figure 3(f)) particularly lymphocytes. No differences were noted with regard to connective tissue changes between samples from khat chewers and khat chewers who smoked tobacco.

4. Discussion

This study compared histopathological changes in biopsies of the buccal mucosa from volunteers who have never chewed khat (controls), chronic khat chewers, and chronic khat chewers who smoked tobacco. Chronicity in khat chewing especially in relation to induction of oral keratotic lesions has previously been defined as a period of khat use exceeding 2 years as well as a high frequency of khat use, but not necessarily the amount of khat consumed per sitting [11, 14, 18]. Biopsies were taken from the most affected site on the buccal

mucosa on clinical evaluation, which always coincided with the buccal mucosa on side of the mouth identified by the patient as the chewing side.

The buccal epithelium is normally nonkeratinizing, and this is consistent with what was observed in tissue samples from nonchewers in this study. However, epithelial tissues from khat chewers were found to be keratinized, with some tissues depicting orthokeratinization and formation of a layer similar to the granular cell layer of skin tissue. These findings are similar to those described in previous clinical studies [14, 18] and one laboratory study in organotypic models of oral mucosa [22]. According to our findings, less than 1% of the superficial cell layer in control samples was keratinized. However, the proportion of the superficial cell layer that was keratinized in khat chewers and khat chewers who smoked tobacco accounted for more than one-third of the thickness of that particular layer. To the best of our knowledge, no previous study has attempted to quantify in this manner the degree of keratinization in the buccal epithelium of chronic khat users in comparison to that from nonchewers. This study did not find any differences in the degree and type of keratinization between khat chewers and khat chewers who smoked tobacco, suggesting that concomitant use of tobacco has only a limited effect on overall appearance.

Normal thickness of epithelium of the oral mucosa varies depending on the site. The thickest epithelium is found in the buccal mucosa where it measures approximately 290 μm [23]. In this study, epithelial thickness in khat chewers was significantly increased in general as well as in specific cell layers of the epithelium when compared to nonchewers. There were pronounced acanthosis and marked intracellular edema particularly in khat chewers who also smoked tobacco. These findings agree with those from a previous study that demonstrated acanthosis and intracellular edema as key features of khat induced mucosal changes [18]. However, contrary to what was observed in organotypic models of oral mucosa [22], the proportion of each of the layers relative to total thickness remained unchanged in all the groups and measured about 10%, 63%, and 27% for the basal, spinous, and superficial layers, respectively. The difference between our findings here and those described within *in vitro* organotypic models could be explained by the abundance of cells with stem-cell properties within *in vivo* epithelium that ensure enhanced compensatory responses leading to epithelial hyperplasia. This view is supported by the observed proportional increase in the thickness of the basal cell layer which suggests a higher capacity of the oral epithelium to replenish itself and to mount compensatory responses when compared to *in vitro* organotypic epithelium.

A point worth noting in this study is that no evidence of dysplasia was observed in any of the tissue samples studied. This is contrary to findings of a previous study [14] in which over 35% of the biopsies from the khat chewers who used tobacco were found to have dysplastic changes, particularly samples taken from the chewing side. Another study by the same author showed that the dysplastic changes were mild and the lesions could not be considered potentially malignant lesions [18]. Khat chewing has also been found to be a risk factor for developing cellular atypia as shown in a cytological assessment of buccal mucosa in chronic chewers [15]. In our view, the differences in the findings in these studies could be due to variations in chronicity of the khat chewing habit among participants in the different studies. The degree of tobacco use and the method of tobacco use among khat chewers in the different studies could also contribute to the observed differences.

Our study found a high concentration of melanin in basal keratinocytes and presence of scattered melanophages and melanin pigment in the submucosa of tissue samples of khat chewers. A higher proportion of tissues from khat chewers also showed fibrosis and many tortuous blood vessels as well as chronic inflammatory cell infiltrate. In this study, correlation between amounts of khat chewed and degree of pathological changes could not be determined due to the fact that we studied only one group (chronic khat chewers) and within group patterns were not detectable and were not presented in the results. There was also a limitation with regard to sample size due to the difficulty in finding volunteers willing to undergo biopsy procedures. There is a need for larger studies with four or more study groups of varying chronicity and khat consumption levels to enable correlation studies.

5. Conclusion

The findings of this study identify acanthosis, intracellular edema, hyperkeratosis, and fibrosis as key histological features of oral lesions induced by chronic chewing of khat. In addition, the study highlights key structural changes for specific layers of the epithelium and identifies increased melanin production as another factor contributing to the overall discoloration of the buccal mucosa in chronic khat chewers. From our findings, it appears that concomitant smoking has only limited effect on the clinical and histological appearance of khat induced oral lesions. As has been suggested before, and in view of the diverse histological and clinical presentation of these lesions, both physical and chemical factors are likely to play a role in their etiology.

Conflict of Interests

The authors declare that there is no conflict of interests regarding the publication of this paper and that there was no other funding for this work besides that from their institution.

Acknowledgments

The authors thank the staff at the Moi University School of Dentistry and Meru District Hospital for their assistance in clinical procedures and the histopathology laboratory staff at Moi Teaching and Referral Hospital for their technical support. This study was funded by Moi University through the Graduate Studies Research and Extension Committee.

References

[1] A. El-Menyar, A. Mekkodathil, H. Al-Thani, and A. Al-Motarreb, "Khat use: history and heart failure," *Oman Medical Journal*, vol. 30, no. 2, pp. 77–82, 2015.

[2] K. A. Sheikh, M. El-setouhy, U. Yagoub, R. Alsanosy, and Z. Ahmed, "Khat chewing and health related quality of life: cross-sectional study in Jazan region, Kingdom of Saudi Arabia," *Health and Quality of Life Outcomes*, vol. 12, no. 1, article 44, 2014.

[3] M. Al-Habori, "The potential adverse effects of habitual use of *Catha edulis* (khat)," *Expert Opinion on Drug Safety*, vol. 4, no. 6, pp. 1145–1154, 2005.

[4] T. M. Al-Qirim, M. Shahwan, K. R. Zaidi, Q. Uddin, and N. Banu, "Effect of khat, its constituents and restraint stress on free radical metabolism of rats," *Journal of Ethnopharmacology*, vol. 83, no. 3, pp. 245–250, 2002.

[5] F. A. Sawair, A. Al-Mutwakel, K. Al-Eryani et al., "High relative frequency of oral squamous cell carcinoma in Yemen: qat and tobacco chewing as its aetiological background," *International Journal of Environmental Health Research*, vol. 17, no. 3, pp. 185–195, 2007.

[6] A. M. Feyissa and J. P. Kelly, "A review of the neuropharmacological properties of khat," *Progress in Neuro-Psychopharmacology and Biological Psychiatry*, vol. 32, no. 5, pp. 1147–1166, 2008.

[7] S. W. Toennes, S. Harder, M. Schramm, C. Niess, and G. F. Kauert, "Pharmacokinetics of cathinone, cathine and norephedrine after the chewing of khat leaves," *British Journal of Clinical Pharmacology*, vol. 56, no. 1, pp. 125–130, 2003.

[8] A. Astatkie, M. Demissie, Y. Berhane, and A. Worku, "Oral symptoms significantly higher among long-term khat (*Catha edulis*) user university students in Ethiopia," *Epidemiology and Health*, vol. 37, Article ID e2015009, 2015.

[9] A. A. Ali, "Qat Habit in Yemen society: a causative factor for oral periodontal diseases," *International Journal of Environmental Research and Public Health*, vol. 4, no. 3, pp. 243–247, 2007.

[10] F. Kassie, F. Darroudi, M. Kundi, R. Schulte-Hermann, and S. Knasmüller, "Khat (*Catha edulis*) consumption causes genotoxic effects in humans," *International Journal of Cancer*, vol. 92, no. 3, pp. 329–332, 2001.

[11] A. A. Ali, A. K. Al-Sharabi, J. M. Aguirre, and R. Nahas, "A study of 342 oral keratotic white lesions induced by qat chewing among 2500 Yemeni," *Journal of Oral Pathology and Medicine*, vol. 33, no. 6, pp. 368–372, 2004.

[12] M. Gorsky, J. B. Epstein, H. Levi, and N. Yarom, "Oral white lesions associated with chewing khat," *Tobacco Induced Diseases*, vol. 2, no. 3, pp. 145–150, 2004.

[13] N. Yarom, J. Epstein, H. Levi, D. Porat, E. Kaufman, and M. Gorsky, "Oral manifestations of habitual khat chewing: a case-control study," *Oral Surgery, Oral Medicine, Oral Pathology, Oral Radiology and Endodontology*, vol. 109, no. 6, pp. e60–e66, 2010.

[14] A. A. Ali, "Histopathologic changes in oral mucosa of Yemenis addicted to water-pipe and cigarette smoking in addition to takhzeen al-qat," *Oral Surgery, Oral Medicine, Oral Pathology, Oral Radiology and Endodontology*, vol. 103, no. 3, pp. e55–e59, 2007.

[15] H. G. E. Ahmed, A. S. A. Omer, and S. A. Abd Algaffar, "Cytological study of exfoliative buccal mucosal cells of Qat chewers in Yemen," *Diagnostic Cytopathology*, vol. 39, no. 11, pp. 796–800, 2011.

[16] H. E. Soufi, M. Kameswaran, and T. Malatani, "Khat and oral cancer," *Journal of Laryngology and Otology*, vol. 105, no. 8, pp. 643–645, 1991.

[17] A. H. Nasr and M. L. Khatri, "Head and neck squamous cell carcinoma in Hajjah, Yemen," *Saudi Medical Journal*, vol. 21, no. 6, pp. 565–568, 2000.

[18] A. A. Ali, A. K. Al-Sharabi, and J. M. Aguirre, "Histopathological changes in oral mucosa due to takhzeen al-qat: a study of 70 biopsies," *Journal of Oral Pathology and Medicine*, vol. 35, no. 2, pp. 81–85, 2006.

[19] E. Stucken, J. Weissman, and J. H. Spiegel, "Oral cavity risk factors: experts' opinions and literature support," *Journal of Otolaryngology—Head & Neck Surgery*, vol. 39, no. 1, pp. 76–89, 2010.

[20] F. Carvalho, "The toxicological potential of khat," *Journal of Ethnopharmacology*, vol. 87, no. 1, pp. 1–2, 2003.

[21] N. N. Al-Hebshi and N. Skaug, "Khat (*Catha edulis*)—an updated review," *Addiction Biology*, vol. 10, no. 4, pp. 299–307, 2005.

[22] O. M. Lukandu, E. Neppelberg, O. K. Vintermyr, A. C. Johannessen, and D. E. Costea, "Khat alters the phenotype of *in vitro*-reconstructed human oral mucosa," *Journal of Dental Research*, vol. 89, no. 3, pp. 270–275, 2010.

[23] S. Prestin, S. I. Rothschild, C. S. Betz, and M. Kraft, "Measurement of epithelial thickness within the oral cavity using optical coherence tomography," *Head and Neck*, vol. 34, no. 12, pp. 1777–1781, 2012.

Effect of EDTA Conditioning and Carbodiimide Pretreatment on the Bonding Performance of All-in-One Self-Etch Adhesives

Shipra Singh,[1] Rajni Nagpal,[1] Shashi Prabha Tyagi,[1] and Naveen Manuja[2]

[1]Department of Conservative Dentistry and Endodontics, Kothiwal Dental College and Research Centre, Moradabad 244001, India
[2]Department of Pediatric Dentistry, Kothiwal Dental College and Research Centre, Moradabad 244001, India

Correspondence should be addressed to Rajni Nagpal; rajni_hisar@yahoo.co.in

Academic Editor: Paulo H. P. D'Alpino

Objective. This study evaluated the effect of ethylenediaminetetraacetic acid (EDTA) conditioning and carbodiimide (EDC) pretreatment on the shear bond strength of two all-in-one self-etch adhesives to dentin. *Methods.* Flat coronal dentin surfaces were prepared on one hundred and sixty extracted human molars. Teeth were randomly divided into eight groups according to two different self-etch adhesives used [G-Bond and OptiBond-All-In-One] and four different surface pretreatments: (a) adhesive applied following manufacturer's instructions; (b) dentin conditioning with 24% EDTA gel prior to application of adhesive; (c) EDC pretreatment followed by application of adhesive; (d) application of EDC on EDTA conditioned dentin surface followed by application of adhesive. Composite restorations were placed in all the samples. Ten samples from each group were subjected to immediate and delayed (6-month storage in artificial saliva) shear bond strength evaluation. Data collected was subjected to statistical analysis using three-way ANOVA and post hoc Tukey's test at a significance level of $p < 0.05$. *Results and Conclusion.* EDTA preconditioning as well as EDC pretreatment alone had no significant effect on the immediate and delayed bond strengths of either of the adhesives. However, EDC pretreatment on EDTA conditioned dentin surface resulted in preservation of resin-dentin bond strength of both adhesives with no significant fall over six months.

1. Introduction

Adhesion to dentin may be achieved either following an "etch-and-rinse" or a "self-etch" approach. Self-etch approach has been claimed to be user-friendlier and less technique-sensitive. Another important clinical benefit of self-etch adhesives is the absence of, or at least lower incidence of postoperative sensitivity [1]. This has been attributed to their less aggressive and more superficial interaction with dentin leaving tubules largely obstructed by smear [2]. However, some studies have shown a potential disadvantage in incorporating the smear layer into the hybrid layer [3–5]. Although the smear layer is reinforced by impregnated resin, bonding defects may be produced [6]. Since such defects may decrease the resistance and stability of the hybridized smear layer, its removal by incorporating a separate etching step may be necessary to obtain reliable, strong resin-dentin bonds [7–9]. Therefore, a conditioning system capable of changing the tooth surface by removing the smear layer and partially removing the surface layer of hydroxyapatite while simultaneously not destroying the organic portion of the dentin may be beneficial as pretreatment for mild self-etch adhesives. Some studies have demonstrated that separate phosphoric acid etching of dentin could decrease the bond strength and durability of self-etch adhesives [10, 11]. Therefore, conditioning with a mild etchant like EDTA may prove to be beneficial for bonding of mild self-etch adhesives to dentin.

Whereas phosphoric acid etching of dentin leads to dissolving both the extra and the intrafibrillar minerals resulting in recession and collapse of the collagen matrix, only partial removal of the smear layer with the maintenance of about 30% of the smear plugs and no morphological alterations of the dentin surface is observed following application of 17% EDTA on dentin for 60 seconds [12]. Phosphoric acid-etching of dentin causes collagen fibrils to become slightly denatured and swollen compared to EDTA-treatment [13].

Jacques and Hebling reported that pretreatment with a mild etchant such as 0.5 M EDTA improved the bond strength of the Clearfil SE bond [14]. Torii et al. also reported that EDTA conditioning was effective in improving dentin bonding for all-in-one adhesives [15]. Therefore, it may be anticipated that EDTA conditioning may improve the bonding efficacy of mild all-in-one self-etch adhesives to dentin [16]. Moreover EDTA has been shown to have a MMP inhibitory effect which may help in improving the durability of resin-dentin bond [17].

Degradation of the resin-dentin bonds, due to hydrolysis of the collagen fibrils, involves the participation of endogenous matrix metalloproteinases (MMPs) which become entrapped within the dentin substrate during tooth development [18, 19]. Therefore, the use of MMP inhibitors and collagen cross-linkers have been suggested as a valid alternative in an attempt to prolong the resin-dentin bond stability by overcoming this self-degradation process [20]. Chlorhexidine (CHX), Galardin (GL), CMT, SB-3 CT, proanthocyanidins (PA), 1-ethyl-3-(3-dimethylaminopropyl) carbodiimide (EDC), tetracycline, and quaternary ammonium methacrylates or benzalkonium chloride have been employed in various studies to improve the durability of resin-dentin bond [21–25].

The potential of cross-linkers is related to the possibility to improve the mechanical strength of the collagen network, improve the resistance to enzymatic degradation, and inactivate exposed MMPs bound to matrix collagen. When acid-etched dentin containing activated matrix-bound MMPs is treated with cross-linking agents, they inactivate the catalytic site of proteases [26]. Carbodiimide [EDC, 1-ethyl-3-(3-dimethylaminopropyl)] has been described as a collagen cross-linker with MMP inhibitory properties. EDC have been used as alternative cross-linking agents to glutaraldehyde, since they contain no potentially cytotoxic aldehyde residuals [27, 28]. EDC effectively improves the durability of resin-dentin bonds by increasing the mechanical properties of the collagen matrix [29]. Most of the research regarding the effect of EDC on dental adhesion has been done using etch-and-rinse adhesives; however the effect of EDC on bonding of contemporary self-etch adhesives needs to be evaluated. Moreover the effect of prior EDTA conditioning on the bonding of specific all-in-one adhesive systems still needs to be determined. Hence, the aim of this study was to investigate the effect of (i) EDTA conditioning, (ii) EDC pretreatment, or (iii) combined effect of EDTA preconditioning and EDC application on the immediate and long-term bonding efficacy of two different all-in-one self-etch adhesives. The null hypothesis tested was that there is no effect of EDTA or EDC pretreatment on the immediate and delayed bond strength of two different all-in-one self-etch adhesives to dentin.

2. Materials and Method

The study was performed in one hundred and sixty freshly extracted noncarious, human molars. The teeth were examined under stereomicroscope (Olympus, Tokyo, Japan) and teeth free of caries, cracks, or any developmental defects were included. Teeth were cleaned of debris. Calculus was removed using ultrasonic scaler and then the teeth were stored in 0.5% Chloramine T Trihydrate (Sigma Aldrich, Bangalore, India)

for no more than 3 months. Tooth crowns were flattened using a low-speed diamond saw (Isomet, Buehler Ltd., Lake Bluff, IL, USA) under water irrigation unless superficial dentin was visible and a standardized smear layer was created with 600-grit silicon-carbide (SiC) paper. The samples were embedded in an autopolymerizing resin at the level of cementoenamel junction with long axis perpendicular to the acrylic resin surface. Teeth were randomly divided into eight groups according to two different self-etch adhesives used (G-Bond (GC Corp., Tokyo, Japan) and OptiBond-All-In-One (KERR, Orange, CA, USA)) (Table 2) and four different surface pretreatments. Each group was further divided into two subgroups for immediate (a) and delayed (b) bond strength evaluation.

Group 1 (GB). G-Bond was applied following manufacturer's instructions.

Group 2 (GB-EDTA). Dentin conditioning with 24% EDTA gel for 1 minute (Trisodium EDTA Gel, Pyrex Pharmaceuticals, Roorkee), followed by rinsing with distilled water, blot dried prior to application of G-bond.

Group 3 (GB-EDC). Application of EDC (0.3 M for 1 minute) on smear covered dentin surface and blot dried before application of G-Bond.

Group 4 (GB-EDTA + EDC). Dentin was conditioned with 24% EDTA gel for 1 minute, rinsed with distilled water, and blot dried. This was followed by application of EDC (0.3 M) for 1 minute and then blot dried, followed by application G-Bond adhesive.

Group 5 (OB). OptiBond-All-In-One was applied following manufacturer's instructions.

Group 6 (OB-EDTA). Dentin conditioning with EDTA (24% gel for 1 minute) followed by rinsing with water blot dried prior to application of OptiBond-All-In-One.

Group 7 (OB-EDC). Application of EDC (0.3 M for 1 minute) on smear covered dentin surface and blot dried before application of OptiBond-All-In-One.

Group 8 (OB-EDTA + EDC). Dentin was conditioned with 24% EDTA gel for 1 minute, rinsed with distilled water, and blot dried. This was followed by application of EDC (0.3 M) for 1 minute and then blot dried, followed by application OptiBond-All-In-One adhesive.

Transparent plastic tubes 54-HL (TYGON Medical tubing, Saint Gobain, Akron, OH, USA) of internal diameter 3 mm and 2 mm height with thickness 0.5 mm were pre-cut and placed perpendicular to the prepared surface. A hybrid resin composite (Filtek Z350 XT, Body Shade A1, Nanohybrid, 3 M ESPE) was filled into the precut tubes. Each bonded specimen was light-cured for 20 seconds using Spectrum 800 (Dentsply, Caulk, Milford, USA) at light intensity of 600 mW/cm^2. The plastic tubes were gently cut and carefully removed with a number 11 surgical blade after polymerization.

Table 1: Mean shear bond strength values both immediate and delayed for G-Bond and OptiBond-All-In-One adhesives.

Groups	Immediate Testing Mean	SD	Groups	Delayed Testing Mean	SD	p value
1a (GB)	33.30[abc]	5.54	1b	23.10[c]	5.53	0.022*
2a (GB-EDTA)	38.40[ab]	9.23	2b	27.90[ab]	8.97	0.018*
3a (GB-EDC)	37.70[abc]	7.72	3b	32.70[ab]	8.11	0.429
4a (GB-EDTA + EDC)	40.80[a]	7.58	4b	34.90[a]	5.49	0.286
5a (OB)	29.00[c]	6.99	5b	20.30[c]	5.83	0.020*
6a (OB-EDTA)	32.30[abc]	4.79	6b	22.30[c]	7.45	0.006*
7a (OB-EDC)	30.20[bc]	5.29	7b	25.60[bc]	5.52	0.344
8a (OB-EDTA + EDC)	31.90[abc]	6.44	8b	27.60[abc]	6.96	0.403

Groups with the same superscripts are not statistically different ($p > 0.05$); * denotes statistically significant groups.

Table 2: Composition and manufacturer's instructions of adhesive systems used in the study.

Adhesive	Composition	Manufacture	Technique
G-Bond	4-MET, phosphate ester monomer, UDMA, acetone, water, microfiller, and photoinitiator	GC Corp.; Tokyo, Japan	(i) Shake the bottle thoroughly prior to dispensing (ii) Immediately apply to the prepared enamel and dentin surfaces using the disposing applicator (iii) Leave undisturbed for 5–10 seconds (iv) Dry thoroughly for 5 seconds with oil free air under maximum air pressure. The final results should be a thin, rough, adhesive film with the appearance of frosted glass and which doesn't visibly move under further air pressure (v) Light cure for 10 seconds
OptiBond-All-In-One	GPDM, GDM, HEMA, Bis-GMA, water, ethanol, acetone, silica, CQ, and sodium hexafluorosilicate	OP; Kerr; Orange, CA, USA	(i) Shake adhesive bottle briefly. (vigorously for 10 seconds) (ii) Using the disposable applicator brush, apply a generous amount of OptiBond-All-In-One adhesive to enamel/dentin surface. Scrub the surface with a brushing motion for 20 seconds (iii) Apply a second application of OptiBond-All-In-One All-In-One adhesive with a brushing motion for 20 seconds (iv) Dry the adhesive with gentle air first and then medium air for at least 5 seconds with oil-free air (v) Light cure for 10 seconds

3. Determination of Dentin Shear Bond Strength

Half of the specimens (1a–8a) were then stored in distilled water at 37°C for 24 hours for immediate testing. The remaining half samples from each group (1b–8b) were stored in artificial saliva (ICPA, Wet Mouth) for 6 months before shear bond strength evaluation [30, 31]. Shear bond strength was determined using a universal testing machine (Instron, ADMET, Enkay Enterprises, New Delhi) using the corresponding computer software. The specimens were placed and stabilized by the jig, while a straight knife-edge rod (2.0 mm) was applied at the tooth restoration interface at a crosshead speed of 1 mm/minute. Load was applied until restoration failure. The mode of failure was determined by observation under a stereomicroscope (Olympus, Tokyo, Japan) at 10x magnification and classified into adhesive (A), mixed (M), and cohesive (C) failures in either dentin or resin. The statistical analysis was done using three-way ANOVA and post hoc Tukey's test SPSS 16.0 version (Statistical Package, SPSS Inc., Chicago, IL, USA) at a significance level of $p < 0.05$.

4. Results

Mean shear bond strength values and standard deviation of all the groups are presented in Table 1. There was no significant difference in bond strengths between the two adhesives when used according to manufacturer's instructions (Table 2). EDTA pre-conditioning had no significant effect on the immediate bond strength of either of the adhesives (Groups 1a and 2a; $p = 0.707$; Groups 5a and 6a; $p = 0.959$). EDC pretreatment alone also had no significant effect on the immediate bond strength of G-Bond (Groups 1a and 3a; $p = 0.836$) and OptiBond-All-In-One (Groups 5a and 7a; $p = 0.999$). Mixed fractures were the most common failure mode in all the groups (Figure 1). There was no significant difference in the mode of failure between the two tested adhesives.

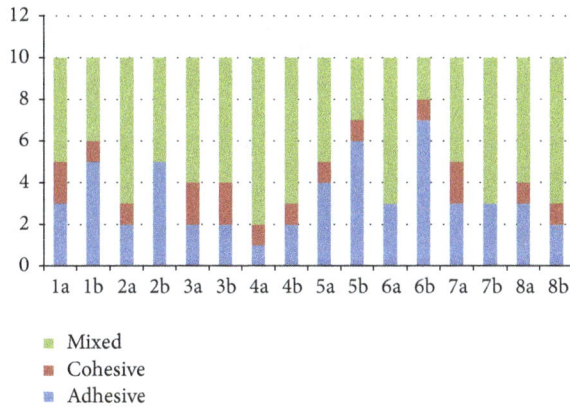

FIGURE 1: Failure modes in different experimental groups.

There was a significant reduction in bond strength for both adhesives G-Bond and OptiBond All-In-One after six months storage (Groups 1a and 1b; $p = 0.022$; Groups 5a and 5b; $p = 0.020$). EDTA preconditioning could not prevent the fall in bond strength over a six-month storage period (Groups 2a and 2b; $p = 0.018$; Groups 6a and 6b; $p = 0.006$). However, EDC pretreatment alone (Groups 3a and 3b; $p = 0.429$; Groups 7a and 7b; $p = 0.344$) or EDC application on EDTA conditioned dentin surface (Groups 4a and 4b; $p = 0.286$; Groups 8a and 8b; $p = 0.403$) resulted in preservation of resin-dentin bond strength of both the adhesives with no significant fall over six months. Failure mode analysis revealed mixed fractures to be the most common in Groups 3b : 4b; 7b and 8b. An increase in adhesive fractures was observed in Groups 1b : 2b; 5b : 6b (Figure 1).

5. Discussion

In the present study, no significant difference was observed between the immediate shear bond strength values of G-Bond and OptiBond-All-In-One adhesives and mixed fractures were the most common failure mode. Bond strength of polymerized adhesives depends upon various factors such as the type of cross-linking monomers, presence and type of filler particles, degree of conversion, and the amount of residual organic solvents. The carboxylic group of 4-MET (4-methacryloyloxyethyl trimellitic acid) renders G-Bond monomers hydrophilic, but less reactive than UDMA (urethane dimethacrylate) in hydrogen bonding with water and it functions as a proton donor that bonds ionically with calcium in hydroxyapatite crystalites [32, 33]. Thus, an extremely thin interface nanointeraction zone (300 nm) is formed as opposed to the traditional hybrid layer appellation that provides resistance to acute debonding stresses and better bond durability and survival of adhesion, minimizing voids. Strong air blowing of the primed surface as suggested in G-Bond accelerates the evaporation of solvent-acetone and the resultant water droplets formed due to phase separation. The excess of nonpolymerizable hydrophilic components (water, acetone, and glutaraldehyde) may give rise to hydration forces that repel water at film boundaries and hence less water

sorption [32]. Aromatic rings present in G-Bond are more stable [34].

OptiBond-All-In-One contains 35 to 45% acetone and 4–9% ethanol. The solvent evaporation from adhesives is influenced by the vapor pressure [35]. As the vapor pressure of acetone is high, it volatilizes rapidly and may dehydrate the dentin. The presence of water in self-etch adhesives is necessary to ensure the ionization of the acidic monomers, but it is not as efficient as acetone or ethanol as a solvent because of its lower vapor pressure [36]. The presence of acetone and ethanol in OptiBond-All-In-One might balance the solvent evaporation without dehydrating dentin, because ethanol ensures the wetness of the substrate, and its vapor pressure is intermediate between acetone and water. Another explanation for the good performance of OptiBond-All-In-One could be the content of glycerol phosphate dimethacrylate monomer in its formulation, a surfactant monomer that may have facilitated the penetration of hydrophobic components into dentin, reducing the phase separation [37, 38]. G-Bond is HEMA (2-hydroxyethyl methacrylate) free adhesive whereas OptiBond-All-In-One is HEMA containing adhesive [33, 39–41]. The hydrophilic monomer, HEMA, in various concentrations is frequently added to one-step self-etch adhesives because of its positive influence on adhesion to dentin, the miscibility of hydrophilic and hydrophobic components in the adhesive blend, and prevention of phase separation. The hydrophilic monomer of HEMA tends to cluster together before polymerization, leading to creation of hydrophilic domains. Moreover, HEMA attracts water even after polymerization. When HEMA is cured in the presence of water, polymerization is incomplete and a porous hydrogel is formed that allows water to permeate through the adhesive layer, compromising bonding effectiveness. It was reported that the amount of water sorption of adhesive polymers increased proportionally to their HEMA concentrations [39]. Some studies have shown that the removal of HEMA from self-etch adhesives would minimize water sorption, while others have observed that the 10% HEMA content would be beneficial for the adhesive system performance [39]. There is still a controversy about the role of HEMA in the bonding performance of adhesives. In the study by Felizardo et al. [39] it was concluded that the influence of HEMA on bond strength to dentin was material dependent.

As there are numerous factors involved in bond degradation, several methods have been proposed (i.e., load cycling, thermal cycling, prolonged water, and artificial saliva incubation) for reproducing clinical situations and simulating the oral environment to test the durability of dentin bonding [42]. In our study, after storage in artificial saliva for six months, both G-Bond and OptiBond-All-In-One depicted significant reduction in the bond strength when used without any pretreatment. Several studies have provided morphological evidence of resin elution and/or hydrolytic degradation of collagen matrices after long-term storage [43]. Accordingly, more adhesive failures were observed after 6-month period.

EDTA is a molecule containing four carboxylic acid groups that can chelate calcium. It has been widely used to dissolve the mineral phase of dentine without altering dentin proteins, thereby avoiding major alterations of the native fibrillar structure of dentin collagen. Further, EDTA has an inhibitory effect on the matrix-bound MMPs of demineralized dentin [17]. In the current study, EDTA preconditioning had no significant effect on the immediate bond strength of the tested self-etch adhesives. Kasraei et al. reported that EDTA application before one-step self-etch adhesive significantly improved the bond strength [44]. However, they used liquid EDTA at 0.5 M concentration for 30 seconds and the adhesives evaluated were also different from our study. Soares et al. also depicted increased bond strength of self-etch adhesive systems used with EDTA preconditioning [45]. However, they conducted the study on bovine incisors using two-step self-etch adhesives whereas, in our study, one-step all-in-one adhesives were used. It has been reported that the efficiency of EDTA depends on many factors: penetration depth of the material, hardness of the dentin, duration of application, pH, form (liquid or gel), and concentration of material [42]. Although EDTA is an excellent MMP inhibitor, it is also water soluble; hence it might be rinsed off EDTA-treated dentin [17]. This might not be able to sustain MMP inhibition for much longer duration. Therefore, in the current study no improvement in durability could be observed after EDTA pretreatment with significant reduction in bond strength after six months, along with an increase in the number of adhesive failures. Another important aspect that must be considered is EDTA delivery form. Even at a higher concentration, a 24% EDTA gel might not be able to etch dentin in the same manner as EDTA in aqueous solution due to its lower wetting capacity. Stape et al. evaluated the effect of 24% EDTA on bond strength of resin cements to dentin and concluded that the effect varied with the different resin cements [46]. Parihar and Pilania also concluded that the effect of EDTA preconditioning on bonding of self-adhesive resin cement was product dependent [47].

EDC, a cross-linking agent with very low cytotoxicity, has shown promising results in eliminating dentin collagen degradation and preserving dentin bond strength with clinically acceptable procedure time [48]. It is the most stable cyanamide isomer, which is able to assemble amino acids into peptides. They are examples of zero length cross-linking agents. However, application of EDC alone in this study, on the dentin surface, without prior EDTA conditioning had no significant effect on the immediate bond strength of both self-etch adhesives. Probably as there was no exposed collagen, EDC was not able to strengthen the collagen matrix by increased cross-linking, whereas most of the studies, which report improved bonding effectiveness with EDC, have been performed using etch and rinse adhesives where EDC is applied to dentin previously demineralized by phosphoric acid which exposes the collagen fibrils.

EDTA removes the smear layer and mildly demineralizes the dentin. Because EDTA does not denature collagen in comparison to phosphoric acid, it creates thinner hybrid layers that are more easily infiltrated with resin [49–52]. Conditioning with 24% EDTA for 1 minute has been shown to demineralize the dentin and expose the collagen fibrils. Subsequent application of EDC promotes cross-linking amongst exposed collagen fibrils. Thus, in the present study, dentin pretreatment with EDC (with and without EDTA) resulted in bond strength preservation after 6 months of storage in artificial saliva for both adhesives used. All EDC treated groups at 6 months revealed mixed fracture patterns to be the most common failure mode. A previous in vitro study also reported that EDC application for 1 minute was effective in inactivating soluble rhMMP-9 and matrix-bound dentin proteinases [53].

Our results are supported by the study of Mazzoni et al., who reported preservation of resin-dentin bond with 1 minute EDC pretreatment and by the study of Bedran-Russo et al. who also reported increased durability of resin-dentin bonds in EDC pretreated group [54, 55]. EDC is capable of cross-linking proteins through covalent peptide bonds by activating the free carboxyl group of glutamic and aspartic acids present in protein molecules to form O-acylisourea intermediate that reacts with the epsilon amino group of lysine or hydroxylysine in an adjacent polypeptide chain to form a stable amide cross-link [56, 57]. Cross-linking increases the mechanical properties of dentin collagen and makes the fibrils more resistant to degradation [55]. Furthermore EDC shows no transdentinal cytotoxicity on odontoblast-like cells and is able to increase the mechanical properties of the collagen matrix [25, 58]. Further studies are required to evaluate the effect of different concentration, time, pH, and form of application of EDTA and EDC on the long-term bonding efficacy of different contemporary adhesive systems to dentin. Effect of incorporation of EDC in the adhesive composition on the resin polymerization also needs to be investigated.

6. Conclusion

Carbodiimide pretreatment of dentin surface resulted in significant preservation of resin-dentin bond over six-month storage period for both all-in-one self-etch adhesives tested. EDTA pretreatment of dentin surface before application of self-etch adhesives had no effect on the durability of resin-dentin bond.

Conflict of Interests

The authors declare that there is no conflict of interests regarding the publication of this paper.

References

[1] M. Unemori, Y. Matsuya, A. Akashi, Y. Goto, and A. Akamine, "Self-etching adhesives and postoperative sensitivity," *American Journal of Dentistry*, vol. 17, no. 3, pp. 191–195, 2004.

[2] J. Perdigão, S. Geraldeli, and J. S. Hodges, "Total-etch versus self-etch adhesive: effect on postoperative sensitivity," *Journal of the American Dental Association*, vol. 134, no. 12, pp. 1621–1629, 2003.

[3] F. R. Tay, R. Carvalho, H. Sano, and D. H. Pashley, "Effect of smear layers on the bonding of a self-etching primer to dentin," *Journal of Adhesive Dentistry*, vol. 2, no. 2, pp. 99–116, 2000.

[4] F. R. Tay, N. M. King, K.-M. Chan, and D. H. Pashley, "How can nanoleakage occur in self-etching adhesive systems that

demineralize and infiltrate simultaneously?" *Journal of Adhesive Dentistry*, vol. 4, no. 4, pp. 255–269, 2002.

[5] H. Koibuchi, N. Yasuda, and N. Nakabayashi, "Bonding to dentin with a self-etching primer: the effect of smear layers," *Dental Materials*, vol. 17, no. 2, pp. 122–126, 2001.

[6] K. Miyasaka and N. Nakabayashi, "Effect of Phenyl-P/HEMA acetone primer on wet bonding to EDTA-conditioned dentin," *Dental Materials*, vol. 17, no. 6, pp. 499–503, 2001.

[7] T. Toida and N. Nakabayashi, "Adhesion of shrunken demineralized dentin—effects of methacrylates with hydrophilic and hydrophobic groups dissolved in primers on recovery of shrunken demineralized dentin," *The Journal of the Japanese Society for Dental Materials and Devices*, vol. 16, no. 3, pp. 232–238, 1997.

[8] B. Van Meerbeek, J. De Munck, Y. Yoshida et al., "Buonocore Memorial Lecture. Adhesion to enamel and dentin: current status and future challenges," *Operative Dentistry*, vol. 28, no. 3, pp. 215–235, 2003.

[9] N. Manuja, R. Nagpal, and S. Chaudhary, "Bonding efficacy of 1-step self-etch adhesives: effect of additional enamel etching and hydrophobic layer application," *Journal of Dentistry for Children*, vol. 79, no. 1, pp. 3–8, 2012.

[10] G. Kato and N. Nakabayashi, "The durability of adhesion to phosphoric acid etched, wet dentin substrates," *Dental Materials*, vol. 14, no. 5, pp. 347–352, 1998.

[11] Y. Torii, K. Itou, Y. Nishitani, K. Ishikawa, and K. Suzuki, "Effect of phosphoric acid etching prior to self-etching primer application on adhesion of resin composite to enamel and dentin," *American Journal of Dentistry*, vol. 15, no. 5, pp. 305–308, 2002.

[12] Z. C. Çehreli and N. Altay, "Etching effect of 17% EDTa and a non-rinse conditioner (NRC) on primary enamel and dentin," *American Journal of Dentistry*, vol. 13, no. 2, pp. 64–68, 2000.

[13] Y. Wang and P. Spencer, "Analysis of acid-treated dentin smear debris and smear layers using confocal Raman microspectroscopy," *Journal of Biomedical Materials Research*, vol. 60, no. 2, pp. 300–308, 2002.

[14] P. Jacques and J. Hebling, "Effect of dentin conditioners on the microtensile bond strength of a conventional and a self-etching primer adhesive system," *Dental Materials*, vol. 21, no. 2, pp. 103–109, 2005.

[15] Y. Torii, R. Hikasa, S. Iwate, F. Oyama, K. Itou, and M. Yoshiyama, "Effect of EDTA conditioning on bond strength to bovine dentin promoted by four current adhesives," *American Journal of Dentistry*, vol. 16, no. 6, pp. 395–400, 2003.

[16] A. Cederlund, B. Jonsson, and J. Blomlöf, "Shear strength after ethylenediaminetetraacetic acid conditioning of dentin," *Acta Odontologica Scandinavica*, vol. 59, no. 6, pp. 418–422, 2001.

[17] J. M. Thompson, K. Agee, S. J. Sidow et al., "Inhibition of endogenous dentin matrix metalloproteinases by ethylenediaminetetraacetic acid," *Journal of Endodontics*, vol. 38, no. 1, pp. 62–65, 2012.

[18] A. J. V. Strijp, D. C. Jansen, J. DeGroot, J. M. Ten Cate, and V. Everts, "Host-derived proteinases and degradation of dentine collagen in situ," *Caries Research*, vol. 37, no. 1, pp. 58–65, 2003.

[19] A. Mazzoni, F. Mannello, F. R. Tay et al., "Zymographic analysis and characterization of MMP-2 and -9 forms in human sound dentin," *Journal of Dental Research*, vol. 86, no. 5, pp. 436–440, 2007.

[20] J. De Munck, P. E. Van Den Steen, A. Mine et al., "Inhibition of enzymatic degradation of adhesive-dentin interfaces," *Journal of Dental Research*, vol. 88, no. 12, pp. 1101–1106, 2009.

[21] J. Hebling, D. H. Pashley, L. Tjäderhane, and F. R. Tay, "Chlorhexidine arrests subclinical degradation of dentin hybrid layers in vivo," *Journal of Dental Research*, vol. 84, no. 8, pp. 741–746, 2005.

[22] R. Nagpal, N. Manuja, and I. K. Pandit, "Effect of proanthocyanidin treatment on the bonding effectiveness of adhesive restorations in pulp chamber," *Journal of Clinical Pediatric Dentistry*, vol. 38, no. 1, pp. 49–53, 2013.

[23] L. Breschi, A. Mazzoni, A. Ruggeri, M. Cadenaro, R. Di Lenarda, and E. D. S. Dorigo, "Dental adhesion review: aging and stability of the bonded interface," *Dental Materials*, vol. 24, no. 1, pp. 90–101, 2008.

[24] D. Scheffel, C. Delgado, D. G. Soares et al., "Increased durability of resin-dentin bonds following cross-linking treatment," *Operative Dentistry*, vol. 40, no. 5, pp. 533–539, 2015.

[25] D. L. S. Scheffel, J. Hebling, R. H. Scheffel et al., "Inactivation of matrix-bound Matrix metalloproteinases by cross-linking agents in acid-etched dentin," *Operative Dentistry*, vol. 39, no. 2, pp. 152–158, 2014.

[26] Y. Liu, L. Tjäderhane, L. Breschi et al., "Limitations in bonding to dentin and experimental strategies to prevent bond degradation," *Journal of Dental Research*, vol. 90, no. 8, pp. 953–968, 2011.

[27] L. L. H. Huang-Lee, D. T. Cheung, and M. E. Nimni, "Biochemical changes and cytotoxicity associated with the degradation of polymeric glutaraldehyde derived cross-links," *Journal of Biomedical Materials Research*, vol. 24, no. 9, pp. 1185–1201, 1990.

[28] H. Petite, J.-L. Dukval, V. Frei, N. Abdul-Malak, M.-F. Sigot-Luizard, and D. Herbage, "Cytocompatibility of calf pericardium treated by glutaraldehyde and by the acyl azide methods in an organotypic culture model," *Biomaterials*, vol. 16, no. 13, pp. 1003–1008, 1995.

[29] D. L. S. Scheffel, L. Bianchi, D. G. Soares et al., "Transdentinal cytotoxicity of carbodiimide (EDC) and glutaraldehyde on odontoblast-like cells," *Operative Dentistry*, vol. 40, no. 1, pp. 44–54, 2015.

[30] A. Panigrahi, K. T. Srilatha, R. G. Panigrahi, S. Mohanty, S. Kbhuyan, and D. Bardhan, "Microtensile bond strength of embrace wetbond hydrophilic sealant in different moisture contamination: an in-vitro study," *Journal of Clinical and Diagnostic Research*, vol. 9, no. 7, pp. ZC23–ZC25, 2015.

[31] R. Subramonian, V. Mathai, J. M. C. Angelo, and J. Ravi, "Effect of three different antioxidants on the shear bond strength of composite resin to bleached enamel: an in vitro study," *Journal of Conservative Dentistry*, vol. 18, no. 2, pp. 144–148, 2015.

[32] B. Poptani, K. S. Gohil, J. Ganjiwale, and M. Shukla, "Microtensile dentin bond strength of fifth with five seventh-generation dentin bonding agents after thermocycling: an in vitro study," *Contemporary Clinical Dentistry*, vol. 3, no. 6, pp. 167–171, 2012.

[33] S. Sauro, D. H. Pashley, F. Mannocci et al., "Micropermeability of current self-etching and etch-and-rinse adhesives bonded to deep dentine: a comparison study using a double-staining/confocal microscopy technique," *European Journal of Oral Sciences*, vol. 116, no. 2, pp. 184–193, 2008.

[34] S. Bouillaguet, P. Gysi, J. C. Wataha et al., "Bond strength of composite to dentin using conventional, one-step, and self-etching adhesive systems," *Journal of Dentistry*, vol. 29, no. 1, pp. 55–61, 2001.

[35] T. Ikeda, J. De Munck, K. Shirai et al., "Effect of air-drying and solvent evaporation on the strength of HEMA-rich versus HEMA-free one-step adhesives," *Dental Materials*, vol. 24, no. 10, pp. 1316–1323, 2008.

[36] K. L. Van Landuyt, J. Snauwaert, J. De Munck et al., "Systematic review of the chemical composition of contemporary dental adhesives," *Biomaterials*, vol. 28, no. 26, pp. 3757–3785, 2007.

[37] X. Guo, P. Spencer, Y. Wang, Q. Ye, X. Yao, and K. Williams, "Effects of a solubility enhancer on penetration of hydrophobic component in model adhesives into wet demineralized dentin," *Dental Materials*, vol. 23, no. 12, pp. 1473–1481, 2007.

[38] C. H. Zanchi, E. A. Münchow, F. A. Ogliari et al., "Development of experimental HEMA-free three-step adhesive system," *Journal of Dentistry*, vol. 38, no. 6, pp. 503–508, 2010.

[39] K. R. Felizardo, L. V. F. M. Lemos, R. V. de Carvalho, A. Gonini Junior, M. B. Lopes, and S. K. Moura, "Bond strength of HEMA-containing versus HEMA-free self-etch adhesive systems to dentin," *Brazilian Dental Journal*, vol. 22, no. 6, pp. 468–472, 2011.

[40] M. Takahashi, M. Nakajima, K. Hosaka, K. Ikeda, R. M. Foxton, and J. Tagami, "Long-term evaluation of water sorption and ultimate tensile strength of HEMA-containing/-free one-step self-etch adhesives," *Journal of Dentistry*, vol. 39, no. 7, pp. 506–512, 2011.

[41] K. L. V. Landuyt, A. Mine, J. D. Munck et al., "Are one-step adhesives easier to use and better performing? Multifactorial assessment of contemporary one-step self-etching adhesives," *The Journal of Adhesive Dentistry*, vol. 11, no. 3, pp. 175–190, 2009.

[42] S. Sauro, F. Mannocci, M. Toledano, R. Osorio, D. H. Pashley, and T. F. Watson, "EDTA or H_3PO_4/NaOCl dentine treatments may increase hybrid layers' resistance to degradation: a microtensile bond strength and confocal-micropermeability study," *Journal of Dentistry*, vol. 37, no. 4, pp. 279–288, 2009.

[43] L. Breschi, A. Mazzoni, A. Ruggeri, M. Cadenaro, R. D. Lenarda, and E. S. S. Dorigo, "Dental adhesion review: aging and stability of the bonded interface," *Dental Materials*, vol. 24, no. 1, pp. 90–101, 2008.

[44] S. Kasraei, M. Azarsina, and Z. Khamverdi, "Effect of Ethylene diamine tetra acetic acid and sodium hypochlorite solution conditioning on microtensile bond strength of one-step self-etch adhesives," *Journal of Conservative Dentistry*, vol. 16, no. 3, pp. 243–246, 2013.

[45] C. J. Soares, C. G. Castro, P. C. F. Santos Filho, and A. S. Da Mota, "Effect of previous treatments on bond strength of two self-etching adhesive systems to dental substrate," *Journal of Adhesive Dentistry*, vol. 9, no. 3, pp. 291–296, 2007.

[46] T. H. S. Stape, M. S. Menezes, B. C. F. Barreto, F. H. B. Aguiar, L. R. Martins, and P. S. Quagliatto, "Influence of matrix metalloproteinase synthetic inhibitors on dentin microtensile bond strength of resin cements," *Operative Dentistry*, vol. 37, no. 4, pp. 386–396, 2012.

[47] N. Parihar and M. Pilania, "SEM evaluation of effect of 37% phosphoric acid gel, 24% EDTA gel and 10% maleic acid gel on the enamel and dentin for 15 and 60 seconds: an in–vitro study," *International Dental Journal of Students' Research*, vol. 1, no. 2, pp. 29–41, 2012.

[48] D. Scheffel, L. Bianchi, D. Soares et al., "Transdentinal cytotoxicity of carbodiimide (EDC) and glutaraldehyde on odontoblast-like cells," *Operative Dentistry*, vol. 40, no. 1, pp. 44–54, 2015.

[49] S. Habelitz, M. Balooch, S. J. Marshall, G. Balooch, and G. W. J. Marshall Jr., "In situ atomic force microscopy of partially demineralized human dentin collagen fibrils," *Journal of Structural Biology*, vol. 138, no. 3, pp. 227–236, 2002.

[50] J. P. S. Blomlöf, L. B. Blomlöf, A. L. Cederlund, K. R. Hultenby, and S. F. Lindskog, "A new concept for etching in restorative dentistry," *International Journal of Periodontics & Restorative Dentistry*, vol. 19, no. 1, pp. 31–35, 1999.

[51] S. Sauro, M. Toledano, F. S. Aguilera et al., "Resin-dentin bonds to EDTA-treated vs. acid-etched dentin using ethanol wet-bonding," *Dental Materials*, vol. 26, no. 4, pp. 368–379, 2010.

[52] S. Sauro, M. Toledano, F. S. Aguilera et al., "Resin–dentin bonds to EDTA-treated vs. acid-etched dentin using ethanol wet-bonding. Part II: effects of mechanical cycling load on microtensile bond strengths," *Dental Materials*, vol. 27, no. 6, pp. 563–572, 2011.

[53] A. Tezvergil-Mutluay, M. M. Mutluay, K. A. Agee et al., "Carbodiimide cross-linking inactivates soluble and matrix-bound MMPs, *in vitro*," *Journal of Dental Research*, vol. 91, no. 2, pp. 192–196, 2012.

[54] A. Mazzoni, V. Angeloni, F. M. Apolonio et al., "Effect of carbodiimide (EDC) on the bond stability of etch-and-rinse adhesive systems," *Dental Materials*, vol. 29, no. 10, pp. 1040–1047, 2013.

[55] A. K. B. Bedran-Russo, C. M. P. Vidal, P. H. Dos Santos, and C. S. Castellan, "Long-term effect of carbodiimide on dentin matrix and resin-dentin bonds," *Journal of Biomedical Materials Research Part B: Applied Biomaterials*, vol. 94, no. 1, pp. 250–255, 2010.

[56] R. Timkovich, "Detection of the stable addition of carbodiimide to proteins," *Analytical Biochemistry*, vol. 79, no. 1-2, pp. 135–143, 1977.

[57] R. Zeeman, P. J. Dijkstra, P. B. Van Wachem et al., "Successive epoxy and carbodiimide cross-linking of dermal sheep collagen," *Biomaterials*, vol. 20, no. 10, pp. 921–931, 1999.

[58] D. L. S. Scheffel, J. Hebling, R. H. Scheffel et al., "Stabilization of dentin matrix after cross-linking treatments, in vitro," *Dental Materials*, vol. 30, no. 2, pp. 227–233, 2014.

3

Transcrestal Sinus Lift Procedure Approaching Atrophic Maxillary Ridge: A 60-Month Clinical and Radiological Follow-Up Evaluation

G. Lo Giudice,[1] G. Iannello,[1] A. Terranova,[1] R. Lo Giudice,[1] G. Pantaleo,[1] and M. Cicciù[2]

[1]*Medical Sciences and Stomatology Department, School of Dentistry, University of Messina, Via Consolare Valeria, 98100 Messina, Italy*
[2]*Human Pathology Department, School of Dentistry, University of Messina, Via Consolare Valeria, 98100 Messina, Italy*

Correspondence should be addressed to M. Cicciù; acromarco@yahoo.it

Academic Editor: Saso Ivanovski

Aim. The aim of this study was to assess the success and the survival rate of dental implants placed in augmented bone after sinus lifting procedures. *Material and Methods.* 31 patients were mainly enrolled for a residual upper jaw crest thickness of 3 mm. CBCT scans were performed before and after the augmentation technique and at the follow-up appointments, at 3, 6, 12, 24, and up to 60 months. The follow-up examination included cumulative survival rate of implants, peri-implant marginal bone loss, and the height of sinus floor augmentation. *Results.* This retrospective study on 31 patients and 45 implants later inserted in a less than 3 mm crest showed excellent survival rates (99.5%), one implant was lost before loading due to an acute infection after 24 days, and two implants did not osteointegrate and were removed after 3 months. The radiological evaluation showed an average bone loss of 0.25 mm (±0.78 mm) at the first follow-up appointment (3 months) up to 0.30 mm (±1.28 mm) after 60-month follow-up. *Conclusion.* In this study it was reported how even in less than 3 mm thick crest a transcrestal technique can predictably be used with a long-term clinical and radiological outcome, giving patients excellent stability of the grafted material and healthy clinical results.

1. Introduction

The jawbone resorption, related to the loose teeth, causes atrophy in the bone volume, by increasing the vertical dimension of occlusion and by reducing the amount of available bone to the implant placement and next prosthesis positioning. In presence of severe postextractive resorption, many techniques have been described to augment the residual bone ridge by using the possibility of the sinus membrane elevation up to 5 mm without any tearing [1]. The sinus lift technique was firstly described by Boyne and James [2] and it was based on a modification of the Caldwell-Luc sinus revision, basically consisting in a lateral approach to the sinus that allows a remarkable bone augmentation >10 mm even in very atrophic ridge [1]; this approach is well documented in literature and has proven to be safe and highly predictable.

In order to reduce morbidity and postoperative discomfort, Tatum Jr., in 1986, proposed a transcrestal approach for the sinus augmentation, using an osteotome sequence to have a controlled fracture of the sinus wall [3]. In 1994 Summers modified this technique, allowing a lateral force compression and increased the lateral bone density. This technique gave the clinicians the opportunity in having the implant site preparation using conical osteotomes [4, 5]. In 2000 Cosci and Luccioli proposed a 1 stage crestal approach using specific drill sequences (Cosci's Technique) and a particular tip able to prevent sinus perforation by using an abrasive removal of the cortical bone, without any fracture [6].

The transcrestal approach is considered the more conservative one and it has several advantages compared to the lateral osteotomy. Even though the transcrestal sinus lifting procedure is blindly performed, the frequency of sinus

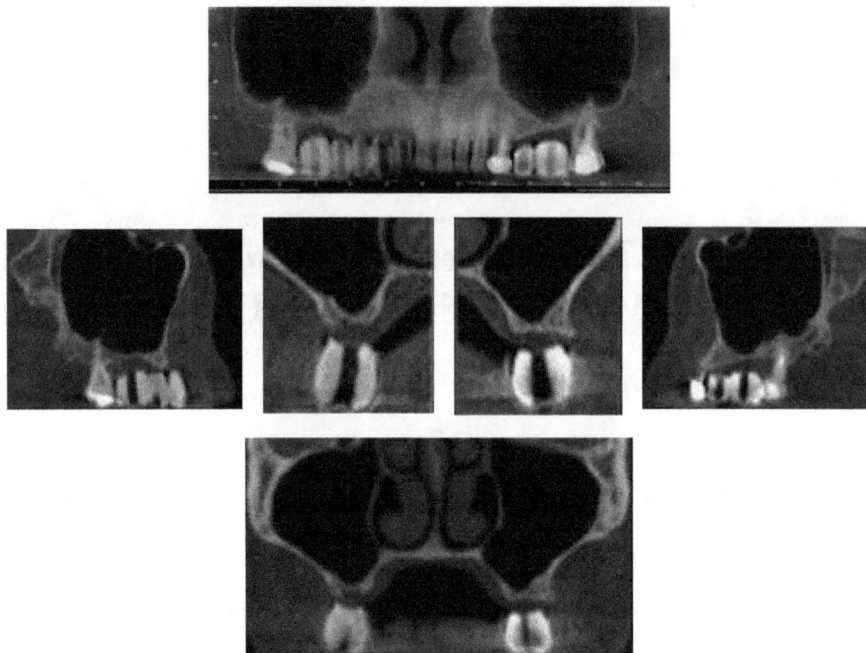

FIGURE 1: Baseline. The CBCT images show the posterior upper jawbone defect.

membrane perforation has been reported as less frequent than the lateral approach [7, 8].

The main goal of this procedure consists in a long time, no subjected to resorption, new bone formation, which allows a high predictable implant survival rate [9, 10].

This technique documented a 5-year survival rate superior to 92.7% for implants placed in less than 5 mm ridge height and 94.9% for implants inserted in more than 5 mm ridge height [11, 12]. These results are strictly linked to the absence of intraoperative and postoperative complication such as membrane perforation, postoperative sinusitis, disturbed wound healing, hematoma, sequestration of bone, and partial or complete graft failure [13, 14]. The absence of membrane perforation can be obtained by either performing a lateral sinus lift approach that allows directly checking the membrane status or, when a crestal approach is performed, gently detaching the membrane and checking, before the graft insertion, its integrity with the Valsalva manoeuvre [15]. Sinusitis might occur due to obstruction of the sinus outflow tract by mucosal edema and particulate graft and can be avoided thanks to a proper radiological evaluation and the absence of membrane perforation [16].

The aim of this retrospective study was to evaluate the survival rate of implants placed in the posterior upper jaw with a residual bone height less than 3 mm using a sequential sinus lift performed by crestal approach. By the five-year follow-up results of the investigations, it was also aimed at highlighting the effectiveness and the predictability of the performing sinus lift by occlusal window. The main limit of the sinus elevation surgery is the long-term follow-up control due to the grafted material resorption after several years. The stability of the grafted material and the clinical outcomes of the treated cases have been also recorded.

2. Materials and Methods

During the period from 2009 to 2014, 256 patients were referred to our Department for having dental implant rehabilitation in the posterior upper jaw region. About those procedures, a number of 64 patients needed bone augmentation by sinus lift surgery. 31 patients were enrolled in this retrospective study as described below.

All the patients, object of our study, 21 men and 10 women (mean age, 51.2), were partially edentulous and necessitate maxillary sinus elevation procedures for the implant placement. Additional inclusion criteria were as follows: residual bone height less than 3 mm, good state of health, absence of disease that affects wound healing or bone metabolism, and no regular medication consumption for >5 months. All the patients subjected to bone regeneration techniques were nonsmokers. Before implant placement, all patients received oral hygiene instruction and all of them were treated with nonsurgical periodontal therapy when considered necessary. All patients signed an informed consent form detailing the study procedures, according to the 2008 Helsinki protocols and the ethical requirements. These patients presented a bone height of 2 mm (±0.5), making sinus lift procedures necessary for the implant placement. The residual bone height was determined for each site by using a Cone Beam Computed Tomography (CBCT).

2.1. Radiographic Analysis. Radiological images (SkyView CBCT Scanner from MyRay) were obtained before implant placement (baseline) (Figure 1), after the sinus augmentation technique (about 6 months post-op) (Figure 2) and the implant positioning (T1), after 3 months (T2), after 6 months

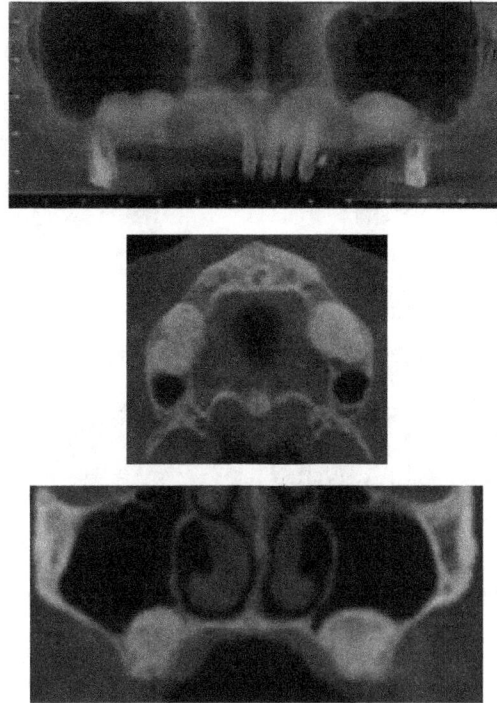

FIGURE 2: The sinus after the augmentation technique. It is possible to underline the material.

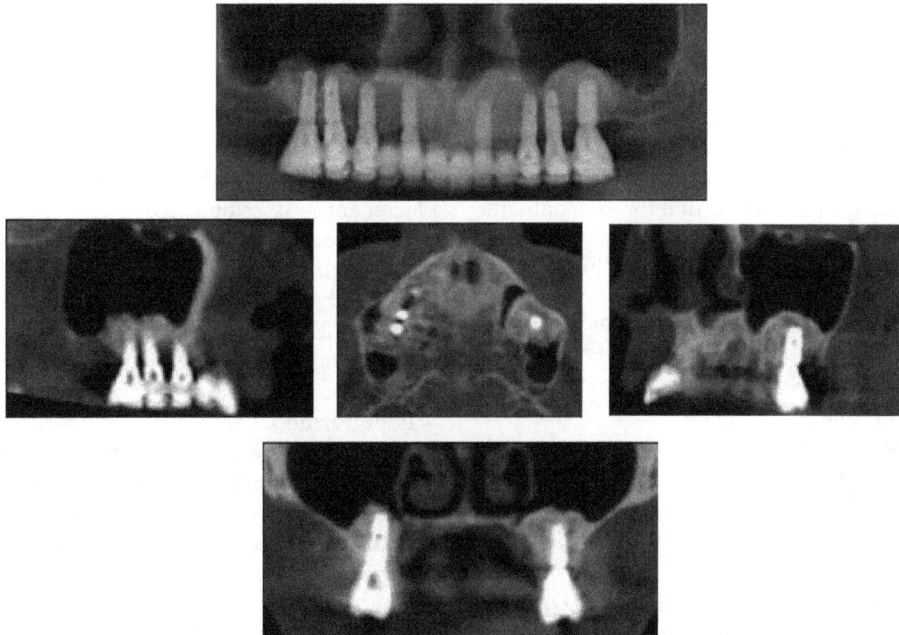

FIGURE 3: 60-month follow-up of the augmented sinus.

(T3), after 12 months (T4), after 24 months (T5), after 48 months (T6), and 60 months (T7) (Figure 3).

The radiographic measurements were made after the 3 d digital reconstruction on the CTs axial section and sagittal or coronal reconstructions, considering the following parameters:

(1) Residual bone height from the alveolar crest to the floor of the maxillary sinus (baseline).

(2) Bone height at T1.

(3) Bone height at follow-up appointments.

The radiological bone augmentation (BA) was calculated using the distance between the sinus floor and the occlusal alveolar ridge at the baseline and comparing it to the same distance at the time of examination (Figure 4).

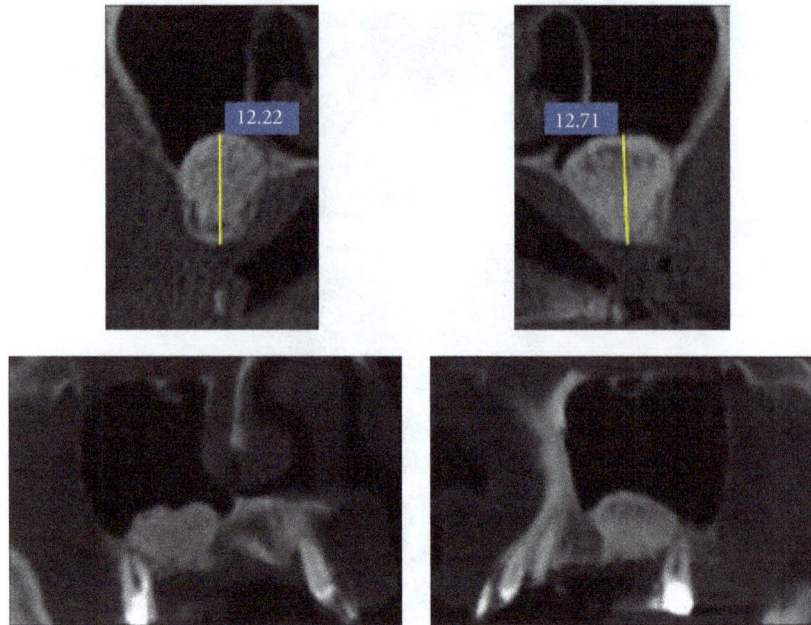

FIGURE 4: Radiological tridimensional evaluation of bone augmentation.

(4) The height of the graft which was calculated measuring from the mesial and distal edges of the graft around the implant to the floor of the sinus.

(5) The graft reduction (GR) which was calculated making the difference between the height of the graft measured at the baseline and the height of the graft at the time of control X-ray analysis. The measure was performed at the same CBCT section for each patient.

Every measurement was calculated as mean value between mesial and distal measurement. A difference of <0.5 mm was considered as a clinically not significant discrepancy.

Peri-implant radiological bone loss, bone resorption, absence of bleeding, and possible signs of inflammation were evaluated during every follow-up appointment by clinical and CBCT evaluation accordingly with the radiological parameters being overstated. The patients included in this clinical study were treated by a single operator and gave their consent to perform the treatment as described in the paper.

2.2. Surgical Procedures. All patients were treated according to the following surgical protocol. All were premedicated with antimicrobial agent (amoxicillin and clavulanic acid 1 gr.) 1 hour before the surgery and continued the therapy for 5 days after, ibuprofen 100 mg twice daily for pain control, if needed, and 0.12% chlorhexidine digluconate mouthwash twice daily for 1 week for plaque control, starting one day after the surgery. A soft diet was recommended, avoiding contact of the surgically involved zone with food for a few days if possible. Patients rinsed their mouth with 0.20% chlorhexidine for 1 minute before surgery and under local anesthesia (mepivacaine 2%); a full-thickness flap was elevated; two vertical releasing incisions were made if necessary. According

TABLE 1: Implant positions ($n = 45$).

Teeth	1.5	1.6	1.7	2.5	2.6	2.7
Implant	3	20	6	5	7	4

to the prosthetic treatment planning, the location for implant placement was established. Bone incision was made with a piezoelectric device (Mectron Piezosurgery) using one cutting bur and dislocating the bone fragment along with the detached Schneiderian membrane into the new upper position. The lifting movement of the membrane without trauma was ensured by using a noncutting divaricator. To ensure the absence of perforation, the Valsalva manoeuvre was performed, confirming the integrity of the membrane, compared to the graft, a mixture of the autologous bone and Geistlich Bio-Oss (Geistlich Biomaterials Italia S.r.l., VI) was gently pushed elevating the already detached membrane, and this step was repeated until the whole site was filled as planned. An intraoral X-ray was made to check the height of the graft. The site was covered with a slow resorbable membrane Geistlich Bio-Gide (Geistlich Biomaterials Italia S.r.l., VI) and sutured with a SUPRAMID NYLON 4/0 nonabsorbable suture (Lorca Marine ES) (Figure 5).

Sutures were removed one week after surgery.

The implants OSSTEM TSIII SA (OSSTEM, KO) were inserted in the first molar position, in the second molar position, and in the second premolar position (Table 1); positioning was made after 6 months, leaving all the implants submerged. After six months the implants were exposed with transmucosal healing abutments and functionally loaded after 2 weeks. All implants had to be in function for a minimum of 48 months.

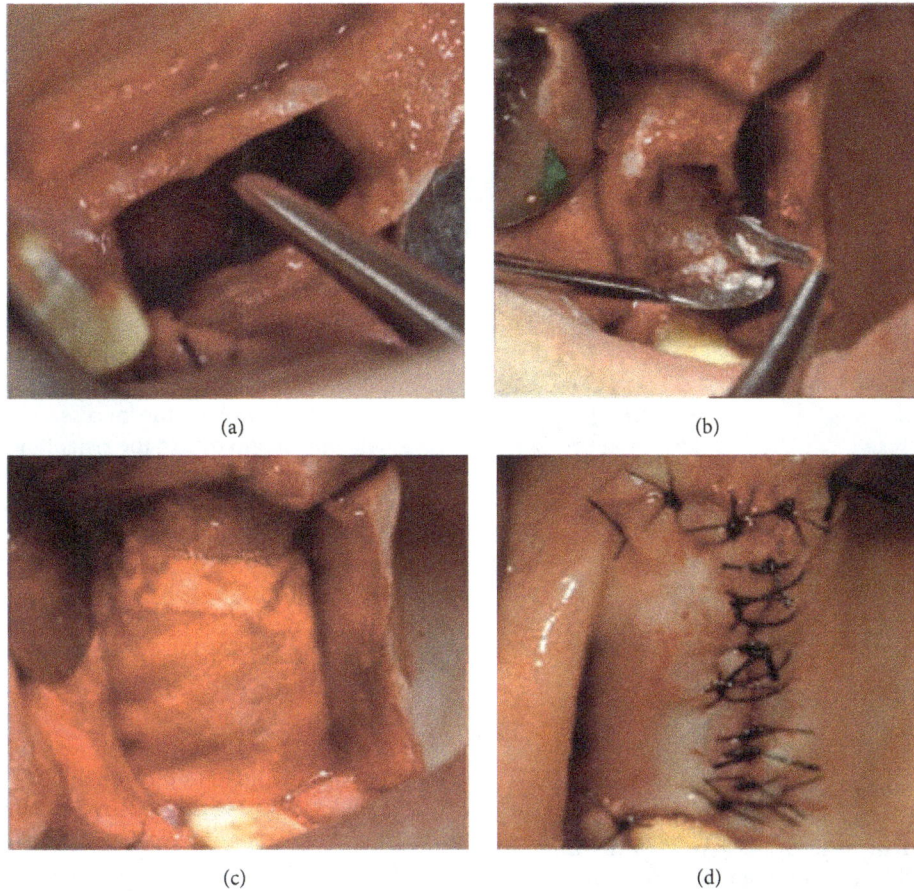

FIGURE 5: Clinical view of the sinus cavity (a). Cavity filled with autologous/heterologous material (b). Collagen sheet placed (c). Suture placed (d).

2.3. Statistical Analysis. The quantitative data (baseline-T7) were expressed as average ± SD. The Student *t*-test (for paired samples) was used to evaluate the statistical difference. Statistical significance was set at $P < 0.05$.

Implant survival was expressed as the percentage of lost implants in relation to the total number of implants inserted. The data were analysed using Kaplan-Meier analysis to provide cumulative survival rates [17, 18] (Figure 6).

3. Results

The first check to the patients was performed at 6 months after the sinus lift surgery performing a new CBCT. The CBCT baselines of each patient and the radiological stents guide have been used for measuring the grafted material presence after the surgery. Moreover, the patient underwent the CBCT by using the same radiologic machine in order to have less bias at the time of the evaluation. During the 5-year period (2009–2014), 45 implants were inserted in 31 patients. The average follow-up time was 52 months (±12 SD; range 0–60 months).

The implants placed were inserted in the first molar position, in the second molar position, and in the second premolar position accordingly with the values recorded on

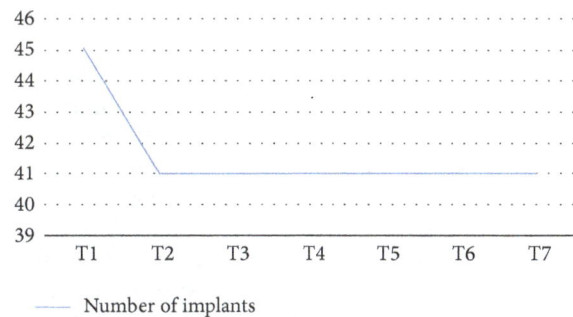

—— Number of implants

FIGURE 6: Implant survival rate.

the Table 1. All the implants used were 4 mm in diameter and number 11 was 8.5 mm in length and number 34 was 10 mm in length (Table 2). The cumulative survival rate of the implants was 99.5%. Of the 45 implants placed, a total of 3 were lost: 1 was lost before loading due to an acute infection after 24 days. Two implants did not osteointegrate and were removed after 3 months (Figure 6). No other adverse effects were observed. The average bone height, considered from the alveolar crest to the bottom of the implant, at the time of implant positioning (T1) was 9.8 mm (±0.86 mm). The measured average bone

TABLE 2: Implant dimension ($n = 45$).

Diameter (mm)	Length (mm)	
	8.5	10
4	11	34

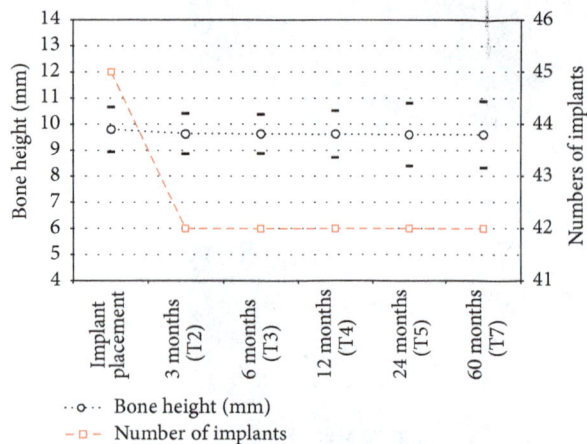

FIGURE 7

height at the first follow-up appointment (T2) was 9.65 mm (± 0.78 mm), with an average bone loss of 0.25 mm. The marginal bone loss of each implant was measured both mesially and distally; the range of loss was from 0 to 2 mm, showing and average value of 0.2 mm (± 0.2 mm) mesially and 0.3 mm (± 0.15 mm) distally (Figure 7 and Table 3).

4. Discussion

The sinus augmentation procedure has been demonstrated as being a reliable and sometimes a mandatory technique when rehabilitating a maxillary atrophic ridge with pneumatized sinuses. The lateral approach proposed by Boyne and James in 1980 allowed a remarkable bone increasing >10 mm, even in atrophic ridges, however resulting in a significant higher postsurgical morbidity and an increased risk of membrane perforation [1, 2, 7]. Crestal approach, osteotome mediated sinus lift surgery, may be performed with different bone grafting material, such as allograft, autogenous bone or heterologous materials, and platelet derivatives themselves or combined with grafting materials, in order to combine the properties of the growth factor to the mechanical presence of soft platelet derivate that allows a better force control during the sinus floor elevation [19–22].

The two augmentation techniques are designed for different clinical situation; Rosen et al. showed how the survival rates for the Summer's technique are strictly linked to the residual bone height, starting from 96% when 5 mm or more of bone is present, dropping to 85% when 4 mm or less is present; however these results may be more linked to the primary stability of the implant than to more biological reasons [23, 24].

The bone height has a relevant influence on the survival rates of implant positioned on augmented bone, decreasing its value with reduced bone height [24, 25].

A decreased bone height resorption rate might be influenced by the osteotomy technique that can maintain a better cellular vitality especially when piezoelectric devices are used instead of rotating instruments [26, 27].

In 1986, Tatum Jr. proposed a transcrestal, more conservative, approach later modified by Summers that first described the use of osteotomes to elevate the membrane and eliminate hammering, making the technique more comfortable for the patient. The crestal technique is nowadays a reliable method allowing contextual implant insertion with good survival rates. However the necessary height of >5 mm of residual bone height due to the risk of membrane perforation and a low implant stability were the main limitation of this technique. In the present retrospective study, the 45 implants later inserted in a 2 mm crest showed excellent survival rates (99.5%), calculated in a significant follow-up period (60 months). This higher result, if compared to other retrospective reports, can be explained thanks to a reduced risk of membrane perforation thanks to the use of piezoelectric device [26]. This outcome is evident considering the bone height gain (7.8 mm, ± 0.86 mm) which is greater than the average of the osteotome technique. This outcome may also be attributed to the nonsmoker selection of patients due to the evidence of the negative impact on bone healing of the nicotine [28].

A reduction of the grafted material has been reported over the first three months of bone remodeling and remained stable over the whole follow-up period (60 months). Other reports showed lower 5-year survival rates of the dental implants placed (97.83, 95.45). However, they consider a higher number of implants [29, 30].

The results observed could be favourably compared with the observation from similar study in which implants were placed into a severely resorbed ridge, with less than 4 mm of residual bone height [31].

Other studies reported lower implant survival rates from 96% to 85.7% when the residual bone height was 4 mm or less, considering the height of bone from the crest of the alveolar ridge to the sinus floor as the most important factor affecting the implant survival rate; this concept is strictly linked to the necessity to insure a high primary stability especially in severe atrophied ridge [12, 23].

More recent studies from Gonzales underlined the good long-term predictability of this technique even in case of simultaneous implant placement in patients with residual bone height of 4 mm or less, confirming that the residual bone height did not increase crestal bone loss or reduce the success rate of the implants and associated prostheses [32].

In particular Mazor et al. showed a 100% implant survival rate at 18-month follow-up, demonstrating the safety and predictability of this minimally invasive sinus lift elevation technique [33].

One of the main aspects that must be considered for a long-term success, especially observed in this study, is linked to the ability to elevate the Schneiderian membrane without any tearing, in addition to a correct anatomy evaluation, a low

TABLE 3: Mean vertical bone heights (mean follow-up 52 ± 12; range, 0–60 months; n = 45 = implants). See Figure 7.

Bone height	Implant placement	3 months (T2)	6 months (T3)	12 months (T4)	24 months (T5)	60 months (T7)
	9.8 mm (±0.86 mm)	9.65 mm (±0.78 mm)	9.63 (±0.75 mm)	9.62 (±0.90)	9.60 (±1.21)	9.60 (±1.28)
n	45	42	42	42	42	42

membrane detachment force, and elasticity and deformation capacity judgment. An increased number of insertion sites can increase the membrane elevation height increasing the elastic properties of the Schneiderian membrane.

The use of grafting materials is, however, debated with several authors describing a consistent bone formation (6.51 mm ± 2.49 mm) even when no grafting material was used after a minimum of 1-year follow-up [34] and others suggest their necessity as the use of a blood clot or platelet concentrates alone may lead to unpredictable results [35]. When grafting materials were used the autologous bone representing nowadays the gold standard however might be subjected to extensive resorption and might be linked to endosinusal contamination due to intraoral pathogens [36, 37].

The height of bone gain is comparable to the one achieved with lateral approach while maintaining the advantage of a less invasive approach with less postoperative morbidity [38].

Our data confirm that the crestal augmentation technique gives the surgeon the possibility of a big bone height augmentation with good long-term survival rates, allowing the insertion of adequate implants per length and diameter, as suggested in literature, even in extreme atrophic ridge.

Further clinical and *in vitro* investigations are needed to measure the mechanical properties of the Schneiderian membrane, minimum force needed for its detachment from the underlying bone and its elasticity and load limits.

5. Conclusion

This analysis suggests that the crestal approach is a successful bone augmentation technique even in a severe atrophic maxilla with 2 mm of crestal bone height.

Conflict of Interests

None of the authors has any conflict of interests to this study.

References

[1] F. Bernardello, D. Righi, F. Cosci, P. Bozzoli, M. Soardi Carlo, and S. Spinato, "Crestal sinus lift with sequential drills and simultaneous implant placement in sites with <5 mm of native bone: a multicenter retrospective study," *Implant Dentistry*, vol. 20, no. 6, pp. 439–444, 2011.

[2] P. J. Boyne and R. A. James, "Grafting of the maxillary sinus floor with autogenous marrow and bone," *Journal of Oral Surgery*, vol. 38, no. 8, pp. 613–616, 1980.

[3] H. Tatum Jr., "Maxillary and sinus implant reconstructions," *Dental clinics of North America*, vol. 30, no. 2, pp. 207–229, 1986.

[4] R. B. Summers, "A new concept in maxillary implant surgery: the osteotome technique," *Compendium*, vol. 15, pp. 154–156, 1994.

[5] R. B. Summers, "The osteotome technique: part 3—less invasive methods of elevating the sinus floor," *Compendium*, vol. 15, no. 6, pp. 698–700, 1994.

[6] F. Cosci and M. Luccioli, "A new sinus lift technique in conjunction with placement of 265 implants: a 6-year retrospective study," *Implant Dentistry*, vol. 9, no. 4, pp. 363–368, 2000.

[7] S. Taschieri, S. Corbella, M. Saita, I. Tsesis, and M. del Fabbro, "Osteotome-mediated sinus lift without grafting material: a review of literature and a technique proposal," *International Journal of Dentistry*, vol. 2012, Article ID 849093, 9 pages, 2012.

[8] I. Woo and B. T. Le, "Maxillary sinus floor elevation: review of anatomy and two techniques," *Implant Dentistry*, vol. 13, no. 1, pp. 28–32, 2004.

[9] M. Beretta, M. Cicciù, E. Bramanti, and C. Maiorana, "Schneider membrane elevation in presence of sinus septa: anatomic features and surgical management," *International Journal of Dentistry*, vol. 2012, Article ID 261905, 6 pages, 2012.

[10] H.-J. Nickenig, M. Wichmann, J. E. Zöller, and S. Eitner, "3-D based minimally invasive one-stage lateral sinus elevation—a prospective randomized clinical pilot study with blinded assessment of postoperative visible facial soft tissue volume changes," *Journal of Cranio-Maxillofacial Surgery*, vol. 42, no. 6, pp. 890–895, 2014.

[11] E. Soardi, F. Cosci, V. Checchi, G. Pellegrino, P. Bozzoli, and P. Felice, "Radiographic analysis of a transalveolar sinus-lift technique: a multipractice retrospective study with a mean follow-up of 5 years," *Journal of Periodontology*, vol. 84, no. 8, pp. 1039–1047, 2013.

[12] M. Del Fabbro, S. Corbella, T. Weinstein, V. Ceresoli, and S. Taschieri, "Implant survival rates after osteotome-mediated maxillary sinus augmentation: a systematic review," *Clinical Implant Dentistry and Related Research*, vol. 14, supplement 1, pp. e159–e168, 2012.

[13] N. M. Timmenga, G. M. Raghoebar, R. Van Weissenbruch, and A. Vissink, "Maxillary sinusitis after augmentation of the maxillary sinus floor: a report of 2 cases," *Journal of Oral and Maxillofacial Surgery*, vol. 59, no. 2, pp. 200–204, 2001.

[14] N. M. Timmenga, G. M. Raghoebar, R. S. B. Liem, R. van Weissenbruch, W. L. Manson, and A. Vissink, "Effects of maxillary sinus floor elevation surgery on maxillary sinus physiology," *European Journal of Oral Sciences*, vol. 111, no. 3, pp. 189–197, 2003.

[15] E. Kfir, V. Kfir, E. Kaluski, Z. Mazor, and M. Goldstein, "Minimally invasive antral membrane balloon elevation for single-tooth implant placement," *Quintessence International*, vol. 42, no. 8, pp. 645–650, 2011.

[16] S. K. Doud Galli, R. A. Lebowitz, R. J. Giacchi, R. Glickman, and J. B. Jacobs, "Chronic sinusitis complicating sinus lift surgery," *American Journal of Rhinology*, vol. 15, no. 3, pp. 181–186, 2001.

[17] E. L. Kaplan and P. Meier, "Nonparametric estimation from incomplete observations," *The Journal of the American Statistical Association*, vol. 53, no. 282, pp. 457–481, 1958.

[18] J. A. Shibli, A. Piattelli, G. Iezzi et al., "Effect of smoking on early bone healing around oxidized surfaces: a prospective, controlled study in human jaws," *Journal of Periodontology*, vol. 81, no. 4, pp. 575–583, 2010.

[19] A. C. Wetzel, H. Stich, and R. G. Caffesse, "Bone apposition onto oral implants in the sinus area filled with different grafting materials. A histological study in beagle dogs," *Clinical Oral Implants Research*, vol. 6, no. 3, pp. 155–163, 1995.

[20] A. Simonpieri, J. Choukroun, M. Del Corso, G. Sammartino, and D. M. D. Ehrenfest, "Simultaneous sinus-lift and implantation using microthreaded implants and leukocyte- and platelet-rich fibrin as sole grafting material: a six-year experience," *Implant Dentistry*, vol. 20, no. 1, pp. 2–12, 2011.

[21] F. Xuan, C. U. Lee, J. S. Son, S. M. Jeong, and B. H. Choi, "A comparative study of the regenerative effect of sinus bone grafting with platelet-rich fibrin-mixed Bio-Oss and commercial fibrin-mixed Bio-Oss: an experimental study," *Journal of Cranio-Maxillofacial Surgery*, vol. 42, no. 4, pp. e47–e50, 2014.

[22] S. Taschieri, S. Corbella, M. Saita, I. Tsesis, and M. Del Fabbro, "Osteotome-mediated sinus lift without grafting material: a review of literature and a technique proposal," *International Journal of Dentistry*, vol. 2012, Article ID 849093, 9 pages, 2012.

[23] P. S. Rosen, R. Summers, J. R. Mellado et al., "The bone-added osteotome sinus floor elevation technique: multicenter retrospective report of consecutively treated patients," *The International Journal of Oral & Maxillofacial Implants*, vol. 14, no. 6, pp. 853–858, 1999.

[24] C. Călin, A. Petre, and S. Drafta, "Osteotome-mediated sinus floor elevation: a systematic review and meta-analysis," *The International Journal of Oral & Maxillofacial Implants*, vol. 29, no. 3, pp. 558–576, 2014.

[25] B. Al-Nawas and E. Schiegnitz, "Augmentation procedures using bone substitute materials or autogenous bone—a systematic review and meta-analysis," *European Journal of Oral Implantology*, vol. 7, supplement 2, pp. S219–234, 2014.

[26] G. Sammartino, O. Trosino, A. E. di Lauro, M. Amato, and A. Cioffi, "Use of piezosurgery device in management of surgical dental implant complication: a case report," *Implant Dentistry*, vol. 20, no. 2, pp. e1–e6, 2011.

[27] C. C. S. Pereira, W. C. Gealh, L. Meorin-Nogueira, I. R. Garcia-Júnior, and R. Okamoto, "Piezosurgery applied to implant dentistry: clinical and biological aspects," *Journal of Oral Implantology*, vol. 40, no. 1, pp. 401–408, 2014.

[28] J. A. Shibli, A. Piattelli, G. Iezzi et al., "Effect of smoking on early bone healing around oxidized surfaces: a prospective, controlled study in human jaws," *Journal of Periodontology*, vol. 81, no. 4, pp. 575–583, 2010.

[29] J. Tetsch, P. Tetsch, and D. A. Lysek, "Long-term results after lateral and osteotome technique sinus floor elevation: a retrospective analysis of 2190 implants over a time period of 15 years," *Clinical Oral Implants Research*, vol. 21, no. 5, pp. 497–503, 2010.

[30] G. B. Bruschi, R. Crespi, P. Capparè, F. Bravi, E. Bruschi, and E. Gherlone, "Localized management of sinus floor technique for implant placement in fresh molar sockets," *Clinical Implant Dentistry and Related Research*, vol. 15, no. 2, pp. 243–250, 2013.

[31] A. A. Winter, A. S. Pollack, and R. B. Odrich, "Placement of implants in the severely atrophic posterior maxilla using localized management of the sinus floor: a preliminary study," *The International Journal of Oral & Maxillofacial Implants*, vol. 17, no. 5, pp. 687–695, 2002.

[32] S. Gonzalez, M.-C. Tuan, K. M. Ahn, and H. Nowzari, "Crestal approach for maxillary sinus augmentation in patients with ≤4 mm of residual alveolar bone," *Clinical Implant Dentistry and Related Research*, vol. 16, no. 6, pp. 827–835, 2013.

[33] Z. Mazor, E. Kfir, A. Lorean, E. Mijiritsky, and R. A. Horowitz, "Flapless approach to maxillary sinus augmentation using minimally invasive antral membrane balloon elevation," *Implant Dentistry*, vol. 20, no. 6, pp. 434–438, 2011.

[34] A. Thor, L. Sennerby, J. M. Hirsch, and L. Rasmusson, "Bone formation at the maxillary sinus floor following simultaneous elevation of the mucosal lining and implant installation without graft material: an evaluation of 20 patients treated with 44 Astra Tech implants," *Journal of Oral and Maxillofacial Surgery*, vol. 65, no. 7, supplement 1, pp. 64–72, 2007.

[35] S.-M. Jeong, C.-U. Lee, J.-S. Son, J.-H. Oh, Y. Fang, and B.-H. Choi, "Simultaneous sinus lift and implantation using platelet-rich fibrin as sole grafting material," *Journal of Cranio-Maxillofacial Surgery*, vol. 42, no. 6, pp. 990–994, 2014.

[36] S. S. Wallace and S. J. Froum, "Effect of maxillary sinus augmentation on the survival of endosseous dental implants. A systematic review," *Annals of Periodontology*, vol. 8, no. 1, pp. 328–343, 2003.

[37] F. Verdugo, A. Castillo, K. Simonian et al., "Periodontopathogen and Epstein-Barr virus contamination affects transplanted bone volume in sinus augmentation," *Journal of Periodontology*, vol. 83, no. 2, pp. 162–173, 2012.

[38] U. Kher, Z. Mazor, P. Stanitsas, and G. A. Kotsakis, "Implants placed simultaneously with lateral window sinus augmentation using a putty alloplastic bone substitute for increased primary implant stability: a retrospective study," *Implant Dentistry*, vol. 23, no. 4, pp. 496–501, 2014.

4

Quality of Root Canals Performed by the Inaugural Class of Dental Students at Libyan International Medical University

Ranya F. Elemam,[1,2] **Ziad Salim Abdul Majid,**[1] **Matt Groesbeck,**[3] **and Álvaro F. Azevedo**[4]

[1]*Department of Restorative Dentistry and Periodontology, School of Dentistry, Libyan International Medical University (LIMU), Benghazi, Libya*
[2]*University of Porto, Porto, Portugal*
[3]*Salt Lake City, UT, USA*
[4]*Faculty of Dentistry, EPIUNIT-ISPUP,, University of Porto, Porto, Portugal*

Correspondence should be addressed to Ranya F. Elemam; ranya_elemam@yahoo.co.uk

Academic Editor: Sema Belli

Objective. The purpose of this study was to radiographically evaluate technical quality of root canal fillings performed by dental undergraduates at Libyan International Medical University in Libya. *Methods.* Root canal cases were treated at university dental clinic from the fall of 2012 to the fall of 2013 by the fourth and fifth year dental students. Students used step-back preparation and cold lateral compaction in the treatment. Radiographs were reviewed over a two-year period from initial procedure to final restoration. Radiographs were evaluated for adequacy or inadequacy by length, density, and taper. Length inadequacy was classified as short or overextended. Overall quality was considered "adequate" based on all three variables. Chi-square tested differences between teeth groupings and adequacy classification. Significant *p* value results were adjusted by Bonferroni correction. *Results.* Adequate length of root canal fillings were observed in roughly half of all samples (48.6%). Density was adequate in 75.8% of the samples. Taper was observed as adequate in 68.8%. Higher quality was evident in anterior teeth (plus premolars) versus molars (65.6% versus 43.3%, resp.; *p* < 0.04). *Conclusion.* Overall quality of endodontic treatment performed by undergraduate dental students was adequate in 53.9% of the cases. Significant opportunity exists to improve the quality of root canals provided by dental students.

1. Introduction

Teaching undergraduate endodontics has been recognized as one of the most formidable challenges across all dental subjects [1]. Educators have had to continuously cope with the discipline's contemporary evolution, which has rapidly spread in the past 2 decades and even outpaced other dental specialties by measures of scholarly research activity [2]. The foremost educational goal of endodontics is to successfully promulgate knowledge as a foundation for graduates to become competent and proficient in actual practice [3]. All endodontic treatment modalities require advanced knowledge and technical skills should be considered essential in pursuing this objective [4].

In contemporary endodontic curricula, educators have devoted special focus to optimize technical quality of root canal procedures. Some studies have demonstrated an association between root canal-specific training during the student's study period and improved quality of root canal fillings performed by dental graduates [5–8]. Further efforts have been made to improve root canal quality via postgraduate interventions, including continuing dental education (CDE) or development of a quality improvement initiative to improve quality of care [6, 9].

The European Society of Endodontology (ESE) has published undergraduate curriculum guidelines updated every decade to encourage the development of high quality undergraduate dental education and acceptable standards of care in clinical endodontic practice [3, 10–12]. These guidelines, widely integrated into endodontic curricula [1], emphasize the necessity for undergraduate students to undertake principles of clinical and theoretical education and apply them to the clinical outcome to reach a minimum competency threshold prior to graduation. Because root canals are widely performed by general dental practitioners as opposed to specialists alone, guiding principles place high expectation for dental students to demonstrate a satisfactory nonsurgical root canal procedure on both single- and multirooted teeth.

We have directly observed endodontic practical sessions in Libya's government-run dental schools and found that they offer abbreviated and very limited exposure to endodontic topics that are inadequate to cultivate knowledge and competence. Reasons for this suboptimal training likely include (1) the vast number of dental students, (2) fewer available patients, (3) a sparsity of endodontic equipment and material availability, (4) limited endodontics staff, and (5) the prevailing belief that endodontics should be a specialist subject. The absence of complete endodontic training in dental education may therefore severely impair a graduate's decision-making and clinical effectiveness, leading to pervasive treatment failures.

In the fall of 2007, the first accredited private medical university in Libya was founded in Benghazi, Libyan International Medical University (LIMU), with the mission to graduate highly qualified graduates in different areas of health. LIMU is the only educational alternative to government-run schools for prospective students in Benghazi. The LIMU dental curricula mandate that endodontic training should be provided to all dental students within five years. A preclinical course is tentatively started in the third year requiring students to perform root canals on at least four anterior human-extracted teeth, two premolars, and two molars. Clinical courses follow, with fourth and fifth year dental students undertaking education in endodontic treatment tailored to specific requirements, including a comprehensive clinical examination informing appropriate diagnosis. During the fourth year, students perform the nonsurgical root canal treatment of four anterior teeth and four premolars. In the fifth year, students are required to complete primary endodontic procedure of three molars in the first semester and a comprehensive case treatment in the second semester. In the sixth year's nine month internship period, students undertake routine orthograde root canal therapy per patient presentation.

Research evaluations of root canal treatment quality have been shown to significantly aid the planning of future endodontic educational programs [13]. While quality evaluations of root canals performed by graduated students during their preclinical and clinical coursework have been widely reported elsewhere, there have been no published reports originating from Libya regarding quality of root canal fillings performed by dental students.

The aim of this study was to evaluate the technical quality of root canal treatment performed by the first undergraduate group during their clinical academic terms in both the fourth and fifth years at LIMU. This effort was also undertaken to gauge the scope of revisions necessary to successfully modify the preclinical program curriculum delivered during the preclinical semesters.

2. Methods

2.1. Patients. Patient cases were treated by thirty-two undergraduate students in the university dental clinic during their fourth and fifth years from the fall of 2012 to the fall of 2013. The study protocol was reviewed and exempted by the institutional review board. All students were supervised by staff specialized in endodontics in the first clinical year. In the final year, a conservative specialist with interest in endodontics was appointed. The ratio of clinical supervisor to student was 1 to 8.

All chart records and radiographs of patients who had received endodontic student treatment at LIMU were collected and reviewed by an investigator from initial procedure time to final restoration, all over the two-year academic period following the group of thirty-two dental students through their clinical course. A total of twenty-seven dental students entered their fifth year, reflecting minor expected attrition. Patients were excluded if they were younger than 16 years of age and if they had records that did not include preoperative and postoperative periapical radiographs, unreadable radiographs due to developing procedures, superimposed anatomical structures, records without complete root canal treatment, or cases of perforation, instrument separation, or missing canals. In year four, the thirty-two students treated a total of 256 teeth. In year five, the twenty-seven remaining students treated 81 teeth. Thus, a total of 337 teeth were treated over the two-year academic period.

2.2. Procedure. After assessing the medical and dental history of each patient, local anesthesia was administered using 2% lignocaine 1:20,000 (Alexandria Co., Alexandria, Egypt). Rubber dam isolation was used for all patients. Access cavity was prepared and the working length was determined using size of 15 K file (Dentsply, Dentsply Ltd., UK). Periapical radiographs were then taken using the paralleling technique with Trophy (France) X-ray unit and the Kodak D-Speed films were exposed at 65 kV, 10 mA. Step-back technique using a stainless steel hand K-files (0.02 taper) was performed and root canals were irrigated using 1% sodium hypochlorite (NaOCl). EDTA 17% gel was used to negotiate calcified canals. All root canals were filled with gutta-percha 0.02 taper (Gapadent co., Ltd., Hamburg, Germany) and zinc oxide-based sealer (Metabiomed Co., Ltd., Korea) using cold lateral condensation technique. An NiTi finger spreader of 2% taper was used to compact the gutta-percha cones and create a space for accessory points. For each root-filled tooth, at least 2 periapical radiographs were taken (preoperative and postobturation). One investigator, a specialist in endodontics, independently examined the radiographs utilizing a magnifying lens (×4) and an X-ray viewer.

2.3. Outcome Variables. Technical quality of root canal fillings was assessed by radiography based on 3 variables: (1) length as compared to the radiographic apex, (2) density of obturation by the presence or absence of voids, and (3) taper. The density and taper of root canal fillings were classified as adequate or inadequate. Length was rated as adequate or short (inadequate) or overextended (also inadequate).

Overall quality was deemed "adequate" if all 3 variables were acceptable according to protocol-specified criteria as presented in Table 2. Postobturation radiographs were captured via paralleling technique, displaying the entire length of the root and 2 to 3 mm beyond it (see sample radiographs in Figures 5(a), 5(b), and 5(c)). Radiographs were assessed for adequate length quality (see the example in Figure 5(a)). Figures 5(b) and 5(c) represented inadequate quality that was either too short in length or of overextended length, respectively.

2.4. Statistical Analysis. Descriptive statistics present categorical variable frequencies and percentages. Chi-square test statistic was performed to determine statistically significant differences between the "adequate" and "inadequate" counted variables. Alpha level was set at .05. If significance was reached, Bonferroni correction was applied to adjust the p value by multiplying it by the number of the comparisons $(2 + 1)$ in each maxillary and mandibular teeth to account for multiple comparisons. Both Excel 2013 (Microsoft, Redmond, WA, USA) and SPSS software v.20 (SPSS Inc., Chicago, IL, USA) were used for all statistical procedures and validation of analysis.

3. Results

After applying inclusion and exclusion criteria, 128 teeth constituted the final sample over the two-year academic period (32 anterior teeth, 29 premolars, and 67 molars).

3.1. Overall Quality (Figure 1)

3.1.1. Maxilla and Mandible Combined. The overall quality was defined by the combination of all three outcome variables that were deemed adequate (length, density, and taper) for all maxillary and mandibular teeth. All measures of adequacy are reported in this results' section and in Figures 1 through 4, whereas inadequate percentages are only reported in the same corresponding figures.

Overall quality was deemed adequate in 53.9% of all maxillary and mandibular teeth. There were statistically significant differences between teeth types, with 65.6% of anterior teeth and premolars classified as adequate compared to 43.3% of molars ($p < 0.04$; Figure 1). By outcome variable for both maxillary and mandibular teeth combined, root canal filling length was observed to be adequate in 48.6% of all teeth, density was adequate in 75.8%, and taper was adequate in 68.8%.

3.2. Length (Figure 2)

3.2.1. Maxilla. Adequate length of root filling was observed in 64.0% of all maxillary teeth. The incisors and molars demonstrated fewer numbers of teeth with adequate length compared to canines and premolars, although this difference was not statistically significant ($p > 0.2$).

3.2.2. Mandible. For mandibular teeth, only premolars and molars were existing and thus analyzed. Adequate length was

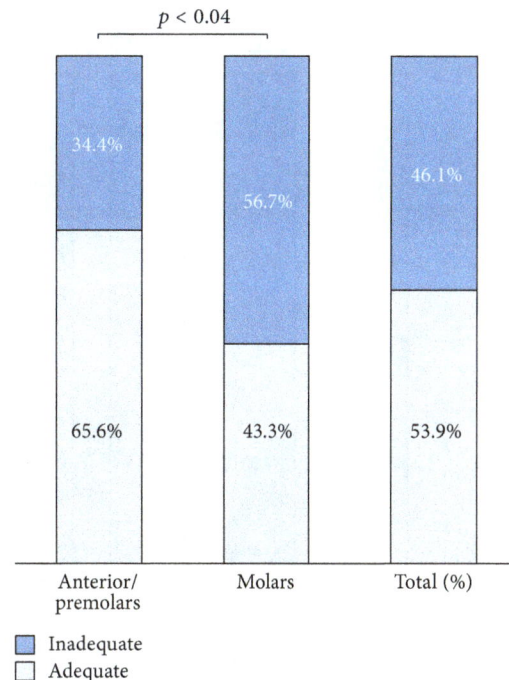

FIGURE 1: Overall quality (%) of root canals in maxillary and mandibular teeth.

observed in 33.3% of all mandibular teeth, of which 37.5% were premolars and 32.4% were molars, but the difference between these groups was not found to be statistically significant ($p > 0.7$).

3.3. Density (Figure 3)

3.3.1. Maxilla. Adequate density of root filling was seen in 82.6% of all maxillary teeth, 57.6% of which were molars and 98.1% were anterior teeth plus premolars. When both groups were compared, the difference was found to be statistically significant ($p < 0.0001$).

3.3.2. Mandible. Adequate density was observed in 69.0% of all mandibular teeth. All premolars were adequate (100%), in contrast to 61.8% of the molars, and the difference was also statistically significant ($p < 0.1$).

3.4. Taper (Figure 4)

3.4.1. Maxilla. Adequate taper was found in 68.6% of all maxillary teeth. The maxillary canines that demonstrated the highest rate of taper (87.5%) compared to the molars were (54.5%), but this difference was not found to be statistically significant ($p > 0.1$).

3.4.2. Mandible. Adequate taper was found in 69.0% of all mandibular teeth, 87.5% of which were premolars and 64.7% were molars, but this difference was also not statistically significant ($p > 0.05$).

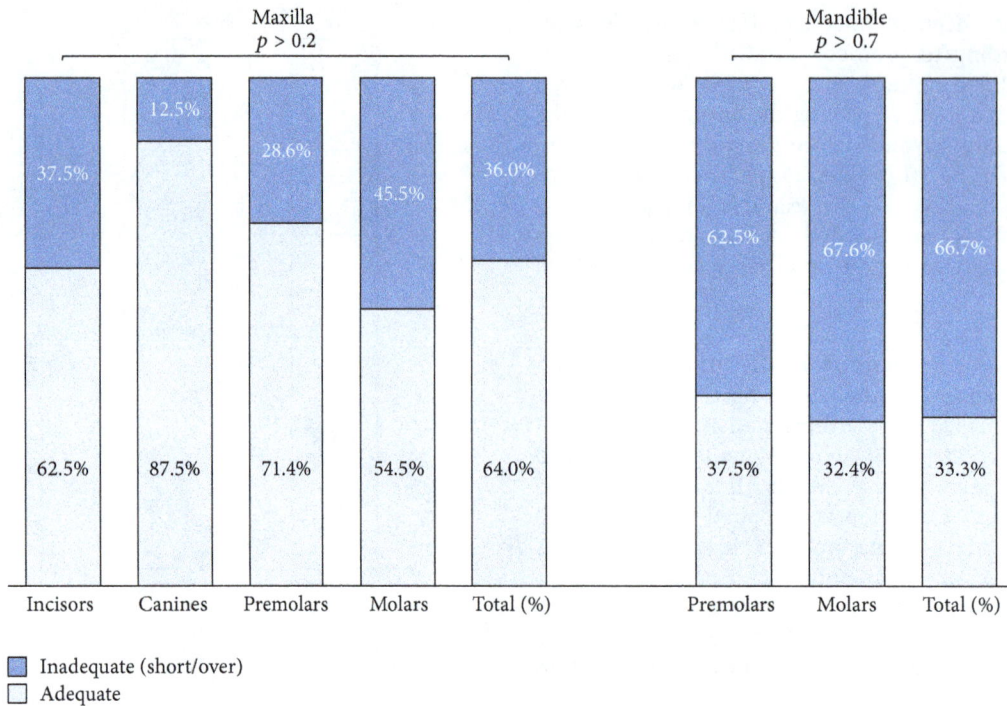

FIGURE 2: Length quality (%) in maxillary and mandibular root canal-filled teeth.

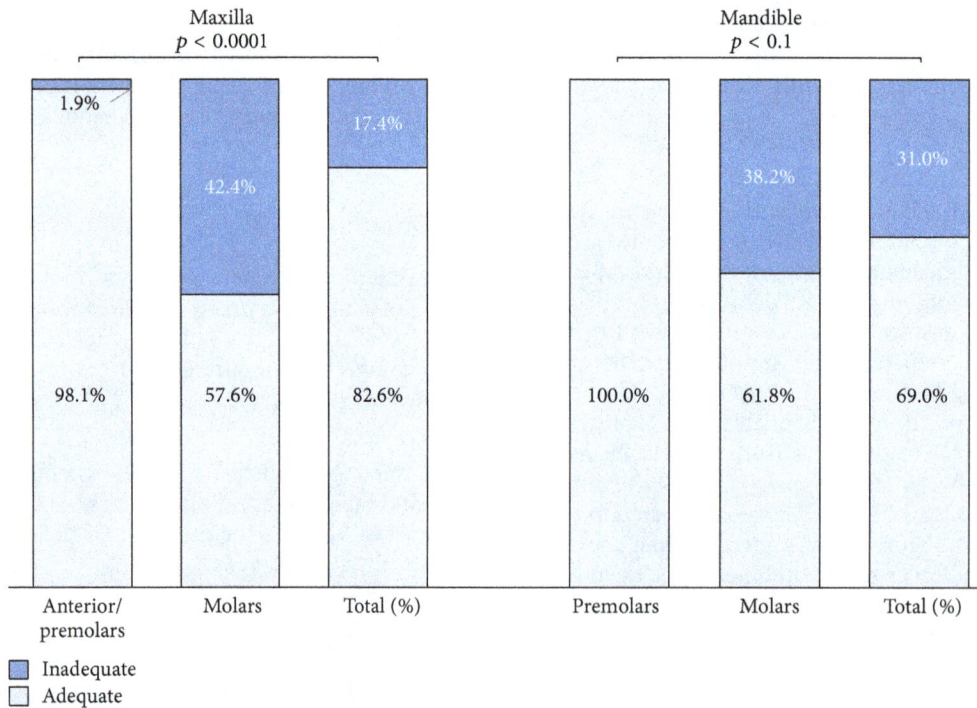

FIGURE 3: Density quality (%) in maxillary and mandibular root canal-filled teeth.

4. Discussion

This is the first endodontic research study of its kind reported from Libya. These data objectively identify the quality of endodontic treatments performed by Libyan dental students, who would shortly be expected to serve the community. Other studies radiographically assessed only the length and density of root canal filling but omitted the taper variable [14–17]. We incorporated the taper variable defined by guidelines [18] and results were comparable to other research studying

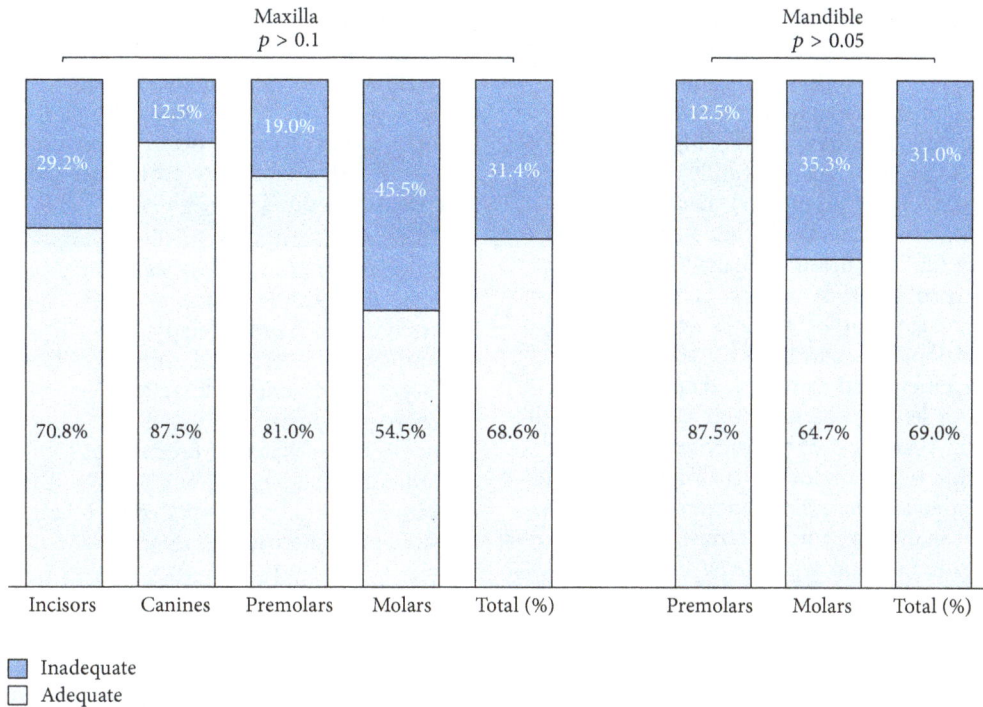

FIGURE 4: Taper quality (%) in maxillary and mandibular root canal-filled teeth.

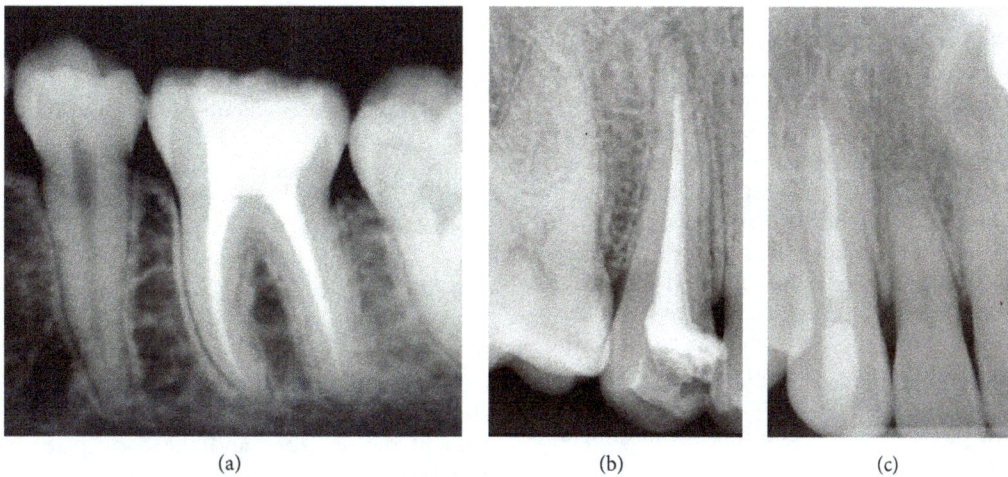

FIGURE 5: Radiographs depicting adequate quality root canal (a), inadequate/short length (b), and inadequate/overextended length (c).

tapers [5, 14, 15, 19]. We observed adequate taper in 68.8% of root canals, a finding slightly less than the 71% reported by Román-Richon and colleagues, in which rotary files were used and 82% were reported by Fonseka and colleagues, of which the latter study only investigated single-rooted molars with wide versus narrow canals [15, 19].

Our percentage of overall quality was 53.9%, less than the reports from Turkey (79.5%), Serbia (74%), and Malaysia (61%) [16, 17, 20], similar to Greece (55%) [21], but greater than reports from Iran (45%), Spain (44%), Sudan (24%), and

Saudi Arabia (23%) [5, 13, 14, 19]. However, inequalities may be difficult to reconcile because of the differences in outcome criteria used, sample sizes, and design. We report a low percentage of adequate molars treated in the second year (43%) compared to the adequately-treated anterior and premolars in the first year (65.6%), which skewed the overall percentage of adequate root fillings to 53.9%. Difficulty in treating molars by undergraduate students was also reported in other studies [13, 14, 20, 21]. In contrast, a Sudanese study showed that the adequacy of posterior teeth was 79.7% versus 20.3% of anterior teeth [5]. One plausible explanation to account for this discrepancy might be attributable to experiential learning and progressive adaptation of individual students.

Overall, inadequate root canal fillings were seen in 46.1% of root canals (Figure 1). Molars showed high percentage of inadequacy 56.7%, which was significantly different from 34.4% of anterior teeth (plus premolars). Difficulty in successfully treating molars was managed by most dental schools [21, 22]. In our study, this significant value may be attributable to the anatomical complexity of molars, lack of specialist supervision during treatment of molars, and insufficient training in time and depth of material devoted to molars and complication management in the preclinical curriculum.

Acceptable filling length was observed in 48.6% of all teeth. This was lower than most of the previous studies [13–17, 19]. This low value may be relevant to a high percentage of fillings with inadequate length in molars. To improve the length of root canal fillings, an electronic apex locator should be used in conjunction with X-ray radiographs. A homogeneous filling was found in 75.8% of root canals. This was less than that reported in other studies from Turkey (92%) [16] and Serbia (92.6%) [17]. In contrast, it was greater than that reported from Saudi Arabia and Iran (34%), Sudan (45%), and Spain (69%) [5, 13, 14, 19]. This might be explained by the fact that LIMU students were using Nitti finger spreaders, which have proven to provide better outcomes for lateral compaction technique, especially in curved canals because of deeper penetration [23].

It is important to recognize that improvements for greater educational impact can likely be bolstered by improved teacher-student alignment, credibility, trust, and a willingness to interact. Knowledge and competency are progressive achievements on the spectrum of learning toward mastery (expertise) [24]. Guidelines have suggested that students be supervised by appropriate endodontic specialists [12]. Our program employs an endodontic specialist in the first clinical year as a supervisor and a restorative specialist in the second. Past guidelines have also recommended an acceptable ratio between supervisor and students [25], which can aid in identifying student weaknesses [26]. Our supervisor-to-student ratio was 1 to 8 for both clinical years; ratios of other studies were 1 to 5 in Iran [13], 1 to 6 in Sudan [5], 1 to 12 in Spain, and 1 to 15 in Greece [27].

Our ratio allowed close monitoring and evaluation, both elements are instrumental in detecting student strengths and weaknesses. However, merely identifying student weaknesses and mishaps without prompt correction may inadvertently reinforce erroneous practices [28]. Even if supervisor feedback is immediate, manner of supervisor feedback is equally important, since competency can only be cultivated in conditions of constructive, directive feedback [12].

In our program and others, there are opportunities to optimize supervisor interaction with students, particularly by training supervisors in tactful approaches to a range of personality types that can ensure that students are motivated to actively participate [29]. Ideally, the supervisor should facilitate reflection of what the student has already learned, encouraged to self-evaluate their own weaknesses and, in opportune moments, remind students of acceptable practice

standards [30]. A 2013 meta-analysis reported that planned, structured debriefings of either individuals alone or in teams can yield up to a 25% increase in performance regardless of it being a real case or a simulated setting [31]. Overall, effective learning is more likely to occur when a student is motivated to acknowledge that they are in need of input ultimately accepting direction [30, 32].

Instead of learning passively by simply being corrected, it is desirable for a student to be as active a learner can be as possible [33, 34]. A 2013 survey of dental students' perspectives reported that 92% preferred dynamic, interactive educational techniques [35]. Active learning can be even achieved by modifying traditionally didactic courses in breakout format for more group- or case-based discussions [36, 37], theater format to better visualize procedures [38], or interacting via an audience response system [18, 39]. It is incumbent upon educators to engage students while it is the responsibility of the students to be willing to participate.

Discerning and addressing student strengths and weaknesses are a key function of formative and summative evaluations, thereby informing educators of their student's needs to effectively model or redesign curricula. These processes are highlighted by both recent guidelines [12] and several studies reporting their use in medical education setting [29, 37, 40, 41] and academic teaching staff should accept the responsibility to employ formative and summative assessment techniques to determine priorities and then revise curricula accordingly just as other programs have to meet the needs of their students [21]. Direct observation of trainees is a vital hallmark of assessment to inform curricula across all specialties of medicine, including endodontic training [29]. As such, the supervisory role of educators, openness to student feedback, and the reporting of that feedback is crucial for actionable evaluations. This is even more important as emerging technologies might at any moment be adopted that could impact diagnosis, treatment, and the dissemination of real clinical skills in clinics or simulators [37, 40]. Qualtrough has estimated that students may be using haptic technology in practical learning applications as early 2020 [1]. Data from our study was compared to other recent published studies and revealed that international agreement related to student performance and the basic principles in applying European endodontics guidelines were followed. However, to improve success with molar teeth, preclinical training must be improved to acquire the clinical skills needed to treat molars. While problems in treating molars were noticed instantly by the endodontic staff at LIMU, a modified curriculum has already been implemented for subsequent groups.

5. New Curriculum Model

Our curriculum has undergone a number of changes and will likely be further revised. The practical sessions of the preclinical course has been divided between two semesters: the first semester of the third year (fifth semester) and the second semester of the fourth year (sixth semester). In the fifth semester, students treat at least four anterior teeth, two premolars and two molars, while in the sixth semester, they treat

TABLE 1: Distribution of teeth and root canals in both jaws.

	Incisors		Canines		Premolars		Molars	
	Teeth	Canals	Teeth	Canals	Teeth	Canals	Teeth	Canals
Maxillary	24	24	8	8	21	36	33	102
Mandibular	0	0	0	0	8	8	34	106

TABLE 2: Criteria for the evaluation of root canal fillings.

Quality variable	Criteria	Definition
Length	Adequate	Filling ends are 0.5 to 2 mm from the radiographic apex
	Overfilled	Filling extends beyond the radiographic apex
	Underfilled	Filling ends are shorter than 2 mm from the radiographic apex
Taper	Adequate	A consistent taper from coronal to apical aspects with good canal shape
	Inadequate	Inconsistent taper
Density	Adequate	Uniform density without clear presence of voids

four molars. The competency-based method [42] was emphasized by ESE around the importance of student quality performance versus quantity [12]. However, there exists diversity between schools regarding minimum requirements of treated cases. The ESE sets minimum number of clinical experiences to be greater than twenty canals, including extracted teeth [43] (Table 1). In the LIMU curriculum, the total number of canals in the preclinical stage was set at 20 to 24.

In this added course, students received a one hour endodontic lecture and gained four hours lab experience per week over sixteen weeks dedicated almost exclusively for molars. During lab sessions, students provided a checklist for self-evaluation for each tooth. They were asked to finish root canal treatment in four extracted molars (two maxillary and two mandibular molars). To enhance their understanding toward the procedural errors and how to avoid them, students were asked to identify and document mishaps as soon as they occurred and to correct simple ledges and perforations. Students also performed treatment in single-rooted teeth using a rotary system for canal preparation. Later, they were asked to present one of their cases to explain the procedure and to detail mishaps and protective actions taken. Because a change took place in the preclinical course, future studies evaluating the clinical performance for this group of students are needed to investigate the impact of this newly-revised curriculum.

6. Conclusion

The quality of root canal fillings performed by undergraduate dental students at the Libyan International Medical University was satisfied in 53.9% of the cases, revealing a substantial gap in unmet educational needs. We must continue to adapt our educational plans to bolster student knowledge and confidence, particularly in treating molars, with the aim of ultimately yielding demonstrated improvements in competency. Testing the effect of the new model and several other education improvement initiatives are required to improve actual clinical performance of subsequent groups of dental students.

Conflict of Interests

The authors declare that there is no conflict of interests regarding the publication of this paper.

References

[1] A. J. E. Qualtrough, "Undergraduate endodontic education: what are the challenges?" *British Dental Journal*, vol. 216, no. 6, pp. 361–364, 2014.

[2] V. R. Vora, *Growth and dissemination of endodontic knowledge [Ph.D. thesis]*, The University of Michigan, 2011.

[3] C. Löst, "Quality guidelines for endodontic treatment: consensus report of the European Society of Endodontology," *International Endodontic Journal*, vol. 39, no. 12, pp. 921–930, 2006.

[4] L.-H. Chueh, S.-C. Chen, C.-M. Lee et al., "Technical quality of root canal treatment in Taiwan," *International Endodontic Journal*, vol. 36, no. 6, pp. 416–422, 2003.

[5] R. O. Elsayed, N. H. Abu-Bakr, and Y. E. Ibrahim, "Quality of root canal treatment performed by undergraduate dental students at the University of Khartoum, Sudan," *Australian Endodontic Journal*, vol. 37, no. 2, pp. 56–60, 2011.

[6] K. S. Al-Fouzan, "A survey of root canal treatment of molar teeth by general dental practitioners in private practice in Saudi Arabia," *Saudi Dental Journal*, vol. 22, no. 3, pp. 113–117, 2010.

[7] A. J. E. Qualtrough, J. M. Whitworth, and P. M. H. Dummer, "Preclinical endodontology: an international comparison," *International Endodontic Journal*, vol. 32, no. 5, pp. 406–414, 1999.

[8] M. Buckley and L. S. W. Spangberg, "The prevalence and technical quality of endodontic treatment in an American subpopulation," *Oral Surgery, Oral Medicine, Oral Pathology, Oral Radiology, and Endodontology*, vol. 79, no. 1, pp. 92–100, 1995.

[9] R. J. G. de Moor, G. M. G. Hommez, J. G. de Boever, K. I. M. Delmé, and G. E. I. Martens, "Periapical health related to the quality of root canal treatment in a Belgian population," *International Endodontic Journal*, vol. 33, no. 2, pp. 113–120, 2000.

[10] European Society of Endodontology, "Consensus report of the European Society of Endodontology on quality guidelines for endodontic treatment," *International Endodontic Journal*, vol. 27, no. 3, pp. 115–124, 1994.

[11] C. Löst, "Undergraduate curriculum guidelines for endodontology," *International Endodontic Journal*, vol. 34, no. 8, pp. 574–580, 2001.

[12] R. De Moor, M. Hülsmann, L.-L. Kirkevang, J. Tanalp, and J. Whitworth, "Undergraduate curriculum guidelines for endodontology," *International Endodontic Journal*, vol. 46, no. 12, pp. 1105–1114, 2013.

[13] S. Moradi and M. Gharechahi, "Quality of root canal obturation performed by senior undergraduate dental students," *Iranian Endodontic Journal*, vol. 9, no. 1, pp. 66–70, 2013.

[14] H. Balto, S. Al Khalifah, S. Al Mugairin, M. Al Deeb, and E. Al-Madi, "Technical quality of root fillings performed by undergraduate students in Saudi Arabia," *International Endodontic Journal*, vol. 43, no. 4, pp. 292–300, 2010.

[15] M. Fonseka, R. Jayasinghe, W. P. M. M. Abeysekara, and K. A. Wettasinghe, "Evaluation of the radiographic quality of roots filling, performed by undergraduates in the Faculty of Dental Sciences, University of Peradeniya, Sri Lanka," *International Journal of Research in Medical Sciences*, vol. 1, no. 3, pp. 12–16, 2013.

[16] G. C. Unal, A. D. Kececi, B. U. Kaya, and A. G. Tac, "Quality of root canal fillings performed by undergraduate dental students," *European Journal of Dentistry*, vol. 5, no. 3, pp. 324–330, 2011.

[17] T. Vukadinov, L. Blažić, I. Kantardžić, and T. Lainović, "Technical quality of root fillings performed by undergraduate students: a radiographic study," *The Scientific World Journal*, vol. 2014, Article ID 751274, 6 pages, 2014.

[18] H. J. Wenz, M. Zupanic, K. Klosa, B. Schneider, and G. Karsten, "Using an audience response system to improve learning success in practical skills training courses in dental studies—a randomised, controlled cross-over study," *European Journal of Dental Education*, vol. 18, no. 3, pp. 147–153, 2014.

[19] S. Román-Richon, V. Faus-Matoses, T. Alegre-Domingo, and V.-J. Faus-Llácer, "Radiographic technical quality of root canal treatment performed ex vivo by dental students at Valencia University Medical and Dental School, Spain," *Medicina Oral, Patologia Oral y Cirugia Bucal*, vol. 19, no. 1, pp. e93–e97, 2014.

[20] P. V. Chakravarthy and J. R. Moorthy, "Radiographic assessment of quality of root fillings performed by undergraduate students in a Malaysian Dental School," *Saudi Endodontic Journal*, vol. 3, no. 2, pp. 77–81, 2013.

[21] M. G. Khabbaz, E. Protogerou, and E. Douka, "Radiographic quality of root fillings performed by undergraduate students," *International Endodontic Journal*, vol. 43, no. 6, pp. 499–508, 2010.

[22] K. M. Barrieshi-Nusair, M. A. Al-Omari, and A. S. Al-Hiyasat, "Radiographic technical quality of root canal treatment performed by dental students at the Dental Teaching Center in Jordan," *Journal of Dentistry*, vol. 32, no. 4, pp. 301–307, 2004.

[23] M. B. Sobhi and I. Khan, "Penetration depth of nickel titanium and stainless steel finger spreaders in curved root canals," *Journal of the College of Physicians and Surgeons Pakistan*, vol. 13, no. 2, pp. 70–72, 2003.

[24] D. W. Chambers, "Competencies: a new view of becoming a dentist," *Journal of Dental Education*, vol. 58, no. 5, pp. 342–345, 1994.

[25] "Undergraduate curriculum guidelines for endodontology. European Society of Endodontology," *International Endodontic Journal*, vol. 25, no. 3, pp. 169–172, 1992.

[26] P. M. Dummer, "Comparison of undergraduate endodontic teaching programmes in the United Kingdom and in some dental schools in Europe and the United States," *International Endodontic Journal*, vol. 24, no. 4, pp. 169–177, 1991.

[27] E. Kelbauskas, L. Andriukaitiene, and I. Nedzelskiene, "Quality of root canal filling performed by undergraduate students of odontology at Kaunas University of Medicine in Lithuania," *Stomatologija*, vol. 11, no. 3, pp. 92–96, 2009.

[28] G. L. Dunnington, K. Wright, and K. Hoffman, "A pilot experience with competency-based clinical skills assessment in a surgical clerkship," *The American Journal of Surgery*, vol. 167, no. 6, pp. 604–607, 1994.

[29] J. R. Kogan, E. S. Holmboe, and K. E. Hauer, "Tools for direct observation and assessment of clinical skills of medical trainees: a systematic review," *The Journal of the American Medical Association*, vol. 302, no. 12, pp. 1316–1326, 2009.

[30] D. R. Sadler, "Formative assessment and the design of instructional systems," *Instructional Science*, vol. 18, no. 2, pp. 119–144, 1989.

[31] S. I. Tannenbaum and C. P. Cerasoli, "Do team and individual debriefs enhance performance? A meta-analysis," *Human Factors*, vol. 55, no. 1, pp. 231–245, 2013.

[32] D. Carless, "Conceptualizing pre-emptive formative assessment," *Assessment in Education: Principles, Policy & Practice*, vol. 14, no. 2, pp. 171–184, 2007.

[33] N. A. Nadershahi, D. J. Bender, L. Beck, and S. Alexander, "A case study on development of an integrated, multidisciplinary dental curriculum," *Journal of Dental Education*, vol. 77, no. 6, pp. 679–687, 2013.

[34] C. F. Shuler, "Keeping the curriculum current with research and problem-based learning," *The Journal of the American College of Dentists*, vol. 68, no. 3, pp. 20–24, 2001.

[35] S. Roopa, M. G. Bagavad, A. Rani, and T. Chacko, "What type of lectures students want?—a reaction evaluation of dental students," *Journal of Clinical and Diagnostic Research*, vol. 7, no. 10, pp. 2244–2246, 2013.

[36] C. J. Miller, J. McNear, and M. J. Metz, "A comparison of traditional and engaging lecture methods in a large, professional-level course," *The American Journal of Physiology—Advances in Physiology Education*, vol. 37, no. 4, pp. 347–355, 2013.

[37] D. L. Cragun, R. D. DeBate, H. H. Severson et al., "Developing and pretesting Case studies in dental and dental hygiene education: using the Diffusion of Innovations model," *Journal of Dental Education*, vol. 76, no. 5, pp. 590–601, 2012.

[38] H. T. Al-Ahmad, "Dental students' perception of theater-based learning as an interactive educational tool in teaching oral surgery in Jordan," *Saudi Medical Journal*, vol. 31, no. 7, pp. 819–825, 2010.

[39] K. M. Satheesh, C. D. Saylor-Boles, J. W. Rapley, Y. Liu, and C. C. Gadbury-Amyot, "Student evaluation of clickers in a combined dental and dental hygiene periodontology course," *Journal of Dental Education*, vol. 77, no. 10, pp. 1321–1329, 2013.

[40] D. C. Johnsen, T. A. Marshall, M. W. Finkelstein et al., "A model for overview of student learning: a matrix of educational outcomes versus methodologies," *Journal of Dental Education*, vol. 75, no. 2, pp. 160–168, 2011.

[41] S. Krasne, P. F. Wimmers, A. Relan, and T. A. Drake, "Differential effects of two types of formative assessment in predicting

performance of first-year medical students," *Advances in Health Sciences Education*, vol. 11, no. 2, pp. 155–171, 2006.

[42] D. W. Chambers, "Toward a competency-based curriculum," *Journal of Dental Education*, vol. 57, no. 11, pp. 790–793, 1993.

[43] S. Gatley, J. Hayes, and C. Davies, "Requirements, in terms of root canal treatment, of undergraduates in the European Union: an audit of teaching practice," *British Dental Journal*, vol. 207, no. 4, pp. 165–170, 2009.

5

Nanomodified Peek Dental Implants: Bioactive Composites and Surface Modification—A Review

Shariq Najeeb,[1] Zohaib Khurshid,[2] Jukka Pekka Matinlinna,[3] Fahad Siddiqui,[4] Mohammad Zakaria Nassani,[1] and Kusai Baroudi[5]

[1]Restorative Dental Sciences, Al-Farabi Colleges, King Abdullah Road, P.O. Box 85184, Riyadh 11891, Saudi Arabia
[2]School of Metallurgy and Materials, University of Birmingham, Edgbaston, Birmingham B15 2TT, UK
[3]Dental Materials Science, Faculty of Dentistry, The University of Hong Kong, 4/F, The Prince Philip Dental Hospital, 34 Hospital Road, Sai Ying Pun, Hong Kong
[4]Division of Oral Health & Society, 2001 McGill College, Suite 500, Montreal, QC, Canada H3A 1G1
[5]Preventive Dental Sciences, Al-Farabi Colleges, King Abdullah Road, P.O. Box 85184, Riyadh 11891, Saudi Arabia

Correspondence should be addressed to Shariq Najeeb; shariqnajeeb@gmail.com

Academic Editor: Dan Boston

Purpose. The aim of this review is to summarize and evaluate the relevant literature regarding the different ways how polyetheretherketone (PEEK) can be modified to overcome its limited bioactivity, and thereby making it suitable as a dental implant material. *Study Selection.* An electronic literature search was conducted via the PubMed and Google Scholar databases using the keywords "PEEK dental implants," "nano," "osseointegration," "surface treatment," and "modification." A total of 16 *in vivo* and *in vitro* studies were found suitable to be included in this review. *Results.* There are many viable methods to increase the bioactivity of PEEK. Most methods focus on increasing the surface roughness, increasing the hydrophilicity and coating osseoconductive materials. *Conclusion.* There are many ways in which PEEK can be modified at a nanometer level to overcome its limited bioactivity. Melt-blending with bioactive nanoparticles can be used to produce bioactive nanocomposites, while spin-coating, gas plasma etching, electron beam, and plasma-ion immersion implantation can be used to modify the surface of PEEK implants in order to make them more bioactive. However, more animal studies are needed before these implants can be deemed suitable to be used as dental implants.

1. Introduction

A dental subgingival implant is a fixture, surgically placed into the alveolar bone, which functions as an artificial root that can stabilize and support a fixed or removable prosthesis [1, 2]. In general, after implantation of a biomaterial, two possible tissue responses can take place. If a fibrous tissue forms between the implant and the bone, the implant fails. However, if a direct intimate bone-implant contact forms, the implant is said to be osseointegrated (a.k.a. osteointegrated) into the alveolar bone [3]. Osseointegration depends on a number of factors. As described by Brånemark [4] and Albrektsson et al. [3], implant material, surgical technique, and healing period are the main factors which govern the success of dental implants. The implant material, usually titanium and its alloys [5], zirconia [6], or, as a potential future material, fiber reinforced composite (FRC) [7] should be biocompatible [8] and should possess suitable surface properties that induce bone formation around the implant. The implant material should have a suitable design [9], high hydrophilicity [10], and an appropriate surface roughness [11]. Coating the implant surface with osteoconductive coatings such as calcium phosphate [12] has been shown to increase the rate of osseointegration of dental implants [11]. Over the last several decades, commercially pure grade 2 or 4 titanium and its alloys have been the material of choice for endosseous implants [13]. However, titanium has been shown to exhibit a variety of problems. Because of the high modulus of elasticity of the titanium alloys, dental implants made from the material can cause stress-shielding [14] which

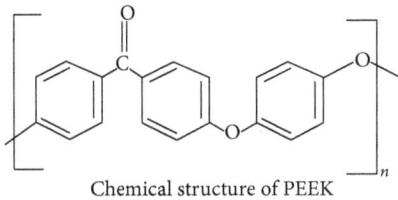

Chemical structure of PEEK

FIGURE 1: The chemical structural formula of polyetheretherketone (PEEK). PEEK is a semicrystalline thermoplastic and it is synthesized via step-growth polymerization by the dialkylation of *bis*-phenolate salts.

may lead to periodontal bone loss [15]. Moreover, studies have documented very rare cases of patients developing hypersensitivity to titanium dental implants [16, 17]. Wear debris and ion leakage [18] can also be of concern with titanium dental implants. Aesthetics can be compromised if the dental implant is visible through a thin biotype gingiva because titanium is a dark material.

Polyetheretherketone (PEEK) is an organic synthetic polymeric tooth coloured material which has the potential to serve as an aesthetic dental implant material [19]. The structure of PEEK is given in Figure 1. It has excellent chemical resistance and biomechanical properties. In its pure form, Young's modulus of PEEK is around 3.6 GPa. Meanwhile, Young's modulus of carbon-reinforced PEEK (CFR-PEEK) is around 18 GPa [7] which is close to that of cortical bone [20, 21]. Hence, it has been suggested that PEEK could exhibit lesser stress-shielding when compared to titanium [22]. However, PEEK has been shown to stimulate less osteoblast differentiation when compared to titanium [23]. This said, PEEK is a bioinert material and it does not possess any inherent osseoconductive properties [24]. PEEK can be coated and blended with bioactive particles to increase the osseoconductive properties and surface roughness. However, high temperatures involved in plasma-spraying can deteriorate PEEK. Furthermore, thick calcium phosphate coatings on PEEK can delaminate because of their limited bond strength when compared to coated titanium implants [25, 26]. Additionally, combining PEEK with particles in the size range of micrometers leads to mechanical properties falling inferior to those of pure PEEK or CFR-PEEK [27]. Therefore, more recently, a significant amount of research has been conducted to modify PEEK by coating or blending it with nanosized particles and producing nanolevel surface topography. The aim of this review is to highlight recent advancements towards producing bioactive nanocomposites and nanolevel surface modifications to ascertain the feasibility of nanomodified PEEK to be used as dental implant material.

2. Bioactive PEEK Nanocomposites

Bioactive particles can be incorporated into PEEK to produce bioactive implants [27]. Hydroxyapatite is a bioceramic with chemistry similar to bone and it is shown to induce bone formation around implants [11]. Hydroxyapatite particles (HAp) of the micrometer size range have been melt-blended

with PEEK producing PEEK-HAp composites but these could be very difficult to be used as dental implants because of the poor mechanical properties produced due to the insufficient interfacial bonding between PEEK and hydroxyapatite particles [27, 28].

Melt-blending PEEK with nanoparticles can be achieved to produce bioactive composite PEEK composite implants and at the same time enhance their mechanical properties [29]. The schematic diagram of the melt-blending process is shown in Figure 2. Melt-blending of PEEK with bioactive nanofillers has been described by Wan et al. [29] and Wu et al. [30]. First, the PEEK powder and nanofillers are codispersed in a suitable solvent to form a uniform suspension. The solvent is then removed by drying in an oven and the powder mixture is placed in suitable moulds in the shape of the implants. The powder mixture and the moulds are preheated to a temperature of about 150°C at 35 MPa pressure. The temperature is then increased to 350°C–400°C at 15 MPa. When the melting point of PEEK is reached, the polymer melts but the bioactive filler particles remain solid. The temperature is maintained for 10 min after which the composite implants are air-cooled to 150°C. Upon cooling, the resultant material is a composite of solid PEEK matrix and the nanofillers dispersed within it (Figure 2).

As shown in Table 1, it can be observed that incorporating nanosized particles to PEEK can produce PEEK composites with enhanced mechanical properties and bioactivity. Wu et al. have suggested that incorporating nanosized TiO_2 particles to PEEK can increase osseointegration [30]. Three-dimensional computerized tomography has shown that a higher amount of bone forms around PEEK/nano-TiO_2 cylindrical implants and they have improved mechanical properties when compared to pure PEEK because of an increased number of nanofiller particles [30]. The effect of free TiO_2 particles on cellular activity has been debated in the literature. Some studies suggest that they can stimulate an inflammatory or carcinogenic response in cells [31] and damage nerve tissue [32]. On the other hand, some studies have suggested that, when used as coatings or solid cores, TiO_2 can increase the rate of cellular proliferation and differentiation [33–35]. However, to date, no studies have investigated the possible release of TiO_2 particles from PEEK/nano-TiO_2 composites after undergoing mechanical loading.

Fluorohydroxyapatite (HAF) has been shown to induce higher bone cell proliferation than conventional hydroxyapatite and it possesses antibacterial properties due to the presence of fluoride ions (F^-) [36–40]. Wang et al. have shown that it can be possible to produce PEEK/nano-HAF implants using the process of melt-blending [29]. These implants possess antimicrobial properties against *Streptococcus mutans*, one of the main causative agents of periodontitis, and can exhibit Young's modulus almost 3 times of that of pure PEEK [29]. This increased modulus is still near to that of bone so PEEK/nano-HAF implants could still produce less stress-shielding than titanium implants. However, no studies have been attempted to investigate this.

Even with the incorporation of bioactive nanoparticles, the water-contact angle of PEEK nanocomposites does not decrease significantly when compared to pure PEEK [29,

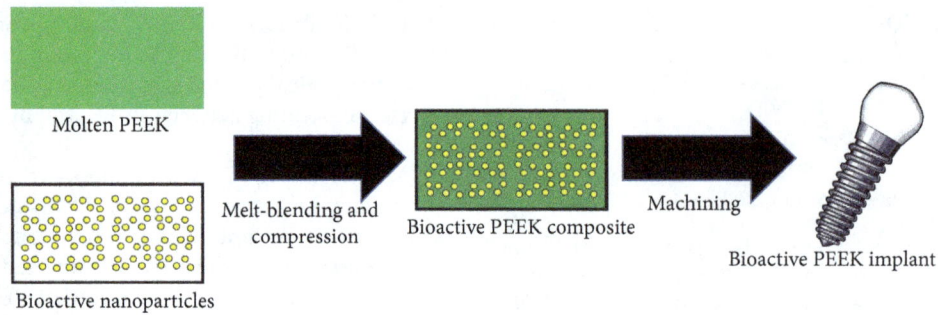

FIGURE 2: A schematic diagram of the process of melt-blending to produce bioactive PEEK composites. First, the PEEK powder and nanofillers are codispersed in a suitable solvent. The solvent is then removed and the mixture is placed in suitable moulds and heated to a temperature above the melting point PEEK under high pressure in a mould (so-called compression moulding). Upon cooling, the resultant material is composite of PEEK and the fillers. The solid composite is then machined to provide shape or surface characteristics suitable for a dental implant.

TABLE 1: Bioactive PEEK nanocomposites and some biomechanical properties.

Material	Particle size	Modulus (GPa)	Tensile strength (MPa)	Contact angle (°)	Animal studies	Reference
PEEK-nTiO$_2$	Not stated	3.8	93	n.d.	Yes	[30]
PEEK-nHAF	Length = 85 ± 10 nm, width: 22 ± 4 nm	12.1 ± 0.4	137.6 ± 9.1	71.5	Yes	[29]
CFR-PEEK-nHAp	<200 nm	n.d.	n.d.	75 (without plasma), 10 (with plasma treatment)	No	[62]

30]. Although gas plasma treatment of PEEK/nano-HAp composite implants does reduce the surface contact angle to as low as 10°, they have not been tested *in vitro* and the effects of plasma gas treatment have been seen to be temporary [41]. As an increased contact angle is an indication of a more hydrophobic implant surface [11], it is still uncertain whether a high contact angle can undermine the long-term biocompatibility of these implants and more research is warranted to investigate this concern.

3. Surface Modifications of PEEK Implants

Different types of surface modifications geared towards making PEEK more bioactive are summarized in Table 2. In contrast to production of nanocomposites of PEEK, surface modification aims to alter the surface of PEEK with little or no effect on the core. To date, four processes have been used to nanomodify the surface of PEEK implants: spin-coating [42–44], gas plasma etching [45–52], electron beam deposition [53–57], and plasma-ion immersion implantation (PIII) [58–62].

3.1. Spin-Coating with Nanohydroxyapatite. Due to the drawbacks of thick hydroxyapatite coatings, research has been conducted and directed to coat implants with thinner coatings [11]. Spin-coating involves the deposition of a thin layer of nano-HA, precipitated in surfactants, organic solvents, and aqueous solution of Ca(NO$_3$)$_2$ and H$_3$PO$_4$, on the implants. During the deposition, the implants are spun at high speeds and are then heat-treated to form the coating [42]. The first study evaluating spin-coated PEEK implants

by Barkarmo et al. [42] showed that the mean removal torque of spin-coated implanted discs was not significantly greater than that of uncoated implants and during the study, several implants failed. However, subsequent studies by Barkarmo et al. [43] and Johansson et al. [44] found higher removal torques compared to uncoated PEEK when the implant design had been modified by adding a threaded, cylindrical design. The findings suggested that an appropriate implant design is a very important factor as well as a suitable bioactive coating for successful PEEK dental subgingival implants. Nevertheless, there have been no studies conducted testing the bond strength of the nanohydroxyapatite coatings and all the current studies on spin-coated nanohydroxyapatite implants have not found any significant differences in the bone-implant contact of the modified and unmodified PEEK.

3.2. Gas Plasma Nanoetching. Nanoetching of PEEK implants can be achieved by exposing them to low power plasma gases like water vapour [45], oxygen/argon, and ammonia [46, 47]. It has been suggested that plasma treatment of PEEK introduces various functional groups on its surface which makes its surface more hydrophilic [48]. The main advantage of using plasma treatment is the ability to produce nanolevel roughness on the implant surface and the extremely low water-contact angle on PEEK surface [46]. Indeed, *in vitro* testing of plasma-etched PEEK implants has been shown to accelerate human mesenchymal cell proliferation [46]. This has been thought to occur because of the increased hydrophilicity [49] and protein adsorption due to nanoroughness [50]. Because there is no coating involved in plasma-etched implants, there is no risk of a coating being

TABLE 2: Various surface modifications for PEEK and some reported properties.

Modification	Surface roughness/pore size	Contact angle (°)	Animal studies	References
Spin-coating				
nHAp	$S_a = 0.686 \pm 0.14\,\mu m$–$0.93 \pm 0.25\,\mu m$	53 ± 4.4	Yes	[42–44]
Gas plasma etching				
O_2/Ar	RMS = 9–19 nm	5–40	No	[46]
NH_3	RMS = 3–7 nm	45–90	No	[46]
O_2	$R_a = 75.33 \pm 10.66$ nm	52	Yes	[47]
E-beam TiO_2				
Conventional	n.d.	54	No	[54]
Anodized	Pore size: 70 nm	≈ 0	Yes	[55]
PIII				
TiO_2	Pore size: 150–200 nm	n.d	No	[45]
Diamond-like carbon	RMS = 5.42 nm	≈ 55	No	[61]

delaminated. Poulsson et al. [47] have produced nanometer level surface roughness on the surface of machined rod shaped PEEK implants using low-pressure oxygen plasma and tested them in sheep. Although the plasma-modified machined implants had a higher surface roughness than uncoated machined and conventional PEEK implants, no significant differences were observed in the bone-implant contact of these implants after being implanted in sheep femurs and tibia after 26 weeks [47]. A recent study by Rochford et al. suggests that oxygen plasma-treated PEEK implants promote adherence of osteoblasts even in the presence of *Staphylococcus epidermidis* [51] but the cellular interaction of these surfaces in the presence of periodontal pathogens is still unknown. It has been observed that the surface properties of plasma-treated PEEK diminish over time [41]. However, it has also been observed and reported that treating PEEK with a pulsed Nd:YAG laser before plasma treating can prolong the effects of plasma [52].

3.3. Electron Beam Deposition. Electron beam deposition is a process used to decompose and deposit nonvolatile fragments on a substrate [53]. A thin titanium coating deposited on PEEK using electron beam deposition has been shown to increase the wettability and promote cellular adhesion [54]. When a titanium coating on PEEK produced by electron beam deposition is anodized, it is converted into a uniformly thick ($2\,\mu m$), crack-free, and highly nanoporous layer of titanium oxide ($nTiO_2$) which can be used to carry BMP-2 [55]. Many published *in vitro* and *in vivo* studies show that BMP-2 is a growth factor which plays a major role in differentiation of stem cells to osteoblasts [56, 57]. Given this, an immobilized growth factor on the surface of the implant could increase the rate of osseointegration around it.

3.4. Plasma Immersion Ion Implantation. A substrate can be coated by a thin film of diverse particles placing the substrate in a plasma of the particles, repeatedly pulsed with high negative voltages which causes the plasma ions to be accelerated and then implanted onto the surface of the

substrate [58, 59]. This process is known as plasma immersion ion implantation (PIII). PEEK can be coated by nano-TiO_2 particles using plasma immersion ion implantation [60]. A study by Lu et al. shows that PIII-coated PEEK implants could exhibit partial antimicrobial activity against *Staphylococcus aureus* and *Escherichia coli* [60]. However, it is not known if these types of surfaces could exhibit similar activity against pathogens more common in the periodontium. Furthermore, these implants have not been tested *in vivo*. Diamond-like carbon coated on PEEK has also been shown to exhibit increased bioactivity *in vitro* but the *in vivo* effects of the surface modification are yet to be evaluated [61].

4. Summary and Conclusion

There are many ways in which PEEK can be modified at a nanometer level to overcome its limited bioactivity. Nanoparticles such as TiO_2, HAF, and HAp can be combined with PEEK through the process of melt-blending to produce bioactive nanocomposites. Moreover, these composites exhibit significantly superior tensile properties when compared to pure PEEK. Additionally, HAF has antibacterial properties which could prevent peri-implantitis and early implant failures. Spin-coating, gas plasma etching, electron beam deposition, and plasma-ion immersion can be used to modify or coat the surface of PEEK implants at a nanometer level. Nanocoatings of materials such as HAp and TiO_2 produced by spin-coating and PIII can impart bioactive properties to the surface. Also, an anodized electron beam-coated TiO_2 nanolayer on PEEK can carry immobilized BMP-2 growth factor which can further enhance cellular activity. However, many of the aforementioned studies have been limited to *in vitro* testing. Using PEEK implants, which have not undergone extensive animal and human testing, yet carries a risk of failing early. Hence, more *in vivo* studies are required before nanomodified PEEK implants can be used broadly in the clinical setting.

Conflict of Interests

The authors have no conflict of interests to declare.

References

[1] M. A. Awad, F. Rashid, and J. S. Feine, "The effect of mandibular 2-implant overdentures on oral health-related quality of life: an international multicentre study," *Clinical Oral Implants Research*, vol. 25, no. 1, pp. 46–51, 2014.

[2] I. Turkyilmaz, A. M. Company, and E. A. McGlumphy, "Should edentulous patients be constrained to removable complete dentures? The use of dental implants to improve the quality of life for edentulous patients," *Gerodontology*, vol. 27, no. 1, pp. 3–10, 2010.

[3] T. Albrektsson, P.-I. Brånemark, H.-A. Hansson, and J. Lindström, "Osseointegrated titanium implants: requirements for ensuring a long-lasting, direct bone-to-implant anchorage in man," *Acta Orthopaedica*, vol. 52, no. 2, pp. 155–170, 1981.

[4] P.-I. Brånemark, "Osseointegrated implants in the treatment of the edentulous jaw. Experience from a 10-year period," *Scandinavian Journal of Plastic and Reconstructive Surgery*, vol. 16, pp. 1–132, 1977.

[5] C. Y. Guo, A. T. H. Tang, and J. P. Matinlinna, "Insights into surface treatment methods of titanium dental implants," *Journal of Adhesion Science and Technology*, vol. 26, no. 1–3, pp. 189–205, 2012.

[6] D. Liu, J. P. Matinlinna, and E. H. N. Pow, "Insights into porcelain to zirconia bonding," *Journal of Adhesion Science and Technology*, vol. 26, no. 8-9, pp. 1249–1265, 2012.

[7] M. Zhang and J. P. Matinlinna, "E-glass fiber reinforced composites in dental applications," *Silicon*, vol. 4, no. 1, pp. 73–78, 2012.

[8] S. K. Mallineni, S. Nuvvula, J. P. Matinlinna, C. K. Yiu, and N. M. King, "Biocompatibility of various dental materials in contemporary dentistry: a narrative insight," *Journal of Investigative and Clinical Dentistry*, vol. 4, no. 1, pp. 9–19, 2013.

[9] M. Esposito, J.-M. Hirsch, U. Lekholm, and P. Thomsen, "Biological factors contributing to failures of osseointegrated oral implants. (I). Success criteria and epidemiology," *European Journal of Oral Sciences*, vol. 106, no. 1, pp. 527–551, 1998.

[10] F. Rupp, L. Scheideler, N. Olshanska, M. de Wild, M. Wieland, and J. Geis-Gerstorfer, "Enhancing surface free energy and hydrophilicity through chemical modification of microstructured titanium implant surfaces," *Journal of Biomedical Materials Research Part A*, vol. 76, no. 2, pp. 323–334, 2006.

[11] L. Le Guéhennec, A. Soueidan, P. Layrolle, and Y. Amouriq, "Surface treatments of titanium dental implants for rapid osseointegration," *Dental Materials*, vol. 23, no. 7, pp. 844–854, 2007.

[12] A. H. Choi, B. Ben-Nissan, J. P. Matinlinna, and R. C. Conway, "Current perspectives: calcium phosphate nanocoatings and nanocomposite coatings in dentistry," *Journal of Dental Research*, vol. 92, no. 10, pp. 853–859, 2013.

[13] P.-I. Brånemark, U. Breine, R. Adell, B. O. Hansson, J. Lindström, and A. Ohlsson, "Intra-osseous anchorage of dental prostheses: I. Experimental studies," *Scandinavian Journal of Plastic and Reconstructive Surgery and Hand Surgery*, vol. 3, no. 2, pp. 81–100, 1969.

[14] J. R. Sarot, C. M. M. Contar, A. C. C. D. Cruz, and R. De Souza Magini, "Evaluation of the stress distribution in CFR-PEEK dental implants by the three-dimensional finite element method," *Journal of Materials Science: Materials in Medicine*, vol. 21, no. 7, pp. 2079–2085, 2010.

[15] R. Huiskes, H. Weinans, and B. Van Rietbergen, "The relationship between stress shielding and bone resorption around total hip stems and the effects of flexible materials," *Clinical Orthopaedics and Related Research*, vol. 274, pp. 124–134, 1992.

[16] A. Sicilia, S. Cuesta, G. Coma et al., "Titanium allergy in dental implant patients: a clinical study on 1500 consecutive patients," *Clinical Oral Implants Research*, vol. 19, no. 8, pp. 823–835, 2008.

[17] A. Siddiqi, A. G. T. Payne, R. K. de Silva, and W. J. Duncan, "Titanium allergy: could it affect dental implant integration?" *Clinical Oral Implants Research*, vol. 22, no. 7, pp. 673–680, 2011.

[18] W. Becker, B. E. Becker, A. Ricci et al., "A prospective multicenter clinical trial comparing one- and two-stage titanium screw-shaped fixtures with one-stage plasma-sprayed solid-screw fixtures," *Clinical implant dentistry and related research*, vol. 2, no. 3, pp. 159–165, 2000.

[19] A. Schwitalla and W.-D. Müller, "PEEK dental implants: a review of the literature," *Journal of Oral Implantology*, vol. 39, no. 6, pp. 743–749, 2013.

[20] H. B. Skinner, "Composite technology for total hip arthroplasty," *Clinical Orthopaedics and Related Research*, no. 235, pp. 224–236, 1988.

[21] J. Y. Rho, R. B. Ashman, and C. H. Turner, "Young's modulus of trabecular and cortical bone material: ultrasonic and microtensile measurements," *Journal of Biomechanics*, vol. 26, no. 2, pp. 111–119, 1993.

[22] H. Yildiz, F.-K. Chang, and S. Goodman, "Composite hip prosthesis design. II. Simulation," *Journal of Biomedical Materials Research*, vol. 39, no. 1, pp. 102–119, 1997.

[23] R. Olivares-Navarrete, R. A. Gittens, J. M. Schneider et al., "Osteoblasts exhibit a more differentiated phenotype and increased bone morphogenetic protein production on titanium alloy substrates than on poly-ether-ether-ketone," *Spine Journal*, vol. 12, no. 3, pp. 265–272, 2012.

[24] A. Rabiei and S. Sandukas, "Processing and evaluation of bioactive coatings on polymeric implants," *Journal of Biomedical Materials Research A*, vol. 101, no. 9, pp. 2621–2629, 2013.

[25] S.-W. Ha, J. Mayer, B. Koch, and E. Wintermantel, "Plasma-sprayed hydroxylapatite coating on carbon fibre reinforced thermoplastic composite materials," *Journal of Materials Science: Materials in Medicine*, vol. 5, no. 6-7, pp. 481–484, 1994.

[26] F. Suska, O. Omar, L. Emanuelsson et al., "Enhancement of CRF-PEEK osseointegration by plasma-sprayed hydroxyapatite: a rabbit model," *Journal of Biomaterials Applications*, vol. 29, no. 2, pp. 234–242, 2014.

[27] M. S. Abu Bakar, M. H. W. Cheng, S. M. Tang et al., "Tensile properties, tension-tension fatigue and biological response of polyetheretherketone-hydroxyapatite composites for load-bearing orthopedic implants," *Biomaterials*, vol. 24, no. 13, pp. 2245–2250, 2003.

[28] K. L. Wong, C. T. Wong, W. C. Liu et al., "Mechanical properties and in vitro response of strontium-containing hydroxyapatite/polyetheretherketone composites," *Biomaterials*, vol. 30, no. 23-24, pp. 3810–3817, 2009.

[29] L. Wang, S. He, X. Wu et al., "Polyetheretherketone/nanofluorohydroxyapatite composite with antimicrobial activity and osseointegration properties," *Biomaterials*, vol. 35, no. 25, pp. 6758–6775, 2014.

[30] X. Wu, X. Liu, J. Wei, J. Ma, F. Deng, and S. Wei, "Nano-TiO$_2$/PEEK bioactive composite as a bone substitute material: in vitro and in vivo studies," *International Journal of Nanomedicine*, vol. 7, pp. 1215–1225, 2012.

[31] S. Huang, P. J. Chueh, Y.-W. Lin, T.-S. Shih, and S.-M. Chuang, "Disturbed mitotic progression and genome segregation are involved in cell transformation mediated by nano-TiO$_2$ long-term exposure," *Toxicology and Applied Pharmacology*, vol. 241, no. 2, pp. 182–194, 2009.

[32] J. Wang, Y. Liu, F. Jiao et al., "Time-dependent translocation and potential impairment on central nervous system by intranasally instilled TiO$_2$ nanoparticles," *Toxicology*, vol. 254, no. 1-2, pp. 82–90, 2008.

[33] Y. Sugita, K. Ishizaki, F. Iwasa et al., "Effects of pico-to-nanometer-thin TiO$_2$ coating on the biological properties of microroughened titanium," *Biomaterials*, vol. 32, no. 33, pp. 8374–8384, 2011.

[34] R. A. Gittens, T. McLachlan, R. Olivares-Navarrete et al., "The effects of combined micron-/submicron-scale surface roughness and nanoscale features on cell proliferation and differentiation," *Biomaterials*, vol. 32, no. 13, pp. 3395–3403, 2011.

[35] N. Wang, H. Li, W. Lü et al., "Effects of TiO$_2$ nanotubes with different diameters on gene expression and osseointegration of implants in minipigs," *Biomaterials*, vol. 32, no. 29, pp. 6900–6911, 2011.

[36] A. Wiegand, W. Buchalla, and T. Attin, "Review on fluoride-releasing restorative materials—fluoride release and uptake characteristics, antibacterial activity and influence on caries formation," *Dental Materials*, vol. 23, no. 3, pp. 343–362, 2007.

[37] I. R. Hamilton, "Biochemical effects of fluoride on oral bacteria," *Journal of Dental Research*, vol. 69, pp. 660–667, 1990.

[38] M. Tahriri and F. Moztarzadeh, "Preparation, characterization, and in vitro biological evaluation of PLGA/nano-fluorohydroxyapatite (FHA) microsphere-sintered scaffolds for biomedical applications," *Applied Biochemistry and Biotechnology*, vol. 172, no. 5, pp. 2465–2479, 2014.

[39] L. Gineste, M. Gineste, X. Ranz et al., "Degradation of hydroxylapatite, fluorapatite, and fluorhydroxyapatite coatings of dental implants in dogs," *Journal of Biomedical Materials Research*, vol. 48, no. 3, pp. 224–234, 1999.

[40] V. Stanić, S. Dimitrijević, D. G. Antonović et al., "Synthesis of fluorine substituted hydroxyapatite nanopowders and application of the central composite design for determination of its antimicrobial effects," *Applied Surface Science*, vol. 290, pp. 346–352, 2014.

[41] C. Canal, R. Molina, E. Bertran, and P. Erra, "Wettability, ageing and recovery process of plasma-treated polyamide 6," *Journal of Adhesion Science and Technology*, vol. 18, no. 9, pp. 1077–1089, 2004.

[42] S. Barkarmo, A. Wennerberg, M. Hoffman et al., "Nano-hydroxyapatite-coated PEEK implants: a pilot study in rabbit bone," *Journal of Biomedical Materials Research Part A*, vol. 101, no. 2, pp. 465–471, 2013.

[43] S. Barkarmo, M. Andersson, F. Currie et al., "Enhanced bone healing around nanohydroxyapatite-coated polyetheretherketone implants: an experimental study in rabbit bone," *Journal of Biomaterials Applications*, vol. 29, no. 5, pp. 737–747, 2014.

[44] P. Johansson, R. Jimbo, P. Kjellin, B. Chrcanovic, A. Wennerberg, and F. Currie, "Biomechanical evaluation and surface characterization of a nano-modified surface on PEEK implants: a study in the rabbit tibia," *International Journal of Nanomedicine*, vol. 9, pp. 3903–3911, 2014.

[45] H. Wang, T. Lu, F. Meng, H. Zhu, and X. Liu, "Enhanced osteoblast responses to poly ether ether ketone surface modified by water plasma immersion ion implantation," *Colloids and Surfaces B: Biointerfaces*, vol. 117, pp. 89–97, 2014.

[46] J. Waser-Althaus, A. Salamon, M. Waser et al., "Differentiation of human mesenchymal stem cells on plasma-treated polyetheretherketone," *Journal of Materials Science: Materials in Medicine*, vol. 25, no. 2, pp. 515–525, 2014.

[47] A. H. C. Poulsson, D. Eglin, S. Zeiter et al., "Osseointegration of machined, injection moulded and oxygen plasma modified PEEK implants in a sheep model," *Biomaterials*, vol. 35, no. 12, pp. 3717–3728, 2014.

[48] C.-M. Chan, T.-M. Ko, and H. Hiraoka, "Polymer surface modification by plasmas and photons," *Surface Science Reports*, vol. 24, no. 1-2, pp. 1–54, 1996.

[49] K. Tsougeni, N. Vourdas, A. Tserepi, E. Gogolides, and C. Cardinaud, "Mechanisms of oxygen plasma nanotexturing of organic polymer surfaces: from stable super hydrophilic to super hydrophobic surfaces," *Langmuir*, vol. 25, no. 19, pp. 11748–11759, 2009.

[50] K. Rechendorff, M. B. Hovgaard, M. Foss, V. P. Zhdanov, and F. Besenbacher, "Enhancement of protein adsorption induced by surface roughness," *Langmuir*, vol. 22, no. 26, pp. 10885–10888, 2006.

[51] E. T. J. Rochford, G. Subbiahdoss, T. F. Moriarty et al., "An in vitro investigation of bacteria-osteoblast competition on oxygen plasma-modified PEEK," *Journal of Biomedical Materials Research A*, vol. 102, no. 12, pp. 4427–4434, 2014.

[52] C. K. Akkan, M. E. Hammadeh, A. May et al., "Surface topography and wetting modifications of PEEK for implant applications," *Lasers in Medical Science*, vol. 29, no. 5, pp. 1633–1639, 2014.

[53] S. J. Randolph, J. D. Fowlkes, and P. D. Rack, "Focused, nanoscale electron-beam-induced deposition and etching," *Critical Reviews in Solid State and Materials Sciences*, vol. 31, no. 3, pp. 55–89, 2006.

[54] C.-M. Han, E.-J. Lee, H.-E. Kim et al., "The electron beam deposition of titanium on polyetheretherketone (PEEK) and the resulting enhanced biological properties," *Biomaterials*, vol. 31, no. 13, pp. 3465–3470, 2010.

[55] C.-M. Han, T.-S. Jang, H.-E. Kim, and Y.-H. Koh, "Creation of nanoporous TiO2 surface onto polyetheretherketone for effective immobilization and delivery of bone morphogenetic protein," *Journal of Biomedical Materials Research—Part A*, vol. 102, no. 3, pp. 793–800, 2014.

[56] B. Wildemann, P. Bamdad, C. Holmer, N. P. Haas, M. Raschke, and G. Schmidmaier, "Local delivery of growth factors from coated titanium plates increases osteotomy healing in rats," *Bone*, vol. 34, no. 5, pp. 862–868, 2004.

[57] M. L. Macdonald, R. E. Samuel, N. J. Shah, R. F. Padera, Y. M. Beben, and P. T. Hammond, "Tissue integration of growth factor-eluting layer-by-layer polyelectrolyte multilayer coated implants," *Biomaterials*, vol. 32, no. 5, pp. 1446–1453, 2011.

[58] J. V. Mantese, I. G. Brown, N. W. Cheung, and G. A. Collins, "Plasma-immersion ion implantation," *MRS Bulletin*, vol. 21, no. 8, pp. 52–56, 1996.

[59] M. A. Lieberman, "Model of plasma immersion ion implantation," *Journal of Applied Physics*, vol. 66, no. 7, pp. 2926–2929, 1989.

[60] T. Lu, X. Liu, S. Qian et al., "Multilevel surface engineering of nanostructured TiO$_2$ on carbon-fiber-reinforced polyetheretherketone," *Biomaterials*, vol. 35, no. 22, pp. 5731–5740, 2014.

[61] H. Wang, M. Xu, W. Zhang et al., "Mechanical and biological characteristics of diamond-like carbon coated poly aryl-ether-ether-ketone," *Biomaterials*, vol. 31, no. 32, pp. 8181–8187, 2010.

[62] A. Xu, X. Liu, X. Gao, F. Deng, Y. Deng, and S. Wei, "Enhancement of osteogenesis on micro/nano-topographical carbon fiber-reinforced polyetheretherketone-nanohydroxyapatite biocomposite," *Materials Science and Engineering C*, vol. 48, pp. 592–598, 2015.

6

Titanium Oxide: A Bioactive Factor in Osteoblast Differentiation

P. Santiago-Medina,[1] **P. A. Sundaram,**[2] **and N. Diffoot-Carlo**[1]

[1]*Department of Biology, University of Puerto Rico, Mayaguez, PR 00680, USA*
[2]*Department of Mechanical Engineering, University of Puerto Rico, Mayaguez, PR 00680, USA*

Correspondence should be addressed to P. A. Sundaram; paul.sundaram@upr.edu

Academic Editor: Tihana Divnic-Resnik

Titanium and titanium alloys are currently accepted as the gold standard in dental applications. Their excellent biocompatibility has been attributed to the inert titanium surface through the formation of a thin native oxide which has been correlated to the excellent corrosion resistance of this material in body fluids. Whether this titanium oxide layer is essential to the outstanding biocompatibility of titanium surfaces in orthopedic biomaterial applications is still a moot point. To study this critical aspect further, human fetal osteoblasts were cultured on thermally oxidized and microarc oxidized (MAO) surfaces and cell differentiation, a key indicator in bone tissue growth, was quantified by measuring the expression of alkaline phosphatase (ALP) using a commercial assay kit. Cell attachment was similar on all the oxidized surfaces although ALP expression was highest on the oxidized titanium alloy surfaces. Untreated titanium alloy surfaces showed a distinctly lower degree of ALP activity. This indicates that titanium oxide clearly upregulates ALP expression in human fetal osteoblasts and may be a key bioactive factor that causes the excellent biocompatibility of titanium alloys. This result may make it imperative to incorporate titanium oxide in all hard tissue applications involving titanium and other alloys.

1. Introduction

Titanium alloys have become the most popular metallic biomaterials in dental applications because of their excellent biocompatibility [1]. This is attributed to the inert nature of the titanium surface due to the formation of a thin native titanium oxide layer [2] which also provides excellent corrosion resistance. Although titanium alloys have virtually replaced other metallic biomaterials in dental implant applications, currently there is little insight into the reasons for this excellent biocompatibility of titanium surfaces. A number of studies have pointed out various factors that contribute to the biocompatibility of titanium or of modified titanium surfaces [3–6]. While these studies have investigated both proliferation and differentiation of osteoblast cell lines evidenced in many instances by gene expression to corroborate biocompatibility, the emphasis has been on physical factors such as roughness, texture, wettability, or substrate microstructural features. Some importance has been paid to the substrate composition, whether Ti or Ti alloy, and the makeup of the surface modified layer. In recent work [3], the

plausible role of titanium oxide in contributing to this outstanding biocompatibility was observed. In studying titanium alloys, it was noticed that ALP activity was higher on oxidized titanium alloys compared to corresponding untreated materials [7, 8]. Despite having a good understanding of the signaling pathways in osteoblast differentiation [4], the effect of titanium oxide on osteoblast differentiation has not been fully researched even though the fact that a thin native titanium oxide layer forms on all titanium alloys is well known and a large amount of research has been conducted on these popular biomaterials.

It is still unclear at the present time whether osteoblast differentiation is affected by titanium oxide or by the oxygen released from the titanium oxide. A recent report suggests that oxygen tension, in and of itself, has a strong effect on osteoblast differentiation and may in fact regulate this process [5], and hypoxic cell cultures demonstrated a lower level of mineralization resulting in a more chondrogenic tissue in comparison to higher levels of oxygen in cell cultures [6]. Healing of fractures has also been reported much earlier to be delayed in the absence of oxygen [9]. In contrast, reactive oxygen species (ROS) has been reported to suppress bone formation and stimulate bone resorption [10]. Osteoblast differentiation involves a complex molecular pathway consisting of various transcription factors and it is well known that many transitional stages comprise the pathway for this process and that several signaling molecules play key roles in overall skeletal development [4]. It is currently unknown if titanium oxide plays a critical role in any step of the signaling cascade. Understanding the manner in which titanium oxide affects osteoblast differentiation may be critical in titanium implantology in terms of reducing hospitalization time and formulating efficient therapeutic procedures.

In this study, hFOB cells were cultured for 10 days on the oxide formed on the surface of two titanium-based alloys from two different methods of oxidation and the degree of osteoblast differentiation was measured through quantification of ALP activity using a commercial assay kit to compare with unoxidized titanium alloy surfaces in an effort to determine if titanium oxide indeed played a role in the differentiation process.

2. Materials and Methods

2.1. Preparation of Titanium Disks. Various samples of the two titanium-based alloys, gamma-TiAl (γ-TiAl [Ti-48Al-2Cr-2Nb (at.%)]) and Ti-6Al-4V (wt.%), were machined in the form of 7 mm diameter cylindrical rods. From these, disks with an approximate thickness of 1 mm were obtained using a slow-speed diamond saw (Buehler). Both surfaces of the disks were ground using 240, 320, 600, and 1200 grit silicon carbide paper in an Ecomet 3 (Buehler). These metal disks were then sonicated in 0.8% Alconox (Fisher, Pittsburgh, Pennsylvania) and 70% ethanol for 10 minutes each, rinsed with deionized water, and dried with a hot-air blow-dryer.

2.2. Thermal Oxidation. Both γ-TiAl and Ti-6Al-4V disks were oxidized in a laboratory furnace (CM Furnaces Inc.) in air at 500°C or 800°C for 1h and later placed in 48-well cell culture plates (Corning). The nomenclature followed in this paper is as follows: γ-TiAl and Ti-6Al-4V disks oxidized at 500°C and 800°C are hereafter referred to as GTi5, GTi8, TiV5, and TiV8, respectively, while untreated disks are designated as GTi and TiV. Atomic force microscopy (AFM) was used to obtain average surface roughness values of the oxidized surfaces. These are given in Table 1.

2.3. Micro Arc Oxidation. Other γ-TiAl and Ti-6Al-4V disk samples were processed using micro arc oxidation (MAO). For the MAO process, a stainless steel beaker was used as the cathode, while the titanium disk (either γ-TiAl or Ti-6Al-4V) was used as the anode. Each sample was mounted in a titanium holder specially designed to allow complete exposure of the sample to the electrolyte [11]. A *Hoefer PS300-B* high voltage power supply (300 V; 500 mA) was operated in galvanostatic mode in order to form the titanium oxide film on the sample surface using the MAO process. Process conditions of sample current of 200 mA and 225 mA for durations of 3 and 4 minutes for each case were utilized based on an earlier study [11]. After treatment, the samples

TABLE 1: Average roughness values (in μm) measured on Ti alloy sample surfaces for various treatments using AFM.

Treatment	Ti-6Al-4V	γ-TiAl
None	51.74	49.30
Oxidation at 500°C	102.40	31.34
Oxidation at 800°C	318.80	65.88
MAO 200 mA, 3 min	246.30	174.50
MAO 200 mA, 4 min	247.60	185.90
MAO 225 mA, 3 min	213.30	137.50
MAO 225 mA, 4 min	301.70	189.80

were rinsed with distilled water and then dried with a blow dryer. The micro arc oxidized samples will be henceforth referred to as MAOGTi for the γ-TiAl samples and the MAOTiV for the Ti-6Al-4V samples, respectively. The oxides formed on both γ-TiAl and Ti-6Al-4V as a result of the MAO treatment for the applied process conditions are mainly rutile and anatase as reported earlier [11, 12]. For thermal oxidation, alumina is the dominant oxide formed on γ-TiAl at 500°C, while rutile is dominant at 800°C [13–16]. For Ti-6Al-4V, thermal oxidation at 500°C produces a combination of an oxide diffused Ti(O) and rutile where the latter phase appears to grow at high temperatures between 650°C and 800°C [17]. The average roughness values of these surfaces were extracted from topography analysis using AFM and presented in Table 1.

2.4. Human Fetal Osteoblast Cell Line. Human osteoblast cells, cell line hFOB 1.19 (ATCC, Manassas, Virginia), were cultured in 90% Dulbecco's Modified Eagle's Medium Nutrient Mixture F-12 Ham (DMEM) (Sigma-Aldrich, St. Louis, Missouri) with 2.5 mM L-Glutamine and 15 mM Hepes, without phenol red, supplemented with 0.3 mg/mL G-418 (Calbiochem, San Diego, California) and 10% Fetal Bovine Serum (FBS) (Hyclone, Logan, Utah). Cells were grown in 25 cm^2 plastic culture flasks (Corning, Corning, New York) and incubated at 33.5°C until confluence. At approximately 100% confluence, cells were washed three times with Phosphate Buffer Saline (PBS) solution (137 mM NaCl, 2.7 mM KCl, 4.3 mM Na$_2$HPO$_4$, and 1.4 mM KH$_2$HPO$_4$) and harvested using 0.25% trypsin-0.53 mM EDTA (Gibco, Gaithersburg, Maryland) at 37°C for 5 min. Cells were then pelleted by low speed centrifugation (3,300 rpm) for 5 minutes and subcultured at a 1 : 3 ratio.

2.5. Alkaline Phosphatase Assay. Cells were seeded in 48-well plates (Becton, Dickinson, Lincoln Park, NJ) at a density of 5×10^4 cells/cm^2 on TiV, TiV5, TiV8, GTi, GTi5, GTi8, MAOTiV, and MAOGTi disks (7 mm in diameter), using the commercial Alkaline Phosphatase Colorimetric Assay Kit (ab83369, Abcam) in order to evaluate osteoblast differentiation quantitatively on thermally oxidized, micro arc oxidized, and untreated γ-TiAl and Ti-6Al-4V disks. Samples were incubated for 3 days at 33.5°C and then for 7 days at 39.5°C to allow osteoblast differentiation. hFOB cells grown on coverslips were used as controls. Modifications to the suggested protocol were made to achieve a more efficient cell lysis, including washing the samples carefully three times with PBS and homogenizing in 60 μL of the Assay Buffer. Also, Triton X-100 (80 μL) was utilized to lyse the cells for an efficient measurement of intracellular ALP. Stop solution (20 μL) was added to terminate ALP activity in the sample. The solution in each well was transferred to a 96-well plate (Becton, Dickinson, Lincoln Park, NJ). pNPP solution (50 μL) was added to each well containing the test samples and background controls. The reaction was incubated for 60 minutes at 25°C, protected from light.

A standard curve was generated to determine the concentration of ALP activity in the sample for which 40 μL of the 5 mM pNPP solution was diluted with 160 μL Assay Buffer to generate a 1 mM pNPP standard. 0, 4, 8, 12, 16, and 20 μL were added to 96-well plate in duplicate to generate 0, 4, 8, 12, 16, and 20 nmol/well pNPP standard. The final volume was brought to 120 μL with Assay Buffer. ALP enzyme solution (10 μL) was added to each well containing the pNPP standard. The reaction was incubated for 60 minutes at 25°C, protected from light. All reactions were stopped by adding 20 μL Stop Solution to each standard and sample reaction except the sample background control reaction (since 20 μL Stop Solution had been added to the background control when prepared previously). The optical density was measured at 405 nm in a microplate reader. The background was corrected by subtracting the value derived from the zero (0) standards from all standards, samples, and sample background control. The pNPP standard curve was plotted and the sample readings were applied to the standard curve to get the amount of pNPP generated. ALP activity of the test samples was calculated using the equation, ALP activity (U/mL) = $A/V/T$, where A is amount of pNPP generated by samples (in μmol), V is volume of sample added to the assay well (in mL), and T is reaction time (in minutes).

2.6. Statistical Analysis. Three independent experiments were performed for each ALP assay, and since each experiment had three replicates, a total of nine replicates per surface were evaluated (MAO γ-TiAl, thermally oxidized γ-TiAl, untreated γ-TiAl, MAO Ti-6Al-4V, thermally oxidized Ti-6Al-4V, untreated Ti-6Al-4V, and control glass coverslips) for a 10-day period of culture. The data from the ALP assay is presented as the mean ± standard deviation (SD) of the optical density of differentiated cells on the different surfaces corresponding to the amount of alkaline phosphatase detected. Each value represents the mean of three measurements of cell differentiation performed on a specific surface as mentioned above. A factorial analysis of variance (ANOVA) was used to assess the significant interactions between type of metal (γ-TiAl or Ti-6Al-4V) and type of surface treatment (micro arc oxidization at 200 mA, 3 min, 200 mA, 4 min, 225 mA, 3 min, and 225 mA, 4 min; thermal oxidization at 500°C and 800°C). All significant interactions were graphically analyzed and, in addition, a randomized block design was performed to reduce the variance in the data. Furthermore, a contrast test was performed to compare the type of metal (γ-TiAl and Ti-6Al-4V) with the surface treatments. Significant differences in cell differentiation on the type of metal and surfaces tested were confirmed using the LSD Fisher test. All analyses were

performed using Infostat (Infostat Inc.). p values < 0.05 were considered to be statistically significant.

3. Results

SEM images of glass coverslips, untreated Ti-6Al-4V and γ-TiAl surfaces (TiV and GTi), micro arc oxidized Ti-6Al-4V and γ-TiAl surfaces (MAOTiV and MAOGTi), and thermally oxidized Ti-6Al-4V and γ-TiAl surfaces (TiV5, TiV8, GTi5, and GTi8), are shown in Figure 1. GTi and TiV (Figures 1(a) and 1(b)) exhibit a smoother surface of the passive oxide layer formed instantaneously on Ti alloys. In contrast, rounded surface structures were visible in TiV5, suggesting clusters of oxide granules. GTi8 and TiV8, on the other hand, exhibited a rougher surface in comparison to the other samples (Figures 1(e) and 1(f)). Larger oxide granules were present on TiV8 (Figure 1(e)) compared to those on GTi8 (Figure 1(f)), conferring an irregular appearance to this surface and suggesting that TiV8 oxide layer could possibly be thicker. The MAO surfaces for Ti-6Al-4V (MAOTiV) (Figure 1(g)) demonstrated a number of large pores on the oxide surface typical of similar treatments on Ti alloys [18, 19]. Although pores were also clearly visible on the surface of MAOGTi, these were smaller and on the average in the submicron range.

SEM images shown in Figure 2 indicate that hFOB 1.19 cells grew normally on the surfaces of untreated γ-TiAl and Ti-6Al-4V disks. Cell attachment and proliferation were similar on both metal surfaces, suggesting normal growth, cell confluence, and attachment under *in vitro* conditions. The osteoblast cells were spread and flattened on the glass coverslips exhibiting such close contact with each other, that detection of cellular boundaries was difficult. Fibrous networks corresponding to fibrillar collagen, the main component of bone ECM, which aid in the adhesion of cells and important for the proper assembly of the extracellular matrix, are visible lending further testimony to the normal growth of osteoblasts on these surfaces. The ECM, which serves as a calcium phosphate reservoir, provides support for the cells, offers protection, and is very important in homeostasis, appears to be forming copiously [20]. Included are nodules of mineralization with a sponge-like morphology and intimately associated with the fibrillar network and scattered throughout the samples [21]. The maturation of the ECM is evidenced by the presence of fibrous networks associated with cells and an increase in nodules of mineralization. On the thermally oxidized Ti-6Al-4V and γ-TiAl alloys at 500°C, cellular attachment and proliferation were similarly observed. A cell multilayer, constituted by elongated and polygonal cells with some round shaped cells (Figure 2), along with the presence of a few small rounded structures which may correspond to mineral nodules, was observed. At higher magnification (Figure 3), the mineral nodules appeared to be in close contact with cells and had a sponge-like appearance. On the thermally oxidized Ti-6Al-4V alloys at 800°C, only irregular structures were observed. There was cell debris indicative of cytotoxicity of the oxide (Figure 3) in agreement with an earlier report [20]. However, on thermally oxidized γ-TiAl alloys, fibrous networks and mineralized nodules

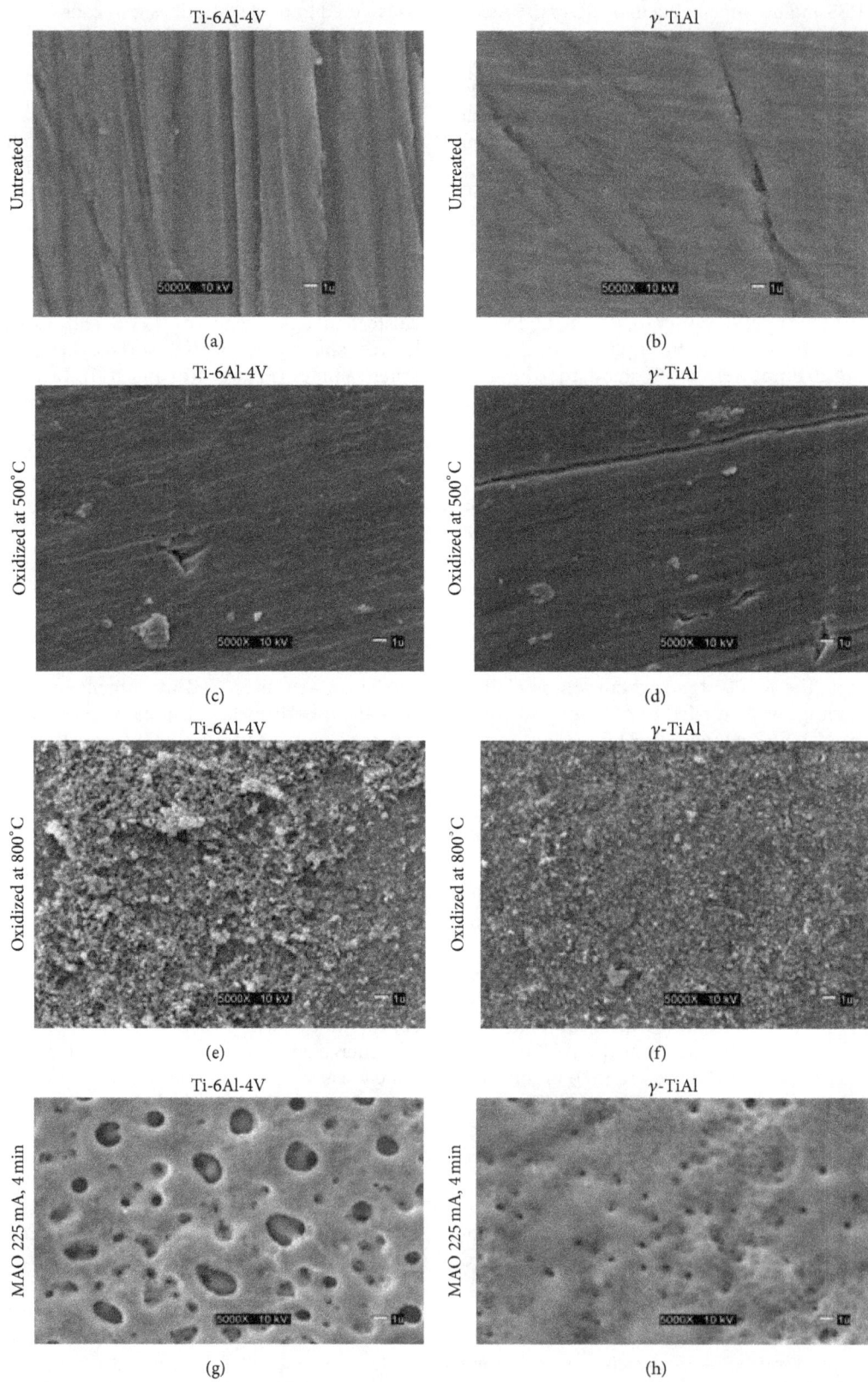

FIGURE 1: SEM images of Ti-6Al-4V and γ-TiAl alloys. (a), (b): untreated, (c), (d): oxidized at 500°C, (e), (f): oxidized at 800°C, and (g), (h): MAO at 225 mA, 4 mins.

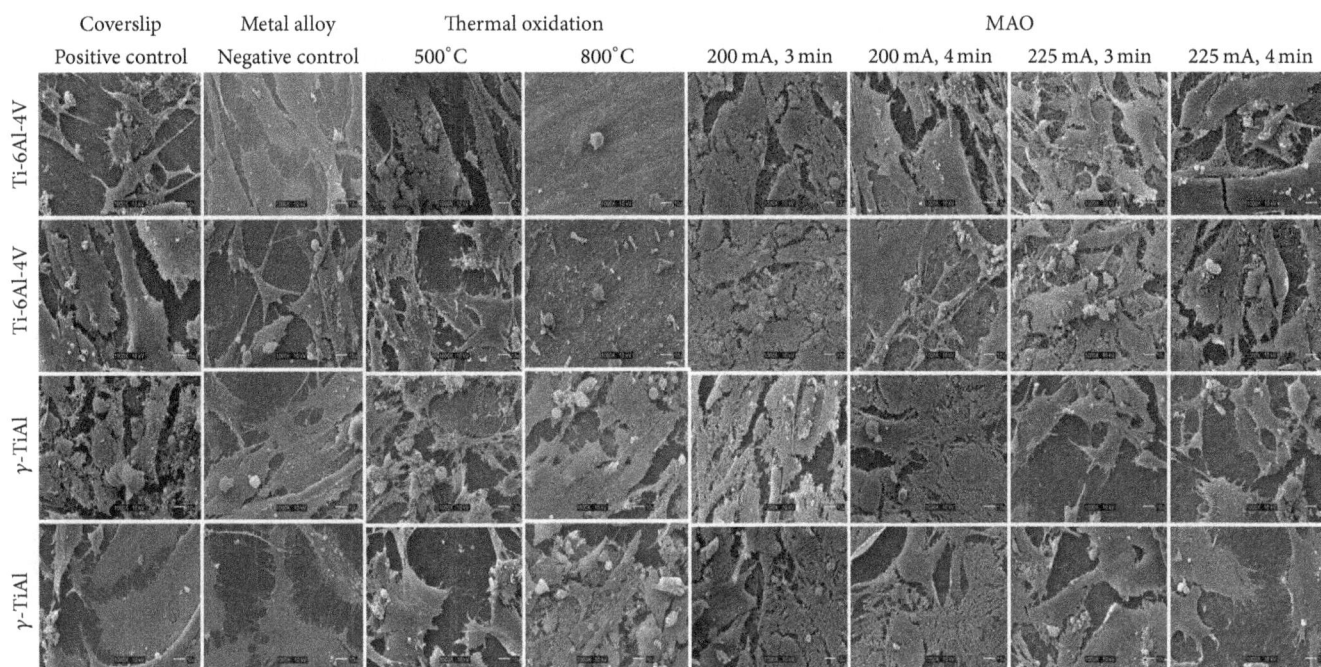

FIGURE 2: SEM micrographs of hFOB 1.19 cells on a glass coverslip (positive control), GTi and TiV (untreated alloys), thermally oxidized TiV5 and GTi5 (500°C), TiV8 and GTi8 (800°C), micro arc oxidized (MAO) TiV (200 mA and 225 mA at 3 min and 4 min), and MAOGTi (200 mA and 225 mA at 3 min and 4 min) disks. Magnification 1000x.

were observed on elongated cells (see Figure 3). Slender cytoplasmic projections (filopodia) extended from the cells in all directions on all micro arc oxidized Ti-6Al-4V and γ-TiAl disks, confirming the biocompatibility of the substrate materials [12]. In addition, sheet-like cytoplasmic protrusions extending from the cell body in all directions suggest the ability of cellular movement, spreading of the cells on the substrate, and/or the fact that cellular division (mitosis) may be occurring. The presence of mineralized nodules again suggests the maturation of the ECM and the formation of bone-like tissue indicating osteoblast differentiation evidenced by a high degree of ALP activity. Taken together, normal cell attachment and proliferation on all the surfaces with the exception of TiV8 indicate the excellent biocompatibility of control, untreated, and treated titanium alloy surfaces.

Standard calibration curves were used to extrapolate the values of alkaline phosphatase (ALP) activity on experimental disks 10 days after seeding based on the alkaline phosphatase assay. The ALP activity, measured as described in Section 2, is plotted in Figure 4 for the various sample surfaces that were utilized in the experiment to measure osteoblast differentiation. It is clear that little ALP activity is observed on the untreated Ti alloy samples while the positive controls (glass coverslips) indicate reasonable ALP activity corresponding to osteoblast differentiation. For the surface treatments of thermal oxidation and MAO, the Ti samples clearly showed relatively higher ALP activity. The highest ALP activity is observed for the Ti alloys subjected to the MAO treatment. As an exception, it must be noted that the ALP activity on Ti-6Al-4V oxidized at 800°C is rather low compared to the other treated samples. ANOVA revealed significant interactions between the factors tested (type of

metal and treatment) and ALP activity. The interaction between the type of metal (γ-TiAl or Ti-6Al-4V) and surface treatment (micro arc oxidation at 200 mA, 3 min, 200 mA, 4 min, 225 mA, 3 min, and 225 mA, 4 min; thermal oxidation at 500°C or 800°C) was significant ($p < 0.05$). There were also significant differences in the amount of alkaline phosphatase detected among these six surfaces studied after 10 days of incubation at 33.5°C and 39.5°C, respectively. Additionally, alkaline phosphatase activity was lower on the positive control (glass coverslips) and even much lower on untreated titanium alloy surfaces in comparison with the micro arc and thermally oxidized alloys. Furthermore, ALP activity increased in γ-TiAl and Ti-6Al-4V alloys and in the MAO treatments where the samples were exposed for longer process times to current density. Although qualitatively there were no significant differences in the number of osteoblast cells attached on the micro arc oxidized or thermally oxidized surfaces collectively, ALP activity was significantly higher on the cell cultures that grew on the micro arc oxidized surfaces in comparison to the thermally oxidized substrates (see Figure 4). Surface roughness of the oxidized surfaces does not appear to show a correlation with ALP activity.

4. Discussion

hFOB adherence is clearly excellent on all surfaces with the exception of TiV8 which may possibly be due to the cellular response to toxic compounds or harmful ions such as vanadium in the oxide layer as a result of thermal oxidation [22]. As such, titanium oxide alone does not pose problems of cytotoxicity since cells did attach and proliferate on surfaces of both alloys subject to oxidation at 500°C and also γ-TiAl

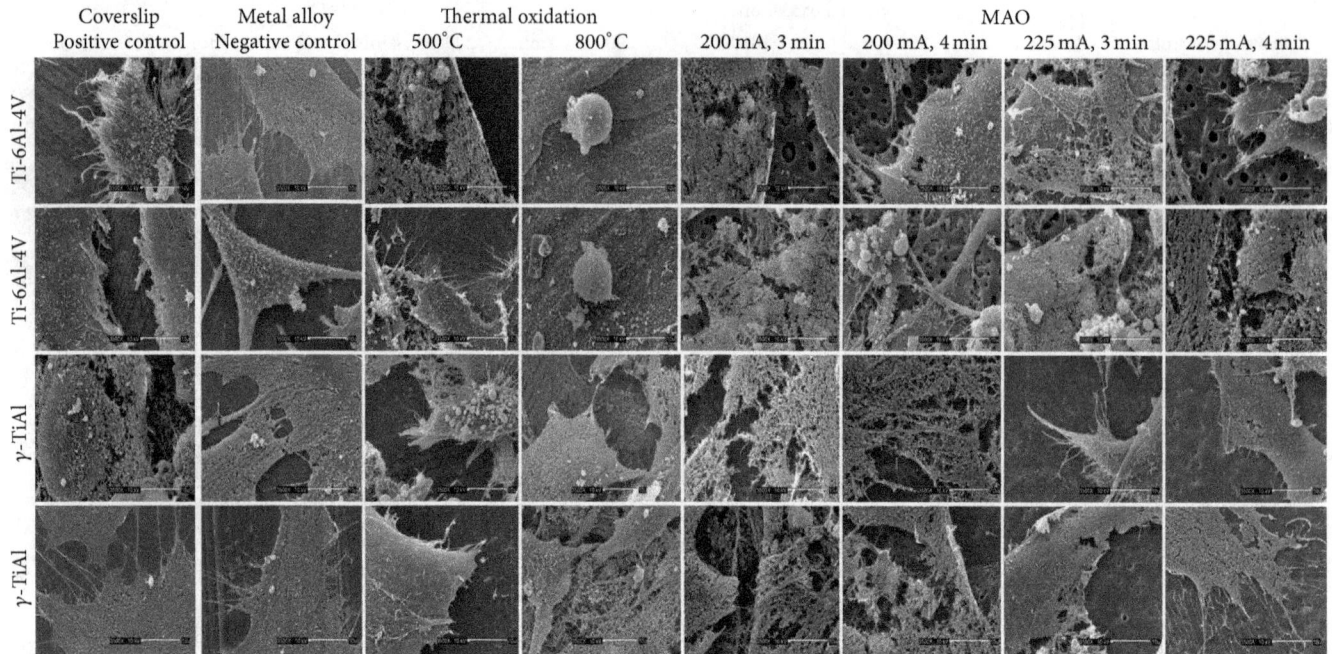

FIGURE 3: SEM micrographs of hFOB 1.19 cells seeded on a glass coverslip (positive control), GTi and TiV (untreated alloys), TiV5 and GTi5 (500°C), TiV8 and GTi8 (800°C), MAOTiV (200 mA and 225 mA at 3 min and 4 min), and MAOGTi (200 mA and 225 mA at 3 min and 4 min) disks and incubated for 10 days (3 days at 33.5°C and subsequently 7 days at 39.5°C). Magnification 3500x.

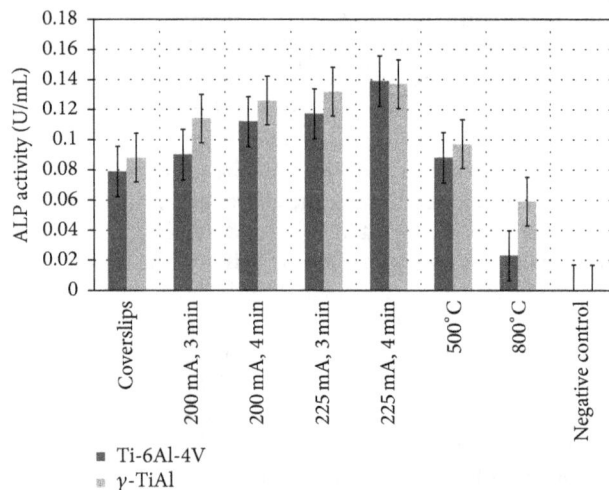

FIGURE 4: Alkaline phosphatase activity on thermally oxidized and MAO treated Ti-6Al-4V and γ-TiAl alloys. ALP activity on positive control (glass coverslips) and untreated Ti alloys is also shown.

oxidized at 800°C where the oxide formed is predominantly composed of titanium oxide in the form of rutile or anatase [23]. An earlier study showed normal cell attachment on TiV8 2 days after seeding but cell debris as a result of subsequent cell death for longer periods of incubation [20].

Osteoblast differentiation, on the other hand, occurred to different extents on all the substrates as measured by ALP activity. Osteoblast differentiation is a well-coordinated physiological process occurring in three stages which include cell proliferation, ECM production and maturation, and matrix mineralization [24]. Correspondingly, proliferative osteoprogenitors such as *Msx2* and *RP59* are expressed in the first stage, followed by *Runx2*, *Osx*, and OC (osteocalcin) during the later stages in this process of differentiation. During proliferation, Col 1 and ALP are detected earlier on followed by the secretion of RGD containing proteins such as bone sialoproteins (BSP) and osteopontin (OP) and culminating in the synthesis of OC in the last stage of differentiation. Bone morphogenetic proteins (BMPs) and various members of TGF-β family are secreted by the osteoblast cells and, once sequestered in the extracellular matrix (ECM), these have also been reported to be critical for osteoblast differentiation [25]. Interaction between Type I collagen and $\alpha2\beta1$ integrin activates a mitogen-activated protein kinase (MAPK) pathway which results in the phosphorylation and activation of *Cbfa1*, in turn stimulating the differentiation of osteoblasts. The ECM which contains BMPs can then induce ALP activity in preosteoblasts [26]. During osteogenesis, the lack of expression of *Runx2* and *Osx* may result in the formation of demineralized bone, although data suggests that these transcription factors act independently of each other [27]. Expression of *Runx2* along with *Cbfβ* and alkaline phosphatase has been found to be critical in the early stage of differentiation while *Osx* becomes very important in the later stage of osteoblast differentiation. While, in the present study, cell attachment and proliferation occur normally on all the substrates, except for TiV8, alkaline phosphatase activity measurements indicate that osteoblast differentiation varies depending on the nature of the substrate. The presence of mineral nodules in the ECM on the titanium sample surfaces provides physical evidence to corroborate the activity of osteoblasts in one of their functional stages after maturation as observed in osteoblast cultures at longer periods of incubation [28]. Ti-6Al-4V and γ-TiAl thermally oxidized disks at 500°C showed both irregular and rounded mineralized structures on the surface. Similar cell morphology and function were observed for the MAO surfaces for both alloys, suggesting the ability of these surfaces to also promulgate differentiation.

The fact that ALP activity was significantly lower on the untreated alloys (TiV, GTi) suggests that the titanium oxide formed on the surface of these alloys may be strongly correlated with the differentiation of the osteoblasts. It was demonstrated in an earlier study that the oxide layer on MAO treated alloys consists of titanium oxide with peaks for both anatase and rutile phases in all the coating conditions applied in this study [11]. Both anatase and rutile have been shown to be beneficial in enhancing nucleation and subsequent hydroxyapatite (HA) precipitation, thereby increasing bioactivity of the titanium surface [29]. The results from the present study also suggest that the incorporation of calcium (Ca) and phosphorus (P) into the titanium oxide may be favorable for cell differentiation. While Ca and P are important in the observation of increased ALP activity on MAO treated surfaces, the Ti alloys samples which were thermally oxidized at 500°C (devoid of Ca and P) also show a reasonably high ALP activity compared to control glass coverslips. A recent study has shown higher elemental oxygen concentration and higher water wettability on TiO_2 surfaces when compared to bare titanium surfaces resulting in a twofold increase in ALP activity and mineralized nodule area [30]. It also appears that the topography of bioengineered titanium surfaces affects gene expression and phenotypic response of osteoprogenitor cells [31]. Higher ALP activity on surfaces containing titanium oxide may possibly be correlated with the surface topography of the substrate which may affect cell proliferation and differentiation [31, 32]. Thus it may be argued that the osteoblast differentiation does not depend solely on Ca and P ions but more so on the presence of titanium oxide. In contrast, another research suggests cell cytotoxicity due to TiO_2 resulting from the interaction between TiO_2 nanoparticles and the lysosomal compartment, independently of the known apoptotic signaling pathways [33]. However, this has not been fully studied. In addition, TiO_2 has been reported to possess antibacterial characteristics in stark contrast to its positive biocompatibility [34].

Although it is clear from this study that titanium oxide increases the ALP activity in osteoblasts, the mechanism associated with this process is still unknown. It was proposed that BMP-2 controls alkaline phosphatase expression and osteoblast mineralization by a Wnt autocrine loop in mesenchymal stem cells (MSCs) [35]. Among the factors that regulate MSC growth and differentiation are soluble factors and cell-substrate interactions, although little is known about the molecular mechanisms by which soluble and substrate signals regulate MSC function. These authors showed that the commitment of human MSCs to the osteogenic and adipogenic lineages *in vitro* involves signaling by mitogen-activated protein kinase (MAPK) pathways. In particular, it was found that dexamethasone, ascorbic acid, and β-glycerophosphate induce MSC differentiation by

regulating the extracellular signal-regulated kinase (ERK1/2) cascade. Furthermore, blocking the ERK1/2 pathway inhibits osteogenic differentiation of MSCs and leads to adipogenesis. Thus MAPK pathways, which are generally activated by growth factors/cytokines and integrin-mediated cell adhesion, play a critical role in directing MSC commitment. MAPK pathways are also activated by physical stimuli to regulate the function of a variety of cell types, including bone cells. In bone, it has been proposed that mature cells such as osteocytes and osteoblasts are responsible for sensing and responding to mechanical stimuli [36]. It is unknown whether the progenitors that give rise to these cells are responsive to mechanical signals. Various signaling pathways, including BMP, Wnt, and notch, regulate bone homeostasis. It is difficult at the present time to determine which of these is affected by titanium oxide to the extent of upregulating ALP activity. While it is clearly demonstrated that hypoxia suppresses osteoblast differentiation and as a consequence bone formation, the mode by which TiO_2 increases ALP activity is not clear cut. One may speculate that a chemical reaction between TiO_2 and the culture medium may somehow result in the release of oxygen and this normoxia has a positive impact on osteoblast differentiation. However, it is clear that TiO_2 is a bioactive factor which indeed upregulates ALP activity, although the manner in which the oxide indeed participates in the biochemical signaling cascade which occurs during differentiation does require further study. This information may be vital in the future of implantology in accelerating fracture healing and other tissue regenerative processes in dental and orthopedic applications. If titanium oxide indeed upregulates osteoblast differentiation, the manufacturers of titanium-based implants would find it advantageous to incorporate titanium oxide as a coating on every surface layer in contact with the tissue side of the implant. Clearly, further research is needed to interrogate the empirical ability of titanium oxide to preferentially favor osteoblast differentiation or at least ALP activity.

5. Conclusions

(1) ALP activity is much higher on oxidized surfaces of both titanium alloys compared to untreated surfaces most probably due to the presence of titanium oxide.

(2) The higher ALP activity on micro arc oxidized surfaces is attributed to the Ca and P content which are not present in the thermally oxidized titanium alloys.

(3) The mechanism for the upregulation of ALP due to titanium oxide needs further study although it is clear that TiO_2 is a bioactive factor in osteoblast differentiation.

Conflict of Interests

There is no financial conflict of interests regarding the data or content of this study.

Acknowledgments

This study was supported by the NIH Grant SO6GM-08103 through the MBRS-SCORE Program at the University of Puerto Rico, Mayaguez Campus. The authors thank Jose Almodovar from the University of Puerto Rico, Mayaguez Campus, who assisted in the acquisition of the immunofluorescence images.

References

[1] H. J. Rack and J. I. Qazi, "Titanium alloys for biomedical applications," *Materials Science and Engineering C*, vol. 26, no. 8, pp. 1269–1277, 2006.

[2] I. Milošev, M. Metikoš-Huković, and H.-H. Strehblow, "Passive film on orthopaedic TiAlV alloy formed in physiological solution investigated by X-ray photoelectron spectroscopy," *Biomaterials*, vol. 21, no. 20, pp. 2103–2113, 2000.

[3] P. Santiago-Medina, P. A. Sundaram, and N. Diffoot-Carlo, "The effects of micro arc oxidation of gamma titanium aluminide surfaces on osteoblast adhesion and differentiation," *Journal of Materials Science: Materials in Medicine*, vol. 25, no. 6, pp. 1577–1587, 2014.

[4] G. L. Lin and K. D. Hankenson, "Integration of BMP, Wnt, and notch signaling pathways in osteoblast differentiation," *Journal of Cellular Biochemistry*, vol. 112, no. 12, pp. 3491–3501, 2011.

[5] C. Nicolaije, M. Koedam, and J. P. T. M. van Leeuwen, "Decreased oxygen tension lowers reactive oxygen species and apoptosis and inhibits osteoblast matrix mineralization through changes in early osteoblast differentiation," *Journal of Cellular Physiology*, vol. 227, no. 4, pp. 1309–1318, 2012.

[6] A. Salim, R. P. Nacamuli, E. F. Morgan, A. J. Giaccia, and M. T. Longaker, "Transient changes in oxygen tension inhibit osteogenic differentiation and Runx2 expression in osteoblasts," *Journal of Biological Chemistry*, vol. 279, no. 38, pp. 40007–40016, 2004.

[7] B. Feng, J. Weng, B. C. Yang, S. X. Qu, and X. D. Zhang, "Characterization of surface oxide films on titanium and adhesion of osteoblast," *Biomaterials*, vol. 24, no. 25, pp. 4663–4670, 2003.

[8] G. Zhao, Z. Schwartz, M. Wieland et al., "High surface energy enhances cell response to titanium substrate microstructure," *Journal of Biomedical Materials Research A*, vol. 74, no. 1, pp. 49–58, 2005.

[9] R. B. Heppenstall, C. W. Goodwin, and C. T. Brighton, "Fracture healing in the presence of chronic hypoxia," *The Journal of Bone and Joint Surgery—American Volume*, vol. 58, no. 8, pp. 1153–1156, 1976.

[10] X.-C. Bai, D. Lu, A.-L. Liu et al., "Reactive oxygen species stimulates receptor activator of NF-κB ligand expression in osteoblast," *Journal of Biological Chemistry*, vol. 280, no. 17, pp. 17497–17506, 2005.

[11] L. Lara Rodriguez, P. A. Sundaram, E. Rosim-Fachini, A. M. Padovani, and N. Diffoot-Carlo, "Plasma electrolytic oxidation coatings on γtiAl alloy for potential biomedical applications," *Journal of Biomedical Materials Research B: Applied Biomaterials*, vol. 102, no. 5, pp. 988–1001, 2014.

[12] L.-H. Li, Y.-M. Kong, H.-W. Kim et al., "Improved biological performance of Ti implants due to surface modification by micro-arc oxidation," *Biomaterials*, vol. 25, no. 14, pp. 2867–2875, 2004.

[13] S. Becker, A. Rahmel, M. Schorr, and M. Schütze, "Mechanism of isothermal oxidation of the intel-metallic TiAl and of TiAl alloys," *Oxidation of Metals*, vol. 38, no. 5-6, pp. 425–464, 1992.

[14] A. Gil, H. Hoven, E. Wallura, and W. J. Quadakkers, "The effect of microstructure on the oxidation behaviour of TiAl-based intermetallics," *Corrosion Science*, vol. 34, no. 4, pp. 615–630, 1993.

[15] N. Zheng, W. Fischer, H. Grübmeier, V. Shemet, and W. J. Quadakkers, "The significance of sub-surface depletion layer composition for the oxidation behaviour of γ-titanium aluminides," *Scripta Metallurgica et Materiala*, vol. 33, no. 1, pp. 47–53, 1995.

[16] J. W. Fergus, "Review of the effect of alloy composition on the growth rates of scales formed during oxidation of gamma titanium aluminide alloys," *Materials Science and Engineering A*, vol. 338, no. 1-2, pp. 108–125, 2002.

[17] S. Kumar, T. S. N. Sankara Narayanan, S. Ganesh Sundara Raman, and S. K. Seshadri, "Thermal oxidation of Ti6Al4V alloy: microstructural and electrochemical characterization," *Materials Chemistry and Physics*, vol. 119, no. 1-2, pp. 337–346, 2010.

[18] P. Whiteside, E. Matykina, J. E. Gough, P. Skeldon, and G. E. Thompson, "In vitro evaluation of cell proliferation and collagen synthesis on titanium following plasma electrolytic oxidation," *Journal of Biomedical Materials Research Part A*, vol. 94, no. 1, pp. 38–46, 2010.

[19] M. Dicu, A. Matei, M. Abrudeanu, and C. Ducu, "Synthesis and properties of the porous titania coatings formed on titanium by plasma electrolytic oxidation for biomedical application," *Journal of Optoelectronics and Advanced Materials*, vol. 13, no. 3, pp. 324–331, 2011.

[20] S. A. Bello, I. de Jesús-Maldonado, E. Rosim-Fachini, P. A. Sundaram, and N. Diffoot-Carlo, "In vitro evaluation of human osteoblast adhesion to a thermally oxidized γ-TiAl intermetallic alloy of composition Ti-48Al-2Cr-2Nb (at.%)," *Journal of Materials Science: Materials in Medicine*, vol. 21, no. 5, pp. 1739–1750, 2010.

[21] M. C. Advincula, F. G. Rahemtulla, R. C. Advincula, E. T. Ada, J. E. Lemons, and S. L. Bellis, "Osteoblast adhesion and matrix mineralization on sol-gel-derived titanium oxide," *Biomaterials*, vol. 27, no. 10, pp. 2201–2212, 2006.

[22] D. R. Haynes, S. D. Rogers, S. Hay, M. J. Pearcy, and D. W. Howie, "The differences in toxicity and release of bone-resorbing mediators induced by titanium and cobalt-chromium-alloy wear particles," *The Journal of Bone & Joint Surgery—American Volume*, vol. 75, no. 6, pp. 825–834, 1993.

[23] C. Delgado-Alvarado and P. A. Sundaram, "Corrosion evaluation of Ti-48Al-2Cr-2Nb (at.%) in Ringer's solution," *Acta Biomaterialia*, vol. 2, no. 6, pp. 701–708, 2006.

[24] T. A. Owen, M. Aronow, V. Shalhoub et al., "Progressive development of the rat osteoblast phenotype in vitro: reciprocal relationships in expression of genes associated with osteoblast proliferation and differentiation during formation of the bone extracellular matrix," *Journal of Cellular Physiology*, vol. 143, no. 3, pp. 420–430, 1990.

[25] G. Xiao, R. Gopalakrishnan, D. Jiang, E. Reith, M. D. Benson, and R. T. Franceschi, "Bone morphogenetic proteins, extracellular matrix, and mitogen-activated protein kinase signaling pathways are required for osteoblast-specific gene expression and differentiation in MC3T3-E1 cells," *Journal of Bone and Mineral Research*, vol. 17, no. 1, pp. 101–110, 2002.

[26] Y. Takeuchi, K. Nakayama, and T. Matsumoto, "Differentiation and cell surface expression of transforming growth factor-β receptors are regulated by interaction with matrix collagen in murine osteoblastic cells," *Journal of Biological Chemistry*, vol. 271, no. 7, pp. 3938–3944, 1996.

[27] K. Nakashima and B. de Crombrugghe, "Transcriptional mechanisms in osteoblast differentiation and bone formation," *Trends in Genetics*, vol. 19, no. 8, pp. 458–466, 2003.

[28] U. Müller, T. Imwinkelried, M. Horst, M. Sievers, and U. Graf-Hausner, "Do human osteoblasts grow into open-porous titanium?" *European Cells and Materials*, vol. 11, pp. 8–15, 2006.

[29] J.-M. Wu, S. Hayakawa, K. Tsuru, and A. Osaka, "Low-temperature preparation of anatase and rutile layers on titanium substrates and their ability to induce in vitro apatite deposition," *Journal of the American Ceramic Society*, vol. 87, no. 9, pp. 1635–1642, 2004.

[30] N. Tsukimura, N. Kojima, K. Kubo et al., "The effect of superficial chemistry of titanium on osteoblastic function," *Journal of Biomedical Materials Research Part A*, vol. 84, no. 1, pp. 108–116, 2008.

[31] J. Isaac, A. Galtayries, T. Kizuki, T. Kokubo, A. Berdal, and J.-M. Sautier, "Bioengineered titanium surfaces affect the gene expression and phenotypic response of osteoprogenitor cells derived from mouse calvarial bones," *European Cells and Materials*, vol. 20, pp. 178–196, 2010.

[32] Z. Huang, R. H. Daniels, R.-J. Enzerink, V. Hardev, V. Sahi, and S. B. Goodman, "Effect of nanofiber-coated surfaces on the proliferation and differentiation of osteoprogenitors *in vitro*," *Tissue Engineering A*, vol. 14, no. 11, pp. 1853–1859, 2008.

[33] Y. Zhu, J. W. Eaton, and C. Li, "Titanium dioxide (TiO_2) nanoparticles preferentially induce cell death in transformed cells in Bak/Bax-independent fashion," *PLoS ONE*, vol. 7, no. 11, Article ID e50607, 2012.

[34] H. Lin, Z. Xu, X. Wang et al., "Photocatalytic and antibacterial properties of medical-grade PVC material coated with TiO_2 film," *Journal of Biomedical Materials Research Part B: Applied Biomaterials*, vol. 87, no. 2, pp. 425–431, 2008.

[35] G. Rawadi, B. Vayssière, F. Dunn, R. Baron, and S. Roman-Roman, "BMP-2 controls alkaline phosphatase expression and osteoblast mineralization by a Wnt autocrine loop," *Journal of Bone and Mineral Research*, vol. 18, no. 10, pp. 1842–1853, 2003.

[36] P. G. Robey and J. D. Termine, "Human bone cells in vitro," *Calcified Tissue International*, vol. 37, no. 5, pp. 453–460, 1985.

7

Quantitative Analysis of Salivary TNF-α in Oral Lichen Planus Patients

T. Malarkodi and S. Sathasivasubramanian

Department of Oral Medicine & Radiology, Faculty of Dental Sciences, Sri Ramachandra University, Porur, Chennai 600116, India

Correspondence should be addressed to T. Malarkodi; tmalarkodi@gmail.com

Academic Editor: Francesco Carinci

Objective. The aim of this study was to quantitatively evaluate the salivary tumor necrosis factor-alpha (TNF-α) level in oral lichen planus patients and to compare the levels of TNF-α between saliva and serum of OLP and controls. *Methods.* Serum and whole saliva from 30 patients with active lesions of oral lichen planus (OLP) and 30 healthy persons were investigated for the presence of TNF-α by enzyme immunoassay. Student's independent t-test and two-sample binomial proportion test were used to calculate significance of the mean values of TNF-alpha in serum and saliva and to determine the proportions of the detected and nondetected samples in both groups. *Results.* Proportion of detection and the mean of detectability between saliva and serum of Group B show an almost equal value, which suggests that saliva can be a good alternate to serum to analyze TNF-α in oral lichen planus patients.

1. Introduction

Lichen planus (LP) is a chronic inflammatory mucocutaneous disease. It was first described by the British physician Erasmus Wilson in 1869. The clinical appearances of these lesions resembled lichens a primitive organism of symbiotic algae and fungi growing on rocks, hence designated as lichen planus [1].

This disease primarily affects the skin and mucosal surfaces including the oral cavity. It can also involve other sites like the scalp and the nails [2]. It is estimated to affect 1% to 2.0% of the general population. The prevalence of oral lichen planus (OLP) in India is around 2.6%. Around 40% of lesions occur on both oral and cutaneous surfaces, 35% occurs on cutaneous surfaces alone, and 25% occur on oral mucosa alone [1]. Oral mucosal involvement can occur concurrently with cutaneous disease or it can be the only manifestation [3]. WHO has grouped this condition under the "potentially malignant disorders" of the oral mucosa [4].

Out of the six clinical forms of OLP the reticular, papular, and plaque type lesions are usually asymptomatic [5] whereas the erosive, atrophic, and bullous type lesions usually present with burning sensation and rarely with pain [3]. Malignant transformation or development of malignancy in the presence of OLP is more likely to occur in atrophic and erosive forms [1]. Majority of studies have reported the rate of malignant transformation of OLP to be between 0.5 and 2% [6].

The exact cause of LP remains unclear; however several predisposing factors like stress, chronic liver disease, and genetics have been implicated in the pathogenesis [3]. Current evidences suggest that LP is a T-cell mediated process. Adhesion molecules, cytokines, chemokine like intracellular adhesion molecules 1 (ICAM-1), vascular adhesion molecule (VCAM-1), interferon gamma (INF-γ) and tumor necrosis factor-alpha (TNF-α) serve to stimulate T-cells, initiate their adhesion to blood vessels, and direct their migration from the blood vessels to the tissues [1].

Tumor necrosis factor-alpha (TNF-α) has been implicated in the pathogenesis of many precancerous, cancerous, autoimmune, and inflammatory diseases including oral submucous fibrosis, oral leukoplakia, oral squamous cell carcinoma, systemic lupus erythematosus, rheumatoid arthritis, psoriasis, and OLP. In addition to being cytotoxic for certain tumor cells, it also acts as an essential mediator in inflammatory and immunologic reactions during host defense by increasing the major histocompatibility complex

(MHC) class I antigen and intercellular adhesion molecule (ICAM) expression on many cells [1, 7].

Saliva as test specimen has several benefits over blood and is increasingly being used in the diagnosis of diseases. It offers distinctive advantages over serum because it can be collected noninvasively. Salivary analysis offers a reliable correlation of various parameters that are routinely evaluated in blood [8]. Early diagnosis and proper treatment are imperative as the oral lesion has the propensity for malignant development [9]. OLP is one of the most frequently encountered mucosal pathology by the dental practitioners. High concentration of TNF-α has a role in the progression of the pathological events in OLP [4] and only few studies are available in the English literature that has evaluated TNF-α in saliva of OLP patients. Hence this study was undertaken to evaluate the salivary and serum TNF-α levels in OLP patients and to probe whether saliva can be used as an alternative to serum in evaluating TNF-α in OLP patients.

The aim of this study was to quantitatively evaluate the salivary TNF-α level in oral lichen planus patients and to compare the levels of TNF-α between saliva and serum of OLP and controls.

2. Materials and Methods

2.1. Subjects. The study group comprised sixty individuals, of which thirty were healthy volunteers and thirty were clinically and histopathologically diagnosed as OLP patients'. Women on oral contraceptives, pregnant women, smokers, alcoholics, and patients with liver disease, renal disease, diabetes mellitus, psoriasis, sjogren syndrome, rheumatoid arthritis, systemic lupus erythematosus, dental diseases, oral mucosal diseases, other infectious diseases, and history of trauma in the last six months, and patients under medications like dexamethasone were not included in the study. The patients' age group for the study ranged from 18 to 75 years with a mean age of 43.5. Out of the thirty oral lichen planus patients 16 were female and 14 were male. The clinical patterns of oral lichen planus were 22 with reticular type, 2 with erosive type, 4 with atrophic, and 2 with papular type. All the patients included in the study were those who had not undergone any form of therapy for their presenting illness. Their details were recorded in a specific case sheet pro forma, which was prepared earlier. Samples from thirty controls who participated in the study were drawn from healthy volunteers who were free of oral and medical illness. The age group for healthy volunteers ranged from 23 to 61 years with the mean age of 42. The patients and healthy controls were given explanation about the study and a written consent was taken. Procedures followed were in accordance with the ethical standards.

2.2. Collection of Samples. Blood samples were collected between 8:00 a.m. and 4:00 p.m. from the subjects. The blood samples were kept undisturbed for 30 min following which the serum was separated from the blood cells by centrifugation. The separated serum was stored in disposable plastic vials at $-80°C$ until the time of analysis. 2 mL of

whole unstimulated saliva were collected simultaneously by drooling method in sterile disposable plastic containers with lid. The salivary samples were transferred to sterile centrifuge tubes. After centrifugation the separated clear salivary fluid was stored in disposable storage vials at $-80°C$ until the time of analysis. Care was taken not to collect sputum.

2.3. Cytokine Assay. All reagents and samples were brought to room temperature (18–25°C) before use. The samples were subjected to analysis and TNF-α concentration was determined using enzyme-linked immunosorbent assay kits (Ray Bio Human TNF-alpha Enzyme Immunoassay) and the results were interpreted by using spectrophotometry at 450 nm. On a linear graph, the optical density values were plotted for each of the calibrators (y-axis) against the corresponding standard concentration of TNF-α (x-axis), and a calibration curve was drawn. The TNF-α concentration of salivary and serum samples were calculated using the optical density and the concentration of the standard. The results were expressed as pg/mL.

2.4. Statistical Analysis. Statistical Package for Social Science (SPSS) software was used to analyze the data. Mean and standard deviation were estimated in each study group. The significance of the mean values of TNF-alpha in serum and saliva between the control and the patients were done using Student's independent t-test. The proportions of the detected and nondetected samples in both groups were determined using two-sample binomial proportion test.

3. Results

Students' independent t-test was used to compare the mean values of Group A (controls) and Group B (OLP) in Tables 1 and 2. As shown in Table 1, the mean value of salivary TNF-α in OLP patients was higher than the control group and it was statistically significant with a P value of 0.039.

As shown in Table 2 the mean serum TNF-α levels in OLP patients was higher than the control group and it was statistically very highly significant with a P value of 0.000697.

Two-sample binomial proportion tests were done to compare the proportion of detectability and nondetectability of TNF-α in salivary and serum samples.

The proportion of detectability of TNF-α in saliva of OLP patients as shown in Table 3 and Figure 1 was high when compared to controls and was statistically significant with a P value of 0.02.

The proportion of detectability of TNF-α in serum of OLP patients as shown in Table 4 and Figure 2 was high when compared to controls and it was statistically very highly significant with a P value of 0.001.

As shown in Table 5 the proportion of detectability of TNF-α in serum of OLP patients was high when compared with saliva from the same group but it was statistically not significant.

Students' independent t-test was used to compare the mean of detectability of TNF-α in saliva and serum of OLP

TABLE 1: Comparison of mean values of TNF-α in saliva of Group A and Group B.

Group	Number of cases	Mean	t-value	P value
A (controls)	30	30.55	2.11	0.039*
B (OLP patients)	30	63.22		

*Significant at $P < 0.05$; **highly significant at $P < 0.01$; ***very highly significant at $P < 0.001$.
TNF: tumor necrosis factor.
OLP: oral lichen planus.

TABLE 2: Comparison of mean values of TNF-α in serum of Group A and Group B.

Group	Number of cases	Mean	t-value	P value
A (controls)	30	16.38	3.6	0.000697***
B (OLP patients)	30	68.44		

*Significant at $P < 0.05$; **highly significant at $P < 0.01$; ***very highly significant at $P < 0.001$.
TNF: tumor necrosis factor.
OLP: oral lichen planus.

TABLE 3: Difference in proportion between detected and nondetected TNF-α values in saliva of Group A and Group B.

Group	Detected	Nondetected	Two-sample binomial proportion test	P value
A (controls)	14 (46.7%)	16 (53.3%)	$Z = 2.38$	0.02*
B (OLP patients)	23 (76.7%)	7 (23.3%)		

*Significant at $P < 0.05$; **highly significant at $P < 0.01$; ***very highly significant at $P < 0.001$.
TNF: tumor necrosis factor.
OLP: oral lichen planus.

TABLE 4: Difference in proportion between detected and nondetected TNF-α values in serum of Group A and Group B.

Group	Detected	Nondetected	Two-sample binomial proportion test	P value
A (controls)	8 (26.7%)	22 (73.3%)	$Z = 3.37$	0.001***
B (OLP patients)	25 (83.3%)	5 (16.7%)		

*Significant at $P < 0.05$; **highly significant at $P < 0.01$; ***very highly significant at $P < 0.001$.
TNF: tumor necrosis factor.
OLP: oral lichen planus.

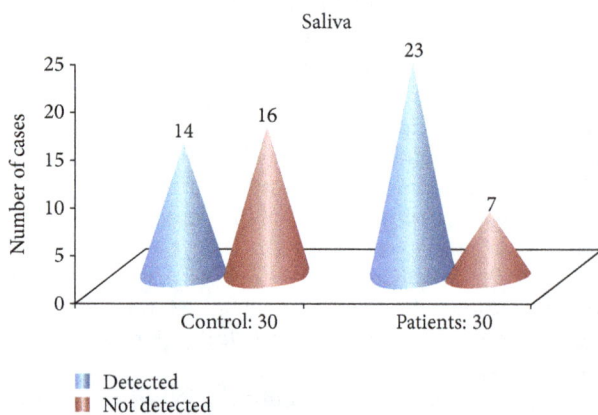

FIGURE 1: Proportion of detectability in saliva of Group A and Group B.

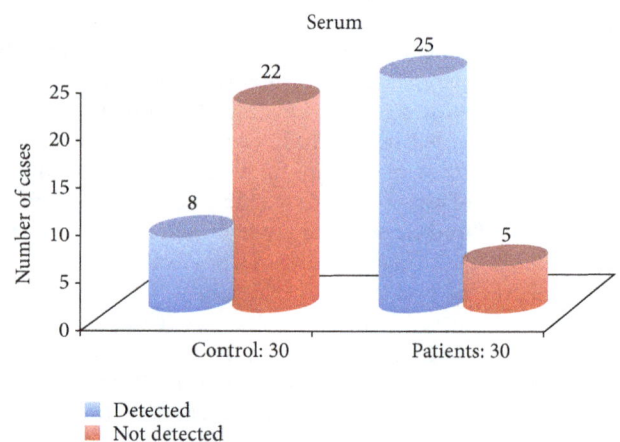

FIGURE 2: Proportion of detectability in serum of Group A and Group B.

patients. As shown in Table 6 the mean of detectability of TNF-α in saliva and serum of OLP patients is same.

Since there is no significant difference between the proportion of detection (Table 5) and the mean of detectability (Table 6) between saliva and serum of Group B, saliva can be used instead of serum to analyze TNF-α in oral lichen planus patients.

TABLE 5: Difference in proportion between detected and nondetected TNF-α values in saliva and serum of Group B.

Group B (OLP patients)	Detected	Nondetected	Two-sample binomial proportion test	P value
Saliva	23 (76.7%)	7 (23.3%)	Z = 0.71	0.52
Serum	25 (83.3%)	5 (16.7%)		

*Significant at $P < 0.05$; **highly significant at $P < 0.01$; ***very highly significant at $P < 0.001$.
TNF: tumor necrosis factor.
OLP: oral lichen planus.

TABLE 6: Comparison of mean values of TNF-α in saliva and serum of Group B.

Group B (OLP patients)	Mean of detected values	Standard deviation	t-test
Saliva	82.46	63.99	t = 0.02
Serum	82.13	61.86	

TNF: tumor necrosis factor.
OLP: oral lichen planus.

4. Discussion

Oral lichen planus (OLP) is a chronic inflammatory disorder. Although the exact etiology of OLP remains unclear, immunological aberration plays a demanding role among the various etiological factors [7]. Though controversies exist around the true malignant potential of OLP, WHO has grouped this lesion under the potentially malignant disorders of the oral mucosa [4]. Previous studies indicate a risk of 0.5–2% for malignant transformation [6]. Accordingly, there is a great need for objective markers to evaluate the prognosis of this condition. Since chronic inflammation has been suggested to be a cofactor for development of oral squamous cell carcinoma (OSCC) in OLP [9], the levels of proinflammatory marker TNF-α in OLP patients were evaluated in this study.

TNF-α is a potentially important and regulatory cytokine in the initiation and progression of OLP, Sugermann et al. [7]. According to Yamamoto et al. [10] and Sklavounou-Andrikopoulou et al. [11] high serum levels of TNF-α were detected in all patients with OLP in comparison with healthy controls. Simultaneously with the expression of other proinflammatory cytokines, OLP lesions have also been shown to contain cells with mRNA for TNF-α [12] and only few studies have measured the salivary levels of TNF-α in OLP patients [13–15]. As there are no studies available which compare the levels of TNF-α in saliva and serum in Indian population, the present study was carried out to evaluate and compare the levels of TNF-α in saliva and serum of oral lichen planus patients. The levels of TNF-α can be quantified using ELISA which is more sensitive, reliable, simple, and widely used and very little sample is required for estimation [16]. In the present study Ray Bio Human TNF-α ELISA kit was used to quantify the levels of TNF-α.

Body fluids that can be used to estimate the TNF-α levels are serum, saliva, and oral tissue transudates. The use of saliva as an adjunctive diagnostic tool has various advantages and supplements the current methodologies. Compared to serum, saliva has significant diagnostic and logistical advantage as a diagnostic fluid as it is less infective, noninvasive, relatively simple collected safely, collected repeatedly without discomfort to the patient, cost effective, easy and safe in disposal; does not require specialized training or special equipment; and lends itself readily for mass screening [17]. These advantages justify that saliva can be used as an easily accessible fluid for research purpose.

TNF-α from a variety of "resident" and "migratory" cells contributes to the total aggregation of bioactive TNF-α in OLP. Within the lesion T lymphocytes, mast cells and keratinocytes are considered to be the plausible cellular source of TNF-α [7]. The exact mechanism by which TNF-α enters saliva is by diffusion, active transport, and leakage through tissue transudates [18].

Unstimulated saliva better represents the physiological state when compared to a stimulated state [8]. Hence in the present study unstimulated saliva was used to determine the levels of TNF-α in saliva.

TNF-α value in Group B (OLP patients) ranged from 0 to 266.67 pg/mL in saliva and 0 to 246 pg/mL in serum. In Group A (controls) it ranged from 0 to 253.33 pg/mL in saliva and 0 to 236 pg/mL in serum.

Results suggested that the mean salivary levels of TNF-α was higher in Group B (OLP patients) when compared to Group A (controls) and it was statistically significant with a P value of 0.039. Similarly in serum, the mean value of TNF-α was higher in Group B (OLP patients) when compared to Group A (controls) and it was statistically very highly significant with a P value of 0.000697. These results were consistent with the previous studies done in saliva [13–15] and serum [10, 11, 19] and signifies that TNF-α plays an important role in the pathogenesis of OLP. The proportion of detectability of TNF-α in saliva of Group B (OLP patients) was significantly high when compared to Group A (controls) with a P value of 0.02. Similarly the proportion of detectability of TNF-α in serum of Group B (OLP patients) was very highly significant when compared to Group A (controls) with a P value of 0.001. The proportion of nondetectable salivary and serum samples for TNF-α was less in Group B (OLP patients) when compared to Group A (controls). Comparing the proportion of detectability between serum and saliva of Group B, (OLP patients) the detectability was marginally high in serum and the mean detectability level of TNF-α in saliva and serum of Group B (OLP patients) was same. This signifies that saliva can be a good alternate for serum to analyze TNF-α in oral lichen planus patients.

23.3% in saliva and 16.7% in serum were not detected for TNF-α in Group B (OLP patients). Diets rich in curcumin and yogurt has been shown to inhibit the activity of TNF-α levels in saliva and serum [20, 21] which can be considered as a reason for nondetectability of TNF-α in saliva and serum of Group B. Gavala et al. have reported that alcohol can inhibit the levels of TNF-α in blood [22]. Although alcoholic patients were excluded from the study, a possible explanation would be that some patients would have voluntarily abstained from revealing the habit. In spite of strictly following the required storage protocols low levels of TNF-α can occur during storage as they were estimated after a specific period of time. This can also be considered as a reason for nondetectability of TNF-α in saliva and serum of OLP patients.

Few salivary and serum samples in Group A (controls) showed elevated levels of TNF-α. Though the exclusion criteria were strictly followed, it can be suggested that these patients would have had a local trauma, aphthous ulcer, upper respiratory tract infection, or any other subclinical infection in the recent past for having high levels of TNF-α in saliva and serum.

Although patients with 5 different clinical manifestations of OLP were enrolled in this study, no subgroups were formed to categorize the clinical types to evaluate and compare the significant difference of TNF-α concentration between them.

This study proves the fact that the expressions of TNF-α in both the test specimens were almost equal. However larger sample size may be required to prove this in a conclusive manner. The study also points to a fact that saliva can be used as a test specimen in the evaluation of TNF-α.

Conflict of Interests

The authors declare that there is no conflict of interests regarding the publication of this paper.

References

[1] S. S. Derossi and K. N. Ciarrocca, "Lichen planus, lichenoid drug reactions, and lichenoid mucositis," *Dental Clinics of North America*, vol. 49, no. 1, pp. 77–89, 2005.

[2] I. Al-Hashimi, M. Schifter, P. B. Lockhart et al., "Oral lichen planus and oral lichenoid lesions: diagnostic and therapeutic considerations," *Oral Surgery, Oral Medicine, Oral Pathology, Oral Radiology and Endodontology*, vol. 103, supplement 1, pp. S25–S31, 2007.

[3] S. B. Ismail, S. K. S. Kumar, and R. B. Zain, "Oral lichen planus and lichenoid reactions: etiopathogenesis, diagnosis, management and malignant transformation," *Journal of Oral Science*, vol. 49, no. 2, pp. 89–106, 2007.

[4] S. Warnakulasuriya, N. W. Johnson, and I. van der Waal, "Nomenclature and classification of potentially malignant disorders of the oral mucosa," *Journal of Oral Pathology and Medicine*, vol. 36, no. 10, pp. 575–580, 2007.

[5] N. Mollaoglu, "Oral lichen planus: a review," *British Journal of Oral and Maxillofacial Surgery*, vol. 38, no. 4, pp. 370–377, 2000.

[6] U. Mattsson, M. Jontell, and P. Holmstrup, "Oral lichen planus and malignant transformation: is a recall of patients justified?" *Critical Reviews in Oral Biology and Medicine*, vol. 13, no. 5, pp. 390–396, 2002.

[7] P. B. Sugermann, N. W. Savage, G. J. Seymour, and L. J. Walsh, "Is there a role for tumor necrosis factor-alpha (TNF-α) in oral lichen planus?" *Journal of Oral Pathology & Medicine*, vol. 25, no. 5, pp. 219–224, 1996.

[8] R. Nishanian, N. Aziz, J. Chung, R. Detels, and J. L. Fahey, "Oral fluids as an alternative to serum for measurement of markers on immune activation," *Clinical and Diagnostic Laboratory Immunology*, vol. 5, no. 4, pp. 507–512, 1998.

[9] M. D. Mignogna, S. Fedele, L. Lo Russo, L. Lo Muzio, and E. Bucci, "Immune activation and chronic inflammation as the cause of malignancy in oral lichen planus: is there any evidence?" *Oral Oncology*, vol. 40, no. 2, pp. 120–130, 2004.

[10] T. Yamamoto, K. Yoneda, E. Ueta, and T. Osaki, "Serum cytokines, interleukin-2 receptor, and soluble intercellular adhesion molecule-1 in oral disorders," *Oral Surgery, Oral Medicine, Oral Pathology*, vol. 78, no. 6, pp. 727–735, 1994.

[11] A. Sklavounou-Andrikopoulou, E. Chrysomali, M. Iakovou, G. A. Garinis, and A. Karameris, "Elevated serum levels of the apoptosis related molecules TNF-α, Fas/Apo-1 and Bcl-2 in oral lichen planus," *Journal of Oral Pathology and Medicine*, vol. 33, no. 7, pp. 386–390, 2004.

[12] M. H. Thornhill, M. N. Pemberton, R. K. Simmons, and E. D. Theaker, "Amalgam-contact hypersensitivity lesions and oral lichen planus," *Oral Surgery, Oral Medicine, Oral Pathology, Oral Radiology, and Endodontics*, vol. 95, no. 3, pp. 291–299, 2003.

[13] S. Pezelj-Ribaric, I. B. Prso, M. Abram, I. Glazar, G. Brumini, and M. Simunovic-Soskic, "Salivary levels of tumor necrosis factor-α in oral lichen planus," *Mediators of Inflammation*, vol. 13, no. 2, pp. 131–133, 2004.

[14] N. L. Rhodus, B. Cheng, S. Myers, L. Miller, V. Ho, and F. Ondrey, "The feasibility of monitoring NF-κB associated cytokines: TNF-α, IL-1α, IL-6, and IL-8 in whole saliva for the malignant transformation of oral lichen planus," *Molecular Carcinogenesis*, vol. 44, no. 2, pp. 77–82, 2005.

[15] N. L. Rhodus, B. Cheng, W. Bowles, S. Myers, L. Miller, and F. Ondrey, "Proinflammatory cytokine levels in saliva before and after treatment of (erosive) oral lichen planus with dexamethasone," *Oral Diseases*, vol. 12, no. 2, pp. 112–116, 2006.

[16] G. R. Adolf and H. R. Lamche, "Highly sensitive enzyme immunoassay for human lymphotoxin (tumor necrosis factor β) in serum," *Journal of Immunological Methods*, vol. 130, no. 2, pp. 177–185, 1990.

[17] M. Gröschl, "Current status of salivary hormone analysis," *Clinical Chemistry*, vol. 54, no. 11, pp. 1759–1769, 2008.

[18] E. Kaufman, "The diagnostic applications of saliva—a review," *Critical Reviews in Oral Biology & Medicine*, vol. 13, no. 2, pp. 197–212, 2002.

[19] E. E. Karagouni, E. N. Dotsika, and A. Sklavounou, "Alteration in peripheral blood mononuclear cell function and serum cytokines in oral lichen planus," *Journal of Oral Pathology and Medicine*, vol. 23, no. 1, pp. 28–35, 1994.

[20] M. M. Lotempio, M. S. Veena, H. L. Steele et al., "Curcumin suppresses growth of head and neck squamous cell carcinoma," *Clinical Cancer Research*, vol. 11, no. 19, pp. 6994–7002, 2005.

[21] S. N. Meydani and W.-K. Ha, "Immunologic effects of yogurt," *The American Journal of Clinical Nutrition*, vol. 71, no. 4, pp. 861–872, 2000.

[22] A. Gavala, K. Venetsanou, C. Kittas et al., "Decreased whole blood TNFα production capacity after acute alcohol exposure and LPS stimulation ex vivo," *Critical Care*, vol. 14, supplement 1, part 13, 2010.

8

Photodynamic Antimicrobial Chemotherapy for Root Canal System Asepsis: A Narrative Literature Review

P. Diogo,[1] T. Gonçalves,[1,2] P. Palma,[1] and J. M. Santos[1]

[1]Faculty of Medicine, University of Coimbra (FMUC), Avenida Bissaya Barreto, 3000-075 Coimbra, Portugal
[2]Centre for Neuroscience and Cell Biology (CNC), University of Coimbra, Coimbra, Portugal

Correspondence should be addressed to P. Diogo; patriciadiogofmed@gmail.com

Academic Editor: Steven Jefferies

Aim. The aim of this comprehensive literature review was to address the question: Does photodynamic therapy (PDT) improve root canal disinfection through significant bacterial reduction in the root canal system? *Methodology.* A comprehensive narrative literature review was performed to compare PDT effect with sodium hypochlorite as the comparative classical irrigant. Two reviewers independently conducted literature searches using a combination of medical subject heading terms and key words to identify relevant studies comparing information found in 7 electronic databases from January 2000 to May 2015. A manual search was performed on bibliography of articles collected on electronic databases. Authors were contacted to ask for references of more research not detected on the prior electronic and manual searches. *Results.* The literature search provided 62 titles and abstracts, from which 29 studies were related directly to the search theme. Considering all publications, 14 (48%) showed PDT to be more efficient in antimicrobial outcome than NaOCl (0.5–6% concentration) used alone and 2 (7%) revealed similar effects between them. Toluidine blue and methylene blue are the most used photosensitizers and most commonly laser has 660 nm of wavelength with a 400 nm diameter of intracanal fiber. *Conclusions.* PDT has been used without a well-defined protocol and still remains at an experimental stage waiting for further optimization. The level of evidence available in clinical studies to answer this question is low and at high risk of bias.

1. Introduction

The main goal of endodontic treatment is to prevent and, when required, to cure apical periodontitis and maintain or reestablish periapical tissue health [1]. To accomplish this objective, it is mandatory to control the microbial load inside the root canal system. The chances of a favourable outcome with endodontic treatment are significantly higher if infection is eradicated effectively by chemomechanical preparation before the root canal is obturated. However, if positive cultures can be obtained from the root canal at the time of root filling, there is a higher risk of treatment failure [2]. In an attempt to improve disinfection, an inter-appointment dressing has been advocated to diminish the percentage of root canals with no cultivable microorganisms in comparison to those only treated with chemomechanical preparation. Nevertheless, the two-visit treatment protocol

did not improve the overall antimicrobial efficacy of the treatment [3]. Indeed, in all cases where viable microorganisms remain in the root canal system, the prognosis for repair is adversely affected [2, 3].

Presence of a *smear layer* after instrumentation reduces effectiveness of irrigants and temporary dressings in disinfecting dentinal tubules. Moreover, complexity of anatomy translated into root canal system with its isthmuses, ramifications, and fins [4] turns complete elimination of bacteria using instrumentation and irrigation into an almost impossible task. Besides, bacteria persisting in biofilms show diverse phenotypes when compared with planktonic cells, including increased resistance to antimicrobial agents [5]. It has been assessed that bacteria in biofilms are approximately 1000-fold less susceptible to effects of commonly used antimicrobial agents than their planktonic equivalents and are highly unaffected with phagocytosis by immune system [6]. There are several mechanisms used by bacteria which allow them to adapt to the environment [7]. Biofilm formation [8], stress response [9], physiological adaptation [7], and the beginning of subpopulations of cells are among some of the adaptive mechanisms used by bacteria along with various systems involving the exchange of genetic material [10] between bacteria. These mechanisms can support bacterial survival under the limiting environments, such as that found in the root canal. One of the most relevant features of adaptation for oral bacteria is the adhesion to surfaces leading to the formation of plaque biofilms, which not only serves to aid in their retention but also results in increased survival rate [11]. Biofilms form when planktonic bacteria in a natural liquid phase are deposited on a surface containing an organic conditioning polymeric matrix or conditioning film [7]. In this dynamic process, several organisms coadhere to the surface [12] and grow with certain cells detaching from the biofilm over time. Biofilm formation in root canals, as postulated by Svensater and Bergenholtz [13], is probably initiated at the moment of the first invasion of the pulp chamber by planktonic oral organisms after some tissue breakdown.

Biofilm disruption and disinfection of root canals are the most critical steps during treatment of an infected root canal system, which are essential to avoid persistence of microbial infection and achieve endodontic success [14]. The mode of action and efficacy of a wide variety of cleaning, antimicrobial, and disinfecting agents such as NaOCl, chlorhexidine, ethylenediamine tetraacetic acid (EDTA), citric acid, hydrogen peroxide, halogens, and ozone have been investigated [15–18]. Disinfecting agents and antimicrobial medicinal products routinely used in endodontics can be inactivated by dentin, tissue fluids, and organic matter [6, 19]. Moreover, some microbial species, such as *Enterococcus faecalis* [20, 21] and *Candida albicans* [22, 23], show resistance to those agents and their efficacy is dependent on the concentration achieved and time of contact [24]. Most of these disinfectants with effective bactericidal activity are used at subtoxic level, but also at concentrations where toxicity is becoming a significant factor. Searching for new methods to provide extra disinfection for root canal system without cytotoxic effects and to improve treatment outcome, innovative techniques including various laser wavelengths [25], hydraulic [26], sonic, and ultrasonic irrigation [27–29], nanoparticles [30], inactivation of efflux pumps [31], and photodynamic therapy (PDT) has been proposed in literature.

PDT was discovered by chance at the very beginning of the twentieth century, when a combination of nontoxic dyes exposed to visible light resulted in microorganism cell death. As reviewed by Henderson and Dougherty in 1992 [32], Oscar Raab, a medical student working with Professor Herman Von Tappeiner in Munich, introduced the concept of microbial cell death induced by interaction of light and chemicals [32]. During the course of Raab's study, he demonstrated that the combination of light and dyes was much more effective in killing the microorganism *Paramecium*.

Those observations were repeated with a diversity of uni- and multicellular organisms. Succeeding work in this laboratory coined the term *photodynamic action* and demonstrated

presence of oxygen as an essential requisite for photosensitization to occur. Years later, Dougherty and coworkers clinically tested PDT in cutaneous/subcutaneous malignant tumours. However, it was John Toth who renamed this therapy as PDT. Combined effect of three elements, *light*, *PS*, and *oxygen*, has been termed *photodynamic antimicrobial chemotherapy* by Wainwright [33] and also recognized as *antimicrobial photodynamic therapy* [34] and *photoactivated disinfection* [35].

PDT uses a nontoxic dye, known as photosensitizer (PS), on a target tissue, which is consequently irradiated with a suitable visible light of the appropriate wavelength to excite the PS molecule to the singlet state in presence of oxygen to produce reactive oxygen species (ROS) [36]. When PS absorbs light, this excited state may then undergo intersystem crossing to the slightly lower energy, but the longer lived, triple state can undergo two kinds of pathways known as Type I (reacting with the substrate) and Type II (reacting with molecular oxygen) photoprocesses. Both pathways require oxygen.

The *type 1 radical and reactive oxygen species* pathway comprises an *electron transfer step* between the triplet PS and a substrate with generation of radical species. The finalist is then intercepted by ground state molecular oxygen yielding a variety of oxidized products. The baseline PS has two electrons in opposite spins (singlet state) in the low energy molecular orbital. Subsequent to the absorption of light, one of these electrons is boosted into a high-energy orbital but keeps its spin (first excited singlet state). This is a short-lived time species, nanoseconds, and can lose its energy by emitting light (fluorescence) or by internal conversion into heat. Type 1 pathway frequently involves initial production of superoxide anion by electron transfer from the triplet PS to molecular oxygen (monovalent reduction) initiating radical-induced damage in biomolecules. Superoxide is not particularly reactive in biological systems and does not by itself cause much oxidative damage but can react with itself to produce hydrogen peroxide and oxygen, a reaction known as *dismutation* that can be catalyzed by the enzyme superoxide dismutase (SOD). The way of the electron relocation between the PS and the substrate is controlled by the relative redox potentials of the two species.

Type 2 pathway, singlet oxygen, involves an electronic *energy transfer process* from the triplet PS to a receptor, most frequently oxygen, which is a triplet in its ground state. The final compound is converted to a highly reactive species, the singlet oxygen ($^1O_2$). The excited singlet state PS may also undergo the process known as *intersystem crossing* whereby the spin of the excited electron inverts to form the relatively long-lived, in terms of microseconds, excited triplet state that has parallel electron spins. The long lifetime of the PS triplet state is explained by the fact that the loss of energy by emission of light (phosphorescence) is a *spin forbidden* process, as the PS would move directly from a triplet to a singlet state. Photosensitized processes of types 1 and 2 depend on the initial involvement of radical intermediates that are subsequently scavenged by oxygen or the generation of the highly cytotoxic singlet oxygen ($^1O_2$) by energy transfer from the photoexcited sensitizer. It is difficult to determine without doubt which of these two mechanisms is more prevalent; both types of reactions can happen simultaneously and the ratio between them depends on three singular features: oxygen, substrate concentration, and PS type [37].

Hamblin and Hasan in 2004 [36] stated that antimicrobial PS can be divided into three categories: (I) those that strongly bind and penetrate the microorganisms (chlorin e6), (II) those that bind weakly as toluidine blue (TB) and methylene blue (MB), and (III) those that do not demonstrate binding at all such as rose bengal (RB). Understanding these mechanisms of action is essential because, in bacterial cells, outer membrane damage plays an imperative role, differently from mammalian cells, where the main targets for PDT are lysosomes, mitochondria, and plasma membranes [38]. Typically, neutral anionic or cationic PS molecules could powerfully destroy Gram-positive bacteria, whereas only cationic PS or strategies which attack the Gram-negative permeability barrier in combination with noncationic PS are able to kill multiple logs of Gram-negative species [39]. This difference in susceptibility between species in the two bacterial types is explained by their cell wall physiology. To understand better the PDT effect in those microorganisms, it is very important to analyse in detail the microbial cell walls. In *Gram-positive bacteria*, the cytoplasmic membrane is surround by a relatively porous peptidoglycan layer and lipoteichoic acid that allows the PS to cross. Different from this, the *Gram-negative bacteria* cell envelope consists of an inner and an outer membrane which are separated by a peptidoglycan layer. The outer membrane forms an effective permeability barrier between the cell and the environment and tends to restrict the binding and penetration of several PS. Fungi are provided with a thick cell wall that includes beta glucan and chitin offering a permeability barrier. In terms of PDT efficacy, in fungal wall, it was described as having an intermediate behavior between Gram-positive and Gram-negative bacteria [40]. On the basis of these considerations, it appears that Gram-negative bacteria represent the most challenging targets for any form of antimicrobial treatment. The mechanism of action of basic polymer PS conjugates is thought to be that of *self-promoted uptake pathway* [41]. In this method, cationic molecules first dislocate the divalent cations, such as calcium (Ca^{2+}) and magnesium (Mg^{2+}), from their position on the outer membrane where they act as an anchor for the negatively charged lipopolysaccharides molecules [40, 41]. The debilitated outer membrane becomes slightly more permeable and allows even more of the cationic PS to gain access thus steadily increasing the disorganizations of the permeability barrier increasing PS uptake with each additional binding. It is thought that host cells only gradually take up cationic molecules by the process of endocytosis, while their uptake into bacteria is relatively fast [39]. Further important observation that has been made about these cationic antimicrobial PS concerns their selectivity for microbial cells compared to host mammalian cells [37]. These findings are relevant, because photoaction occurs in direct contact with membranes [42]. The PS efficiency in generating ROS within membranes is dependent on the intrinsic characteristics of the PS in aqueous solution as well as their partition in the membrane [42]. The early attack of singlet oxygen in membranes lipids is by the specific reaction with double bonds to form allylic hydroperoxides; the efficiency of this reaction is dependent on the lowest ionization potential of the olefins and also on the availability of allylic hydrogens [42]. *Photodynamic lipid peroxidation* is an oxidative degradation of cell membrane lipids, also known as *photoperoxidation*, and it has been related to several microbial cytotoxic effects, such as increased ion permeability, fluidity loss, inactivation of membrane proteins, and cross-linking, which disrupts the intracellular homeostasis. Consequently, necrosis is induced as a cell death process. A probable explanation is that PS bound to the membrane and generates most of the singlet oxygen, $^1O_2$, involved in photoperoxidation [43] highlighting the double selectivity (light and PS cellular localization) and the fact that it works in multiresistant strains and does not encourage resistance [42]. PDT's lethal action is based on photochemical production of ROS and not thermal and cavitation effects, as is the case with high power laser therapy [44]. One of several PDT's advantages clinically is the absence of thermal side effects in periradicular tissues [45] and this property of PDT aspect makes it highly effective in eradicating microorganisms such as bacteria [45], viruses [46], and fungi [47] without causing damage of adjacent tissues due to overheating [45].

In recent years, PDT has been applied in several areas, particularly in periodontology [48–50], in general dentistry [51] and also in endodontic field as an adjunct of classical irrigation solutions in root canal disinfection [52, 53]. These studies suggest PDT's potential as a therapeutic weapon, which aims to support endodontic antimicrobial treatment, especially enhancing irrigation solutions effect. The purpose of this narrative comprehensive literature review is to answer the focused question, "*Is antimicrobial PDT efficacy better than that of sodium hypochlorite's in root canal treatment?*" For this analysis of the literature, we selected and analysed 29 studies using antimicrobial PDT in endodontic field, highlighting methodologies used and their reported effectiveness and efficacy.

2. Materials and Methods

2.1. Criteria in Selection of Studies. For this comprehensive narrative literature review [54], eligibility criteria were (I) articles published in English language; (II) original papers; (III) experimental studies (*in vitro* and *ex vivo*); (IV) clinical studies (*in vivo*); and finally (V) scientific reports of PDT efficacy in root canal disinfection/asepsis. The exclusion criteria were (I) unpublished data, (II) conference papers, (III) historic reviews, (IV) letters to editor, and (V) papers due to PDT outcomes in other fields (outside of endodontics).

As a first step, the aim was to investigate the terms "Endodontic", "Photodynamic Therapy", and "Antimicrobial Disinfection". Briefly, we used PubMed to identify Medical Subject Headings (MeSH) terms corresponding to each term. Nevertheless, MeSH terms use is not common to all articles, making this search method infeasible. Then, exhaustive automated searches of Cochrane Collaboration, Evidence Based Dentistry (EBD), Journal of Evidence-Based Dental Practice (JEBDP), NHS Evidence, and PubMed (Figure 1) were performed from January 2000 up to and including May 2015

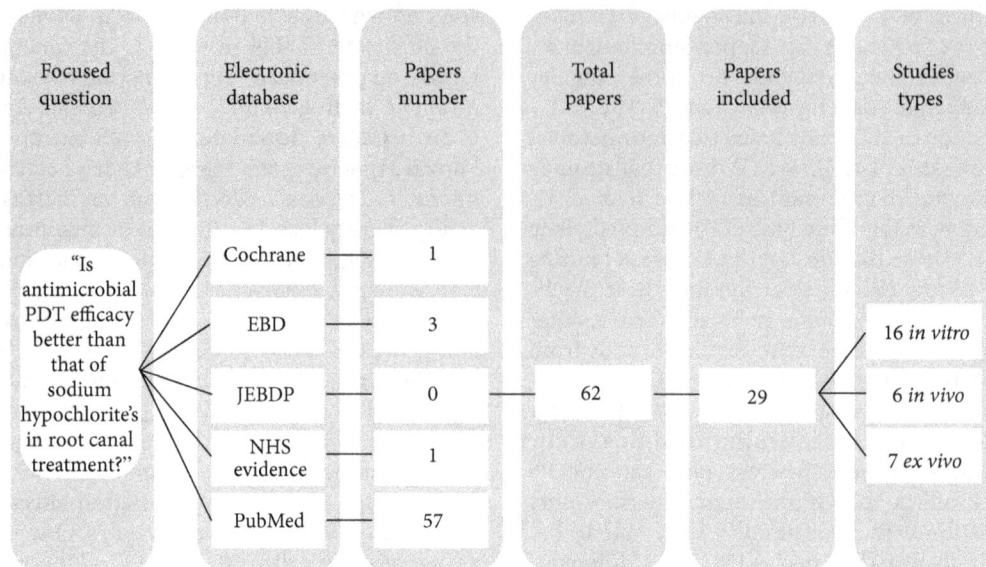

FIGURE 1: Identification of studies used in this narrative review.

using various combinations of the following key indexing terms: (a) *endodontic photodynamic therapy*; (b) *antimicrobial photodynamic therapy*; (c) *photo-activated disinfection*; (d) *light-activated disinfection*; (e) *laser-assisted photosensitization*; (f) *root canal disinfection*; and (g) *endodontic lasers*.

Titles and abstracts of all articles resulting from electronic search were screened independently and in duplicate by 2 reviewers. The review itself was performed to reject articles that did not meet inclusion criteria. Any disagreement between reviewers was solved via debate, although in specific cases of disagreement that were not resolved with discussion, opinion of a senior commentator was required. Hand searching of reference lists of original and reviewed articles that were found to be relevant was also performed.

In a second step, full-text copies of all remaining articles were obtained and further meticulous assessment was performed independently by each reviewer to determine whether or not they were eligible for this study based on the specific inclusion and exclusion criteria cited above and proven for agreement.

Quality evaluation of randomized clinical trials and observational studies was performed using STROBE [55] (strengthening the reporting of observational studies in epidemiology) and CONSORT [56] (consolidated standards of reporting trials) statement criteria, respectively.

3. Results

3.1. PDT Antimicrobial Efficacy in Included Studies. Literature search provided 62 titles and abstracts; from those, 29 studies concerned this theme: 16 were performed in *in vitro* conditions, 6 were *in vivo* studies, and the last 7 readings were *ex vivo*. From all 29 papers included in this review, 16 (55.2%) were *in vitro* studies (Table 1).

In data processing, authors classified all studies in three categories: *category I, in vitro*; *category II, in vivo*; and finally, *category III, ex vivo*, to describe and clarify studies' details. In category I, 16 *in vitro* studies, only 5 (31%) [57–61] reveal best antimicrobial PDT outcomes when compared with sodium hypochlorite (NaOCl) in range of 0.5 to 6%. Only one study performed by Nagayoshi et al. [62] reveals equal results between PDT and NaOCl; the remaining 10 (62.5%) studies [63–72] showed PDT outcomes unhelpful when compared with NaOCl as a classical irrigant solution, in concentration range of 0.5 to 6%. In category II, 6 (21%) papers [35, 58, 73–76] were analysed (Table 2).

All were performed in the human dentition, five [35, 58, 73, 74, 76] were performed in permanent dentition, and only one was achieved in deciduous teeth by Prabhakar et al. [75]. All studies in category II (100%) presented that PDT efficacy overthrew (0.5–2.5%) NaOCl. Considering tooth type and its influence in PDT efficacy outcomes, Garcez et al. group [58, 74] and Jurič et al. [76] tested only permanent uniradicular human teeth (incisors and canines) as samples. However, Prabhakar et al. [75] considered deciduous molars as a prerequisite for his study. Finally, Bonsor et al. [35, 73] used not only uniradicular but also permanent multiradicular teeth. In terms of endodontic diagnosis, Garcez et al. [58] in his first study used patients with necrotic pulps and periapical lesion; then, in 2010, his group [74] performed a second study to assess PDT efficacy in teeth with previous endodontic treatment, endodontic retreatment. Jurič et al. [76] in 2014 evaluated PDT antimicrobial outcomes efficacy applied also in endodontic retreatment. Both studies [74, 76] revealed PDT outcomes near 100% effective.

In category III (*ex vivo*), 7 (24%) papers [5, 77–82] were analysed (Table 3).

Based on this, 3 (43%) studies [5, 78, 79] revealed superior PDT outcomes compared to 0.5–6% of NaOCl and in one study by Xhevdet et al. group [81] showed 2.5% NaOCl

TABLE 1: *In vitro* studies compilation.

Study type	Groups	% NaOCl	Substracte	Photosensitizer	Laser	Parameters evaluated	Conclusion
			In vitro, 16 studies				
Seal et al. 2002 [63]	*Test groups:* Group #1: PDT with 20 combinations of 4 TBO concentrations and 5 laser energy doses ($n = 4$). TBO (12.5, 25, 50, and 100 mg mL^{-1}) incubated for 30 s. Laser (60, 90, 120, 300, and 600 s). Energy dose (2.1, 3.2, 4.2, 10.5, and 21 J). *Control group:* Group #2: NaOCl ($n = 4$). Light source: Canals ($n = 4$) were filled with reduced transport fluid (RTF) for 30 s followed by application of various laser light doses (60, 90, 120, 300, or 600 s). TBO only: Canals ($n = 4$) were filled with TBO at various concentrations (12.5, 25, 50, or 100 mg mL^{-1}) and incubated for 30 s. No treatment: Canals ($n = 17$) were filled with RTF and incubated for 30 s.	3	*S. intermedius* (strain NS)	TBO [12.5, 25, 50, 100 μg mL^{-1}] Preincubation time (PIT): 30 s	Helium-neon [λ632.8 nm] Irradiation time (IT): 60 s, 90 s, 120 s, 300 s, and 600 s	Cell viability Colony-forming-unit – CFU (log$_{10}$)	PDT is bactericidal to *S. intermedius* biofilms in root canals but is not as effective as irrigation with 3% NaOCl.
	Sample: 35 root canals from human uniradicular teeth						
Silva Garcez et al. 2006 [57]	*Test groups:* Group #1: L$^-$ AZ$^-$ Group #2: L$^+$ AZ$^-$ Group #3: L$^-$ AZ$^+$ Group #4: L$^+$ AZ$^+$ Group #5: NaOCl *Control group:* Canals filled with BHI broth and incubated for 24 h.	0.5	*Enterococcus faecalis* (ATCC1494)	AZ paste [0.01%] PIT: 300 s Paste composition: urea peroxide 10%, detergent 15% (Tween 80) and vehicle 75% (carbowax).	GaAlAs diode [λ685 nm] IT: 180 s	Cell viability CFU (log$_{10}$)	In root canals, PDT showed 99.2% *E. faecalis* reduction, whereas 0.5% NaOCl achieved 93.25%.
	Sample: 30 root canals from human uniradicular teeth (upper central incisors and upper canines)						
Garcez et al. 2007 [34]	*Test groups:* Group #1: PDT Group #2: RCT (root canal treatment) with NaOCl Group #3: Combined treatment (PDT + ET with NaOCl) *Control group:* Teeth with 3-day biofilms + BHI for 24 h	2.5	*Proteus mirabilis* (XEN44) *Pseudomonas aeruginosa* (XEN5)	PEI/e6 [NS] PIT: 600 s	MMOptics [λ660 nm] IT: NS	Bioluminescence imaging Cell viability CFU (log$_{10}$)	NaOCl reduced bacteria by 90% while PDT alone reduced bioluminescence by 95%.
	Sample: 10 root canals from uniradicular human teeth (upper central incisors and upper canines)						

TABLE 1: Continued.

Study type	Groups	% NaOCl	Substracte	Photosensitizer	Laser	Parameters evaluated	Conclusion
George and Kishen 2008 [59, 103] In vitro Ex vivo	Test groups: Group #1: RCT with NaOCl; Group #2: PDT; Group #3: RCT + PDT in an emulsion of H_2O_2:triton-XI00 in the ratio 75:24.5:0.5; Group #4: RCT + an emulsion of H_2O_2:triton-XI00 in the ratio 75:24.5:0.5; Control group: Root canal not subject to any treatment	IV:1 EV: 5.2	E. faecalis (strain NS)	MB [1, 5, 10, 15, 20, 25 µM] PIT: 600 s (in the dark) Dark toxicity was evaluated; Perfluorodecahydronaphthalene (oxygen carrier); H_2O_2 (oxider); Triton-XI00 (nonionic detergent)	Power Technology Inc. [λ664 nm] IT: NS	CSLM; Photooxidation activity; Singlet oxygen generation; Cell viability; CFU ($\log_{10}$)	NaOCl showed no viable bacteria after 4 h, but 60% of the root canal shavings confirmed bacterial growth after 24 h. PDT alone or + NaOCl showed the absence of bacteria even after 24 h.

Sample: in vitro: E. faecalis biofilms grown on a glass coverslip that was fixed covering a grove (6 mm diameter) made at the bottom part of a Petri dish; Ex vivo (16–24 years): 30 root canals from human uniradicular teeth (anterior teeth)

Study type	Groups	% NaOCl	Substracte	Photosensitizer	Laser	Parameters evaluated	Conclusion
Meire et al. 2009 [64] In vitro Ex vivo	Test groups: Group #1: Nd:YAG laser (n = 10); Group #2: KTP laser (n = 10); Group #3: PDT (n = 10); Group #4: NaOCl (n = 10); Control group: Group #5: teeth with no treatment (n = 20) – positive control; Group #6: uninoculated teeth (n = 3) – negative control	2.5	E. faecalis (ATCC10541)	TBO [12.7 mg mL^{-1}] PIT: 120 s	Denfotex [λ635 nm] IT: 150 s	Cell viability; CFU ($\log_{10}$); Solid phase cytometry; Epifluorescence microscopy	PDT was less effective than NaOCl (15 min) in reducing E. faecalis, both in aqueous suspension and in the infected tooth model.

Sample: 60 uniradicular human teeth

Study type	Groups	% NaOCl	Substracte	Photosensitizer	Laser	Parameters evaluated	Conclusion
Souza et al.2010 [65]	Test groups: Group #1: PDT with MB + NaOCl (n = 16); Group #2: PDT with TBO + NaOCl (n = 16); Group #3: PDT with MB + NaCl (n = 16); Group #4: PDT with TBO + NaCl (n = 16); Control groups: Ø	2.5	E. faecalis (MB35)	MB/TBO [15/15 µg mL^{-1}] PIT: 120 s	MMOptics [λ660 nm] IT: 240 s	SEM; Cell viability; CFU ($\log_{10}$)	PDT did not significantly enhance disinfection after chemomechanical preparation using NaOCl as irrigant.

Sample: 70 uniradicular human teeth

Study type	Groups	% NaOCl	Substracte	Photosensitizer	Laser	Parameters evaluated	Conclusion
Nagayoshi et al. 2011 [62]	Test groups: Group #1: 5 W, 30 s, PS (+); Group #2: 5 W, 60 s, PS (+); Group #3: 5 W, 120 s, PS (+); Group #4: 5 W, 120 s, PS (−); Control groups: Group #5: NaCL: negative control; Group #6: NaOCl: positive control	2.5	E. faecalis (ATCC29212)	Indocyanine green [12. mg mL^{-1}] PIT: 60 s	P-Laser [λ805 nm] IT: 30, 60, 120 s	Cell viability; CFU ($\log_{10}$); Temperature	PDT had nearly the same antimicrobial effect as 2.5% NaOCl.

Sample: in vitro model of apical periodontitis in resin blocks

TABLE 1: Continued.

Study type	Groups	% NaOCl	Substracte	Photosensitizer	Laser	Parameters evaluated	Conclusion
Nunes et al. 2011 [66]	Test groups: Group #1: OF/IT90 (n = 10) Group #2: OF/IT180 (n = 10) Group #3: NOF/IT90 (n = 10) Group #4: NOF/IT180 (n = 10) Control groups: Group #5: untreated (n = 10) Group #6: NaOCl: positive control (n = 10)	1	E. faecalis (ATCC29212)	MB [100 $\mu g\,mL^{-1}$] PIT: 300 s	Thera Lase [λ660 nm] IT: 90, 180 s	Cell viability CFU ($\log_{10}$)	The highest percentage of E. faecalis reduction was achieved with NaOCl. The use of intracanal fiber during PDT does not reveal improvement.
						Sample: 60 uniradicular human teeth	
Poggio et al. 2011 [67]	Test groups: Group #1: PDT (n = 10) Group #2: PDT + NaOCl (n = 10) Group #3: TBO (n = 10) Group #4: PDT (n = 10) – more time than in group 1 Control groups: Group #5: NaOCl: positive control (n = 10)	0.5 5	Streptococcus mutans (CCUG35176) E. faecalis (ATCC19433) Streptococcus sanguis (CCUG7826)	TBO [100 $\mu g\,mL^{-1}$] PIT: 60 s	FotoSan [λ628 nm] IT: 30, 60 s	Cell viability	In vitro antimicrobial efficacy of 5% NaOCl is higher than PDT.
						Sample: 100 root canals from human uniradicular teeth	
Rios et al. 2011 [68]	Test groups: Group #1: NaOCl Group #2: TBO Group #3: Light Group #4: PDT Group #5: PDT + NaOCl Control groups: The experimental conditions were repeated seven independent times with 15 total experimental samples. Both negative (no growth) and positive (growth without any treatment) controls were done for each independent experiment.	6	E. faecalis (OG1X) A derivative of an oral isolate that has been shown to be cariogenic	TBO [NS] PIT: 30 s	FotoSan [λ628 nm] IT: 30 s	SEM Cell viability CFU ($\log_{10}$)	The bacterial survival rate of the NaOCl/PDT group (0.1%) was significantly lower than the NaOCl (0.66%) and PDT groups (2.9%).
						Sample: uniradicular human teeth (total number of teeth unknown)	
Cheng et al. 2012 [69]	Test groups: Group #1: Nd:YAG Group #2: Er:YAG/NaOCl/NS/DW Group #3: Er:YAG/NS/DW Group #4: Er,Cr:YSGG Group #5: PDT Control groups: Group #6: NaOCl: positive control Group #7: normal saline: negative control	5.25	E. faecalis (ATCC4083)	MB [50 $\mu g\,mL^{-1}$] PIT: 60 s	Nd:YAG [λ1064 nm] IT: 16 s Er:YAG [λ2940 nm] IT: 20 s Er,Cr:YSGG [λ2780 nm] IT: 4 s Lit-601 [λ660 nm] IT: 60 s	SEM Cell viability CFU ($\log_{10}$)	PDT was less effective than NaOCl at surface of the root and 100, 200, and 300 μm inside the dentinal tubule.
						Sample: 220 uniradicular human teeth	

TABLE 1: Continued.

Study type	Groups	% NaOCl	Photosensitizer	Substracte	Laser	Parameters evaluated	Conclusion
Vaziiri et al. 2012 [70]	*Test groups:* Group #1: NaOCl ($n=15$); Group #2: Laser + NaOCl ($n=15$); Group #3: PDT ($n=15$); Group #4: PDT + NaOCl ($n=15$); Group #5: chlorhexidine ($n=15$); *Control groups:* Group #6: no treatment: positive control; Group #7: without inoculation of bacterium: negative control	2.5	TBO [15 μg mL^{-1}] PIT: 300 s	*E. faecalis* (ATCC29212)	FotoSan [λ625 nm] IT: 60 s	Cell viability CFU (log$_{10}$)	NaOCl showed better results than PDT. However, PDT + NaOCl showed the best result.

Sample: 90 root canals from 90 uniradicular human teeth

Pileggi et al. 2013 [60]	*Test groups:* Group #1: PDT (Eosin-Y) with Light+ and L−; Group #2: PDT (Rose bengal) with Light+ and L−; Group #3: PDT (Curcumin) with Light+ and L−; *Control groups:* Group #4: NaOCl positive control	3	Eosyn-Y/RB/curcumin [50 μg mL^{-1}] PIT: 1800 s	*E. faecalis* (135737)	Optilux 501 [λ380–500 nm] IT: 240 s	Cell viability CFU (log$_{10}$)	In BS, PDT significantly reduced *E. faecalis* viability. For biofilm, PDT completely suppressed *E. faecalis*.

Sample: *E. faecalis* 135737 culture collection of the University Hospitals of Geneva; CH was used for the inactivation assays because of its prominent role in endodontic infections

Bumb et al. 2014 [61]	*Test groups:* Group #1: PDT (MB) with Light+; *Control groups:* Group #2: no treatment ($n=10$); Positive control	3	MB [25 mg mL^{-1}] PIT: 600 s	*E. faecalis* (ATCC29212)	Diode laser [λ910 nm] IT: NS	SEM Cell viability CFU (log$_{10}$)	Bacterial reduction in PDT group was 96.70%. PDT potential to be used as an adjunctive antimicrobial procedure.

Sample: 20 uniradicular human teeth

TABLE 1: Continued.

Study type	Groups	% NaOCl	Substracte	Photosensitizer	Laser	Parameters evaluated	Conclusion
Gergova et al. 2015 [71]	Test groups:Group #1: lasers (n = 40) #1.1: Nd:YAG (n = 20) #1.2: diode (n = 20) Group #2: PDT (n = 60) #2.1: FotoSan (n = 20) #2.2: without laser – dark control (n = 20) #2.3: without PS – light control (n = 20) Group #3: iontophoresis (n = 120) #3.1: Cupral (n = 40) #3.2: Ca(OH)$_2$ (n = 40) #3.3: I$_2$/KI$_2$ (n = 40) Group #4 (n = 60) #4.1: 2% Chx (n = 20) #4.2: 2.5% NaOCl (n = 20) #4.3: 30% H$_2$O$_2$ (n = 20) Control groups: Group #5: PBS (n = 20) Positive control	2.5	Two control strains from the American Type Culture Collection (ATCC): Methicillin sensitive Staphylococcus aureus (ATCC29213) E. faecalis (ATCC29212) Clinical isolates served as multidrug-resistant: S. pyogenes S. intermedius E. coli K. pneumonia E. cloacae S. marcescens M. morganii P. aeruginosa A. baumannii C. albicans	TBO [15 μg mL^{-1}] PIT: NS	FotoSan [λ625 nm] IT: 300 s	SEM Cell viability CFU (log$_{10}$) X-ray laser particle sizer	2.5% NaOCl is the most satisfactory result; however, PDT with FotoSan, H$_2$O$_2$, and all tested types of iontophoresis all showed strong disinfection potential without statistical significance.
	Sample: 300 uniradicular human teeth						
Wang et al. 2015 [72]	Test groups:Group #1: PDT (n = 10) Group #2: ultrasonic irrigation + NaOCl #2.1: US + 0.5% NaOCl (n = 10) #2.2: US + 1% NaOCl (n = 10) #2.3: US + 2% NaOCl (n = 10) #2.4: US + 2.5% NaOCl (n = 10) #2.5: US + 5.25% NaOCl (n = 10) Group #3: ultrasonic irrigation + PDT + NaOCl #3.1: US + PDT + 0.5% NaOCl (n = 10) #3.2: US + PDT + 1% NaOCl (n = 10) #3.3: US + PDT + 2% NaOCl (n = 10) #3.4: US + PDT + 2.5% NaOCl (n = 10) #3.5: US + PDT + 5.25% NaOCl (n = 10) Control groups: Group #4: ultrasonic irrigation with 0.9% NaCl (n = 10) Negative control	0.5 1 2 2.5 5.25	E. faecalis (ATCC33186)	MB [100 μM] PIT: 600 s	Diode laser [λ670 nm] IT: 300 s	SEM Cell viability CFU (log$_{10}$)	PDT alone is less efficient than even the 0.5% NaOCl ultrasonic irrigation under the condition of this experiment.
	Sample: 120 intact bovine incisors						

TABLE 2: *In vivo* studies collection.

Study type	Groups	% NaOCl	Substracte	Photosensitizer	Laser	Parameters evaluated	Conclusion
			In vivo, 6 studies				
Bonsor et al. 2006 [35, 73]. Private general dental practice in Scotland by the same operator, UK.	Group #1 (73% molars): Three samples (n = 32): (1.1) After gaining access to the root canal. (1.2) After apex location and PDT process carried out. (1.3) After completion of the canal preparation using citric acid and NaOCl. Group #2 (76% molars): Three samples (n = 32): (2.1) After gaining access to the root canal. (2.2) After conventional preparation using 20% citric acid and NaOCl. (2.3) After a subsequent PDT. *Control groups:* Ø Random allocation? Yes Sample (16–70 years): 64 root canals with closed apices randomly selected from uni- and multiradicular teeth of 14 healthier patients presented with symptoms of irreversible pulpitis or periradicular periodontitis	2.25	Human dentine of the canal's walls. No attempt was made to identify the specific bacterial flora during the culturing process.	TBO [12.7 mg L^{-1}] PIT: 60 s	SaveDent Diode laser [λ633 ± 2 nm] IT: 120 s	Scores for levels of infection	PDT showed best results (93%) when compared to conventional irrigants solutions like NaOCl and acid citric (76%).
Bonsor et al. 2006 [35, 73]. Private general dental practice in Scotland by the same operator, UK.	Group #1: Three samples (n = 30) (1.1) After gaining access to the root canal. (1.2) After conventional endodontic therapy with NaOCl. (1.3) After PDT. *Control groups:* Ø Random allocation? Yes Sample (16–70 years): 64 root canals with closed apices randomly selected from uni- and multiradicular teeth of 14 healthier patients presented with symptoms of irreversible pulpitis or periradicular periodontitis	2.25	Human dentine of the canal's walls. No attempt was made to identify the specific bacterial flora during the culturing process.	TBO [NS] PIT: 60 s	SaveDent Diode laser [λ633 ± 2 nm] IT: 60, 120 s	Scores for levels of infection	PDT showed best results when compared to conventional irrigant solutions.
Garcez et al. 2008 [58]. Private dental practice in São Paulo by the same operator, Brazil.	Group #1: Three samples (n = 30) (1.1) After gaining access to the root canal. (1.2) After conventional endodontic therapy with NaOCl. (1.3) After PDT. Group #2: Two samples after 1 week with Ca(OH)$_2$. (2.1) After 2nd conventional endodontic therapy with NaOCl. (2.2) After 2nd PDT. *Control groups:* Ø Random allocation? Yes Sample (21–35 years): 20 selected cases of patients presenting with symptoms of irreversible pulpitis or periradicular periodontitis in anterior teeth (incisors and canines) selected at random	2.5	Human dentine of the canal's walls. No attempt was made to identify the specific bacterial flora during the culturing process.	PEI/e6 [60 μmol L^{-1}] PIT: 120 s	MMOptics Diode laser [λ660 nm] IT: 240 s	Cell viability CFU (log$_{10}$)	The use of PDT leads to a significant further reduction of bacterial load, and a second appointment PDT is even more effective than the first.

TABLE 2: Continued.

Study type	Groups	% NaOCl	Substracte	Photosensitizer	Laser	Parameters evaluated	Conclusion
Garcez et al. 2010 [74]. Private dental practice in São Paulo by the same operator, Brazil.	Group #1: Three samples (n = 30) (1.1) After gaining access to the root canal. (1.2) After conventional endodontic therapy with NaOCl. (1.3) After PDT. *Control groups:* Ø Random allocation? No	2.5	Biofilms At least 1 microorganism resistant to antibiotic medication.	PEI/e6 [≈19 μg mL^{-1}] PIT: 120 s	MMOptics Diode laser [λ660 nm] IT: 240 s	Microbiological identification Antibiogram analyses Cell viability CFU (log$_{10}$)	NaOCl reduced to 0.8 species per root canal. After PDT, microorganism growth was not detected on any of the samples.
	Sample (17–52 years): 30 anterior uniradicular human teeth with previous endodontic treatment from 21 patients without random allocation						
Prabhakar et al. 2013 [75]. Department of Pedodontics and Preventive Dentistry, Bapuji Dental College and Hospital, Davangere, Karnataka, India.	Group #1: Three samples (n = 12) (1.1) After gaining access to the root canal. (1.2) After conventional endodontic therapy with NaOCl. (1.3) After PDT. *Control groups:* Ø Random allocation? No	0.5	Culture samples	MB [50 μg mL^{-1}] PIT: 300 s	Silberbauer low level laser Diode laser [λ660 nm] IT: NS	Cell viability CFU (log$_{10}$)	PDT showed best results than NaOCl.
	Sample (4–7 years): 12 human deciduous molars with caries lesions affecting the pulp and diagnosed as necrotic pulps (pulpectomies) from twelve children without random allocation						
Jurič et al. 2014 [76]	Group #1: Three samples (n = 21) (1.1) After gaining access to the root canal (initial) (1.2) After chemomechanical preparation (1.3) After chemomechanical preparation + PDT. *Control groups:* Ø Random allocation? Yes	2.5	Biofilms	Helbo blue PS [10 mg mL^{-1}] PIT: 120 s Phenothiazinium chloride	Helbo system Diode laser [λ660 nm] IT: 60 s	Microbiological identification Cell viability CFU (log$_{10}$)	Although endodontic re-treatment (ERT) alone produced a significant reduction in the number of bacteria species, the combination of ERT + PDT was statistically more effective.
	Sample (20–45 years): 21 anterior uniradicular human teeth (incisors or canines) with previous endodontic treatment from 21 patients with random allocation						

TABLE 3: *Ex vivo* studies compilation.

Study type	Groups	% NaOCl	Substracte	Photosensitizer	Laser	Parameters evaluated	Conclusion
			Ex vivo, 7 studies				
Lim et al. 2009 [77]	*Experiment #1* *Test groups:*Group #1: laser ($n = 10$) Group #2: PDT + PS in water ($n = 10$) Group #3: NaOCl ($n = 10$) Group #4: PDT + PS in Mix ($n = 10$) *Control groups:*Group #5: no treatment ($n = 15$): positive control *Experiment #2* *Test groups:* Group #1: PDT + PS in water ($n = 6$) Group #2: PDT + PS in Mix ($n = 6$) Group #3: cleaning and shaping ($n = 6$) Group #4: PDT + PS in Mix + cleaning and shaping ($n = 6$) *Control groups:* Group #5: no treatment ($n = 6$): positive control	5.25	*E. faecalis* (ATCC29212)	MB [$100 \ \mu$M] PIT: NS Dissolved in water and MIX	Model PPM35 [$\lambda 660$ nm] IT: 1200 s	Cell viability CFU ($\log_{10}$)	NaOCl showed best results that conventional PDT.
			Sample: 85 freshly extracted uniradicular human teeth				
Ng et al. 2011 [78]	*Test groups:*Group #1: chemomechanical debridement with NaOCl ($n = 26$) Group #2: PDT + chemomechanical debridement with NaOCl ($n = 26$) *Control groups:* ∅	6	Human intracanal dentinal shavings	MB [$50 \ \mu$g mL^{-1}] PIT: 300 s	BWTEK Inc. [$\lambda 665$ nm] IT: 150 s–break 150 s–150 s	DNA probes Cell viability CFU ($\log_{10}$)	PDT + NaOCl showed better results when compared to NaOCl alone.
			Sample: 52 freshly extracted human teeth with pulpal necrosis (9 incisors, 5 canines, 12 premolars, and 26 molars)				

TABLE 3: Continued.

Study type	Groups	% NaOCl	Substracte	Photosensitizer	Laser	Parameters evaluated	Conclusion
Stojicic et al. 2013 [5]	Test groups:Group #1: 0.1% EDTA + 0.1% H₂O₂ (1 min) Group #2: 0.1% EDTA + 0.1% Chx (1 min) Group #3: MB 15 (PIT = 5 min) 1 min LASER Group #4: MB 100 (no PIT) 1 min LASER Group #5: MB 100 (PIT = 5 min) 1 min LASER Group #6: MB 100 (PIT = 5 min) + 0.1% EDTA + 0.1% H₂O₂ 1 min LASER Group #7: MB 100 (PIT = 5 min) + 0.1% EDTA + 0.1% Chx 1 min LASER Group #8: 2% CHX 1 min Group #9: 1% NaOCl 1 min Group #10: 2% NaOCl 1 min Control groups: Group #11: 1 mL of sterile water for 6 min: positive control	1.0 2.0	$E.\ faecalis$ (VP3-181, VP3-180, Gel 31, and Gel 32)	MB BS – [15 μmol L^{-1}] Biofilm – [100 μmol L^{-1}] PIT: 300 s	Twin Laser (MMOptics) [λ660 nm] IT: 30 s, 60 s, 180 s	Viability staining CLSM	Modified PDT killed 20 times more than conventional PDT and up to 8 times more than 2% CHX and 1% NaOCL
	Sample: Bacterial plaque from 3 adult volunteers used in 4 strains of $E.\ faecalis$ (originally isolated from root canals of the teeth with periapical lesions)						
Bago et al. 2013 [79]	Test groups:Group #1: NaOCl (n = 20) Group #2: EndoActivator + NaOCl (n = 20) Group #3: Diode laser (n = 20) Group #4: PDT (n = 20) Group #5: PDT + 3D Endoprobe (n = 20) Control groups: Group #6: NaCl (n = 10): positive control	2.5	$E.\ faecalis$ (ATCC29212)	Phenothiazine chloride/TBO [10 mg mL^{-1}]/[155 μg mL^{-1}] PIT: 60, 120 s	Helbo and Laser HF [λ660 nm] IT: 60 s The 2 lasers have the same wavelength.	SEM Cell viability CFU (log₁₀) PCR	PDT using both laser systems and the sonic activated NaOCl irrigation were significantly more effective than diode irradiation and single NaOCl.
	Sample: 120 uniradicular human teeth (mandibular incisors and maxillary second premolar extracted because of periodontal disease or extensive carious lesions without root caries or previous endodontic treatment)						
Hecker et al. 2013 [80]	Test groups:Group #1: NaOCl (0.5%, 1.0% or 3.0%) for 30, 60, or 600 s (n = 10) Group #2: NaOCl (0.5%, 1.0% or 3.0%) for 30, 60, or 600 s + neutralizing solution (n = 10) Group #3: PDT (n = 10) Control groups Group #4: TBO (only) (n = 10) Group #5: laser (only) (n = 10) Group #6: apical section as sterile control: negative control Group #7: middle section to confirm successful infection: positive control	0.5 1.0 3.0	$E.\ faecalis$ (ATCC29212)	TBO [NS] PIT: 60 s	Pact 200 system [λ635 nm] IT: 240, 360 s	Cell viability CFU (log₁₀) SEM	The antibacterial PDT system did not achieve sufficient disinfection when compared to NaOCL
	Sample: roots of freshly extracted permanent bovine mandibular incisors (total number of teeth unknown)						

TABLE 3: Continued.

Study type	Groups	% NaOCl	Substracte	Photosensitizer	Laser	Parameters evaluated	Conclusion
Muhammad et al. 2014 [82]	Test groups:Group #1: PDT with Aseptim Plus - LED disinfection system (n = 10); Group #2: PDT with diode laser; Group #3: PUI + 17% EDTA + 2.6% NaOCl; Control groups; Group #4: no inoculation (n = 2): negative control; Group #5: with inoculation (n = 2): positive control	2.6	E. faecalis; S. salivarius (ATCC7073); P. gingivalis (ATCC 33277); P. intermedia	TBO [15 μg mL^{-1}] PIT: 60 s	LED [λ635 nm] Diode laser [λ650 nm] IT$_{(LED/DIODE)}$: 120 s	SEM; Scores for levels of infection (Bonsor et al. 2006 [35, 73])	The group treated with PUI + 2.5% NaOCl + 17% EDTA solution has the best results when compared to PDT with 2 different light sources.
	Sample: 30 roots obtained from 50 extracted human single and multirooted teeth						
Xhevdet et al. 2014 [81]	Experiment #1; E. faecalis (n = 78); Test groups:Group #1: PDT (1 min) (n = 13); Group #2: PDT (3 min) (n = 13); Group #3: PDT (5 min) (n = 13); Group #4: NaOCl + PBS (n = 13); Group #5: NaOCl + 10 sec passive ultrasonic irrigation (PUI) (n = 13); Control groups; Group #6: no treatment (n = 13): positive control; Experiment #2; C. albicans (n = 78); Test groups: Group #1: PDT (1 min) (n = 13); Group #2: PDT (3 min) (n = 13); Group #3: PDT (5 min) (n = 13); Group #4: NaOCl + PBS (n = 13); Group #5: NaOCl + 10 sec PUI (n = 13); Control groups; Group #6: no treatment (n = 13): positive control	2.5	E. faecalis (ATCC29121); Candida albicans (ATCC60193)	Phenothiazine chloride [10 mg mL^{-1}] PIT: 60 s	HELBO [λ660 nm] IT: 60, 180, 300 s	Flow cytometry; SEM; Cell viability; CFU ($\log_{10}$)	Irrigation with NaOCl showed similar results to 5 min irradiation of PDT.
	Sample: 156 extracted uniradicular human teeth						

TABLE 4: PDT microbial reduction outcomes.

Author	Study type	Microorganisms	Efficacy (% or $\log_{10}$)
Seal et al. 2002 [63]	*In vitro*	*S. intermedius*	$5\log_{10}$
Bonsor et al. 2006 [35, 73]	*In vivo*	Polymicrobial infected teeth	96.7
Bonsor et al. 2006 [35, 73]	*In vivo*	Polymicrobial infected teeth	91
Silva Garcez et al. 2006 [57]	*In vitro*	*E. faecalis*	99.2
Garcez et al. 2007 [34]	*In vitro*	*P. mirabilis* and *P. aeruginosa*	98
Garcez et al. 2008 [58]	*In vivo*	Polymicrobial human dentine of the canal's walls	99.9
George and Kishen 2008 [59, 103]	*In vitro/ex vivo*	*E. faecalis*	100
Lim et al. 2009 [77]	*Ex vivo*	*E. faecalis*	99.99
Meire et al. 2009 [64]	*In vitro/ex vivo*	*E. faecalis*	1–$1.5\log_{10}$
Souza et al. 2010 [65]	*In vitro*	*E. faecalis*	99.48
Garcez et al. 2010 [74]	*In vivo*	Polymicrobial infected teeth	100
Nagayoshi et al. 2011 [62]	*In vitro*	*E. faecalis*	99.99
Ng et al. 2011 [78]	*Ex vivo*	Human intracanal dentinal shavings	70
Nunes et al. 2011 [66]	*In vitro*	*E. faecalis*	99.41
Poggio et al. 2011 [67]	*In vitro*	*S. mutans*; *E. faecalis*, and *S. sanguis*	91.49
Rios et al. 2011 [68]	*In vitro*	*E. faecalis*	99.9
Bago et al. 2013 [79]	*Ex vivo*	*E. faecalis*	99.99
Cheng et al. 2012 [69]	*In vitro*	*E. faecalis*	96.96
Pileggi et al. 2013 [60]	*In vitro*	*E. faecalis*	96.7
Stojicic et al. 2013 [5]	*Ex vivo*	*E. faecalis*	100
Vaziri et al. 2012 [70]	*In vitro*	*E. faecalis*	82.3%
Hecker et al. 2013 [80]	*Ex vivo*	*E. faecalis*	Not specified
Prabhakar et al. 2013 [75]	*In vivo*	Polymicrobial infected teeth	99.99
Bumb et al. 2014 [61]	*In vitro*	*E. faecalis*	96.7
Gergova et al. 2015 [71]	*In vitro*	*S. aureus*; *E. faecalis*; *S. pyogenes*; *S. intermedius*; *E. coli*; *K. pneumonia*; *E. cloacae*; *S. marcescens*; *M. morganii*; *P. aeruginosa*; *A. baumannii*; *C. albicans*	42–54
Jurič et al. 2014 [76]	*In vivo*	Polymicrobial infected teeth	100
Muhammad et al. 2014 [82]	*Ex vivo*	*E. faecalis*; *S. salivarius*; *P. gingivalis*; *P. intermedia*	Not specified
Xhevdet et al. 2014 [81]	*Ex vivo*	*E. faecalis* and *C. albicans*	71.59
Wang et al. 2015 [72]	*In vitro*	*E. faecalis*	$5.20\log_{10}$

irrigation showed similar results to 5 min irradiation of PDT, $10\,mg\,mL^{-1}$ phenothiazine chloride as PS irradiated with 660 nm light source.

Considering all 29 publications, 14 of them (48%) [5, 34, 35, 57–61, 73–76, 78, 79] showed best PDT antimicrobial outcome compared to (0.5–6%) NaOCl used alone; 2 (7%) [62, 81] papers reveal similar effects between them and the last 13 (45%) [63–72, 77, 80, 82] studies revealed supremacy of sodium hypochlorite (0.5–6%).

3.2. Antimicrobial PDT Outcomes.
The present narrative literature review was based on hypothesis that antimicrobial PDT efficacy was better than sodium hypochlorite in root canal asepsis. Considering all studies chronologically organized in Table 4, 48% (14 papers) showed PDT is more efficient than NaOCl (0.5–6% concentration) used alone and 7% (2 papers) reveal similarity in antimicrobial outcome effects between them.

On the other hand, 45% (13 studies) of studies reveal supremacy of sodium hypochlorite. From all studies, it must be observed that 55.2% (16 studies) were conducted at *in vitro* conditions, revealing preferential experimental phase where PDT remains in the last two decades. This must be taken into consideration, when comparing with clinical PDT studies, in which evidence reveals unanimous evidence supremacy of PDT over NaOCl.

3.3. Evaluation Parameters.
The 29 studies analysed for this review revealed assessment of antimicrobial PDT efficacy was done through several parameters, from microbiological evaluation (classical analysis) to recent advanced imaging approaches. At the beginning, bacteriological experimental *in vitro* studies presented results through colony-forming units (CFU). This approach overcomes limitation of direct microscopic counting of bacterial cells, where all cells, dead and live, are counted; CFU estimates only viable cells of each

group, before and after treatment, in planktonic suspensions and biofilms. Results are given as CFU/mL (colony-forming units per millilitre) for liquids. This approach was used in 24 studies (83%) [34, 57–66, 68–72, 74–81]; Bonsor et al. [35, 73] used bacterial load scores, instead of the usual CFU, to evaluate PDT antimicrobial efficacy in clinical studies. Muhammad et al. [82] in 2014 over an *ex vivo* study elected the same evaluation unit as in Bonsor et al. studies, repeating bacterial score, complemented with microbiological identification.

Scanning electron microscopic (SEM) *in vitro* investigations have demonstrated the penetration of bacteria up to 1000 μm into dentinal tubules and hence it is very difficult for normal irrigants to penetrate till this depth. NaOCl can penetrate in a range of 60–150 μm into dentinal tubules and of Nd:YAG laser at a range of 400–850 μm. *Enterococcus faecalis* is known to colonize dentinal tubules up to depth of 600–1000 μm and conventional irrigants cannot penetrate more than 100 μm [83]. With SEM, Bumb et al.'s [61] *in vitro* study revealed bacteria found till the depth of 980 μm (control group) and in PDT group achieved a depth of 890–900 μm free from microorganisms, which revealed PDT as a promising root canal disinfection approach. SEM is a remarkably versatile technique, which reproduces the exact morphology of structures, but as the main disadvantage of dehydration of the sample. It was used in 10 (34%) studies [61, 65, 68, 69, 71, 72, 79–82] and ESEM (environmental scanning electron microscope) [84] which allows preservation of the sample before and after light irradiation was not used in any study. CSLM was used only in one study of George and Kishen [59] showing capability of obtaining in-focus images from selected depths allowing three-dimensional reconstruction of topologically complex objects with a specific hardware analysis. The same study [59] also evaluated dark toxicity (detail described in photosensitizers subchapter) and ROS production. PDT antimicrobial killing can be mediated by type I and type II reactions, although singlet oxygen is the predominant chemical entity causing cell death. Analysis and quantification of singlet/reactive oxygen species detection seem to be an excellent methodology to quantify antimicrobial PDT outcomes. However, of all studies analysed, only George and Kishen [59] performed ROS quantification and state that the increased photooxidation potential and singlet oxygen generation were thought to have collectively contributed towards the biofilm matrix disruption [59] and bacterial inactivation.

3.4. Photosensitizers. Photosensitizers (PS), which were preferentially located at the bacterial cytoplasmic membrane, have been found to be very potent photoantimicrobial agents. One important exception is represented by acridines [36], such as proflavine or acridine orange, which mostly interpolate with DNA bases. Highest modifications of cell functions and morphology, triggered by photodynamic inactivation, are typically due to damaged membranous domains [36]. This pattern of photoinduced subcellular damage is in agreement with lack of mutagenic effects [85], as well as with absence of selection of photoresistant microbial strains even after several photosensitization treatments.

Methylene blue (MB), a well-established PS, has been used in PDT for targeting endodontic bacteria since 2007 [34]

and remains as one of the most used; but the first PS used in endodontic field was toluidine blue (TBO) [63]. Hydrophilicity of MB, along with its low molecular weight and positive charge, allows it to cross outer membrane of Gram-negative bacteria through porin channels [33, 86]. MB predominantly interacts with anionic macromolecule lipopolysaccharide, resulting in generation of MB dimers, which participate in the photosensitization process. From all studies evaluated, 12 (41%) [35, 63–65, 67, 68, 70, 71, 73, 79, 80, 82] used TBO as PS, while 10 (34%) [5, 59, 61, 65, 66, 69, 75, 77, 78, 87] studies used MB. One study, elaborated by Souza et al. [65], used both TBO and MB as PS. The best antimicrobial PDT results were achieved with TBO and MB as PS in the same concentration, 15 μg mL^{-1} [5, 65, 70, 71, 82]. All concentration variations are studied first in preliminary findings to obtain fluorescence characteristics [45] in ultraviolet-visible absorption spectra on a diode-array spectrophotometer to understand absorption pattern and to establish final concentration. In designing criteria for definition of second generation PS, an essential feature has been evaluated, *dark toxicity* [88]. It is clearly desirable that PS has zero or very low cytotoxicity in total absence of light and this indicates antimicrobial PDT efficacy results strictly from combination between PS and light source. Reviewing literature in this aspect, only one study from George and Kishen [59] had this aspect in mind.

The period of intimate contact between PS and substrate without irradiation, known as preincubation time (PIT), diverges in terms of PS used. It is also important that PIT is fixed in total absence of light, even natural light [88]. The most used TBO PIT was 60 seconds (s) [35, 67, 73, 80, 82] from a range of 30–300 s (mean = 95.5 s) and MB PIT most used was 300 s [5, 66, 75, 78] from a range of 60–600 s (mean = 353.3 s).

3.5. Light. Phototherapy describes use of light in treatment of disease; photochemotherapy, on the other hand, involves a combination of administration of a photosensitizing agent followed by action of light on tissues in which the agent is located [89]. PDT kills microorganisms by combined action of visible light and a photosensitizing dye. From all 29 studies evaluated, laser wavelength gap referred to in literature was between 380 [60] and 910 nm [61] (mean = 650.8 nm), while most used light source was a diode laser of 660 nm [5, 34, 58, 65, 66, 69, 74–77, 79, 81] wavelength. Some orthodox photosensitizers have lost their proficiency because they needed specific light source for each one and combination between them triggers the costs. Several examples can illustrate this aspect: Azpaste (685 nm) [57]; indocyanine green (805 nm) [62]; eosin-Y, and curcumin (380–500 nm) [60] which make them, nowadays, outdated.

In terms of commercial light sources, there are three diode lasers that authors would like to remark: *Denfotex* of 635 nm (SaveDent; Denfotex, Inverkeithing, UK) [64, 90, 91], *Helbo* of 660 nm (Helbo Photodynamic Systems, Grieskirchen, Austria) [91], and *FotoSan* emitting in the red spectrum with a power peak at 628 nm (FotoSan; CMS Dental, Copenhagen, Denmark) [67, 68, 71]. Delivery of PDT treatment with Denfotex, according to the manufacturer's recommendations, includes TBO as PS at a concentration of 12.7 mg L^{-1}, applied in 120 s as preincubation time (PIT); followed by an irradiation time (IT) of 150 s with a laser output power of 100 mW using the spherical tip. Helbo system advocates Helbo Endo Blue PS, a MB dye, at a concentration of $10 \, mg \, L^{-1}$ fully covering the root canal with a PIT of 180 s; after this time, according to the manufacturer's recommendations, excess PS dye should be removed and light source applied for an IT of 120 s and an output power of 75 mW with an attached 2D spot probe Helbo Photodynamic Systems. Meire et al. in 2012 [91] performed an *in vitro* study comparing Denfotex with Helbo. The same team [91] reported that log reduction with Helbo system was higher than with Denfotex; however, the best results were achieved with 2.5% NaOCl for 300 s. Several differences between the two systems were described and might account for the distinctive reduction outcomes in viable cells [91]. First, the PS dyes are chemically different; secondly, Helbo Blue PS is much more concentrated than Denfotex PS. Thirdly, following the PS application and the recommended PIT, the PS excess has to be removed with the Helbo system, dried canal [91], but not with the two other systems: Denfotex and FotoSan, where fiber is inserted in the liquid [67, 68, 71, 91]. In the three PDT systems, all probes are different. While the Helbo systems 2D spot probe is designed for two-dimensional exposure, Denfotex and FotoSan tips emit in three dimensions and this has strong implications for energy densities at the target. Also the lasers wavelengths are slightly different. It seems that there is also a clear reduction in light exposure as irradiation time (IT): Denfotex (150 s) [91], Helbo (120 s) [91], and FotoSan (30 s) [67, 68, 71].

FotoSan uses only TBO as a FotoSan PS, available in three types of viscosities (low, medium, and high), all at the same concentration ($100 \, \mu g \, mL^{-1}$) and the light source with an output power of 100 mW. FotoSan was evaluated in 3 (10.3%) studies [67, 68, 71], curiously all conducted in *in vitro* conditions with FotoSan protocol IT of 30 s.

Poggio et al. [67] tested 30 s and also 90 s of IT and declared that with the longer light exposure, it results in an increased percentage of bacterial reduction for different groups of *Enterococcus faecalis*, *Streptococcus mutans*, and *Streptococcus sanguis* strains. For this reason, this group admits that FotoSan needs to be applied into canal for at least 90 s, because 30 s of irradiation showed lower performance when compared to PDT with IT of 90 s, although the same group reveals that the best outcomes were achieved with PDT 30 s of IT combined with 5% NaOCl.

Irradiation time (IT) is an important issue to considerer and, in this parameter, PDT studies outcomes are very dissimilar with a range between 30 s [63, 68] and 1800 s [60]. Considering the most used wavelength of 660 nm, preference irradiation time is in the range between 30 s [5] and 1200 s [77] (mean = 223 s).

The last aspect considered in laser literature is the need for an intracanal fiber tip to spread light into root dentinal walls as well as within biofilms. From all studies analysed, only Nunes et al. [66] explored *in vitro* effectiveness of PDT with and without use of an intracanal optical fiber. Nunes et al. [66] concluded that, under experimental conditions, PDT was effective against *E. faecalis*, regardless of whether or not

it is applied through an intracanal fiber. Considering the use of intracanal fiber, only 4 (13.8%) studies [63, 70, 75, 80] were not performed with intracanal fiber (Table 5).

Prabhakar et al. [75], in these particular conditions, revealed in a clinical study that antimicrobial PDT performance is better than 0.5% NaOCl. When PDT is implemented in planktonic suspensions established in multiwells, light source was applied 20 mm [60] away from well. Considering intracanal fiber, fiber tip diameter most used was 400 nm [59, 62, 64, 72, 77]. In terms of intracanal fiber location inside root, it varies from full working length (WL) [34, 58, 62, 64, 66, 71, 76, 79, 81, 82], the most prevalent, to WL-1 millimeters (mm) [57, 74], WL-2 mm [61, 68], WL-3 mm [67–69], and WL-4 mm [35, 73]. Contemplating the same device, intracanal fiber, in terms of applying movements to itself or inserting endodontic tip static inside root canal to improve the best light diffusion through root canal [66]. The former was applied in 5 studies [34, 58, 65, 66, 79] with spiral movements from apical to cervical and latter maintained static [64, 76, 77] inside root canal orifice [77] or at WL [64, 76].

3.6. Disinfection Protocol. In literature, when PDT studies are accomplished in teeth, the majority of them are performed in human single rooted tooth specimens with no evidence of caries or defects and radicular pathology. Considering tooth type, there is only one study performed in deciduous teeth [75]; the majority was achieved in permanent uniradicular human teeth. However, four studies used not only uniradicular but also multiradicular teeth [35, 73, 78, 82]. Besides, decayed teeth are also studied in deciduous [75] and permanent teeth [79].

Slaughterhouse bovine teeth [80] are convenient to use in antimicrobial PDT studies because of their match with human dentine; more precisely, their dentinal tubules are very similar to human teeth in quantity, size, diameter, morphology, and density. Moreover, bovine teeth [12] are simple to acquire and reduced size makes handling easier; in this term, they were used in 2 (7%) studies [72, 80]. Only one study, performed by Nagayoshi et al. [62], was executed in a resin block which attempts to mimic an *in vitro* model of apical periodontitis.

In the most common experimental model, dental specimens are decoronated to a standard length of 12 mm [67, 68, 78, 79] although gap value is very wide, from 8 [59, 77] to 15 mm [66, 81] or complete root canal length. Patency of apical foramina is established and then mechanical [35, 58, 61, 63–68, 70, 71, 73, 74, 76, 78, 79, 81, 82] instrumentation is performed using nickel-titanium rotary files, predominantly in a coronoapical (crown-down) technique [35, 58, 61, 63–68, 70, 71, 73, 74, 76, 78, 79, 81, 82] from canal orifice to apical third, until it reaches the value of master apical file (MAF) of K (Kerr) file 40 [58, 59, 68, 70]. However, other MAF have been described, such as 35 [57, 79, 81] and 30 [34].

In terms of irrigation with disinfecting agents, those are used for smear layer (SL) removal, lubrication, debris removal, and antimicrobial effects. SL is composed of organic and inorganic components like vital or necrotic pulp tissue, microorganisms, saliva, blood cells, and tooth structure. Among irrigation solutions, sodium hypochlorite (NaOCl)

TABLE 5: Studies compilation: laser, photosensitizer, and fiber applied.

Study type	Year	Author	Wavelength (nm)	Diameter of fiber (μm) Working length (WL) EL	Laser Power of output (mW)	Power of density (mW/cm²)	Energy fluence (J/cm²)	Photosensitizer Type	Concentration (μg/mL)	PDT outcomes +	−
In vitro, 16 studies	2002	Seal et al. [63]	632.8	*Without fiber* Light at the orifice of the access cavity 365	35	—	42.9, 63.3, 85.7, 214.3, 428.6	TBO	12.5, 25, 50, 100	+	—
	2006	Silva Garcez et al. [57]	685	WL-1 mm Helicoidal movements, from apical to cervical 200	50	—	—	AZpaste	0.01% AZ paste	+	
	2007	Garcez et al. [34]	660	WL Spiral movements, from apical to cervical 400	40	—	5, 10, 20 e 40	PEI/e6	NS	+	
	2008	George and Kishen [59, 103]	664	NS NS 400 WL IV: static spherical tip in the centre of the liquid	30	—	63.69	MB	1, 5, 10, 15, 20, 25 μM	+	
	2009	Meire et al. [64]	635	EV: 70% of the light radially as a cylinder uniformly and 30% at the tip; moved up and down in the canal 300	100	—	—	TBO	12.7 mg mL⁻¹		—
		Souza et al. [65]	660	NS Spiral movements from apical to cervical 400	40	—	—	MB/TBO	15/15		—
	2011	Nagayoshi et al. [62]	805	WL NS	5000	—	—	Indocyanine green	12. mg mL⁻¹		R
	2011	Nunes et al. [66] Study with and without fiber	660	*Without fiber* Handpiece placed in root canal orifice 216 WL Spiral movements from apical to cervical 500	90	300	—	MB	100		—
		Poggio et al. [67]	628	WL-3 mm Endotip guide to the apical parts	—	—	—	TBO	100		—

TABLE 5: Continued.

Study type	Year	Author	Wavelength (nm)	Diameter of fiber (μm) Working length (WL)	Power of output (mW)	Power of density (mW/cm^2)	Energy fluence (J/cm^2)	Photosensitizer Type	Concentration (μg/mL)	PDT outcomes +	PDT outcomes −
		Rios et al. [68]	628	EL NS; WL-2/3 mm; NS	—	—	—	TBO	NS	+	−
		Cheng et al. [69]	*Nd:YAG* [λ1064 nm]	*Nd:YAG* 200; WL-1; Spiral movement	—	—	—	MB	50		−
			Er:YAG [λ2940 nm]	*Er:YAG* 300; Orifice of root canal; NS							
	2012		*Er,Cr:YSGG* [λ2780 nm]	*Er,Cr:YSGG* 415; WL-1; NS							
			Diode [λ660 nm]	*Diode* 2000; WL-3 mm; NS							
		Vaziri et al. [70]	625	*Without fiber*	—	200	12	TBO	15 [BS] All 1 μM		−
		Pileggi et al. [60]	380–500	10.4 mm Light source 20 mm away from the bacteria NS	—	450	108	Eosin-Y RB Curcumin	*Biofilms* Eosin-Y 100 μM RB/curcumin 10 μM	+	
	2014	Bumb et al. [61]	910	NS; WL-2 mm; Circular movements, from apical to cervical 200; WL	1000	—	—	MB	25 mg mL^{-1}	+	
	2015	Gergova et al. [71]	660	Helicoidal traction movements, from apical to cervical 400	100	—	—	TBO	0.1 mg mL^{-1}		−
	2015	Wang et al. [72]	670	NS; NS	50	—	—	MB	60 μM		−

TABLE 5: Continued.

Study type	Year	Author	Wavelength (nm)	Diameter of fiber (μm) Working length (WL) EL	Laser Power of output (mW)	Power of density (mW/cm²)	Energy fluence (J/cm²)	Photosensitizer Type	Concentration (μg/mL)	PDT outcomes
In vivo, 6 studies		Bonsor et al. [35, 73]	633	Flexible hollow tube WL-4 mm Moved up and down about 3 mm at 20 s	100	—	—	TBO	12.7 mg mL⁻¹	+
	2006	Bonsor et al. [35, 73]	633	Flexible emitter tip WL-4 mm Moved up and down about 3 mm at 20 s 300	100	—	—	TBO	NS	+
	2008	Garcez et al. [58]	660	WL Spiral movements, from apical to cervical 200	40	—	—	PEI/e6	60 μmol L⁻¹	+
	2010	Garcez et al. [74]	660	WL-1 mm Spiral movements	40	—	—	PEI/e6	≈19	+
	2013	Prabhakar et al. [75] Deciduous teeth	660	Without fiber	30	—	8.6	MB	50	+
	2014	Jurič et al. [76]	660	450 WL Static 400	100	—	—	Phenothiazinium chloride		+
Ex vivo, 7 studies	2009	Lim et al. [77]	660	Root canal orifice Static 250	30	—	—	MB	100 μM	–
		Ng et al. [78]	665	10 mm 360° NS [BS]	—	100	30	MB	50 μg mL⁻¹	+
	2011	Stojicic et al. [5]	660	Long optical fiber with a diameter 0.4 mm Biofilm Conical frustum tip with the end diameter of 5 mm NS 320	40	—	—	MB	[BS] 15 μmol L⁻¹ Biofilm 100 μmol L⁻¹	+
		Bago et al. [79]	660	WL Spiral movements, from apical to cervical	100	—	—	Phenothiazine chloride/TBO	10 mg mL⁻¹/155	+

TABLE 5: Continued.

Study type	Year	Author	Wavelength (nm)	Diameter of fiber (μm) Working length (WL) EL	Power of output (mW)	Power of density (mW/cm²)	Energy fluence (J/cm²)	Type	Concentration (μg/mL)	+	−
									Laser	**Photosensitizer**	**PDT outcomes**
	2013	Hecker et al. [80]	635	*Without fiber* 300 WL	200	—	—	TBO	NS		—
		Muhammad et al. [82]	650	Moved all along the canals NS	20	—	—	TBO	15 μg mL⁻¹		—
	2014	Xhevdet et al. [81]	660	WL Light at the tip and from the lateral sides	100	100	—	Phenothiazine chloride	10 mg mL⁻¹		≀

is the classical irrigant most used in endodontic therapy as a powerful antibacterial organic tissue dissolving agent.

NaOCl penetrates to a depth of approximately 130 μm [92] to 160 μm into dentinal tubules whereas tubular infection may occur closer to cementum-dentin junction (up to 1000 μm) [93]. Bumb et al. [61] demonstrated in scanning electron microscope (SEM) penetration up to 1000 μm into dentinal tubules of *E. faecalis* and compared penetrating power between a high power laser (Nd:YAG) that can go to a range of 400–850 μm and PDT group that reaches as deep as 890–900 μm.

Considering NaOCl as an unquestionable irrigation solution, its universal effective minimal concentration remains unclear. Apart from various outcomes reported by previous studies on comparative effectiveness of hypochlorite at different concentrations, it is regularly accepted that effectiveness of NaOCl is proportional to its concentration [24, 72, 94]. In antimicrobial PDT studies, NaOCl concentration range is between 0.5 [57, 67, 75, 80] and 6% [68, 78] and mainstream of studies used 2.5% NaOCl concentration [34, 58, 62, 64, 65, 70, 71, 74, 76, 79, 81]. Due to the fact that NaOCl has an influence upon only organic components of SL, it should be used with demineralizing agents, which can remove inorganic component of smear layer. Concerning SL elimination, only 3 readings [35, 70, 73] reported citric acid as a SL deletion, one at 10% [70] and two at 20% from the same author, Bonsor et al. [35, 73]. But the most popular SL removal is by far 17% ethylenediamine tetraacetic acid (EDTA) [34, 57–59, 61, 63, 65–69, 71, 74, 76–78, 81, 82].

3.7. Microorganisms. Reviewing literature on use of several microorganisms in PDT studies, authors could not evaluate *in vivo* studies in those terms, because no attempt was made to identify bacterial flora during culture process [35, 58, 73, 75] in four of six studies. Only Garcez et al., 2010 [74], and Jurič et al., 2014 [76], established microbiological identification.

Among all studies, we analysed 23 studies (all *in vitro* and *ex vivo*), and from those, 20 (87%) elected *Enterococcus faecalis* as substract to quantify antimicrobial PDT effectiveness. *E. faecalis* is a Gram-positive facultative anaerobe commonly detected in asymptomatic, persistent endodontic infections. Its prevalence in such infections ranges from 24% to 77% [95]. This finding can be explained by various survival and virulence factors [95] expressed by *E. faecalis*, including its ability to compete with other microorganisms, invade dentinal tubules, and resist nutritional deprivation.

E. faecalis was used not only in planktonic suspensions, but also in form of biofilms and the most common strain selected was ATCC29212. However, biofilm maturation time did not follow a linear pattern; besides, a huge discrepancy exists. Some authors used young biofilms with range of 2 [60, 68], 4 [60], and 7 days [81, 82] very distinct from mature biofilms performed with biofilms of 21 [61, 66], 28 [5, 69, 72, 77], and 70 days [59]. According to Kishen and Haapasalo 2010 [12], a mature biofilm is considered when maturation period is equal to or higher than 21 days and only 7 (30%) studies [5, 59, 61, 66, 69, 72, 77] respected this mature biofilm criteria. Apart from *E. faecalis*, other microorganisms were reviewed. Of note, in literature, the first PDT *in vitro* study

was performed by Seal et al. 2002 [63] in root canals infected with *Streptococcus intermedius* (Gram-positive facultative anaerobe) biofilm with 2 days of maturation using TBO as PS and a helium-neon laser as light source.

4. Discussion

PDT, a technique with potentially significant antimicrobial properties, is a fairly recent approach in endodontic disinfection protocols. While the oral applications of PDT have been extensively tested, variations in study type and design limits the ability to synthesize or pool the available quantitative data, thereby permitting a formal meta-analysis and a systematic review.

Furthermore, many of the studies quantitatively measuring the degree of bacterial kill fail to report baseline bacterial counts or concentrations, thus limiting the ability to assess the bactericidal efficacy of PDT. Considering this apparent variation in reporting results among the studies analysed, it is difficult to provide a definitive assessment of the research question posed in this review. It is important to mention that PDT efficacy is shown in CFU or in percentage and logarithm (in form of $\log_{10}$); nonetheless, authors state this is pointless without the perception of the initial concentration. As an example, if we have an initial sample from a root canal of 10^7 microorganisms and if after PDT approach we had 10^5, statistically, 99% were killed, but there are still 100000 microorganisms left inside the root canal. Considering the variation in units at outcomes, the final results analysis is difficult.

Even though PDT has significant advantages (cited in Section 1), potential adverse events as tooth discoloration have been reported previously in root canal treatment when MB and TBO were used as PS [96]. It is also important that future clinical studies clearly report adverse events associated with PDT so that an estimation of the benefit-to-risk ratio from the use of PDT is feasible. Nonetheless, there were no adverse effects mentioned in the included studies of the current review.

PDT outcomes in literature have been reported by the dual combination of PS and a visible light source in the presence of oxygen; however, recently, Lins de Sousa et al. [97] analysed that twice-daily blue light of 420 nm, energy density of 72 Jcm^{-2}, and irradiation time of 776 s without PS are a promising approach in the inhibition of five days' *Streptococcus mutans* matrix-rich biofilm development. It has remarkably inhibited the production of insoluble EPS, which is responsible for the scaffold of the extracellular biofilm matrix. The authors suggest that this evidence is very important to improve standardization in PDT procedures in the total absence of light as the evaluation of PS dark toxicity in some studies reviewed did not address this important issue.

In the literature, residual systemic photosensitization has also been reported as a potentially adverse event associated with the use of intravenous PS [98]; but this effect appears to not be associated with oral applications of PDT [99]. The role of PDT in root canal disinfection has been tested using several combinations of PS and light sources and has shown divergent results and these studies have revealed several limitations associated with antimicrobial PDT. For successful

PDT to affect significant reduction or eradication of microorganisms, a PS is required which will show enough affinity for microorganisms without catalyzing photodamage to host tissues, a light source at a wavelength that can penetrate tissues (630–700 nm), and sufficient oxygenation to produce a level of reactive oxygen species (ROS) necessary to induce photodynamic lipid peroxidation and, as a consequence, necrosis and cell death. If there is photodamage to both tissues and microorganisms, efficacy will be suboptimal.

Microorganisms in the root canal flora and their growth mode were found to influence their susceptibility to PDT in a dose-dependent manner [100] and biofilms can be difficult to eradicate not only because of their effect as barriers to PS uptake, but also their ability to diffuse or attenuate light in the root canal dentinal tubules. Even dentin, dentin matrix, pulp tissue, bacterial lipopolysaccharides, and bovine serum albumin were found to significantly decrease PDT antimicrobial efficacy [101] and, as a consequence, an effort to enhance the PDT by nanoparticle-based technology appears promising [102]. Other strategies include the use of a PS solvent [103], efflux pump inhibitors [100], or photoactivated functionalized chitosan nanoparticles for disinfection and stabilization of the dentin matrix [104]. Because the application of PDT for additional reduction of the microbial load of root canal systems seems promising, it would be beneficial to identify the ideal combination of PS and light wavelength in preclinical studies and conduct future randomized controlled trials to test the effect of PDT on root canal disinfection in various indications.

5. Conclusion

PDT has been used thus far without a consensus-based, well-defined protocol, and therefore still remains at an experimental stage waiting for further optimization. Limited clinical information is currently available on the use of PDT in root canal disinfection. Currently, the level of evidence of available clinical studies to answer this question is low. Nevertheless, the results of this review suggest, based primarily on available *in vivo* studies, that PDT could perform well as an antimicrobial adjuvant. PDT appears to be a promising antimicrobial platform so further studies are warranted to optimize protocols using standardized laser and PS parameters to assess the PDT efficacy. Therefore, within the limits of the present review, one may conclude that the efficacy of PDT remains questionable, but promising. It is further suggested that an additional potential benefit from the use of PDT in root canal disinfection may exist where highly resistant bacteria are present in the root canal space, thus affecting the treatment prognosis. Further research is necessary to establish the appropriate PDT parameters allowing adequate antimicrobial action without harmful host side effects.

Conflict of Interests

The authors declare that there is no conflict of interests regarding the publication of this paper.

References

[1] S. Friedman, "Considerations and concepts of case selection in the management of post-treatment endodontic disease (treatment failure)," *Endodontic Topics*, vol. 1, no. 1, pp. 54–78, 2002.

[2] U. Sjögren, D. Figdor, S. Persson, and G. Sundqvist, "Influence of infection at the time of root filling on the outcome of endodontic treatment of teeth with apical periodontitis," *International Endodontic Journal*, vol. 30, no. 5, pp. 297–306, 1997.

[3] T. Waltimo, M. Trope, M. Haapasalo, and D. Ørstavik, "Clinical efficacy of treatment procedures in endodontic infection control and one year follow-up of periapical healing," *Journal of Endodontics*, vol. 31, no. 12, pp. 863–866, 2005.

[4] J. F. Siqueira Jr., M. C. Araújo, P. F. Garcia, R. C. Fraga, and C. J. Dantas, "Histological evaluation of the effectiveness of five instrumentation techniques for cleaning the apical third of root canals," *Journal of Endodontics*, vol. 23, no. 8, pp. 499–502, 1997.

[5] S. Stojicic, H. Amorim, Y. Shen, and M. Haapasalo, "Ex vivo killing of *Enterococcus faecalis* and mixed plaque bacteria in planktonic and biofilm culture by modified photoactivated disinfection," *International Endodontic Journal*, vol. 46, no. 7, pp. 649–659, 2013.

[6] Y.-G. Qiang, C. M. N. Yow, and Z. Huang, "Combination of photodynamic therapy and immunomodulation: current status and future trends," *Medicinal Research Reviews*, vol. 28, no. 4, pp. 632–644, 2008.

[7] L. C. De Paz, "Redefining the persistent infection in root canals: possible role of biofilm communities," *Journal of Endodontics*, vol. 33, no. 6, pp. 652–662, 2007.

[8] J. W. Costerton, K. J. Cheng, G. G. Geesey et al., "Bacterial biofilms in nature and disease," *Annual Review of Microbiology*, vol. 41, pp. 435–464, 1987.

[9] G. Svensäter, B. Sjögreen, and I. R. Hamilton, "Multiple stress responses in *Streptococcus mutans* and the induction of general and stress-specific proteins," *Microbiology*, vol. 146, no. 1, pp. 107–117, 2000.

[10] K. Lewis, "Persister cells and the riddle of biofilm survival," *Biochemistry*, vol. 70, no. 2, pp. 267–274, 2005.

[11] G. H. W. Bowden and I. R. Hamilton, "Survival of oral bacteria," *Critical Reviews in Oral Biology & Medicine*, vol. 9, no. 1, pp. 54–85, 1998.

[12] A. Kishen and M. Haapasalo, "Biofilm models and methods of biofilm assessment," *Endodontic Topics*, vol. 22, no. 1, pp. 58–78, 2010.

[13] G. Svensater and G. Bergenholtz, "Biofilms in endodontic infections," *Endodontic Topics*, vol. 9, no. 1, pp. 27–36, 2004.

[14] M. Zehnder, "Root Canal Irrigants," *Journal of Endodontics*, vol. 32, no. 5, pp. 389–398, 2006.

[15] J. M. Santos, P. J. Palma, J. C. Ramos, A. S. Cabrita, and S. Friedman, "Periapical inflammation subsequent to coronal inoculation of dog teeth root filled with Resilon/Epiphany in 1 or 2 treatment sessions with chlorhexidine medication," *Journal of Endodontics*, vol. 40, no. 6, pp. 837–841, 2014.

[16] A. Bystrom, R. Claesson, and G. Sundqvist, "The antibacterial effect of camphorated paramonochlorophenol, camphorated phenol and calcium hydroxide in the treatment of infected root canals," *Endodontics & Dental Traumatology*, vol. 1, no. 5, pp. 170–175, 1985.

[17] J. F. Siqueira Jr., T. Guimarães-Pinto, and I. N. Rôças, "Effects of chemomechanical preparation with 2.5% sodium hypochlorite and intracanal medication with calcium hydroxide on cultivable

bacteria in infected root canals," *Journal of Endodontics*, vol. 33, no. 7, pp. 800–805, 2007.

[18] R. D. Morgental, A. Singh, H. Sappal, P. M. P. Kopper, F. V. Vier-Pelisser, and O. A. Peters, "Dentin inhibits the antibacterial effect of new and conventional endodontic irrigants," *Journal of Endodontics*, vol. 39, no. 3, pp. 406–410, 2013.

[19] I. Portenier, H. Haapasalo, A. Rye, T. Waltimo, D. Ørstavik, and M. Haapasalo, "Inactivation of root canal medicaments by dentine, hydroxylapatite and bovine serum albumin," *International Endodontic Journal*, vol. 34, no. 3, pp. 184–188, 2001.

[20] M. Evans, J. K. Davies, G. Sundqvist, and D. Figdor, "Mechanisms involved in the resistance of *Enterococcus faecalis* to calcium hydroxide," *International Endodontic Journal*, vol. 35, no. 3, pp. 221–228, 2002.

[21] W. L. Chai, H. Hamimah, S. C. Cheng, A. A. Sallam, and M. Abdullah, "Susceptibility of *Enterococcus faecalis* biofilm to antibiotics and calcium hydroxide," *Journal of Oral Science*, vol. 49, no. 2, pp. 161–166, 2007.

[22] T. M. T. Waltimo, E. K. Sirén, H. L. K. Torkko, I. Olsen, and M. P. P. Haapasalo, "Fungi in therapy-resistant apical periodontitis," *International Endodontic Journal*, vol. 30, no. 2, pp. 96–101, 1997.

[23] M. A. Al-Fattani and L. J. Douglas, "Biofilm matrix of Candida albicans and Candida tropicalis: chemical composition and role in drug resistance," *Journal of Medical Microbiology*, vol. 55, no. 8, pp. 999–1008, 2006.

[24] J. F. Siqueira Jr. and I. N. Rôças, "Clinical implications and microbiology of bacterial persistence after treatment procedures," *Journal of Endodontics*, vol. 34, no. 11, pp. 1291–1301, 2008.

[25] A. Kuştarci, Z. Sümer, D. Altunbaş, and S. Koşum, "Bactericidal effect of KTP laser irradiation against *Enterococcus faecalis* compared with gaseous ozone: an ex vivo study," *Oral Surgery, Oral Medicine, Oral Pathology, Oral Radiology and Endodontology*, vol. 107, no. 5, pp. e73–e79, 2009.

[26] C. Heilborn, K. Reynolds, J. D. Johnson, and N. Cohenca, "Cleaning efficacy of an apical negative-pressure irrigation system at different exposure times." *Quintessence International*, vol. 41, no. 9, pp. 759–767, 2010.

[27] R. J. G. De Moor, M. Meire, K. Goharkhay, A. Moritz, and J. Vanobbergen, "Efficacy of ultrasonic versus laser-activated irrigation to remove artificially placed dentin debris plugs," *Journal of Endodontics*, vol. 36, no. 9, pp. 1580–1583, 2010.

[28] A. Halford, C.-D. Ohl, A. Azarpazhooh, B. Basrani, S. Friedman, and A. Kishen, "Synergistic effect of microbubble emulsion and sonic or ultrasonic agitation on endodontic biofilm in vitro," *Journal of Endodontics*, vol. 38, no. 11, pp. 1530–1534, 2012.

[29] R. G. Macedo, B. Verhaagen, D. F. Rivas, M. Versluis, P. Wesselink, and L. van der Sluis, "Cavitation measurement during sonic and ultrasonic activated irrigation," *Journal of Endodontics*, vol. 40, no. 4, pp. 580–583, 2014.

[30] A. Shrestha, S. Zhilong, N. K. Gee, and A. Kishen, "Nanoparticulates for antibiofilm treatment and effect of aging on its antibacterial activity," *Journal of Endodontics*, vol. 36, no. 6, pp. 1030–1035, 2010.

[31] M. Kvist, V. Hancock, and P. Klemm, "Inactivation of efflux pumps abolishes bacterial biofilm formation," *Applied and Environmental Microbiology*, vol. 74, no. 23, pp. 7376–7382, 2008.

[32] B. W. Henderson and T. J. Dougherty, "How does photodynamic therapy work?" *Photochemistry and Photobiology*, vol. 55, no. 1, pp. 145–157, 1992.

[33] M. Wainwright, "Photodynamic antimicrobial chemotherapy (PACT)," *Journal of Antimicrobial Chemotherapy*, vol. 42, no. 1, pp. 13–28, 1998.

[34] A. S. Garcez, M. S. Ribeiro, G. P. Tegos, S. C. Núñez, A. O. C. Jorge, and M. R. Hamblin, "Antimicrobial photodynamic therapy combined with conventional endodontic treatment to eliminate root canal biofilm infection," *Lasers in Surgery and Medicine*, vol. 39, no. 1, pp. 59–66, 2007.

[35] S. J. Bonsor, R. Nichol, T. M. S. Reid, and G. J. Pearson, "Microbiological evaluation of photo-activated disinfection in endodontics (an in vivo study)," *British Dental Journal*, vol. 200, no. 6, pp. 337–341, 2006.

[36] M. R. Hamblin and T. Hasan, "Photodynamic therapy: a new antimicrobial approach to infectious disease?" *Photochemical and Photobiological Sciences*, vol. 3, no. 5, pp. 436–450, 2004.

[37] A. P. Castano, T. N. Demidova, and M. R. Hamblin, "Mechanisms in photodynamic therapy: part one—photosensitizers, photochemistry and cellular localization," *Photodiagnosis and Photodynamic Therapy*, vol. 1, no. 4, pp. 279–293, 2004.

[38] A. C. Trindade, J. A. P. De Figueiredo, L. Steier, and J. B. B. Weber, "Photodynamic therapy in endodontics: a literature review," *Photomedicine and Laser Surgery*, vol. 33, no. 3, pp. 175–182, 2015.

[39] T. Dai, Y.-Y. Huang, and M. R. Hamblin, "Photodynamic therapy for localized infections-state of the art," *Photodiagnosis and Photodynamic Therapy*, vol. 6, no. 3-4, pp. 170–188, 2009.

[40] A. Minnock, D. I. Vernon, J. Schofield, J. Griffiths, J. H. Parish, and S. B. Brown, "Mechanism of uptake of a cationic water-soluble pyridinium zinc phthalocyanine across the outer membrane of *Escherichia coli*," *Antimicrobial Agents and Chemotherapy*, vol. 44, no. 3, pp. 522–527, 2000.

[41] S. George, M. R. Hamblin, and A. Kishen, "Uptake pathways of anionic and cationic photosensitizers into bacteria," *Photochemical and Photobiological Sciences*, vol. 8, no. 6, pp. 788–795, 2009.

[42] J. P. Tardivo, A. Del Giglio, C. S. De Oliveira et al., "Methylene blue in photodynamic therapy: from basic mechanisms to clinical applications," *Photodiagnosis and Photodynamic Therapy*, vol. 2, no. 3, pp. 175–191, 2005.

[43] Y. R. Kim, S. Kim, J. W. Choi et al., "Bioluminescence-activated deep-tissue photodynamic therapy of cancer," *Theranostics*, vol. 5, no. 8, pp. 805–817, 2015.

[44] T. J. Dougherty, C. J. Gomer, B. W. Henderson et al., "Photodynamic therapy," *Journal of the National Cancer Institute*, vol. 90, no. 12, pp. 889–905, 1998.

[45] N. S. Soukos, P. S.-Y. Chen, J. T. Morris et al., "Photodynamic therapy for endodontic disinfection," *Journal of Endodontics*, vol. 32, no. 10, pp. 979–984, 2006.

[46] M. Wainwright, "Local treatment of viral disease using photodynamic therapy," *International Journal of Antimicrobial Agents*, vol. 21, no. 6, pp. 510–520, 2003.

[47] J. M. Bliss, C. E. Bigelow, T. H. Foster, and C. G. Haidaris, "Susceptibility of *Candida* species to photodynamic effects of Photofrin," *Antimicrobial Agents and Chemotherapy*, vol. 48, no. 6, pp. 2000–2006, 2004.

[48] A. Azarpazhooh, P. S. Shah, H. C. Tenenbaum, and M. B. Goldberg, "The effect of photodynamic therapy for periodontitis: a systematic review and meta-analysis," *Journal of Periodontology*, vol. 81, no. 1, pp. 4–14, 2010.

[49] F. Vohra, M. Q. Al-Rifaiy, G. Lillywhite, M. I. Abu Hassan, and F. Javed, "Efficacy of mechanical debridement with adjunct

antimicrobial photodynamic therapy for the management of peri-implant diseases: a systematic review," *Photochemical and Photobiological Sciences*, vol. 13, no. 8, pp. 1160–1168, 2014.

[50] A. A. Takasaki, A. Aoki, K. Mizutani et al., "Application of antimicrobial photodynamic therapy in periodontal and peri-implant diseases," *Periodontology 2000*, vol. 51, no. 1, pp. 109–140, 2009.

[51] H. Gursoy, C. Ozcakir-Tomruk, J. Tanalp, and S. Yilmaz, "Photodynamic therapy in dentistry: a literature review," *Clinical Oral Investigations*, vol. 17, no. 4, pp. 1113–1125, 2013.

[52] S. H. Siddiqui, K. H. Awan, and F. Javed, "Bactericidal efficacy of photodynamic therapy against *Enterococcus faecalis* in infected root canals: a systematic literature review," *Photodiagnosis and Photodynamic Therapy*, vol. 10, no. 4, pp. 632–643, 2013.

[53] V. Chrepa, G. A. Kotsakis, T. C. Pagonis, and K. M. Hargreaves, "The effect of photodynamic therapy in root canal disinfection: a systematic review," *Journal of Endodontics*, vol. 40, no. 7, pp. 891–898, 2014.

[54] B. N. Green, C. D. Johnson, and A. Adams, "Writing narrative literature reviews for peer-reviewed journals: secrets of the trade," *Journal of Chiropractic Medicine*, vol. 5, no. 3, pp. 101–117, 2006.

[55] V. Elm, D. G. Altman, M. Egger, S. J. Pocock, C. Gøtzsche, and J. P. Vandenbroucke, "The strengthening the reporting of observational studies in epidemiology (STROBE) statement: guidelines for reporting observational studies," *The British Medical Journal*, vol. 335, no. 7624, pp. 806–808, 2033.

[56] P. Jüni, D. G. Altman, and M. Egger, "Assessing the quality of controlled clinical trials," *The BMJ*, vol. 323, no. 7, pp. 42–46, 2001.

[57] A. Silva Garcez, S. C. Núñez, J. L. Lage-Marques, A. O. C. Jorge, and M. S. Ribeiro, "Efficiency of NaOCl and laser-assisted photosensitization on the reduction of *Enterococcus faecalis* in vitro," *Oral Surgery, Oral Medicine, Oral Pathology, Oral Radiology and Endodontology*, vol. 102, no. 4, pp. 93–98, 2006.

[58] A. S. Garcez, S. C. Nuñez, M. R. Hamblin, and M. S. Ribeiro, "Antimicrobial effects of photodynamic therapy on patients with necrotic pulps and periapical lesion," *Journal of Endodontics*, vol. 34, no. 2, pp. 138–142, 2008.

[59] S. George and A. Kishen, "Augmenting the antibiofilm efficacy of advanced noninvasive light activated disinfection with emulsified oxidizer and oxygen carrier," *Journal of Endodontics*, vol. 34, no. 9, pp. 1119–1123, 2008.

[60] G. Pileggi, J. C. Wataha, M. Girard et al., "Blue light-mediated inactivation of *Enterococcus faecalis* in vitro," *Photodiagnosis and Photodynamic Therapy*, vol. 10, no. 2, pp. 134–140, 2013.

[61] S. Bumb, D. Bhaskar, C. Agali et al., "Assessment of photodynamic therapy (PDT) in disinfection of deeper dentinal tubules in a root canal system: an in vitro study," *Journal of Clinical and Diagnostic Research*, vol. 8, no. 11, pp. 67–71, 2014.

[62] M. Nagayoshi, T. Nishihara, K. Nakashima et al., "Bactericidal effects of diode laser irradiation on *Enterococcus faecalis* using periapical lesion defect model," *ISRN Dentistry*, vol. 2011, Article ID 870364, 6 pages, 2011.

[63] G. J. Seal, Y.-L. Ng, D. Spratt, M. Bhatti, and K. Gulabivala, "An in vitro comparison of the bactericidal efficacy of lethal photosensitization or sodium hyphochlorite irrigation on *Streptococcus intermedius* biofilms in root canals," *International Endodontic Journal*, vol. 35, no. 3, pp. 268–274, 2002.

[64] M. A. Meire, K. De Prijck, T. Coenye, H. J. Nelis, and R. J. G. De Moor, "Effectiveness of different laser systems to kill *Enterococcus faecalis* in aqueous suspension and in an infected tooth model," *International Endodontic Journal*, vol. 42, no. 4, pp. 351–359, 2009.

[65] L. C. Souza, P. R. R. Brito, J. C. Machado de Oliveira et al., "Photodynamic therapy with two different photosensitizers as a supplement to instrumentation/irrigation procedures in promoting intracanal reduction of *Enterococcus faecalis*," *Journal of Endodontics*, vol. 36, no. 2, pp. 292–296, 2010.

[66] M. R. Nunes, I. Mello, G. C. N. Franco et al., "Effectiveness of photodynamic therapy against *Enterococcus faecalis*, with and without the use of an intracanal optical fiber: an in vitro study," *Photomedicine and Laser Surgery*, vol. 29, no. 12, pp. 803–808, 2011.

[67] C. Poggio, C. R. Arciola, A. Dagna et al., "Photoactivated disinfection (PAD) in endodontics: an in vitro microbiological evaluation," *International Journal of Artificial Organs*, vol. 34, no. 9, pp. 889–897, 2011.

[68] A. Rios, J. He, G. N. Glickman, R. Spears, E. D. Schneiderman, and A. L. Honeyman, "Evaluation of photodynamic therapy using a light-emitting diode lamp against enterococcus faecalis in extracted human teeth," *Journal of Endodontics*, vol. 37, no. 6, pp. 856–859, 2011.

[69] X. Cheng, S. Guan, H. Lu et al., "Evaluation of the bactericidal effect of Nd:YAG, Er:YAG, Er,Cr:YSGG laser radiation, and antimicrobial photodynamic therapy (aPDT) in experimentally infected root canals," *Lasers in Surgery and Medicine*, vol. 44, no. 10, pp. 824–831, 2012.

[70] S. Vaziri, A. Kangarlou, R. Shahbazi, A. Nazari Nasab, and M. Naseri, "Comparison of the bactericidal efficacy of photodynamic therapy, 2.5% sodium hypochlorite, and 2% chlorhexidine against *Enterococcous faecalis* in root canals; an in vitro study," *Dental Research Journal*, vol. 9, no. 5, pp. 613–618, 2012.

[71] R. T. Gergova, T. Gueorgieva, M. S. Dencheva-Garova et al., "Antimicrobial activity of different disinfection methods against biofilms in root canals," *Journal of Investigative and Clinical Dentistry*, 2015.

[72] Y. Wang, S. Xiao, D. Ma, X. Huang, and Z. Cai, "Minimizing concentration of sodium hypochlorite in root canal irrigation by combination of ultrasonic irrigation with photodynamic treatment," *Photochemistry and Photobiology*, vol. 91, no. 4, pp. 937–941, 2015.

[73] S. J. Bonsor, R. Nichol, T. M. S. Reid, and G. J. Pearson, "An alternative regimen for root canal disinfection," *British Dental Journal*, vol. 201, no. 2, pp. 101–105, 2006.

[74] A. S. Garcez, S. C. Nuñez, M. R. Hamblim, H. Suzuki, and M. S. Ribeiro, "Photodynamic therapy associated with conventional endodontic treatment in patients with antibiotic-resistant microflora: a preliminary report," *Journal of Endodontics*, vol. 36, no. 9, pp. 1463–1466, 2010.

[75] A. Prabhakar, C. Yavagal, S. Agarwal, N. Basappa, and S. Pradhan, "Antimicrobial effects of laser-assisted photodynamic therapy in pediatric endodontic treatment: a new clinical horizon," *International Journal of Laser Dentistry*, vol. 3, no. 3, pp. 77–81, 2013.

[76] I. B. Jurič, V. Plečko, D. G. Panduric, and I. Anič, "The antimicrobial effectiveness of photodynamic therapy used as an addition to the conventional endodontic re-treatment: a clinical study," *Photodiagnosis and Photodynamic Therapy*, vol. 11, no. 4, pp. 549–555, 2014.

[77] Z. Lim, J. L. Cheng, T. W. Lim et al., "Light activated disinfection: an alternative endodontic disinfection strategy," *Australian Dental Journal*, vol. 54, no. 2, pp. 108–114, 2009.

[78] R. Ng, F. Singh, D. A. Papamanou et al., "Endodontic photodynamic therapy ex vivo," *Journal of Endodontics*, vol. 37, no. 2, pp. 217–222, 2011.

[79] I. Bago, V. Plečko, D. G. Panduric, Z. Schauperl, A. Baraba, and I. Anić, "Antimicrobial efficacy of a high-power diode laser, photo-activated disinfection, conventional and sonic activated irrigation during root canal treatment," *International Endodontic Journal*, vol. 46, no. 4, pp. 339–347, 2013.

[80] S. Hecker, K.-A. Hiller, K. M. Galler, S. Erb, T. Mader, and G. Schmalz, "Establishment of an optimized ex vivo system for artificial root canal infection evaluated by use of sodium hypochlorite and the photodynamic therapy," *International Endodontic Journal*, vol. 46, no. 5, pp. 449–457, 2013.

[81] A. Xhevdet, D. Stubljar, I. Kriznar et al., "The disinfecting efficacy of root canals with laser photodynamic therapy," *Journal of Lasers in Medical Sciences*, vol. 5, no. 1, pp. 19–26, 2014.

[82] O. H. Muhammad, M. Chevalier, J.-P. Rocca, N. Brulat-Bouchard, and E. Medioni, "Photodynamic therapy versus ultrasonic irrigation: interaction with endodontic microbial biofilm, an ex vivo study," *Photodiagnosis and Photodynamic Therapy*, vol. 11, no. 2, pp. 171–181, 2014.

[83] S. George, A. Kishen, and K. P. Song, "The role of environmental changes on monospecies biofilm formation on root canal wall by *Enterococcus faecalis*," *Journal of Endodontics*, vol. 31, no. 12, pp. 867–872, 2005.

[84] L. Bergmans, P. Moisiadis, W. Teughels, B. Van Meerbeek, M. Quirynen, and P. Lambrechts, "Bactericidal effect of Nd:YAG laser irradiation on some endodontic pathogens ex vivo," *International Endodontic Journal*, vol. 39, no. 7, pp. 547–557, 2006.

[85] M. Wainwright, "The development of phenothiazinium photosensitisers," *Photodiagnosis and Photodynamic Therapy*, vol. 2, no. 4, pp. 263–272, 2005.

[86] M. Wainwright, D. A. Phoenix, J. Marland, D. R. A. Wareing, and F. J. Bolton, "A study of photobactericidal activity in the phenothiazinium series," *FEMS Immunology and Medical Microbiology*, vol. 19, no. 1, pp. 75–80, 1997.

[87] Z. Wang, Y. Shen, and M. Haapasalo, "Effectiveness of endodontic disinfecting solutions against young and old *Enterococcus faecalis* biofilms in dentin canals," *Journal of Endodontics*, vol. 38, no. 10, pp. 1376–1379, 2012.

[88] P. F. C. Menezes, C. A. S. Melo, V. S. Bagnato, H. Imasato, and J. R. Perussi, "Dark cytotoxicity of the photoproducts of the photosensitizer photogem after photobleaching induced by a laser," *Laser Physics*, vol. 15, no. 3, pp. 435–442, 2005.

[89] R. Ackroyd, C. Kelty, N. Brown, and M. Reed, "The history of photodetection and photodynamic therapy," *Photochemistry and Photobiology*, vol. 74, no. 5, pp. 656–669, 2001.

[90] L. Bergmans, P. Moisiadis, B. Huybrechts, B. Van Meerbeek, M. Quirynen, and P. Lambrechts, "Effect of photo-activated disinfection on endodontic pathogens ex vivo," *International Endodontic Journal*, vol. 41, no. 3, pp. 227–239, 2008.

[91] M. A. Meire, T. Coenye, H. J. Nelis, and R. J. G. De Moor, "Evaluation of Nd: YAG and Er: YAG irradiation, antibacterial photodynamic therapy and sodium hypochlorite treatment on *Enterococcus faecalis* biofilms," *International Endodontic Journal*, vol. 45, no. 5, pp. 482–491, 2012.

[92] E. Berutti, R. Marini, and A. Angeretti, "Penetration ability of different irrigants into dentinal tubules," *Journal of Endodontics*, vol. 23, no. 12, pp. 725–727, 1997.

[93] L. B. Peters, P. R. Wesselink, J. F. Buijs, and A. J. Van Winkelhoff, "Viable bacteria in root dentinal tubules of teeth with apical periodontitis," *Journal of Endodontics*, vol. 27, no. 2, pp. 76–81, 2001.

[94] B. P. F. A. Gomes, C. C. R. Ferraz, M. E. Vianna, V. B. Berber, F. B. Teixeira, and F. J. de Souza-Filho, "*In vitro* antimicrobial activity of several concentrations of sodium hypochlorite and chlorhexidine gluconate in the elimination of *Enterococcus faecalis*," *International Endodontic Journal*, vol. 34, no. 6, pp. 424–428, 2001.

[95] C. H. Stuart, S. A. Schwartz, T. J. Beeson, and C. B. Owatz, "*Enterococcus faecalis*: its role in root canal treatment failure and current concepts in retreatment," *Journal of Endodontics*, vol. 32, no. 2, pp. 93–98, 2006.

[96] R. A. Figueiredo, L. C. Anami, I. Mello, E. D. S. Carvalho, S. M. Habitante, and D. P. Raldi, "Tooth discoloration induced by endodontic phenothiazine dyes in photodynamic therapy," *Photomedicine and Laser Surgery*, vol. 32, no. 8, pp. 458–462, 2014.

[97] D. Lins de Sousa, R. Araújo Lima, I. C. Zanin et al., "Effect of twice-daily blue Light treatment on matrix-rich biofilm development," *PLoS ONE*, vol. 10, no. 7, Article ID e0131941, 2015.

[98] K. Konopka and T. Goslinski, "Photodynamic therapy in dentistry," *Journal of Dental Research*, vol. 86, no. 8, pp. 694–707, 2007.

[99] M. Wilson, "Lethal photosensitisation of oral bacteria and its potential application in the photodynamic therapy of oral infections," *Photochemical and Photobiological Sciences*, vol. 3, no. 5, pp. 412–418, 2004.

[100] M. H. Upadya and A. Kishen, "Influence of bacterial growth modes on the susceptibility to light-activated disinfection," *International Endodontic Journal*, vol. 43, no. 11, pp. 978–987, 2010.

[101] A. Shrestha and A. Kishen, "The effect of tissue inhibitors on the antibacterial activity of chitosan nanoparticles and photodynamic therapy," *Journal of Endodontics*, vol. 38, no. 9, pp. 1275–1278, 2012.

[102] T. C. Pagonis, J. Chen, C. R. Fontana et al., "Nanoparticle-based endodontic antimicrobial photodynamic therapy," *Journal of Endodontics*, vol. 36, no. 2, pp. 322–328, 2010.

[103] S. George and A. Kishen, "Influence of photosensitizer solvent on the mechanisms of photoactivated killing of *Enterococcus faecalis*," *Photochemistry and Photobiology*, vol. 84, no. 3, pp. 734–740, 2008.

[104] A. Shrestha, M. R. Hamblin, and A. Kishen, "Photoactivated rose bengal functionalized chitosan nanoparticles produce antibacterial/biofilm activity and stabilize dentin-collagen," *Nanomedicine: Nanotechnology, Biology, and Medicine*, vol. 10, no. 3, pp. 491–501, 2014.

9

Clinical Advantages and Limitations of Monolithic Zirconia Restorations Full Arch Implant Supported Reconstruction: Case Series

Joao Carames,[1] **Loana Tovar Suinaga,**[2] **Yung Cheng Paul Yu,**[2] **Alejandro Pérez,**[2] **and Mary Kang**[2]

[1]*Faculty of Dental Medicine at the University of Lisbon, Lisbon, Portugal*
[2]*Ashman Department of Periodontology and Implant Dentistry, New York University College of Dentistry, 345 East 24th Street, Suite 3W, New York, NY 10010, USA*

Correspondence should be addressed to Alejandro Pérez; apa270@nyu.edu

Academic Editor: Sang-Choon Cho

Purpose. The purpose of this retrospective case series is to evaluate the clinical advantages and limitations of monolithic zirconia restorations for full arch implant supported restorations and report the rate of complications up to 2 years after insertion. *Materials and Methods.* Fourteen patients received implant placement for monolithic zirconia full arch reconstructions. Four implants were placed in seven arches, eleven arches received six implants, two arches received seven implants, two arches received eight implants, and one arch received nine implants. *Results.* No implant failures or complications were reported for an implant survival rate of 100% with follow-up ranging from 3 to 24 months. *Conclusions.* Monolithic zirconia CAD-/CAM-milled framework restorations are a treatment option for full arch restorations over implants, showing a 96% success rate in the present study. Some of the benefits are accuracy, reduced veneering porcelain, and minimal occlusal adjustments. The outcome of the present study showed high success in function, aesthetics, phonetics, and high patient satisfaction.

1. Introduction

Full arch implant supported restorations have been documented to have high success rates [1–6]. Many combinations of materials have been used for this type of restorations such as metal alloy-acrylic, metal alloy-composite, and metal alloy-ceramic [1, 5, 7]. However, complications including fractured or debonded acrylic resin teeth, wear of opposing surfaces, ceramic chipping, difficulty in shade matching of acrylic and pink ceramic, lack of passive fit, and extensive work for repair after framework breakage have encouraged dentists to look for other material options [1, 5, 7]. The use of zirconia for frameworks is an option that has been proposed [2, 7, 8].

Zirconium oxide is a material that has shown increased popularity in contemporary dentistry [3, 9]. Many studies have shown excellent physical, mechanical, biological, and chemical properties of this material [3, 5, 9, 10]. Fixed dental prostheses were designed and milled in a one-piece zirconia substructure and veneering porcelain was then directly fired onto the substructure [3, 4]. Nevertheless, some reports have documented veneering ceramic fractures (chipping) [1–12] and fractures of the zirconia substructure [1, 3–5].

To overcome these problems, CAD/CAM one-block milled monolithic zirconia was introduced as an alternative for the treatment of implant supported full arch reconstructions [3–5, 12]. The fabrication of the structure in one block reduces breakage possibilities and avoids chipping [4, 5]. Moreover, high strength, minimal occlusal adjustment, and accuracy are some of its advantages [3, 4, 6, 13].

Short-term available data indicates that full contour zirconia framework can be used successfully in implant dentistry [3, 7]. Seven articles involving full contour zirconia restorations have been published (Table 1). Five articles were

TABLE 1: Literatures of monolithic zirconia.

Author	Publication date	Study type	N (number of arches)
Papaspyridakos and Lal [12]	2008	Case report	1
Lazetera [13]	2009	Case report	1
Papaspyridakos and Lal [9]	2010	Case report	1
Larsson et al. [11]	2010	Prospective study	10
Rojas-Vizcaya [1]	2011	Case report	2
Sadid-Zadeh et al. [5]	2013	Case report	1
Pozzi et al. [10]	2013	Retrospective study	26

case reports [1, 5, 9, 12, 13]. One retrospective study with 3- to 5-year follow-up was published in 2013 [10], and one prospective study with 3-year follow up was published in 2010 [11]. Further research is required to evaluate the long-term outcome of monolithic zirconia restorations. Studies of material inherent accelerated aging [3] and wear of opposing dentition are necessary [5].

The purpose of this retrospective case series was to evaluate the clinical advantages and limitations of monolithic zirconia restorations for full arch implant supported restorations and report the rate of complications up to 2 years after insertion.

2. Materials and Methods

Clinical data in this study was obtained from the implant database (ID) in the Ashman Department of Periodontology and Implant Dentistry at New York University College of Dentistry. This dataset was extracted as deidentified information from the routine treatment of patients in the department. The ID was certified by the Office of Quality Assurance at NYUCD. This study is in compliance with the health insurance portability and accountability act (HIPAA).

2.1. Study Subjects. Patients which referred to New York University Ashman Department of Periodontology and Implant Dentistry in need of prosthetic full arch fixed reconstruction in maxilla, mandible, or both were consecutively selected. The inclusion criteria included patients at least 21 years old, with edentulous maxilla and/or mandible and at least four to nine implants needed to be placed and osseointegrated. Fourteen patients (Four females and ten males with a mean age of 56 years old, range: 37–67) met the inclusion criteria. Each subject selected for this study from the ID had undergone the fabrication of monolithic zirconia frameworks for full arch implant supported reconstructions. Twelve of these patients required maxillary and mandibular full arch reconstruction, and two involved only the maxillary arch. In the two maxillary reconstructions the opposing dentition was in one patient natural teeth and a fixed prosthesis and in the other a complete mandibular denture. A total of twenty-six edentulous arches were restored: fourteen maxillary and twelve mandibular arches. Patients were informed about the prosthetic protocol, risks, and alternatives of treatment.

All complications after delivery were recorded at each follow-up visit up to 3 years. Failures were defined as any defect in the restorations that required the fabrication of

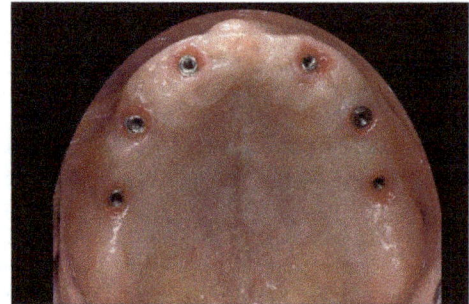

FIGURE 1: Maxillary occlusal view after tissue healing.

a new restoration such as fracture and misfitting. Complications were defined as any defect in the restorations that required repair by laboratory technicians or correction of clinicians such as chipping of veneers (lab) and screw loosening (clinician).

2.2. Procedures

(1) Diagnostic alginate impressions (Jeltrate Plus, Denstply, Milford, DE, USA) were made and poured with model stone (Microstone ISO type 3, WhipMix, Louisville, KY, USA). Occlusal rims were fabricated and adjusted intraorally. Interocclusal records, face bow registration, and centric relation records were taken. Casts were articulated and artificial teeth arrangements (ATA) were performed. Additionally, ATA were duplicated to obtain radiographic and surgical guides. Patients were sent for Cone Beam Computed Tomography (CBCT) scans to evaluate bone dimension and implant positioning (Figures 2 and 3).

(2) Four to nine dental implants were placed in the edentulous arches using surgical guides. A one-stage surgical procedure was performed according to the implant planning. The surgical protocol followed the manufacturer's instructions. External connection implants were placed in twenty-three arches, and internal connection implants with intermediate abutments were placed in three arches. The healing time prior to the prosthetic phase was 12 weeks. (Figure 1).

(3) During the healing period and until the prosthetic phase was completed, patients wore transitional complete dentures.

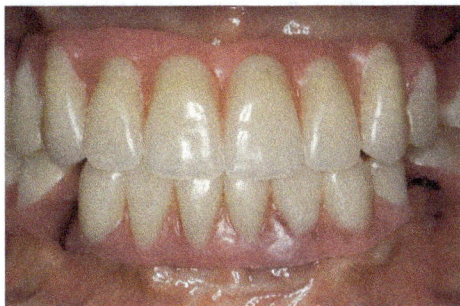

FIGURE 2: Intraoral frontal view of artificial teeth arrangement.

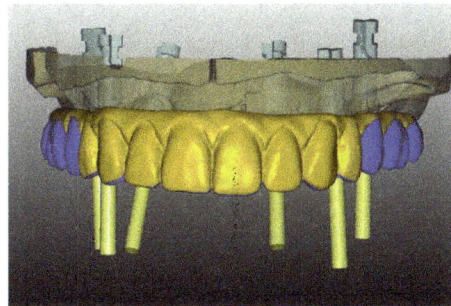

FIGURE 4: Digital preview of the maxillary monolithic prosthesis.

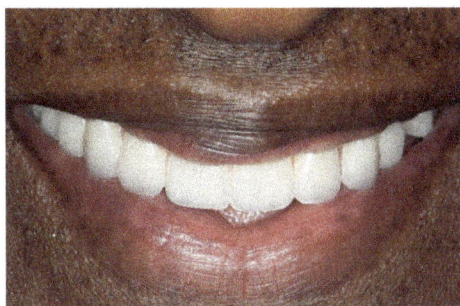

FIGURE 3: Smile view with artificial teeth arrangement.

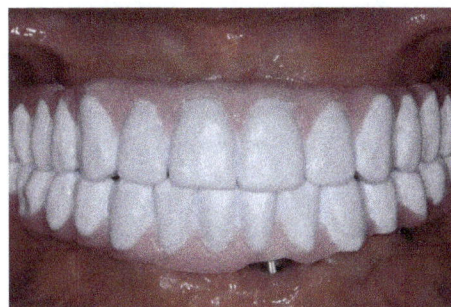

FIGURE 5: Intraoral frontal view with the epoxy resin prototype.

(4) Fixture level impressions were made of polyether impression material (Impregum, 3M ESPE, St. Paul, MN, USA) in custom light cure resin trays (TRIAD Blue TruTray Visible Light Cure, Dentsply, York, PA, USA). The master cast was made of a reproduction of the gingival soft tissue using a polyvinylsiloxane, addition-type silicone (GI-Mask, Coltene/Whaledent, Cuyahoga Falls, OH, USA) and resin fortified, low expansion die stone (ResinRock ISO Type 4, WhipMix, Louisville, KY, USA). In two patients, in which opposing arches were not restored as full arch reconstructions, alginate impressions were made (Jeltrate Plus, Dentsply, Milford, DE, USA) with stock disposable perforated trays (COE Spacer trays, GC America Inc, Chicago, IL, USA). Interocclusal registrations were made with wax rims (TRIAD Pink Denture Base Regular Pink Fibered, York, PA, USA and Pink Wax Bite Blocks, Keystone, Cherry Hill, NJ, USA). Face bow registration and centric relation record were taken. Artificial teeth arrangements with acrylic dentures teeth (Portrait IPN Dentsply, Milford, DE, USA) were placed in an adequate position to achieve esthetics, phonetics, and vertical dimension in occlusion. Bite registration was taken with vinyl polysiloxane material (BLU Bite HP, Henry Schein, Melville, NY, USA).

(5) The laboratory procedures were performed according to the manufacturer's instructions (Zirconia Prettau, Zirkonzahn, Neuler, Germany) at an authorized laboratory. The master cast, opposing cast articulated, and artificial teeth arrangement were scanned to determine the interocclusal relationship to the software (Zirkonzahn.software, Zirkonzahn, Neuler, Germany). According to the corresponding implant type, connectors are milled in titanium to fit in the master cast and scanned again. The prostheses were designed on the software. An epoxy resin prototype was milled and sent for try-in to ensure adequate fit, function, esthetics, and phonetics. After some minor adjustments, the restoration was milled in a monolithic zirconia block. Sixteen of the 26 full arch restorations were digitally cut back on the anterior area to improve esthetics. Characterizations of teeth were made in the monolithic framework (Colour Liquid Prettau, Zirkonzahn, Neuler, Germany). The final restorations were sintered in the oven (Keromikofen 1500, Zirkonzahn, Neuler, Germany). Framework fitting was verified in the master cast. Soft tissue ceramic (ICE Zirkon Keramik Tissue Shades, Zirkonzahn, Neuler, Germany) and ceramic (ICE Zirkon Ceramics and Stains Prettau, Zirkonzahn, Neuler, Germany) according to the shade selection was applied on the framework for esthetic results. Additionally, the prosthesis was sintered overnight. Last working step was placement and bonding of the titanium sleeves into the milled zirconia framework. Finally, prostheses were glaze-fired and sent for delivery. (Figures 4, 5, 6, 7,8, and 9).

(6) The final full arch prostheses were clinically verified with one screw test for passive fit. Moreover, periapical radiographs were taken for radiographic examination. All patients approved and agreed with shape and shade of finals restorations. (Figures 10, 11, and 12).

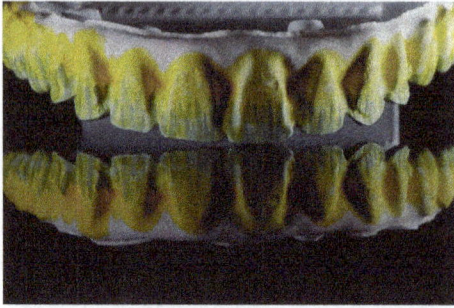

FIGURE 6: Maxillary monolithic prosthesis with teeth characterization.

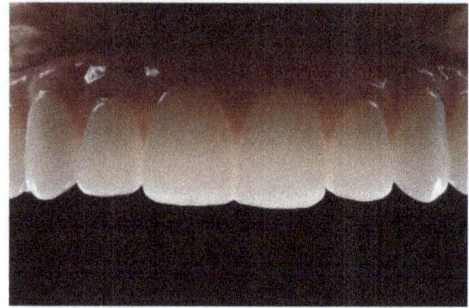

FIGURE 9: Translucency effect in the anterior maxilla after application of ceramics in the digital cut back.

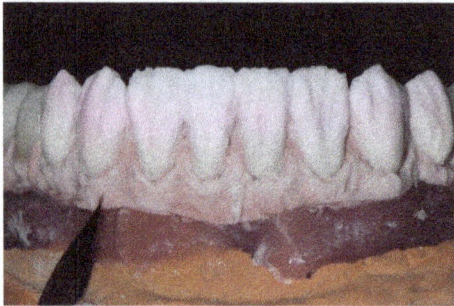

FIGURE 7: Ceramic application for gingiva colors and teeth ceramic.

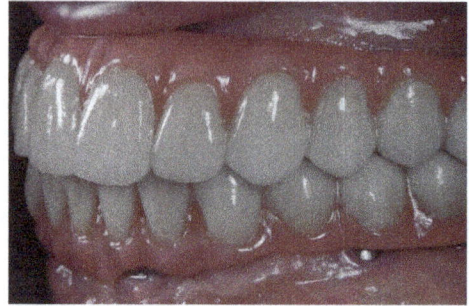

FIGURE 10: Intraoral lateral view of the final prostheses.

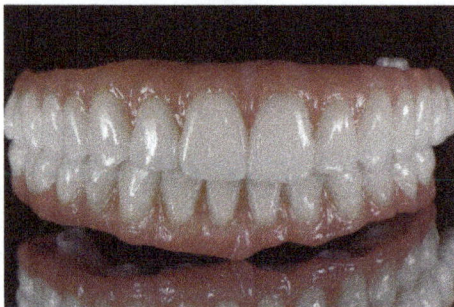

FIGURE 8: Prostheses after final sintering.

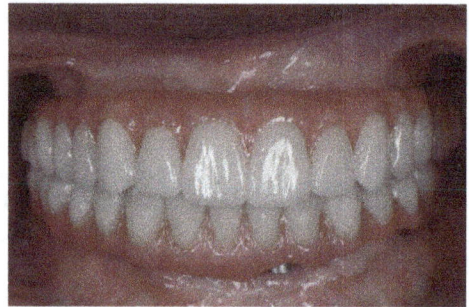

FIGURE 11: Intraoral frontal view of the final prostheses.

(7) Occlusal screws were torqued following manufacturer's instructions. Gutta-percha was placed in all access holes. In screw-retained restorations, a light-cure microhybrid composite (Z100 Restorative, 3M, St Paul, MN, USA) with proper shade was used to close the access hole. In screw-/cement-retained, fixed prostheses were cemented with temporary cement (TempBond, Kerr, Orange, CA, USA) and excesses were cleaned. The importance of removing the temporary cement and recementing every year, to avoid cement wear and loosening of the prostheses, was explained to the patients.

(8) On the day of delivery, alginate impressions were made to fabricate full-cover maxillary night guards. A week later, patients received the night guards and were instructed to wear them at night.

(9) Recall appointments were performed after 2 weeks and 3 months after insertion. A yearly appointment is required for clinical and radiographic examination.

3. Results

Fourteen patients received implant placement for monolithic zirconia full arch reconstructions. Four implants were placed in seven arches, eleven arches received six implants, two arches received seven implants, two arches received eight implants, and one arch received nine implants. No implant failures or complications were reported for an implant survival rate of 100% with follow-up ranging from 3 to 24 months (Table 2).

Previous restorations of the total arches were as follows: sixteen had nonrestorable teeth or previously failed fixed prostheses, five arches with teeth and removable partial

TABLE 2: Results of 14 cases in which monolithic zirconia framework for full arch implant supported reconstruction was used.

Subjects	Location	Number of implants	Type of restoration	Time of follow-up	Complications
1	Mandible	4	Screw-retained	10 months	None
	Maxilla	6	Screw-retained	10 months	None
2	Mandible	4	Screw-retained	1 year, 10 months	None
	Maxilla	7	Screw-retained	1 year, 10 months	None
3	Mandible	6	Screw-retained	1 year, 8 months	None
	Maxilla	6	Screw-retained	1 year, 8 months	None
4	Mandible	4	Screw-retained	5 months	None
	Maxilla	6	Screw-retained	5 months	None
5	Mandible	6	Screw-retained	1 year	None
	Maxilla	6	Screw-retained	1 year	None
6	Mandible	4	Screw-retained	7 months	None
	Maxilla	6	Screw-retained	7 months	None
7	Mandible	4	Screw-retained	3 months	None
	Maxilla	4	Screw-retained	3 months	None
8	Mandible	4	Screw-retained	1 year, 3 months	None
	Maxilla	8	Screw-retained	1 year, 3 months	Chipping #9, at 1-year follow-up
9	Mandible	6	Screw-retained	10 months	None
	Maxilla	7	Screw-retained	10 months	None
10	Mandible	6	Screw-retained	2 years	None
	Maxilla	8	Screw-retained	2 years	None
11	Mandible	7	Screw- and cement-retained	3 years, 6 months	None
	Maxilla	8	Screw- and cement-retained	3 years, 6 months	None
12	Maxilla	8	Screw-retained	3 years, 6 months	None
13	Maxilla	9	Screw-retained	1 year	None
14	Maxilla	6	Screw-retained	4 months	None
	Mandible	6	Screw-retained	4 months	None

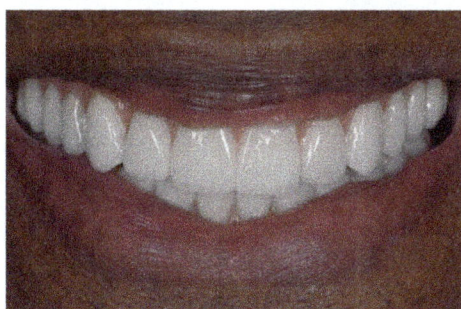

FIGURE 12: Smile view of the final prostheses.

dentures, three complete dentures, and two metal alloy-acrylic prostheses.

Of the twenty-six full arches, twenty-four were implant supported screw-retained, and two full arches were combined implant supported screw-/cement-retained (Table 2). Seventeen full arch restorations were digitally cut back on the buccal surface of the anterior area to improve esthetics. Nine full arch restorations were designed without veneering porcelain. All prostheses were in function at the time of the follow-up, which was from 3 months up to 3 years and 6 months, whereas fourteen arches were followed up up to 1 year. All monolithic zirconia prostheses were clinically and radiographically examined. No defects of the prosthesis were detected and no frameworks needed to be remade. However, a chip-off fracture of the ceramic veneer occurred in 1 of 26 restorations (Table 2, case #8), giving a prosthetic success rate of 96%. The only chip-off fracture occurred in the buccal surface of the veneer in a left central incisor after one year of insertion. A ceramic laminate was used to restore the chip-off. No fracture of the monolithic zirconia frameworks or any other mechanical complications such as screw loosening or decementation of the prostheses were reported. No patient complaints regarding their prosthesis esthetic or function were record.

4. Discussion

Improved clinical performance can be expected to be achieved by using monolithic zirconia restorations [2, 10, 11]. Clinical studies have shown increased values of strength and toughness for monolithic zirconia compared to zirconia frameworks with laminate veneering [3, 5]. It has also been shown to result in high standards of esthetics and a reduced amount of metal used in the oral cavity [5, 10]. Full arch monolithic zirconia restorations have shown similar overall survival when compared with high-nobel alloy-based metal ceramic restorations [14]. No bulk fractures or failures in the framework had been reported in the literature with a follow-up of 8 years [2]. The result of the present retrospective case series is in accordance with these trends as no flaws in the monolithic framework occurred during the follow-up examinations.

Several different complications have been related to the use of hybrid prostheses with implants, such as fractures of titanium framework and gold alloys over 5 years [15] and fracture or wear of acrylic teeth due to poor bonding of acrylic to the framework [16]. With ceramometal restorations, chipping or fracture of the ceramic is due to different factors. These include impact and fatigue load, occlusal forces, differences in thermal expansion coefficients, low elastic modulus of the metal, improper design, microdefects, and trauma. Extensive work for repair is required after framework failures [1]. A full monolithic zirconia occlusal contour appears to be a solution to this complication [5, 9, 11, 12]. The present study supports these findings, as twenty-five of 26 monolithic zirconia restorations presented no complications during the follow-up period.

However, chipping of veneering ceramic is a frequent complication of zirconia-based restorations on teeth and implants [3, 4, 7, 9, 11] and sometimes cannot be solved by ceramic polishing [10]. The exact reason for veneer chipping in zirconia core restorations is unclear. Three factors generally play an important role such as interfacial bonding, match of the core-veneer materials, and strength of the veneering ceramic. Also the veneering technique has a potential effect on the chipping of the ceramic due to the processing methods of ceramic, which include repeated sintering in the oven [4]. To overcome chipping fractures of veneered zirconia restorations, laboratory technicians and clinicians should follow precise steps in manufacturing zirconia-based restorations with the knowledge that zirconia as a framework material is highly susceptible to surface modifications and improper laboratory and clinical handling technique [3]. Chip-off fractures of the veneering ceramics have been associated with roughness of the veneering ceramic because of grinding or occlusal function [3, 11]. Analysis of crack propagation direction showed that the chipping failure had originated from roughness of the ceramic at the occlusal region of the cusps. Occlusal adjustments should only be performed with fine grain diamonds, followed by thorough polishing sequence [3]. The use of digital cut back in the monolithic zirconia prevents roughness on the surface that produces the crack propagation and chipping of the veneering. In reference to the present study, of the seventeen arches that were digitally cut back in the anterior area, only one veneer chipping was recorded at 1-year follow-up.

Translucency has been considered one of the primary factors in controlling the esthetic outcome of ceramic restorations. Zirconia has been considered an opaque material compared to other dental ceramic. A recent report has shown some degree of translucency in the zirconia, which was less sensitive to thickness compared to lithium disilicate and leucite-free porcelain. However, translucency of the zirconia ceramics also increased exponentially as the thickness decreased [17]. The digital cut back in the monolithic zirconia allows the restorations to have some degree of translucency. One of the problems with glass ceramics for monolithic restorations is that due to low flexural strength values (360–400 MPa for lithium disilicate) frameworks are prone to fracture when subjected to occlusal loads. Moreover, the use of zirconia frameworks with glass ceramic veneers has been described to have high rates of chipping. In our study zirconia veneers in monolithic restorations resulted in high esthetic, good mechanical properties, and less complications.

Wear rates of the enamel opposing zirconia ceramic have been reported, showing cracks or even fractures in all the ridges. The hardness and thickness of enamel, chewing behavior, parafunctional habits, and neuromuscular forces as well as abrasive nature of food can influence clinical wear. Due to the elasticity modulus of 210 GPa of zirconia and hardness of 1200 Vickers Hardness, some enamel wear is expected. Moreover, some reports have shown that polished monolithic zirconia has the lowest wear rate on an enamel antagonist compared to veneered zirconia, glazed zirconia using a glaze spray, monolithic base alloy, or glazed zirconia using glaze ceramic [18, 19]. However, the use of night guard is recommended after the delivery of the final monolithic zirconia to prevent wear of the opposing dentition.

Screw-retained implant restorations are often chosen because they offer better retrievability, decreased space requirements, and healthier soft tissue. On the other hand, cement-retained restorations offer improved occlusal accuracy, enhanced esthetics, increased chances of achieving a passive fit, and decreased instances of retention loss [18]. Moreover, some systematic reviews have shown that differences between cement- and screw-retained restorations are not statistically significant. These reports concluded that screw-retained restorations are equally suitable [18–20]. However, the preferred technique in this study was screw-retained implant restoration due to their retrievability, less biological complications, and easy repair of technical complications. In accordance to this idea, 88% of the restorations in this study were screw-retained. No complications such as screw loosening or decementation were reported in the present study. And only one veneer chipping was found after 1-year follow-up.

5. Conclusions

(1) Monolithic zirconia CAD/CAM-milled framework restorations are a treatment option for full arch restorations over implants, showing a 96% success rate in the present study. Some of the benefits are accuracy, reduced veneering porcelain, and minimal occlusal adjustments. The outcome of the present study showed high success in function, aesthetics, phonetics, and high patient satisfaction.

(2) A full occlusal contour monolithic framework can diminish chipping of the veneered porcelain. However, the fabrication is technique sensitive and should follow the appropriate steps discussed in this study.

(3) The digital cut back for veneer placement in the monolithic zirconia was an effective option to avoid surface roughness that can produce crack propagation and veneer chipping.

(4) Twenty-three of 26 restorations were screw-retained due to their retrievability, less biological complications, and easy repair of technical complications. Only, one veneer chipping was found in one these restorations. Of the three cement-retained restorations no complications were reported.

(5) Within the limitations of the present study monolithic zirconia CAD/CAM milled prosthetic restorations were a successful treatment option for full arch implants supported restorations.

(6) More long-term data studies are required for the full arch monolithic zirconia restorations in order to evaluate success and complications over the time.

Conflict of Interests

The authors reported no conflict of interests related to this study.

References

[1] F. Rojas-Vizcaya, "Full zirconia fixed detachable implant-retained restorations manufactured from monolithic zirconia: clinical report after two years in service," *Journal of Prosthodontics*, vol. 20, no. 7, pp. 570–576, 2011.

[2] C. Larsson and P. V. von Steyern, "Implant-supported full-arch zirconia-based mandibular fixed dental prostheses. Eight-year results from a clinical pilot study," *Acta Odontologica Scandinavica*, vol. 71, no. 5, pp. 1118–1122, 2013.

[3] P. C. Guess, W. Att, and J. R. Strub, "Zirconia in fixed implant prosthodontics," *Clinical Implant Dentistry and Related Research*, vol. 14, no. 5, pp. 633–645, 2012.

[4] B. Kanat, E. M. Çömlekoğlu, M. Dündar-Çömlekoğlu, B. Hakan Sen, M. Özcan, and M. Ali Güngör, "Effect of various veneering techniques on mechanical strength of computer-controlled zirconia framework designs," *Journal of Prosthodontics*, vol. 23, no. 6, pp. 445–455, 2014.

[5] R. Sadid-Zadeh, P. R. Liu, R. Aponte-Wesson, and S. J. O'Neal, "Maxillary cement retained implant supported monolithic zirconia prosthesis in a full mouth rehabilitation: a clinical report," *Journal of Advanced Prosthodontics*, vol. 5, no. 2, pp. 209–217, 2013.

[6] H. H. Zaghloul and J. F. Younis, "Marginal fit of implant-supported all-ceramic zirconia frameworks," *Journal of Oral Implantology*, vol. 39, no. 4, pp. 417–424, 2013.

[7] B. Limmer, A. E. Sanders, G. Reside, and L. F. Cooper, "Complications and patient-centered outcomes with an implant-supported monolithic zirconia fixed dental prosthesis: 1 year results," *Journal of Prosthodontics*, vol. 23, no. 4, pp. 267–275, 2014.

[8] J. Oliva, X. Oliva, and J. D. Oliva, "All-on-three delayed implant loading concept for the completely edentulous maxilla and mandible: a retrospective 5-year follow-up study," *The International Journal of Oral & Maxillofacial Implants*, vol. 27, no. 6, pp. 1584–1592, 2012.

[9] P. Papaspyridakos and K. Lal, "Immediate loading of the maxilla with prefabricated interim prosthesis using interactive planning software, and CAD/CAM rehabilitation with definitive zirconia prosthesis: 2-year clinical follow-up," *Journal of Esthetic and Restorative Dentistry*, vol. 22, no. 4, pp. 223–234, 2010.

[10] A. Pozzi, S. Holst, G. Fabbri, and M. Tallarico, "Clinical reliability of CAD/CAM cross-arch zirconia bridges on immediately loaded implants placed with computer-assisted/template-guided surgery: a retrospective study with a follow-up between 3 and 5 years," *Clinical Implant Dentistry and Related Research*, 2013.

[11] C. Larsson, P. Vult von Steyern, and K. Nilner, "A prospective study of implant-supported full-arch yttria-stabilized tetragonal zirconia polycrystal mandibular fixed dental prostheses: three-year results," *The International Journal of Prosthodontics*, vol. 23, no. 4, pp. 364–369, 2010.

[12] P. Papaspyridakos and K. Lal, "Complete arch implant rehabilitation using subtractive rapid prototyping and porcelain fused to zirconia prosthesis: a clinical report," *Journal of Prosthetic Dentistry*, vol. 100, no. 3, pp. 165–172, 2008.

[13] A. Lazetera, "Extreme class II full arch zirconia implant bridge," *Australasian Dental Practice*, vol. 7, pp. 170–174, 2009.

[14] S. D. Heintze and V. Rousson, "Survival of zirconia- and metal-supported fixed dental prostheses: a systematic review," *The International Journal of Prosthodontics*, vol. 23, no. 6, pp. 493–502, 2010.

[15] B. Bergendal and S. Palmqvist, "Laser-welded titanium frameworks for implant-supported fixed prostheses: a 5-year report," *The International Journal of Oral & Maxillofacial Implants*, vol. 14, no. 1, pp. 69–71, 1999.

[16] A. Ortorp and T. Jemt, "Clinical experiences of CNC-milled titanium frameworks supported by implants in the edentulous jaw: 1-year prospective study," *Clinical Implant Dentistry and Related Research*, vol. 2, no. 1, pp. 2–9, 2000.

[17] F. Wang, H. Takahashi, and N. Iwasaki, "Translucency of dental ceramics with different thicknesses," *Journal of Prosthetic Dentistry*, vol. 110, no. 1, pp. 14–20, 2013.

[18] S. Sherif, H. K. Susarla, T. Kapos, D. Munoz, B. M. Chang, and R. F. Wright, "A systematic review of screw-versus cement-retained implant-supported fixed restorations," *Journal of Prosthodontics*, vol. 23, no. 1, pp. 1–9, 2014.

[19] J. Nissan, D. Narobai, O. Gross, O. Ghelfan, and G. Chaushu, "Long-term outcome of cemented versus screw-retained implant-supported partial restorations," *The International Journal of Oral & Maxillofacial Implants*, vol. 26, no. 5, pp. 1102–1107, 2011.

[20] I. Sailer, S. Mühlemann, M. Zwahlen, C. H. F. Hämmerle, and D. Schneider, "Cemented and screw-retained implant reconstructions: a systematic review of the survival and complication rates," *Clinical Oral Implants Research*, vol. 23, no. 6, pp. 163–201, 2012.

10

Association between IFN-γ +874A/T and IFN-γR1 (-611A/G, +189T/G, and +95C/T) Gene Polymorphisms and Chronic Periodontitis in a Sample of Iranian Population

Zahra Heidari,[1,2] **Hamidreza Mahmoudzadeh-Sagheb,**[1,2] **Mohammad Hashemi,**[3,4]
Somayeh Ansarimoghaddam,[5] **Bita Moudi,**[1,2] **and Nadia Sheibak**[2]

[1]*Infectious Diseases and Tropical Medicine Research Center, Zahedan University of Medical Sciences,*
 Zahedan 98167-43175, Iran
[2]*Department of Histology, School of Medicine, Zahedan University of Medical Sciences, Zahedan 98167-43175, Iran*
[3]*Cellular and Molecular Research Center, Zahedan University of Medical Sciences, Zahedan 98167-43175, Iran*
[4]*Department of Clinical Biochemistry, School of Medicine, Zahedan University of Medical Sciences and Health Services,*
 Zahedan 98167-43175, Iran
[5]*Department of Periodontology, School of Dentistry, Zahedan University of Medical Sciences, Zahedan 98167-43175, Iran*

Correspondence should be addressed to Hamidreza Mahmoudzadeh-Sagheb; histology@ymail.com

Academic Editor: Tommaso Lombardi

Background. Interferon gamma (IFN-γ) is an immune regulatory cytokine that acts through its receptor and plays important role in progression of inflammatory disease such as chronic periodontitis (CP). The purpose of this study was to determine the differences in the distribution of IFN-γ (+874A/T) and IFN-γR1 (-611A/G, +189T/G, and +95C/T) gene polymorphisms among CP and healthy individuals and to investigate relationships between these polymorphisms and susceptibility to CP. *Materials and Methods.* 310 individuals were enrolled in the study including 210 CP patients and 100 healthy controls. Single nucleotide polymorphisms at IFN-γ (+874A/T) and IFN-γR1 (-611A/G, +189T/G, and +95C/T) were analyzed by ARMS-PCR and PCR-RFLP methods. *Results.* The significant difference was found in genotype and allele frequency of IFN-γ (+874A/T) gene polymorphism in chronic periodontitis patients and healthy controls. The distribution of genotypes and allele frequencies for IFN-γR1 (-611A/G, +189T/G, and +95C/T) were similar among the groups and no differences in the frequencies of alleles or genotypes of IFN-γR1 genetic polymorphisms variants between case and control groups were detected. *Conclusion.* The finding of this study showed that IFN-γ +874A/T gene polymorphism may affect susceptibility to CP, whereas IFN-γR1 genetic polymorphisms at -611A/G, +189T/G, and +95C/T were not associated with this disease.

1. Introduction

Chronic periodontitis (CP) is a multifactorial inflammatory disease that is initiated by the accumulation of dental plaque and destroys the dental attachment apparatus. The interaction of this bacterial biofilm with the host immune system induces inflammation and immune responses, which lead to progressive attachment loss, bone loss, and eventually tooth loss. This common complex infectious disease affects 10–15 percent of the adult population [1–4].

The host inflammatory immune reaction, genetic factors, and environmental factors affect the risk of developing periodontitis. Recent studies have demonstrated that elevated levels of inflammatory biomarkers and genetic variants of some cytokines could cause susceptibility to periodontitis [4–7].

Increase of cytokines such as interferons (IFNs) has been found in infected human periodontium and their levels can be associated with progression of lesions and severity of inflammatory diseases. Interferons are a large family of cytokines that acts against viruses, tumors, and cell proliferation and acts as immunomodulatory factors [8–10].

Type II IFN (interferon-gamma) that is encoded by the interferon-gamma (IFN-γ) gene has stronger imunomodulatory effects than type I IFN (interferon-alpha) and plays important roles in periodontal tissue destruction [10].

IFN-γ also activates macrophages and is a regulatory cytokine in the process of immune reaction. Although interferon-α and interferon-β can be secreted by all cells, IFN-γ is expressed by CD4+ Th1 cells, cytotoxic CD8 cells, activated NK cells, mononuclear cells, and dendritic cells found in periodontal tissues. The molecular signaling pathways that lead to chronic elevation of IFN-γ expression in periodontal diseases are still the subject of investigation [8, 9].

Binding of IFN-γ to its heterodimeric receptor complex induces cellular activation and upregulation of specific genes [11–13].

This complex consists of two or more subunits IFN-γR1 (ligand-binding subunit) and IFN-γR2 (transmembrane accessory factor) that are encoded by chromosome 21. It is believed that both parts of the receptor complex are necessary for normal signaling. Dimerization of IFN-γR1 is facilitated by binding of homodimeric IFN-γ with association of IFN-γR2. Based on the evidence interaction of IFN-γ with both subunits of the receptor causes association of these parts. Cellular activation of IFN-γ may be induced in lower levels through an additional receptor, which is still unknown [12, 13].

The place of IFN-γR expression is on nucleated cells such as some immune cells, endothelial cells, and fibroblasts [14].

The producing cell type, the nature of the stimulus, and the genetic background may influence cytokine secretion levels [7, 15].

The expression of IFN-γ is considerable because of its elevated transcriptional and translational expression in inflamed gingival tissues and gingival crevicular fluid (GCF). Reports have demonstrated that genetic factors may play an important role in the risk of periodontal diseases [7, 9, 16].

Focus of most genetic research in periodontitis is on gene polymorphisms. Polymorphisms, probably occurring at regulatory regions of cytokine genes, may increase susceptibility to some infectious diseases and influence the course and prognosis of the disease [7, 17].

The IFN-γ gene is located on chromosome 12q24 and contains four exons [8, 18].

There is a single nucleotide polymorphism +874A/T that is located at the 5′-end of a CA repeat in the first intron of the human IFN-γ gene. The +874 T allele is connected to the 12 CA repeats, whereas the A allele is linked with the non-12 CA repeats. The +874 T allele is associated with high IFN-γ expression in opposition to low expression of the A allele [8].

IFN-γR1 gene is located on chromosome 6p23.3 with seven exons [14, 18, 19].

The minimal promoter region of IFN-γR1 is highly polymorphic [20].

There is an association between mycobacterial infections and mutations of IFN-γRs genes. It is demonstrated that the mutations prevalently occur in IFN-γR1 more than IFN-γR2.

Total lack of IFN-γR1 expression on the cell surface results in recessive IFN-γR1 defect or loss of IFN-γ binding completely [12].

As a result, the level of IFN-γR1 expression is probably the main factor of IFN-γ responsiveness [20].

Polymorphisms in the genes that encode involving enzymes in the biotransformation of carcinogens have been related to cancer development [19].

Published reports have focused on the correlation of IFN-γR1 promoter polymorphism and susceptibility to infectious disease [20].

Effects of IFN-γR1 -611 (rs1327474) single nucleotide polymorphisms (SNPs) on the promoter activity are stronger than SNP at position -56 of IFN-γR [13].

Rosenzweig et al. used a luciferase reporter system and found that G-611 carrier constructs are stronger in promoter activity than constructs carrying -611A [20].

IFN-γR1 (+95C/T) SNP (rs7749390) seems to control the intron-exon splicing process and is mapped on the exon/intron splice site [18].

Similar studies on periodontal disease mainly have focused on the potentially functional polymorphisms of IFN-γ like +874A/T [8].

Considering the critical role of IFN-γ and IFN-γR1 in immunity, we performed a population-based case-control study to explore the effects of genetic polymorphisms of IFN-γ and IFN-γR1 in the risk of CP.

In present study, we examined the effects of IFN-γ (+874A/T) and IFN-γR1 (-611A/G, +189T/G, and +95C/T) gene polymorphisms on prevalence of chronic periodontitis.

2. Materials and Methods

2.1. Subject Population. This case-control study was done on 210 CP patients and 100 healthy individuals. All subjects were exclusively Iranian ethnicities from the region of Sistan and Baluchistan.

Patients with chronic periodontitis were examined at the Periodontology Department, Dentistry Clinic of Zahedan University of Medical Sciences (ZUMS). The average age of individuals was 28.33 ± 5.765 (95 female and 115 male). All subjects had at least 20 teeth and were of good general health.

The disease diagnosis was based on physical examination, medical and dental history, probing depth (measured as the distance from the gingival margin to the bottom of the pocket), and assessment of clinical attachment loss (as the distance from the cement-enamel junction to the bottom of the periodontal pocket). Probing was performed at six sites around each tooth using a WHO periodontal probe and recording the maximum values, tooth mobility, and radiographs. The loss of alveolar bone was determined radiographically [21, 22].

The control group consisted of 100 unrelated healthy individuals who had no clinical history of periodontal disease. Controls were selected from subjects referred to the Dentistry Clinic for reasons other than periodontal disease and were matched for age, ethnicity, and gender (29.22 ± 3.597, 52 female and 48 male).

TABLE 1: The primers sequences used for detection of IFN-γ (+874A/T), IFN-γR1 (-611A/G), (+189T/G), and (+95C/T) gene polymorphisms using ARMS-PCR and RFLP-PCR.

Gene	Polymorphisms	Primers	Sequence
IFN-γR1	-611A/G	Forward	AGAGCAGACCTCTTCATGAGAGGCTGTCT
	rs1327474	Reverse	ACATTTTTAGAAGAGAATGAGACTTCAAA
	+95C/T	Forward	GCCATTTGGTGGTCCATTAC
	rs7749390	Reverse	TCCAGACAGCTGGAATCAGT
	+189T/G	Forward	CTCTTTCTCCTACCCCTTGTCAT
	rs11914	Reverse	CAGCGCATAATCGTATTTAAAAGTG
IFN-γ	+874A/T	Forward (T allele)	TTCTTACAACACAAAATCAAATCT
	rs62559044	Forward (A allele)	TTCTTACAACACAAAATCAAATCA
		Reverse	TCAACAAAGCTGATACTCCA

2.2. Exclusion Criteria. Smokers, pregnant women, and persons with history of or current cardiovascular disorders, systemic disorders such as diabetes, immunodeficiency, HIV infection, hepatitis, and viral infections, long-term use of anti-inflammatory drugs, malignant diseases, chemotherapy, and orthodontic instruments were excluded from the study.

2.3. Sample Collection. The study was performed with the approval of the Committees for Ethics of Zahedan University of Medical sciences (number 6210). Written informed consent was obtained from all participants.

2 mL peripheral blood was collected from all participants in Na-EDTA tubes.

2.4. DNA Extraction and Genetic Analysis. DNA for genetic analysis was extracted from peripheral blood samples using salting out method according to Hashemi et al. [23].

The primers that were used for genotyping were listed in Table 1.

Genotyping for the +874A/T polymorphism (rs62559044) in IFN-γ gene was performed by using the amplification refractory mutation system-polymerase chain reaction (ARMS-PCR) as was described previously by Pravica et al. [24].

PCR was performed using 2X Prime Taq Premix (Genet Bio, Korea). For each sample, we used two tubes, one for A allele and another tube for T allele. In each 0.20 mL reaction, 1 μL of each primer, 1 μL of genomic DNA (~100 ng/mL) and 10 μL of 2X Prime Taq Premix (Genet Bio, Korea), and 7 μL ddH$_2$O were added. A-allele tube contained forward primer for A allele and reverse primer and T allele tube contained forward primer for T allele and reverse primer. PCR reaction was performed according to the following protocol: initial denaturation at 95°C for 5 min, 30 cycles of denaturation at 95°C for 30 s, annealing at 57.1°C for 30 s, extension at 72°C for 30 s, and final extension at 72°C for 5 min. The amplified products were separated by electrophoresis on a 2% agarose gels stained with 0.5 μg/mL ethidium bromide and observed under UV light. Two sample products were available for each subject (1 for each specific A or T allele of the IFN-γ +874A/T variant) (Table 3, Figure 1).

(-611A/G) rs1327474, (+189T/G) rs11914, and (+95C/T) rs7749390 polymorphisms in IFN-γR1 gene were genotyped

TABLE 2: The restriction enzymes used for digestion of IFN-γR1 (-611A/G), (+189T/G), and (+95C/T) gene polymorphisms using RFLP-PCR.

Position	Restriction enzyme	PCR product
-611	Hpy188I	G allele: 204 bp and 29 bp
		A allele: 233 bp
+189	TaqI	G allele: 286 bp and 210 bp
		T allele: 496 bp
+95	BstC8I	C allele: 87 bp, 121 bp, and 158 bp
		T allele: 208 bp and 158 bp

using the polymerase chain reaction restriction fragment length polymorphism (PCR-RFLP) technique by specific primers and enzymes (Tables 1 and 2).

For genetic analysis of IFN-γR1 (-611A/G) rs1327474 polymorphism PCR was performed using 2X Prime Taq Premix (Genet Bio, Korea). In each 0.20 mL reaction, 1 μL of each primer, 1 μL of genomic DNA (~100 ng/mL) and 10 μL of 2X Prime Taq Premix (Genet Bio, Korea), and 7 μL ddH$_2$O were added. PCR reaction was performed according to the following protocol: initial denaturation at 95°C for 5 min, 30 cycles of denaturation at 95°C for 30 s, annealing at 62°C for 30 s, extension at 72°C for 30 s, and final extension at 72°C for 5 min. The PCR product (10 μL) was digested using Hpy188I restriction enzyme. The G allele was digested and produced 204 bp and 29 bp fragments while the A allele was undigested and produced a 233 bp fragment. The PCR and fragments were verified on 3% agarose gels containing 0.5 μg/mL ethidium bromide and were visualized under UV light (Figure 1).

Genotyping of IFN-γR1 (+189T/G) rs11914 polymorphism was performed by PCR reaction containing 2X Prime Taq Premix (Genet Bio, Korea). In each 0.20 mL reaction, 1 μL of each primer, 1 μL of genomic DNA (~100 ng/mL) and 10 μL of 2X Prime Taq Premix (Genet Bio, Korea), and 7 μL ddH$_2$O were added. PCR reaction was performed according to the following protocol: initial denaturation at 95°C for 5 min, 30 cycles of denaturation at 95°C for 30 s, annealing at 63.7°C for 30 s, extension at 72°C for 30 s, and final extension at 72°C for 5 min. The PCR product (10 μL) was digested using TaqI restriction enzyme. The G allele was digested and produced

TABLE 3: The PCR protocols for genetic analysis of IFN-γ (+874A/T), IFN-γR1 (-611A/G), (+189T/G), and (+95C/T) gene polymorphisms using ARMS-PCR and RFLP-PCR.

Gene	Polymorphisms	Denaturation	Annealing	Extension	Final extension
IFN-γR1	-611A/G rs1327474	95°C for 30 s	62°C for 30 s	72°C for 30 s	72°C for 5 min
	+95C/T rs7749390	95°C for 30 s	62°C for 30 s	72°C for 30 s	72°C for 5 min
	+189T/G rs11914	95°C for 30 s	63.7°C for 30 s	72°C for 30 s	72°C for 5 min
IFN-γ	+874A/T rs62559044	95°C for 30 s	57.1°C for 30 s	72°C for 30 s	72°C for 5 min

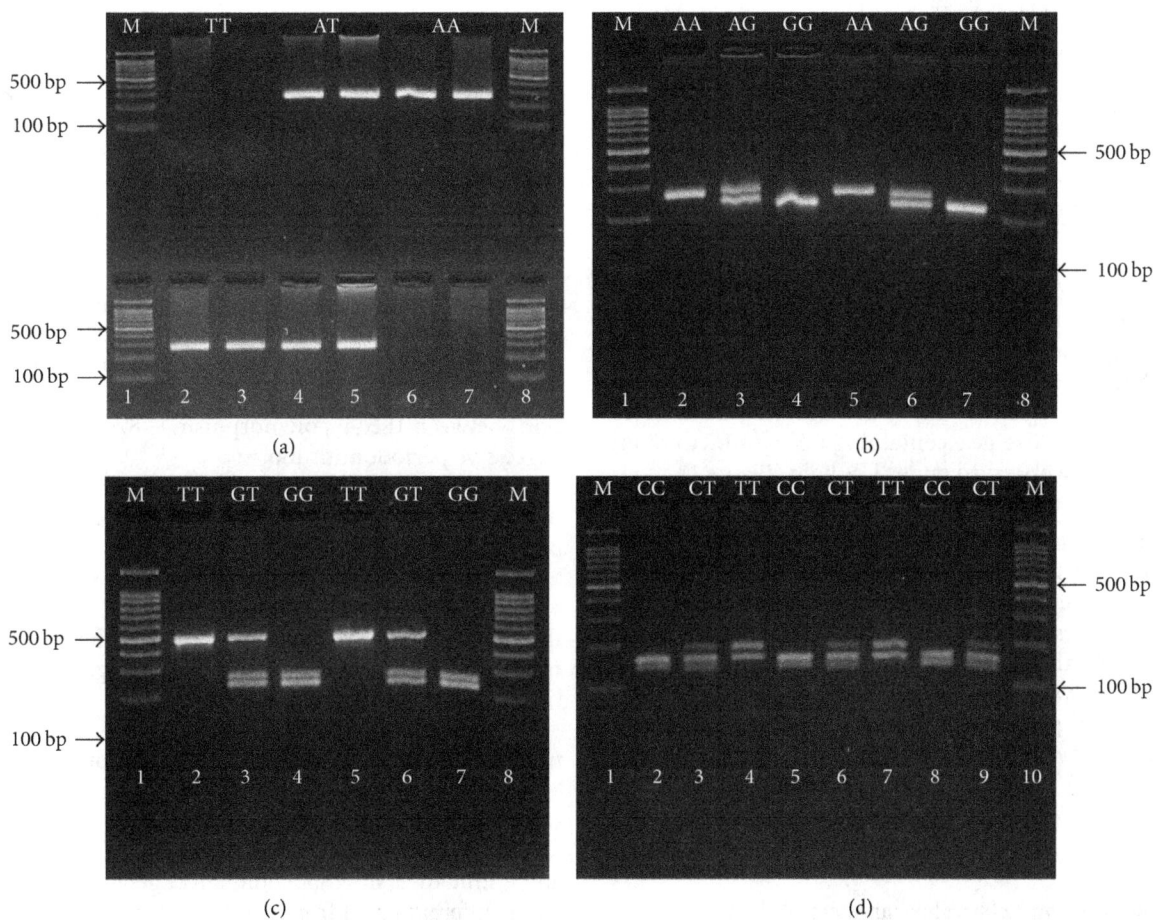

FIGURE 1: Electrophoresis pattern of ARMS-PCR for detection of IFN-γ (+874A/T) (a) and RFLP-PCR IFN-γR1 (-611A/G), (+189T/G), and (+95C/T) gene polymorphism (resp., (b), (c), and (d)). (a) Lines 1 and 8: marker 100 bp; Lines 2 and 3: product sizes were 264 bp for forward T allele primer (FT) and reverse primer (R); Homozygote TT; Lines 6 and 7: product sizes were 264 bp for forward A allele primer (FA) and reverse primer (R); Homozygote AA; Lines 4 and 5: product sizes were 264 bp for FT, FA, and R; Heterozygote AT; (b) Lines 1 and 8: marker 100 bp; Lines 2 and 5: Homozygote AA; Lines 4 and 7: Homozygote GG; Lines 3 and 6: Heterozygote AG; (c) Lines 1 and 8: marker 100 bp; Lines 2 and 5: Homozygote TT; Lines 4 and 7: Homozygote GG; Lines 3 and 6: Heterozygote GT; (d) Lines 1 and 10: Marker 100 bp, Lines 2, 5, and 8: Homozygote CC; Lines 4 and 7: Homozygote TT; Lines 3, 6, and 9: Heterozygote CT.

286 bp and 210 bp fragments while the T allele was undigested and produced a 496 bp fragment. Each reaction was verified on 2% agarose gels containing 0.5 μg/mL ethidium bromide and observed under UV light (Figure 1).

PCR for genetic analysis of IFN-γR1 (+95C/T) rs7749390 polymorphism was performed using 2X Prime Taq Premix (Genet Bio, Korea). In each 0.20 mL reaction, 1 μL of each primer, 1 μL of genomic DNA (~100 ng/mL) and 10 μL of 2X Prime Taq Premix (Genet Bio, Korea), and 7 μL ddH$_2$O were added. PCR reaction was performed according to the following protocol: initial denaturation at 95°C for 5 min, 30 cycles of denaturation at 95°C for 30 s, annealing at 62°C for

TABLE 4: Demographic data in patients with chronic periodontitis (CP) and controls.

	Patients with CP	Controls
Age		
Mean age	28.33 ± 5.765	29.22 ± 3.597
Age range	16–42	24–37
Gender		
Female	95 (45.2%)	52 (52%)
Male	115 (54.8%)	48 (48%)
Race		
Sistani	82 (39%)	42 (42%)
Baluch	71 (33.8%)	24 (24%)
Other	57 (27.1%)	34 (34%)
Clinical parameters		
BOP index (%)	85.86 ± 3.68	—
Mean PD (mm)	5.58 ± 0.63	1.50 ± 0.86
CAL (mm)	5.44 ± 0.58	—

"—" means bleeding and attachment loss were not seen in controls.
Data are n (%) or mean ± SD.

30 s, extension at 72°C for 30 s, and final extension at 72°C for 5 min. The PCR product (10 μL) was digested using BstC8I restriction enzyme. The G allele was digested and produced 87 bp, 121 bp, and 158 bp fragments and the T allele produced 208 bp and 158 fragment. The PCR and fragments were verified on 3% agarose gels containing 0.5 μg/mL ethidium bromide and were observed under UV light (Figure 1).

2.5. Statistical Analysis. The significance of the differences in the observed frequencies of IFN-γ and IFN-γR1 polymorphisms in the control and patient groups was computed by Chi-square test with software SPSS ver.20.0. Only the values of P less than 0.05 were considered significant. The risk associated with individual alleles or genotypes was as calculated by performing a multiple logistic regression analysis to estimate the odds ratio (OR) and confidence interval 95% (CI).

3. Results

The demographic and clinical parameters of the CP patients and healthy controls were shown in Table 4. The CP group exhibited a significantly greater mean of PD (5.58 ± 0.63 mm versus 1.50±0.86 mm) and CAL (5.44±0.58 mm) and a higher percentage of sites with BOP (85.86 ± 3.68%) than the control group ($P < 0.05$).

The demographic data showed that the mean ages for patients with CP and healthy subjects did not differ between the two groups (resp., 28.33 ± 5.765 and 29.22 ± 3.597, $P < 0.05$). There were no significant differences between subjects with periodontitis and controls regarding the ethnicity and gender (Table 4).

The genotype and allele frequencies distributions among cases and controls have been shown in Table 5.

Significant difference in the genotype and allele frequencies of the IFN-γ gene polymorphism at positions +874A/T

between CP patients and healthy subjects was found ($P = 0.038$).

The IFN-γR1 polymorphisms at positions -611A/G, +189T/G, and +95C/T were not significantly different between subjects with chronic periodontitis and controls ($P > 0.05$).

To explore the potential higher-order gene-gene interactions, we performed haplotype analysis. We found 14 haplotypes (Table 6). The findings showed that haplotypes were not significantly different between subjects with CP and controls ($P = 0.774$).

4. Discussion

The present study investigated the association of four gene polymorphisms with CP in a sample of Iranian population. Our study was the first one to explore the polymorphism at this locus on the susceptibility to CP.

Our findings showed that IFN-γR1 (+95C/T, -611A/G, and +189T/G) polymorphisms are not associated with the risk of CP in our population, whereas we found significant association for alleles and genotypes of IFN-γ (+874A/T) SNP between patients with CP and controls.

On the contrary, Holla et al. [8] found no significant correlation for alleles and genotypes of IFN-γ +874A/T polymorphism between patients with CP and controls.

Data of Erciyas et al. [25] studies showed no associations between IFN-γ polymorphism (+874) and generalized aggressive periodontitis too.

Loo et al. [16] study did not find any significant difference in gene investigation (IL-1b, IL-6, IFN-γ, and IL-10) in the CP patients and healthy subjects.

One reason for the conflicting results is various genotype and allele frequencies between different ethnic populations that confirm heterogeneity of populations; therefore a genetic risk factor in one population may not change disease susceptibility in another population [26, 27].

Different findings probably are results of the complex nature of periodontitis, which is because of the interaction between many factors such as pathogens, host immune response, and role of environment [8].

Difference in the sample size, criteria of subject selection, and ethnic diversity that could affect genetic variations may cause different result from similar studies [28].

According to the fact that a single genetic polymorphism has weak effect on immunity reactions, interactions of other genes and environment are concerned and can possibly change observed phenotype [8, 18].

The correlation between IFN-γ levels and variation in experimental periodontitis is clear, but the molecular mechanisms of its connection to inflammation of periodontium have not been found [8].

Interaction between some factors such as age, sex, ethnic background, and geography can potentially change disease prevalence. In other words, these elements may lead to various effects of cytokine gene polymorphisms in different population samples [7, 26].

IFN-γ is an immune regulator and for its binding and signaling the IFN-γR1 subunit is essential [16, 29].

TABLE 5: The genotypes and allele distribution of IFN-γ/IFN-γR1 polymorphisms in chronic periodontitis (CP) patients and controls.

Polymorphism	CP $n = 210$	Controls $n = 100$	OR 95% (CI)	P value
		IFN-γ +874A/T		
AA	71 (33.8%)	20 (20%)	2.420 (CI = 1.063–5.511)	0.035
AT	117 (55.7%)	65 (65%)	1.227 (CI = 0.596–2.529)	0.579
TT	22 (10.5%)	15 (15%)	—	Ref = 1
Alleles				
A	259 (61.7%)	105 (52.5%)	1.455 (CI = 1.036–2.045)	0.031
T	161 (38.3%)	95 (47.5%)	—	Ref = 1
		IFN-γR1 -611A/G		
AA	67 (31.9%)	33 (33%)	0.883 (CI = 0.452–1.726)	0.715
GA	97 (46.2%)	47 (47%)	0.923 (CI = 0.450–1.893)	0.826
GG	46 (21.9%)	20 (20%)	—	Ref = 1
Alleles				
A	231 (55%)	113 (56.5%)	0.941 (CI = 0.670–1.321)	0.725
G	189 (45%)	87 (43.5%)	—	Ref = 1
		IFN-γR1 +189T/G		
GG	23 (11%)	8 (8%)	1.426 (CI = 0.603–3.370)	0.419
GT	62 (29.5%)	30 (30%)	1.025 (CI = 0.602–1.744)	0.927
TT	125 (59.5%)	62 (62%)	—	Ref = 1
Alleles				
G	108 (25.7%)	46 (23%)	1.159 (CI = 0.780–1.721)	0.465
T	312 (74.3%)	154 (77%)	—	Ref = 1
		IFN-γR1 +95C/T		
CC	54 (25.7%)	24 (24%)	—	Ref = 1
TC	95 (45.2%)	48 (48%)	0.880 (CI = 0.486–1.592)	0.672
TT	61 (29%)	28 (28%)	0.968 (CI = 0.502–1.867)	0.923
Alleles				
C	203 (48.3%)	96 (48%)	—	Ref = 1
T	217 (51.7%)	104 (52%)	0.987 (CI = 0.704–1.382)	0.938

OR: odd ratio; CI: confidence interval.

According to published reports, IFN-γ has essential role in initiation and progression of inflammatory diseases [18, 30].

Reports have demonstrated that IFN-γ +874A/T polymorphism is related to different levels of this cytokine and can affect the immune response and susceptibility to inflammatory diseases [8].

The T allele of the IFN-γ (+874A/T) found in increased producers of this cytokine indicated that polymorphism in IFN-γ gene causes differences in the immunoregulatory role of its molecules [16].

Findings have indicated that the +874 IFN-γ polymorphism was associated with two important autoimmune processes: Systemic Lupus Erythematosus and arthritis [31].

It has been demonstrated that IFN-γ (+874A/T) allele can change the susceptibility to tuberculosis (TB) [27, 32].

Mutations in IFN-γR1 coding gene cause excessive susceptibility to mycobacterial infection and can be disruptive [16, 29].

Correlation between two IFN-γR1 promoter polymorphisms and immunity against malaria in West Africa is emerging evidence that prevalent IFN-γR1 variants may affect incidence of infection in the population [29].

There is emerging evidence that genetic polymorphisms of rs1327475 (-611A/G) and rs7749390 (+95C/T) were correlated with an altered risk of tuberculosis (TB) [18].

Lee et al. [33] study suggested that IFN-γR1 (83G/A) polymorphism may be associated with increased predisposition to leprosy [33].

These findings confirmed that IFN-γ probably is a regulatory key in immune response and inflammation process.

Any number of gene polymorphisms that have any function in IFN-γ dependent inflammatory responses could be essential in determining susceptibility or resistance to periodontitis [32, 34].

Complex diseases genetically have heterogeneous nature. These common diseases may be caused by several genotypes at various positions on a chromosome that lead to moderate, increased, or reduced effects [32].

There are few longitudinal studies that have focused on the relationship between IFN-γ genotype and periodontal disease severity, alveolar bone loss, tooth loss, and response to CP treatment. There is no longitudinal study concerning the putative role of IFN-γ in periodontal disease outcome. Therefore, we do not know the functional consequences of these polymorphisms in our subjects [8, 25].

TABLE 6: The haplotype analysis for IFN-γ/IFN-γR1 polymorphisms.

Haplotypes	CP group n (%)	Control group n (%)	P
AATT	62 (29.5)	31 (31.0)	P = 0.774 > 0.05
AGTG	16 (7.6)	9 (9)	
AGCT	5 (2.4)	4 (4.0)	
TGCG	2 (1.0)	—	
TACT	2 (1.0)	1 (1.0)	
TACG	—	1 (1.0)	
TGTT	4 (1.9)	2 (2.0)	
AACT	29 (13.8)	15 (15.0)	
AATG	46 (21.9)	19 (19.0)	
AGTT	15 (7.1)	4 (4.0)	
AACG	11 (5.2)	2 (2.0)	
AGCG	4 (1.9)	1 (1.0)	
TATT	7 (3.3)	6 (6.0)	
TATG	7 (3.3)	5 (5.0)	
Total	210 (100.0)	100 (100.0)	

Undoubtedly, further investigations about serum level of IFN-γ, gene expression, RNA expression, stereological analysis of tissue destruction, and immunohistochemical changes in patients with these polymorphisms are necessary for interpretation of histological changes.

Additional insight into the biology of chronic periodontitis and stratified phenotypic analysis of CP would be provided by further studies and would assist in a better comprehension of molecular impression of polymorphisms.

The limitation of this study is its relatively small sample size and lack of observance of specific bacteria. Consequently, subgroup analysis was not possible. Replications in larger populations are needed to conclusively confirm or reject our findings. Subject selection with high accuracy and exact matching between groups were strengths of our study.

5. Conclusion

Taken together, our results suggest that IFN-γ +874A/T genetic polymorphism has association with susceptibility to CP in Iranian population, but IFN-γR1 gene (in -611A/G, +189T/G, and +95C/T positions) is not associated with the risk of CP in this population. Larger studies are needed to confirm these findings on the relationships of genetic variations to the pathogenesis of CP.

Conflict of Interests

The authors declare that there is no conflict of interests regarding the publication of this paper.

Acknowledgments

The project was funded by Zahedan University of Medical Sciences, Grant no. 6210, and a portion of the master's thesis of Anatomical sciences no. 90/K. The authors acknowledge the patients and healthy participants who willingly participated in the study.

References

[1] Z. Heidari, H. Mahmoudzadeh-Sagheb, M. Hashemi, and M. A. Rigi-Ladiz, "Quantitative analysis of interdental gingiva in patients with chronic periodontitis and transforming growth factor-β1 29C/T gene polymorphisms," Journal of Periodontology, vol. 85, no. 2, pp. 281–289, 2014.

[2] Z. Armingohar, J. J. Jørgensen, A. K. Kristoffersen, K. Schenck, and Z. Dembic, "Polymorphisms in the interleukin-1 gene locus and chronic periodontitis in patients with atherosclerotic and aortic aneurysmal vascular diseases," Scandinavian Journal of Immunology, vol. 79, no. 5, pp. 338–345, 2014.

[3] P. L. Preethi, S. R. Rao, B. T. Madapusi, and M. Narasimhan, "Immunolocalization of Ki-67 in different periodontal conditions," Journal of Indian Society of Periodontology, vol. 18, no. 2, pp. 161–165, 2014.

[4] Z. Heidari, "The association between proinflammatory gene polymorphisms and level of gingival tissue degradation in chronic periodontitis," Gene, Cell and Tissue, vol. 1, no. 2, Article ID e21898, 2014.

[5] F. Mesa, F. O'Valle, M. Rizzo et al., "Association between COX-2 rs 6681231 genotype and Interleukin-6 in periodontal connective tissue. A pilot study," PLoS ONE, vol. 9, no. 2, Article ID e87023, 2014.

[6] G. Ribeiro Souto, C. M. Queiroz Jr., M. H. N. G. de Abreu, F. Oliveira Costa, and R. Alves Mesquita, "Pro-inflammatory, Th1, Th2, Th17 cytokines and dendritic cells: a cross-sectional study in chronic periodontitis," PLoS ONE, vol. 9, no. 3, Article ID e91636, 2014.

[7] Z. Heidari, H. Mahmoudzadeh-Sagheb, M. A. Rigi-Ladiz, M. Taheri, A. Moazenni-Roodi, and M. Hashemi, "Association of TGF-β1 − 509 C/T, 29 C/T and 788 C/T gene polymorphisms with chronic periodontitis: a case-control study," Gene, vol. 518, no. 2, pp. 330–334, 2013.

[8] L. I. Holla, B. Hrdlickova, P. Linhartova, and A. Fassmann, "Interferon-γ +874A/T polymorphism in relation to generalized chronic periodontitis and the presence of periodontopathic bacteria," Archives of Oral Biology, vol. 56, no. 2, pp. 153–158, 2011.

[9] S. Zhang, A. Crivello, S. Offenbacher, A. Moretti, D. W. Paquette, and S. P. Barros, "Interferon-gamma promoter hypomethylation and increased expression in chronic periodontitis," Journal of Clinical Periodontology, vol. 37, no. 11, pp. 953–961, 2010.

[10] M. H. Tanaka, E. M. A. Giro, L. B. Cavalcante et al., "Expression of interferon-γ, interferon-α and related genes in individuals with Down syndrome and periodontitis," Cytokine, vol. 60, no. 3, pp. 875–881, 2012.

[11] M. J. Newport, C. M. Huxley, S. Huston et al., "A mutation in the interferon-γ-receptor gene and susceptibility to mycobacterial infection," The New England Journal of Medicine, vol. 335, no. 26, pp. 1941–1949, 1996.

[12] S. D. Rosenzweig and S. M. Holland, "Defects in the interferon-γ and interleukin-12 pathways," Immunological Reviews, vol. 203, no. 1, pp. 38–47, 2005.

[13] L. Xiang, O. U. Elci, K. E. Rehm, and G. D. Marshall, "Associations between cytokine receptor polymorphisms and variability in laboratory immune parameters in normal humans," Human Immunology, vol. 75, no. 1, pp. 91–97, 2014.

[14] S. Jüliger, M. Bongartz, A. J. F. Luty, P. G. Kremsner, and J. F. J. Kun, "Functional analysis of a promoter variant of the gene encoding the interferon-gamma receptor chain I," *Immunogenetics*, vol. 54, no. 10, pp. 675–680, 2003.

[15] P. R. Moreira, P. M. A. Lima, K. O. B. Sathler et al., "Interleukin-6 expression and gene polymorphism are associated with severity of periodontal disease in a sample of Brazilian individuals," *Clinical & Experimental Immunology*, vol. 148, no. 1, pp. 119–126, 2007.

[16] W. T. Y. Loo, C.-B. Fan, L.-J. Bai et al., "Gene polymorphism and protein of human pro- and anti-inflammatory cytokines in Chinese healthy subjects and chronic periodontitis patients," *Journal of Translational Medicine*, vol. 10, no. 1, article 8, 2012.

[17] A. R. Ebadian, M. Radvar, J. T. Afshari et al., "Gene polymorphisms of TNF-α and IL-1β are not associated with generalized aggressive periodontitis in an Iranian subpopulation," *Iranian Journal of Allergy, Asthma and Immunology*, vol. 12, no. 4, pp. 345–351, 2013.

[18] J. Lü, H. Pan, Y. Chen et al., "Genetic polymorphisms of IFNG and IFNGR1 in association with the risk of pulmonary tuberculosis," *Gene*, vol. 543, no. 1, pp. 140–144, 2014.

[19] R. M. S. de Araújo, C. F. V. de Melo, F. M. Neto et al., "Association study of SNPs of genes IFNGR1 (rs137854905), GSTT1 (rs71748309), and GSTP1 (rs1695) in gastric cancer development in samples of patient in the northern and northeastern Brazil," *Tumor Biology*, vol. 35, no. 5, pp. 4983–4986, 2014.

[20] S. D. Rosenzweig, A. A. Schäffer, L. Ding et al., "Interferon-γ receptor 1 promoter polymorphisms: population distribution and functional implications," *Clinical Immunology*, vol. 112, no. 1, pp. 113–119, 2004.

[21] G. C. Armitage, "Periodontal diagnoses and classification of periodontal diseases," *Periodontology*, vol. 34, pp. 9–21, 2004.

[22] G. C. Armitage, "Development of a classification system for periodontal diseases and conditions," *Annals of Periodontology*, vol. 4, no. 1, pp. 1–6, 1999.

[23] M. Hashemi, A. K. Moazeni-Roodi, A. Fazaeli et al., "Lack of association between paraoxonase-1 Q192R polymorphism and rheumatoid arthritis in southeast Iran," *Genetics and Molecular Research*, vol. 9, no. 1, pp. 333–339, 2010.

[24] V. Pravica, C. Perrey, A. Stevens, J.-H. Lee, and I. V. Hutchinson, "A single nucleotide polymorphism in the first intron of the human IFN-γ gene: absolute correlation with a polymorphic CA microsatellite marker of high IFN-γ production," *Human Immunology*, vol. 61, no. 9, pp. 863–866, 2000.

[25] K. Erciyas, S. Pehlivan, T. Sever, M. Igci, A. Arslan, and R. Orbak, "Association between TNF-α, TGF-βi, IL-10, IL-6 and IFN-γ gene polymorphisms and generalized aggressive periodontitis," *Clinical & Investigative Medicine*, vol. 33, no. 2, pp. 85–91, 2010.

[26] M. L. Laine, W. Crielaard, and B. G. Loos, "Genetic susceptibility to periodontitis," *Periodontology 2000*, vol. 58, no. 1, pp. 37–68, 2012.

[27] J. Wang, S. Tang, and H. Shen, "Association of genetic polymorphisms in the IL12-IFNG pathway with susceptibility to and prognosis of pulmonary tuberculosis in a Chinese population," *European Journal of Clinical Microbiology and Infectious Diseases*, vol. 29, no. 10, pp. 1291–1295, 2010.

[28] Ö. Ö. Yücel, E. Berker, L. Mesci, K. Eratalay, E. Tepe, and İ. Tezcan, "Analysis of TNF-α (-308) polymorphism and gingival crevicular fluid TNF-α levels in aggressive and chronic periodontitis: a preliminary report," *Cytokine*, vol. 72, no. 2, pp. 173–177, 2015.

[29] O. Koch, D. P. Kwiatkowski, and I. A. Udalova, "Context-specific functional effects of IFNGR1 promoter polymorphism," *Human Molecular Genetics*, vol. 15, no. 9, pp. 1475–1481, 2006.

[30] I. Niedzielska and S. Cierpka, "Interferon γ in the etiology of atherosclerosis and periodontitis," *Thrombosis Research*, vol. 126, no. 4, pp. 324–327, 2010.

[31] J. L. Bidwell, N. A. P. Wood, H. R. Morse, O. O. Olomolaiye, L. J. Keen, and G. J. Laundy, "Human cytokine gene nucleotide sequence alignments," *European Journal of Immunogenetics*, vol. 26, no. 2-3, pp. 135–223, 1999.

[32] A. G. Pacheco, C. C. Cardoso, and M. O. Moraes, "*IFNG* + 874T/A, *IL10* -1082G/A and *TNF*-308G/A polymorphisms in association with tuberculosis susceptibility: a meta-analysis study," *Human Genetics*, vol. 123, no. 5, pp. 477–484, 2008.

[33] S.-B. Lee, B. C. Kim, S. H. Jin et al., "Missense mutations of the interleukin-12 receptor beta 1(*IL12RB1*) and interferon-gamma receptor 1 (*IFNGR1*) genes are not associated with susceptibility to lepromatous leprosy in Korea," *Immunogenetics*, vol. 55, no. 3, pp. 177–181, 2003.

[34] D. A. Fraser, B. G. Loos, U. Boman et al., "Polymorphisms in an interferon-γ receptor-1 gene marker and susceptibility to periodontitis," *Acta Odontologica Scandinavica*, vol. 61, no. 5, pp. 297–302, 2003.

11

Effect of Nd:YAG Low Level Laser Therapy on Human Gingival Fibroblasts

Andreas S. Gkogkos, Ioannis K. Karoussis, Ioannis D. Prevezanos, Kleopatra E. Marcopoulou, Kyriaki Kyriakidou, and Ioannis A. Vrotsos

Department of Periodontology, School of Dentistry, University of Athens, 2 Thivon Street, Goudi, 115 27 Athens, Greece

Correspondence should be addressed to Ioannis A. Vrotsos; ivrotsos@dent.uoa.gr

Academic Editor: Yoshitaka Hara

Aim. To evaluate the effect of Low Level Laser Therapy (LLLT) on human gingival fibroblasts in terms of proliferation and growth factors' secretion (EGF, bFGF, and VEGF). *Materials and Methods.* Primary cultures of keratinized mucosa fibroblasts were irradiated by a Nd:YAG laser 1064 nm with the following energy densities: 2.6 J/cm^2, 5.3 J/cm^2, 7.9 J/cm^2, and 15.8 J/cm^2. Controls were not irradiated. Cultures were examined for cell proliferation and growth factors' secretion after 24, 48, and 72 hours. All experimental procedures were performed in duplicate. Data were analyzed by Student's t-test ($p < 0.05$). *Results.* All laser-irradiation doses applied promoted a higher cell proliferation at 48 hours in a dose-response relationship compared to controls. This difference reached statistical significance for the cultures receiving 15.8 J/cm^2 ($p = 0.03$). Regarding EGF, all laser irradiation doses applied promoted a higher secretion at 48 hours in a reverse dose-response pattern compared to controls. This difference reached statistical significance for the cultures receiving 2.6 J/cm^2 ($p = 0.04$). EGF levels at the other time points, bFGF, and VEGF showed a random variation between the groups. *Conclusion.* Within the limits of this study, LLLT (Nd:YAG) may induce gingival fibroblasts' proliferation and upregulate the secretion of EGF. Further studies are needed to confirm these results.

1. Introduction

Laser devices, almost 50 years after their introduction, find numerous applications in health sciences and are used successfully in several dental specialties. At a high output power, lasers cause thermomechanical ablation used for incisions and hard or soft tissue removal. However, at a low output power (0.2–0.5 W), referred to as Low Level Laser Therapy (LLLT), they may present a stimulatory effect, via a photobiologic phenomenon (photobiomodulation), promoting tissue healing, reducing inflammation, and inducing analgesia [1]. The exact biological mechanisms that explain LLLT's effect are still a matter of research.

It has been reported that irradiation with red or near-infrared light can lead to the activation of mitochondrial respiratory chain components and the initiation of a signaling cascade which promotes mitosis and growth factors' secretion [2]. Growth factors represent keystones in the wound healing procedures. Specially, blood-derived fibroblast growth factor

(bFGF) has anti-inflammatory effect [3], vascular endothelial growth factor (VEGF) plays a role in angiogenesis, inflammation, and wound healing [4, 5], and epidermal growth factor (EGF) promotes a dose-dependent migratory response in gingival fibroblasts accelerating wound healing [6].

It has been shown that LLLT may influence the proliferation of various cells participating in oral wound healing process, such as gingival fibroblasts [7], gingival epithelial cells [8], periodontal ligament cells [9], osteoblasts [10], and bone mesenchymal stem cells [11]. Although several studies support the stimulating effect of LLLT on gingival fibroblasts, the vast majority of them used diode lasers [7, 12–14]. Literature data using neodymium-doped yttrium aluminum garnet (Nd:YAG) 1064 nm lasers are very rare. Additionally, the aforementioned studies present heterogeneity in terms of wavelengths, output powers, time of application, energy densities, and technical parameters such as the type of optical fiber and the distance between optical fiber and targeting cells. The determination of parameters that could optimize

LLLT's impact on wound healing of periodontal tissues is very important. A positive upgrowth stimulation effect of LLLT on gingival fibroblasts could have clinical applications in both nonsurgical and surgical periodontal therapy.

Thus, the aim of this *in vitro* study was to evaluate the effect of various energy densities of LLLT, performed with a Nd:YAG laser (1064-nm) on human gingival fibroblasts in terms of cells' proliferation and specific growth factors' secretion (EGF, bFGF, and VEGF), at certain time points after irradiation.

2. Materials and Methods

2.1. Biopsy Collection. For the purpose of this *in vitro* study, connective tissue specimens were obtained by two healthy nonsmoking donors (1 female 30 ys, 1 male 30 ys). Biopsies were performed during second-stage implant surgeries at the Postgraduate Clinic, Department of Periodontology, National and Kapodistrian University of Athens. Immediately after flap elevation, 6×6 mm specimens were collected from the connective tissue part of the flap. All tissue collections were carried out according to the approved guidelines set by the Human Ethics Board of Kapodistrian University of Athens, School of Dentistry.

2.2. Cell Cultures. Specimens were carefully sliced into 3 mm slides. Explants plated on 35 mm dishes, produced outgrowths composed of fibroblasts, after culture in Dulbecco's Modified Eagle's Medium (DMEM; Gibco Grand Island, NY) supplemented with 10% bovine calf serum (Grand Island, NY), 100 U/mL penicillin G sodium, 100 mg/mL streptomycin sulfate, and 250 pg/mL amphotericin B (Gibco, Grand Island, NY). The obtained fibroblasts grew on standard conditions ($37°C$, 85% humidity, and 5% CO_2). After the first passage (cells reached 80%–85% confluence), cultures were subjected to immunomagnetic cell sorting using STRO-1 (BioLegend, San Diego, CA, USA) and anti-IgM MicroBeads (Miltenyi Biotec, Bergisch Gladbach, Germany) according to the manufacturers' instructions (MACS; Miltenyi Biotec, Bergisch Gladbach, Germany), in order to determine the cells' type (fibroblasts). The experiment took place at the third passage. After cultures' growth, cells were trypsinized and seeded at 12-well multiwall (3.8 cm^2) plates (10000 cells/mL) in DMEM 10% fetal bovine serum (FBS). Before laser irradiation the medium of samples and controls was completely removed and replaced with serum-free DMEM.

2.3. Laser Irradiation. The irradiation was performed with a Nd:YAG laser (1064-nm, DEKA Smart File) and a prefabricated, commercially available, handpiece (manipolo per terapia N40601). The laser beam was directed perpendicularly to the cell level from a distance of 5 mm. Cells were irradiated for 20, 40, 60, or 120 seconds (Figure 1).

The irradiation settings were power 0.5 W, frequency 10 Hz, energy 50 mJ, and pulse duration ≥ 700 μsec. The corresponding energy densities were 2.6 J/cm^2, 5.3 J/cm^2, 7.9 J/cm^2, and 15.8 J/cm^2, respectively (Table 1). A wide range of energy densities was selected, to investigate all the possible

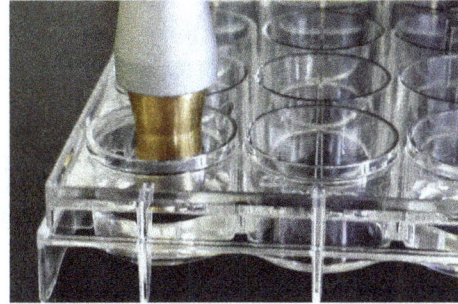

FIGURE 1: The irradiation was carried out with manipolo per terapia N4060 handpiece, approximately 5 mm above cell level.

TABLE 1: Laser parameters used during irradiation.

Laser	Nd:YAG			
Wavelength	1064 nm			
Spectrum	Near-infrared			
Irradiation mode	Pulsed wave, long pulse (≥ 700 μsec)			
Settings	Power 0,5 W, frequency 10 Hz, and energy 50 mJ			
Duration	20 s	40 s	60 s	120 s
Energy density	2.6 J/cm^2	5.3 J/cm^2	7.9 J/cm^2	15.8 J/cm^2
Irradiation	Single treatment at day 0			
Spot area	0,785 cm^2 (manipolo per terapia N40601)			
Distance of irradiation	5 mm			

effects of LLLT with Nd:YAG laser on gingival fibroblasts, either positive or negative. Control cultures were not irradiated. All experiments were performed in duplicate.

2.4. Proliferation Assessment. Cells were counted after trypsinization (0,05% trypsin/EDTA in PBS for 5 minutes) at day 0 (baseline levels), 24, 48, and 72 hours after irradiation for both irradiated and control groups. The proliferation was assessed with an optical method. In an inverted optical microscope (Zeis), cell counting was performed over a hemocytometer, by an experienced blinded (the examiner was not aware of the treatment for each culture) biologist.

2.5. Growth Factors Assay. Growth factors' secretion was assessed with Luminex technology. Luminex's xMAP technology is based on a combination of flow cytometry, microspheres, lasers, digital signal processing, and traditional chemistry. The technique involves Luminex's 100 distinct sets of tiny color-coded beads, called microspheres. Each bead set can be coated with a specific capture probe or Anti Tag to allow the capture and detection of specific targets. The technology allows rapid and precise analysis of several protein molecules, within a single reaction.

Supernatants were collected at day 0 (baseline levels), 24, 48, and 72 hours after irradiation. A quantitative analysis of EGF, bFGF, and VEGF levels was performed, according to the

(a)

(b)

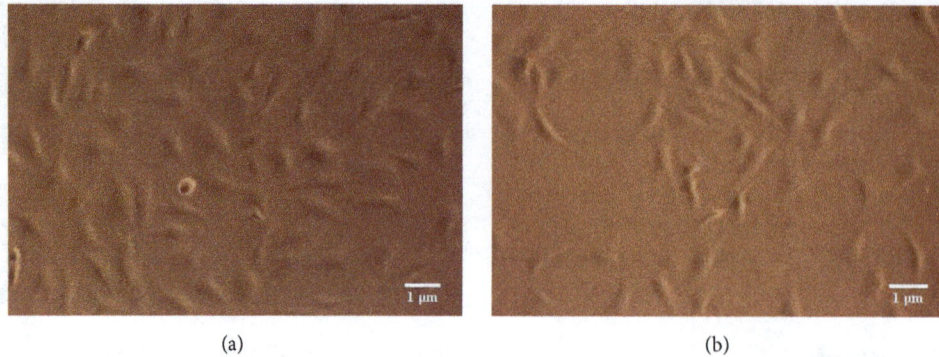

FIGURE 2: Human gingival fibroblasts at 48 hours. (a) Irradiated with Nd:YAG laser for 120 (120 s group) (original magnification, ×100). (b) Nonirradiated (Ctrl group), (original magnification, ×100).

TABLE 2: Cell counts of control and test groups for the different time points.

Cells	N	Mean (SD)	Median (range)	p value[*]
24 hours				
Controls	4	39500 (10116)	41000 (28000, 48000)	
20 s	4	35250 (8382)	37000 (24000, 43000)	0.54
40 s	4	37000 (11605)	38000 (22000, 50000)	0.76
60 s	4	41000 (13216)	40000 (26000, 58000)	0.86
120 s	4	38750 (8539)	37500 (30000, 50000)	0.91
48 hours				
Controls	4	44000 (15144)	38000 (34000, 66000)	
20 s	4	45500 (5972)	44000 (40000, 54000)	0.86
40 s	4	51500 (9849)	51000 (40000, 64000)	0.43
60 s	4	61500 (5972)	60000 (56000, 70000)	0.07
120 s	4	68000 (6325)	69000 (60000, 74000)	**0.03**
72 hours				
Controls	4	72750 (10500)	69500 (64000, 88000)	
20 s	4	58000 (17205)	57000 (40000, 78000)	0.19
40 s	4	79500 (22531)	81000 (52000, 104000)	0.60
60 s	4	81500 (13796)	83000 (64000, 96000)	0.35
120 s	4	83500 (17388)	86000 (60000, 102000)	0.33

[*]Versus control.

manufactures' recommendations (Luminex Human Growth Factor 4-plex Panel Kit, Invitrogen, CA).

2.6. Statistical Analysis. To investigate differences in cells' number between each test group and controls, we used *Student's t-test*. For the comparison of growth factors (EGF, VEGF, and bFGF) we first calculated the change from the baseline measurement for each group and we compared those changes using *t-test*, at every time point. All tests were two-sided at $\alpha = 5\%$ level of statistical significance.

3. Results

All laser-irradiation doses applied promoted a higher cell proliferation at 48 hours compared to control group. This difference reached statistical significance for the group irradiated for 120 s versus control group (mean: 68000, SD:

6324.555, 95% CI: 57936.22–78063.78, and $p = 0.03$) (Figures 2(a) and 2(b)).

A dose-response relationship, at 48 h may be implied. At 72 hours, all laser-irradiated groups (except 20 s) cells' number was higher than controls. The growth curves are shown in Table 2 and Figure 4.

Growth factors' secretion results are presented in Table 3. Regarding EGF, all laser-irradiation doses applied promoted a higher secretion at 48 hours compared to control group. This difference reached statistical significance for the group irradiated for 20 s versus control group (mean: 16.7, SD: 5.608923, 95% CI: 7.774953–25.62505, and $p = 0.04$) (Figure 3). A reverse dose-response relationship, at 48 h, may be implied. As far as VEGF, at 48 h, values were higher or equal to controls. EGF and VEGF values, at the other time points (24 and 72 hours) and bFGF as well, showed a random variation between the groups.

TABLE 3: Mean (SD) change from the baseline measurement for each group at every time point.

	N	EGF Mean (SD)	p value*	N	VEGF Mean (SD)	p value*	N	bFGF Mean (SD)	p value*
					24 h				
Ctrl	4	3.9 (3.8)		4	2.9 (2.1)		4	−0.8 (3.6)	
20 s	4	−0.9 (8.8)	0.36	4	1.3 (0.3)	0.18	4	−2.9 (3.1)	0.41
40 s	4	−3.4 (11.2)	0.27	4	1.6 (1.3)	0.34	4	−1.9 (3.1)	0.65
60 s	4	−6.4 (8.6)	0.07	4	1.5 (0.4)	0.25	4	−0.4 (2.4)	0.87
120 s	4	11.3 (19.3)	0.48	4	4.9 (1.5)	0.18	4	−0.4 (1.8)	0.86
					48 h				
Ctrl	4	−9.6 (19.3)		4	3.3 (3.0)		4	−0.4 (1.9)	
20 s	4	16.7 (5.6)	**0.04**	4	7.0 (4.2)	0.20	4	1.3 (2.4)	0.33
40 s	4	9.9 (18.2)	0.19	4	4.0 (3.8)	0.77	4	−0.6 (1.4)	0.84
60 s	4	2.5 (22.9)	0.45	4	3.3 (2.2)	0.51	4	−0.3 (2.7)	0.94
120 s	4	−1.1 (4.8)	0.43	4	6.0 (7.4)	0.42	4	0.4 (1.1)	0.52
					72 h				
Ctrl	4	−0.1 (11.4)		4	3.8 (6.1)		4	0.4 (3.4)	
20 s	4	7.9 (7.7)	0.29	4	4.5 (4.4)	0.85	4	1.1 (2.3)	0.73
40 s	4	10.4 (11.5)	0.24	4	5.3 (5.7)	0.73	4	1.0 (1.1)	0.74
60 s	4	−5.3 (12.7)	0.57	4	2.6 (2.9)	0.75	4	−2.1 (3.3)	0.34
120 s	4	−1.9 (3.4)	0.78	4	3.6 (4.6)	0.98	4	−0.6 (2.3)	0.65

*t-test versus control.

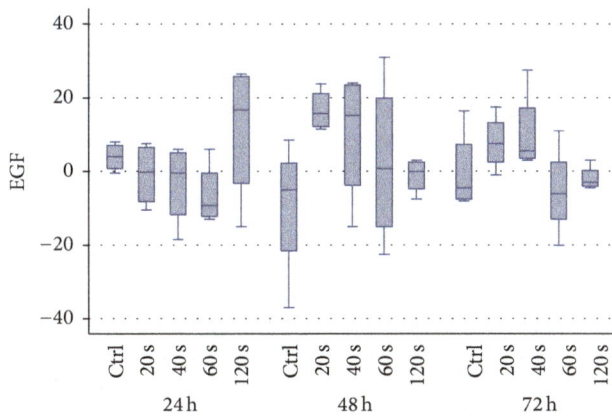

FIGURE 3: Boxplot of EGF values differences from baseline for each radiation time and control, after 24, 48, and 72 hours.

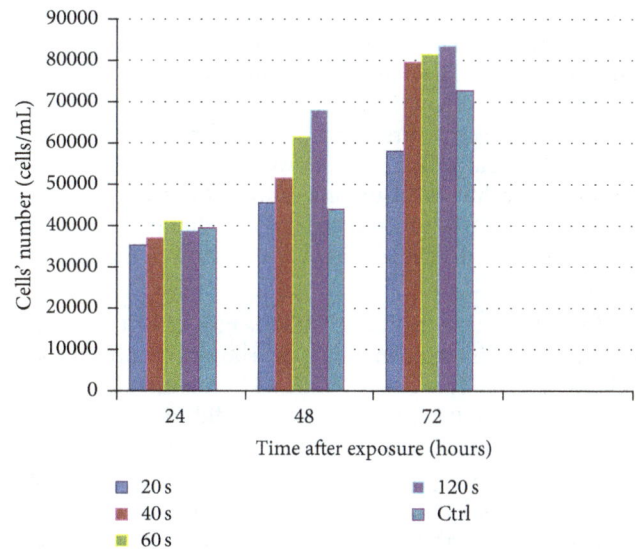

FIGURE 4: Cells' number of control and test groups 24, 48, and 72 hours after irradiation.

4. Discussion

4.1. LLLT and Cells Proliferation. Within the limitations of this study (sample size and arbitrary energy densities), it appeared that treatment with low power laser (LLLT) using Nd:YAG laser, specifically in irradiation time of 120 s (energy density: 15.8 J/cm^2), resulted in a statistically significant increase of cells' population ($p = 0.03$), compared to the control group, 48 hours after irradiation. In the international literature, some publications on the effect of laser devices on gingival fibroblasts, skin fibroblasts, and animal fibroblasts can be found [3, 15–19]. The heterogeneity, among these studies, regarding the type of laser devices used and their settings (wavelength, energy density), does not allow a direct comparison between them and exportation of a detailed conclusion. However, it is generally supported, in most of the studies, that LLLT increases the cell population of gingival fibroblasts [7, 13, 20–22]. A recent systematic review, about the effect of LLLT in various human and animal cell cultures, showed the ability of laser to modulate cellular proliferation. However, finding the most appropriate irradiation settings is still an important piece of research [23].

It is worth mentioning that there is no equivalent study in the literature, concerning the settings of Nd:YAG laser and irradiation time. However, three studies researched the effect of Nd:YAG laser on gingival fibroblasts [15–17]. Specifically, Chen et al., in 2000, noticed evidence of a decrease in the vitality of human gingival fibroblasts (cell damage zone 2.2~4.2 mm in diameter), after irradiation (1.0–3.0 W), for 10 sec. However, when defocused irradiation was applied (2 mm from the cell level), no significant decrease in cell vitality was observed. The main difference between Chen's study and ours is the irradiation power (1–3 W versus 0.5 W). It seems that these power values cause cells' death. Furthermore, Chen et al. used a 400 μm diameter fiber in contact or in 2 mm distance from cell level, in contrast with the present study, where a defocused handpiece (which ensured a uniform distribution of radiation on cells across the surface of the well) from the distance of 5 mm was used. Possibly the minus spot size (increased energy density) led to cells' death [15]. Moreover, Gutknecht et al. reported cellular (L-929 fibroblast cell cultures) damage with a necrotic zone of 8.1~10.0 mm in diameter after Nd:YAG laser irradiation (2.1~3.0 W) for 30 seconds [16]. It is obvious that at these two studies examined the possible hazard effect of Nd:YAG laser irradiation on gingival fibroblasts' vitality. In our study, the aim was to investigate the possible beneficial effects of Nd:YAG laser, using low level settings.

In another *in vitro* study, in skin fibroblasts, it appeared that the application of the Nd:YAG laser and KTP laser at high doses (10–40 J/cm^2 and 3–12 J/cm^2, resp.) resulted in structural damage to the DNA of cells [24]. In corresponding results, Hawkins and Abrahamse using high doses of irradiation with a HeNe laser (632.8-nm) observed a deterioration of structural components of the membrane and the DNA of the cells. They showed better results in skin fibroblasts' proliferation and migration after irradiation with HeNe laser (632.8-nm), relative to the diode 830 nm and Nd:YAG (1064 nm) (irradiation with 5 J/cm^2 on the first and fourth day) [25].

The other study, using Nd:YAG laser for LLLT (1.5 J/cm^2), was from Chellini et al. in 2010, who showed that fibroblasts' (cell line derived from mice NIH/3T3 fibroblasts) irradiation did not alter the vitality of cells, but it did not enhance cell proliferation too, 24 and 48 hours after irradiation. Instead, LLLT resulted in significant production of type I collagen. Results indicated the possible regulator role of LLLT with Nd:YAG laser in this particular cell culture [17]. Between this study and ours are many differences (primary culture versus cell line, frequency, energy, optic fiber diameter, time, and distance of irradiation), so a direct comparison cannot be implied. However, regarding energy densities (1.5 J/cm^2 versus 2.6 to 15.8 J/cm^2), it can be postulated that energy densities higher than 2.6 J/cm^2 should be used in LLLT with Nd:YAG laser to achieve gingival fibroblast proliferation.

In literature, there are studies using other laser wavelengths in LLLT. Specifically, Kreisler et al. found a statistically significant difference in gingival fibroblasts proliferation, 24 and 48 hours after irradiation with a diode laser (809 nm, 7.84 J/cm^2) [26]. The same biostimulatory effect of LLLT in gingival fibroblasts in *in vitro* studies was found by Basso et al. in 2012 with a diode laser (780±3 nm, 0.5 and 3 J/cm^2) [13],

Vinck et al. in 2003 with a diode laser (830 nm, 1 J/cm^2) [27], Azevedo et al. in 2006 with a diode laser (660 nm, 2 J/cm^2) [7], and Pourzarandian et al. in 2005 with a Er:YAG laser (3.37 J/cm^2) [20].

4.2. LLLT and Growth Factors' Secretion. In this study, we found that all laser-irradiation doses applied promoted a higher secretion of EGF, at 48 hours, compared to control group. This difference reached statistical significance for the group irradiated for 20 s versus the control group ($p = 0.04$). A reverse dose-response relationship, at 48 h, may be implied. Potentially, this trend exists, in the other groups, like VEGF at 48 h, where all laser-irradiated group's values of VEGF were higher or equal to controls. However, due to the small sample, this claim remains to be confirmed by future studies. EGF and VEGF values at the other time points (24 and 72 hours) and bFGF as well showed a random variation between the groups.

It should be emphasized that in the literature there is no study to date to examine the secretion of EGF and VEGF from gingival fibroblasts after irradiation with Nd:YAG laser. The only relative reference is EGF secretion and LLLT, done by Mvula et al. in 2009, who studied the synergistic action of the growth factor with LLLT (636 nm, diode laser), which led to the proliferation of stem cells of adipose tissue [28].

In an experimental study on gingival fibroblast culture, it was found that irradiation with diode laser caused increased production of VEGF and TGF-b mRNA and the corresponding mRNA for the synthesis of type I collagen [29]. Also, Kipshidze et al., in 2001, showed that LLLT (He:Ne, 632 nm, 2.1 J/cm^2) resulted in a statistically significant increase of VEGF secretion in culture of myocardium fibroblasts [30]. Dourado et al. in 2011, in an *in vitro* study in endothelial and nonendothelial cells of mice gastrocnemius, showed that LLLT with HeNe (632.8 nm) or GaAs (904 nm) laser increased angiogenesis and the proliferation of regenerating cells and decreased polymorphonuclear neutrophils [31]. Furthermore, in an *in vivo* animal (rat) study, it was found that LLLT with diode laser radiation in two different lengths (with energy density of 35 and 5 J/cm^2, resp.) resulted in a statistically significant reduction of expression of mRNA transcripting VEGF, after injury of the rats' tongue [32]. These data suggest that LLLT accelerates wound healing.

In the present study, no difference was observed in the secretion of bFGF between groups. Safavi et al. in 2008 led to similar results while LLLT with HeNe laser (7.51 J/cm^2) in mice gingiva showed a statistically significant increase in secretion of PDGF and TGF-b genes, 30 minutes after irradiation, but no influence to bFGF [3]. Indeed, Hawkins and Abrahamse reported that LLLT with Nd:YAG laser (1064 nm, 16 J/cm^2) resulted in reduced secretion of TGF-b ($p \leq 0.05$). In contrast, irradiation with HeNe laser (632.8-nm, 5 J/cm^2) resulted in marginally significant increase in secretion of bFGF ($p = 0.05$) [25]. Moreover, Saygun et al. found a statistical significance ($p \leq 0.01$) in bFGF expression after irradiation with a diode laser (685 nm for 140 s, 2 J/cm^2) [21]. Damante et al. concluded similar results in an *in vitro* study with a diode laser (660 nm, 3 J/cm^2 and 5 J/cm^2) [14]. Finally, it has been showed that LLLT with KTP laser (532 nm,

$0.8 \, J/cm^2$) in human skin fibroblasts led to statistically significant increase of bFGF gene expression [18]. These studies show that LLLT with diode laser, KTP, or HeNe laser possibly have an advantage compared to Nd:YAG laser, concerning bFGF secretion. On the other hand, Usumez et al. in an animal study found that Nd:YAG and 980 nm diode laser therapy ($8 \, J/cm^2$) accelerated the wound healing process by changing the expression of PDGF and bFGF [33].

Finally it is transpired that LLLT with Nd:YAG laser, at the settings used in this study (energy densities 2.6 to $15.8 \, J/cm^2$), promoted both keratinized mucosa fibroblasts' proliferation and EGF secretion, 48 hours after irradiation. It could be postulated that a repetition of LLLT (with Nd:YAG laser) every 48 hours could possibly induce growth factors' secretion and cells proliferation after each irradiation.

5. Conclusion

Within the limitations of this experimental study (sample size and arbitrary energy densities), the results indicated that LLLT (Nd:YAG 1064 laser) did not cause cell death for the settings used. It appears that these settings of Nd:YAG laser are safe. Moreover, the cell proliferation of primary cultured gingival fibroblasts increased after laser irradiation, presenting a potentially dose-dependent action. LLLT (Nd:YAG, 1064 laser) contributes probably to the secretion of EGF in a reverse dose-response pattern. Finally, it becomes clear that more studies with larger sample sizes are needed, in order to draw solid conclusions. Future studies should consider evaluating growth factors, irradiation parameters, and/or laser wavelengths.

Conflict of Interests

The authors declare that there is no conflict of interests regarding the publication of this paper.

Acknowledgment

This study was funded by the authors.

References

[1] J. D. Carroll, M. R. Milward, P. R. Cooper, M. Hadis, and W. M. Palin, "Developments in low level light therapy (LLLT) for dentistry," *Dental Materials*, vol. 30, no. 5, pp. 465–475, 2014.

[2] X. Gao and D. Xing, "Molecular mechanisms of cell proliferation induced by low power laser irradiation," *Journal of Biomedical Science*, vol. 16, no. 1, article 4, 2009.

[3] S. M. Safavi, B. Kazemi, M. Esmaeili, A. Fallah, A. Modarresi, and M. Mir, "Effects of low-level He-Ne laser irradiation on the gene expression of IL-1β, TNF-α, IFN-γ, TGF-β, bFGF, and PDGF in rat's gingiva," *Lasers in Medical Science*, vol. 23, no. 3, pp. 331–335, 2008.

[4] J. E. Janis, R. K. Kwon, and D. H. Lalonde, "A practical guide to wound healing," *Plastic and Reconstructive Surgery*, vol. 125, no. 6, pp. 230e–244e, 2010.

[5] D. I. R. Holmes and I. C. Zachary, "Vascular endothelial growth factor regulates stanniocalcin-1 expression via neuropilin-1-dependent regulation of KDR and synergism with fibroblast growth factor-2," *Cellular Signalling*, vol. 20, no. 3, pp. 569–579, 2008.

[6] F. Nishimura and V. P. Terranova, "Comparative study of the chemotactic responses of periodontal ligament cells and gingival fibroblasts to polypeptide growth factors," *Journal of Dental Research*, vol. 75, no. 4, pp. 986–992, 1996.

[7] L. H. Azevedo, F. de Paula Eduardo, M. S. Moreira, C. de Paula Eduardo, and M. M. Marques, "Influence of different power densities of LILT on cultured human fibroblast growth: a pilot study," *Lasers in Medical Science*, vol. 21, no. 2, pp. 86–89, 2006.

[8] K. Ejiri, A. Aoki, Y. Yamaguchi, M. Ohshima, and Y. Izumi, "High-frequency low-level diode laser irradiation promotes proliferation and migration of primary cultured human gingival epithelial cells," *Lasers in Medical Science*, vol. 29, no. 4, pp. 1339–1347, 2014.

[9] J.-Y. Wu, C.-H. Chen, L.-Y. Yeh, M.-L. Yeh, C.-C. Ting, and Y.-H. Wang, "Low-power laser irradiation promotes the proliferation and osteogenic differentiation of human periodontal ligament cells via cyclic adenosine monophosphate," *International Journal of Oral Science*, vol. 5, no. 2, pp. 85–91, 2013.

[10] V. Aleksic, A. Aoki, K. Iwasaki et al., "Low-level Er:YAG laser irradiation enhances osteoblast proliferation through activation of MAPK/ERK," *Lasers in Medical Science*, vol. 25, no. 4, pp. 559–569, 2010.

[11] J. Wang, W. Huang, Y. Wu et al., "MicroRNA-193 pro-proliferation effects for bone mesenchymal stem cells after low-level laser irradiation treatment through inhibitor of growth family, member 5," *Stem Cells and Development*, vol. 21, no. 13, pp. 2508–2519, 2012.

[12] W. Lim, J. Kim, S. Kim et al., "Modulation of lipopolysaccharide-induced NF-κB signaling pathway by 635 nm irradiation via heat shock protein 27 in human gingival fibroblast cells," *Photochemistry and Photobiology*, vol. 89, no. 1, pp. 199–207, 2013.

[13] F. G. Basso, T. N. Pansani, A. P. S. Turrioni, V. S. Bagnato, J. Hebling, and C. A. De Souza Costa, "In vitro wound healing improvement by low-level laser therapy application in cultured gingival fibroblasts," *International Journal of Dentistry*, vol. 2012, Article ID 719452, 6 pages, 2012.

[14] C. A. Damante, G. De Micheli, S. P. H. Miyagi, I. S. Feist, and M. M. Marques, "Effect of laser phototherapy on the release of fibroblast growth factors by human gingival fibroblasts," *Lasers in Medical Science*, vol. 24, no. 6, pp. 885–891, 2009.

[15] Y. J. Chen, J. H. Jeng, B. S. Lee, H. F. Chang, K. C. Chen, and W. H. Lan, "Effects of Nd:YAG laser irradiation on cultured human gingival fibroblasts," *Lasers in Surgery and Medicine*, vol. 27, no. 5, pp. 471–478, 2000.

[16] N. Gutknecht, S. Kanehl, A. Moritz, C. Mittermayer, and F. Lampert, "Effects of Nd:YAG-laser irradiation on monolayer cell cultures," *Lasers in Surgery and Medicine*, vol. 22, no. 1, pp. 30–36, 1998.

[17] F. Chellini, C. Sassoli, D. Nosi et al., "Low pulse energy Nd:YAG laser irradiation exerts a biostimulative effect on different cells of the oral microenvironment: 'an in vitro study,'" *Lasers in Surgery and Medicine*, vol. 42, no. 6, pp. 527–539, 2010.

[18] V. K. M. Poon, L. Huang, and A. Burd, "Biostimulation of dermal fibroblast by sublethal Q-switched Nd:YAG 532 nm

laser: collagen remodeling and pigmentation," *Journal of Photochemistry and Photobiology B: Biology*, vol. 81, no. 1, pp. 1–8, 2005.

[19] Y. Weng, Y. Dang, X. Ye, N. Liu, Z. Zhang, and Q. Ren, "Investigation of irradiation by different nonablative lasers on primary cultured skin fibroblasts," *Clinical and Experimental Dermatology*, vol. 36, no. 6, pp. 655–660, 2011.

[20] A. Pourzarandian, H. Watanabe, S. M. P. M. Ruwanpura, A. Aoki, and I. Ishikawa, "Effect of low-level Er:YAG laser irradiation on cultured human gingival fibroblasts," *Journal of Periodontology*, vol. 76, no. 2, pp. 187–193, 2005.

[21] I. Saygun, S. Karacay, M. Serdar, A. U. Ural, M. Sencimen, and B. Kurtis, "Effects of laser irradiation on the release of basic fibroblast growth factor (bFGF), insulin like growth factor-1 (IGF-1), and receptor of IGF-1 (IGFBP3) from gingival fibroblasts," *Lasers in Medical Science*, vol. 23, no. 2, pp. 211–215, 2008.

[22] I. S. Feist, G. De Micheli, S. R. S. Carneiro, C. P. Eduardo, S. P. H. Miyagi, and M. M. Marques, "Adhesion and growth of cultured human gingival fibroblasts on periodontally involved root surfaces treated by Er:YAG laser," *Journal of Periodontology*, vol. 74, no. 9, pp. 1368–1375, 2003.

[23] P. V. Peplow, T.-Y. Chung, and G. D. Baxter, "Laser photobiomodulation of proliferation of cells in culture: a review of human and animal studies," *Photomedicine and Laser Surgery*, vol. 28, no. 1, pp. S3–S40, 2010.

[24] N. Senturk, A. Bedir, B. Bilgici et al., "Genotoxic effects of 1064-nm Nd:YAG and 532-nm KTP lasers on fibroblast cell cultures: experimental dermatology," *Clinical and Experimental Dermatology*, vol. 35, no. 5, pp. 516–520, 2010.

[25] D. H. Hawkins and H. Abrahamse, "Time-dependent responses of wounded human skin fibroblasts following phototherapy," *Journal of Photochemistry and Photobiology B: Biology*, vol. 88, no. 2-3, pp. 147–155, 2007.

[26] M. Kreisler, A. B. Christoffers, H. Al-Haj, B. Willershausen, and B. D'Hoedt, "Low level 809-nm diode laser-induced in vitro stimulation of the proliferation of human gingival fibroblasts," *Lasers in Surgery and Medicine*, vol. 30, no. 5, pp. 365–369, 2002.

[27] E. M. Vinck, B. J. Cagnie, M. J. Cornelissen, H. A. Declercq, and D. C. Cambier, "Increased fibroblast proliferation induced by light emitting diode and low power laser irradiation," *Lasers in Medical Science*, vol. 18, no. 2, pp. 95–99, 2003.

[28] B. Mvula, T. J. Moore, and H. Abrahamse, "Effect of low-level laser irradiation and epidermal growth factor on adult human adipose-derived stem cells," *Lasers in Medical Science*, vol. 25, no. 1, pp. 33–39, 2010.

[29] S. S. I. Hakki and S. B. Bozkurt, "Effects of different setting of diode laser on the mRNA expression of growth factors and type i collagen of human gingival fibroblasts," *Lasers in Medical Science*, vol. 27, no. 2, pp. 325–331, 2012.

[30] N. Kipshidze, V. Nikolaychik, M. H. Keelan et al., "Low-power helium: neon laser irradiation enhances production of vascular endothelial growth factor and promotes growth of endothelial cells in vitro," *Lasers in Surgery and Medicine*, vol. 28, no. 4, pp. 355–364, 2001.

[31] D. M. Dourado, S. Fávero, R. Matias, P. D. T. C. Carvalho, and M. A. Da Cruz-Höfling, "Low-level laser therapy promotes vascular endothelial growth factor receptor-1 expression in endothelial and nonendothelial cells of mice gastrocnemius exposed to snake venom," *Photochemistry and Photobiology*, vol. 87, no. 2, pp. 418–426, 2011.

[32] T. C. Silva, T. M. Oliveira, V. T. Sakai et al., "In vivo effects on the expression of vascular endothelial growth factor-A$_{165}$ messenger ribonucleic acid of an infrared diode laser associated or not with a visible red diode laser," *Photomedicine and Laser Surgery*, vol. 28, no. 1, pp. 63–68, 2010.

[33] A. Usumez, B. Cengiz, S. Oztuzcu, T. Demir, M. H. Aras, and N. Gutknecht, "Effects of laser irradiation at different wavelengths (660, 810, 980, and 1,064 nm) on mucositis in an animal model of wound healing," *Lasers in Medical Science*, vol. 29, no. 6, pp. 1807–1813, 2014.

12

Computer-Guided Implant Surgery in Fresh Extraction Sockets and Immediate Loading of a Full Arch Restoration: A 2-Year Follow-Up Study of 14 Consecutively Treated Patients

M. Daas,[1,2] **A. Assaf,**[3,4] **K. Dada,**[2,5] **and J. Makzoumé**[6]

[1]*Department of Prosthodontics, René Descartes University, Paris, France*
[2]*Private Practice, 62 Boulevard de la Tour Maubourg, 75007 Paris, France*
[3]*Department of Prosthodontics, Beirut Arab University, Beirut, Lebanon*
[4]*Department of Prosthodontics, Lebanese University, Beirut, Lebanon*
[5]*Former Clinical Associate, Louis Mournier Hospital, Colombes, France*
[6]*Department of Removable Prosthodontics, Saint-Joseph University, Beirut, Lebanon*

Correspondence should be addressed to A. Assaf; dr.andre.assaf@gmail.com

Academic Editor: Andreas Stavropoulos

Statement of Problem. Low scientific evidence is identified in the literature for combining implant placement in fresh extraction sockets with immediate function. Moreover, the few studies available on immediate implants in postextraction sites supporting immediate full-arch rehabilitation clearly lack comprehensive protocols. *Purpose.* The purpose of this study is to report outcomes of a comprehensive protocol using CAD-CAM technology for surgical planning and fabrication of a surgical template and to demonstrate that immediate function can be easily performed with immediate implants in postextraction sites supporting full-arch rehabilitation. *Material and Methods.* 14 subjects were consecutively rehabilitated (13 maxillae and 1 mandible) with 99 implants supporting full-arch fixed prostheses followed between 6 and 24 months (mean of 16 months). Outcome measures were prosthesis and implant success, biologic and prosthetic complications, pain, oedema evaluation, and radiographic marginal bone levels at surgery and then at 6, 12, 18, and 24 months. Data were analyzed with descriptive statistics. *Results.* The overall cumulative implant survival rate at mean follow-up time of 16 months was 97.97%. The average marginal bone loss was 0,9 mm. *Conclusions.* Within the limitations of this study, the results validate this treatment modality for full-arch rehabilitations with predictable outcomes and high survival rate after 2 years.

1. Introduction

For 40 years, the use of osseointegrated implants has shown to be a supplementary modality for treating full or partial edentulism [1]. Since the early 1990s, providing shorter treatment periods to patients has become a major focus first via the one-stage surgical technique [2] and then through the immediate loading protocol [3]. Delivering a fixed prosthesis on the same day of the last extractions supported by immediate implants has quickly become a major challenge. Patients can therefore never be left without teeth and the treatment length is ultimately shortened.

These protocols provide multiple benefits [4]: (1) only one surgical session, (2) immediate loading of a temporary prosthesis allowing for a reduction of the patient's discomfort and facilitating his return to social and professional life, (3) avoiding the resorption of hard tissues, the two-thirds of this reduction occurring during the first 3 months, (4) guiding the soft tissue healing for an optimal aesthetic environment and minimal recession, and (5) taking advantage of the extraction socket healing potential.

Nevertheless, if treatments by immediate implants associated with deferred loading have a long clinical history [5] and offer good results [6], low scientific evidence exists for their combination with immediate function.

The published clinical results are somewhat unsettled. Balshi and Wolfinger 1997 [7] and then Chaushu et al. 2001 [8] obtained success rates of 80% and 82.4%, respectively, for immediately loaded implants in postextraction sites. More encouraging results were reported by Cooper et al. 2002 [9] as well as by Grunder 2001 [10] with survival rates of 100% and 97.3%, respectively, for similar protocols in the mandible. However, it was reported by de Sanctis et al. 2009 [11] that in spite of achieving predictable osteointegration when implants were placed in fresh extraction sockets, the occurrence of buccal bone resorption may limit the use of this surgical approach.

More recently, Villa and Rangert 2005 [12] reported a 100% success rate for the treatment of 20 patients with 97 implants placed in postextraction sites and combined with early function. They demonstrated that, with an appropriate biomechanical, surgical, and medical protocol considering preservation of high implant stability and controlled inflammatory response, implants may be successfully osseointegrated when immediately placed and early-loaded in postextraction sites.

Moreover, the few studies available on immediate implants in postextraction sites supporting immediate full-arch rehabilitation are focused on the surgical part of the procedure and clearly lacked comprehensive prosthetic protocols whereas the NobelGuide concept (NobelBiocare AB) presents a step by step treatment procedure that is known to be meticulous and successful [13]. The purpose of this study is to evaluate the effectiveness of a protocol combining a computed tomographic scan-derived surgical template with an immediate implant placement in postextraction sites together with immediate temporization and loading.

2. Materials and Methods

In this prospective case series study, clinical and radiological data analysis were carried out over a two and half years period, on a total of 14 consecutively treated subjects (mean age 58.14 years) to be restored with fixed full arches prosthesis: 6 women and 8 men were treated via immediate implantation combined to CAD-CAM technology (NobelGuide, Nobel-Biocare AB).

2.1. Inclusion Criteria. The authors defined the following inclusion criteria in patient selection:

(1) noncontributory medical history such as uncontrolled diabetes, and osteoporosis.

(2) adequate bone volume and density for conventional dental implant placement as determined by CBCT without the need for bone or soft-tissue grafts,

(3) patients requiring clearance of all remaining maxillary teeth,

(4) no infected sockets.

2.2. Exclusion Criteria. Consider the following:

(1) heavy smokers and/or confirmed bruxing subjects,

TABLE 1: Quantitative data concerning size and number of the successful and failed implants used in 14 subjects.

Implant type	Length (mm)	Number	Failed
NobelSpeedy NP	13	4	0
NobelSpeedy RP	11.5	2	0
	13	55	1
	15	21	0
NobelSpeedy WP	7	1	0
	8.5	2	1
	10	7	0
	13	7	0

(2) the total or partial lack of the above 4 inclusion criteria.

During preliminary evaluation, medical history and subjects' consent were collected. Preliminary screenings, including intraoral and panoramic radiographs, were performed. Eligible subjects received oral hygiene instructions. A total of 99 implants with external hexagon (NobelSpeedy and NobelBiocare AB) and oxidized surface (Ti-unite Groovy and NobelBiocare AB) were inserted and loaded immediately after surgery via previously manufactured lab-made prosthesis (Table 1). All surgeries were performed by one clinician and procedures were preplanned according to the collected data. Outcome measures were prosthesis and implant success, biologic and prosthetic complications, pain, oedema, and radiographic marginal bone levels evaluation at surgery and then at 6, 12, 18, and 24 months.

2.3. Protocol. Impressions were made as for conventional partial removable denture, followed by intermaxillary relation registration. A trial denture was fabricated, tried in subject's mouth to validate the accuracy of the interarch relationship, and then processed to obtain a radiographic template according to the NobelGuide protocol (e.g., with at least 6 radiographic markers) (Figure 1). A first cone beam computed tomography (CBCT) was made with the radiographic template in place.

The remaining teeth were removed from the master model. Ridge (shape and volume) were regularized according to both the clinical findings and the CBCT findings (Figure 2). Two parameters were of particular consideration, the data collected during the periodontal examination and the prosthetic needs. The clinical findings included the probing depth, initial radiographic survey, and the preliminary planning following the first CBCT. In case of reduced prosthetic space, an additional osteotomy was performed but with caution, as resorption inevitably follows any surgical procedure. Still, a subcrestal leveling of the implants at the planning phase was programmed with implant platform positioned 2 mm under the coronal part of the vestibular alveolar crest.

Teeth that have been removed on the modified master model were replaced with denture teeth. The radiographic template was also altered so to be used for a second CBCT (e.g., scanning of the prosthesis itself) without any modification of the radiographic markers' position.

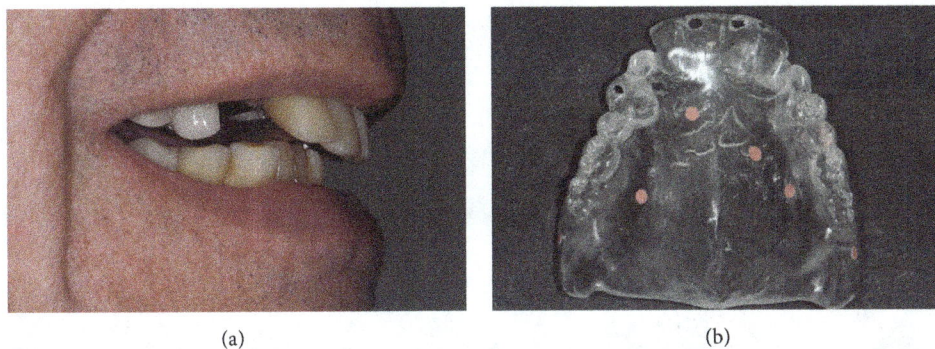

(a)

(b)

FIGURE 1: (a) Preoperative view demonstrating failing maxillary dentition. The treatment plan includes immediate implants in combination with CAD-CAM technology and their immediate loading with a prefabricated fixed prosthesis. (b) A radiographic template is realized according to the protocol for partially edentulous patient: verification windows to assess correct seating of radiographic template and radiopaque markers placed below gingival plane.

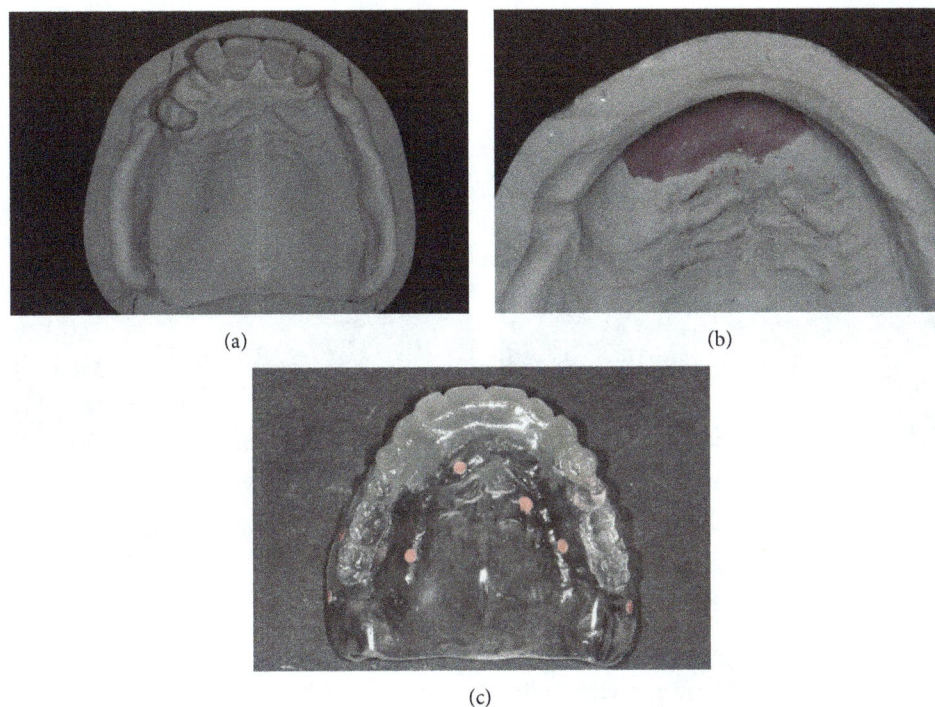

(a)

(b)

(c)

FIGURE 2: ((a) and (b)) Teeth are cut off from the master model according to the periodontal probing data. In this case, an additional osteotomy has been planned according to the prosthetic needs. (c) The radiographic template is repositioned on the master model and an additional set-up is done. This additional set-up is then polymerized. Observe that the location of the radiographic markers at this stage must remain the same.

Finally, subject's data and prosthesis data were loaded into the Procera software (ProceraCadDesign, NobelBiocare AB) and a high resolution 3D model was then created. Planning was performed according to conventional protocols. However, it seemed to be more effective with this immediate implants procedure (Figure 3) for the following reasons: (1) implant's length and diameter were easier to choose to assure enough primary bone anchorage, (2) remaining bone areas could be used more effectively, and (3) implant positioning was made according to the prosthetic project which was perhaps the most difficult objective to fulfill in such procedures. Otherwise, the implant placement would be more dependent on the remaining bone volume than on the prosthetic project and the procedure a hands-free one. The surgical template was ordered and data were also used to prepare a master model that allows for the fabrication of an all-acrylic resin fixed prosthesis (Figure 4) before the surgical session.

2.4. Surgery. The surgical procedure was performed under local anesthesia with articaine chlorhydrate containing epinephrine 1:100,000 (Alpha spe, Dentsply). All subjects

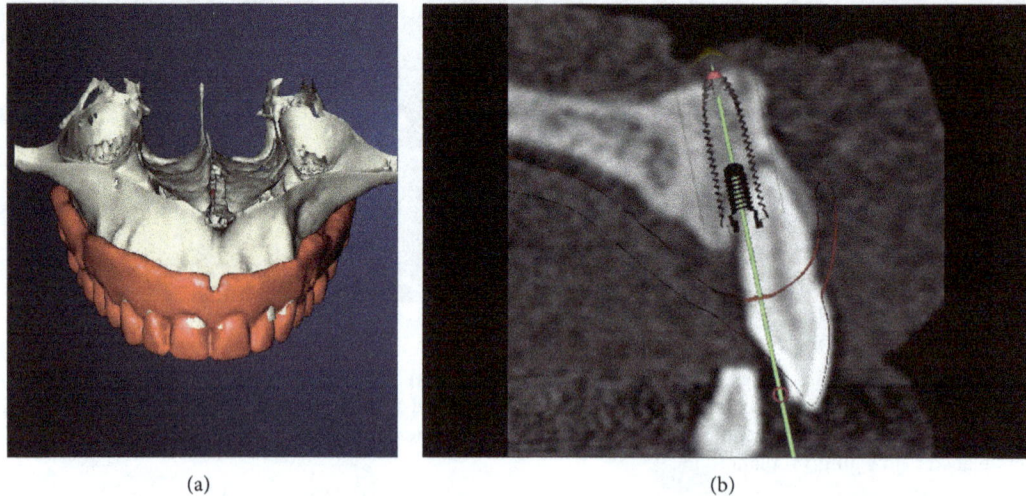

(a)   (b)

FIGURE 3: (a) Even if this template has never been worn by the patient, it can be merged to the patient CT data because of the radiographic markers. (b) Respect of the prosthetic project is easier with the computer-aided technology than in conventional hands-free procedure for immediate implants.

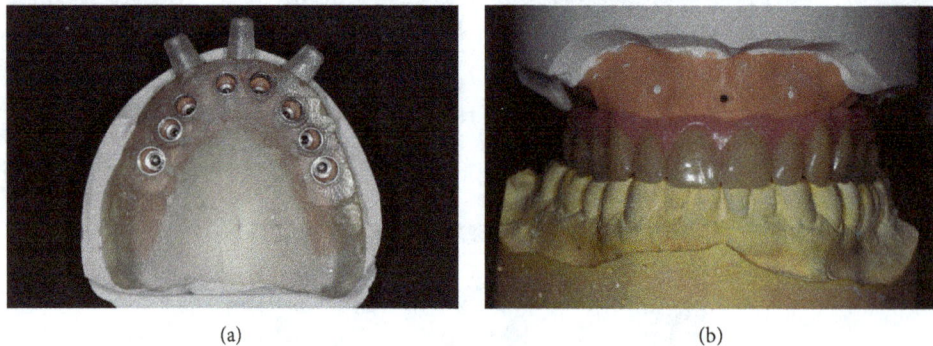

(a)   (b)

FIGURE 4: (a) Implant replicas are combined with the surgical template to obtain a master model. (b) The full-arch rehabilitation is realized on this model before the surgical session.

were sedated with diazepam (Valium 10 mg, Roche, Basel, Switzerland). Antibiotics amoxicillin 875 mg and clavulanic acid 125 mg (Augmentin 2 g, Glaxo Smith Kline) were given 1 hour prior to surgery and daily for 6 days thereafter. Corticoids (Solupred 60 mg, Sanofi Aventis) were administered daily from the day of surgery until 4 days postoperatively. Analgesics, 500 mg mefenamic acid (Ponstan Forte, Wilton ParkHouse, Wilton Place, Dublin 2, Ireland), were given on the day of surgery and postoperatively for the first 4 days if needed.

Three stages were followed in the procedure (Figure 5).

(1) As with immediate complete denture cases, the remaining teeth were extracted, followed by osteotomy and/or soft tissue management when needed [14]. This regularization allowed for correct repositioning of the soft tissues close to the conditions of an edentulous ridge. It was reported from the master cast to the mouth via a transparent replica of the surgical stereolithographic guide (NobelGuide), fabricated in

occlusion. Once made, these corrections secured an exact repositioning of the stereographic guide on the ridge.

(2) Positioning of the surgical template in the correct interarch relationship. The difficulties of repositioning the vestibular flap were countered by a strict positioning of the surgical guide(s) in the correct interarch relation for a precise transfer of the surgical planning.

(3) Implant placement per se. Implant length ranged from 7 to 13 mm.

2.5. Prosthetic Procedure. Expandable abutments (Guided Abutments, NobelBiocare AB) were mounted in the provisional restoration. The bridge was then positioned over the implants and screw-retained by manual tightening. The correct abutment connection was checked visually (Figure 5) and assessed radiographically. The correct centric relation was verified and minor occlusal adjustments were performed

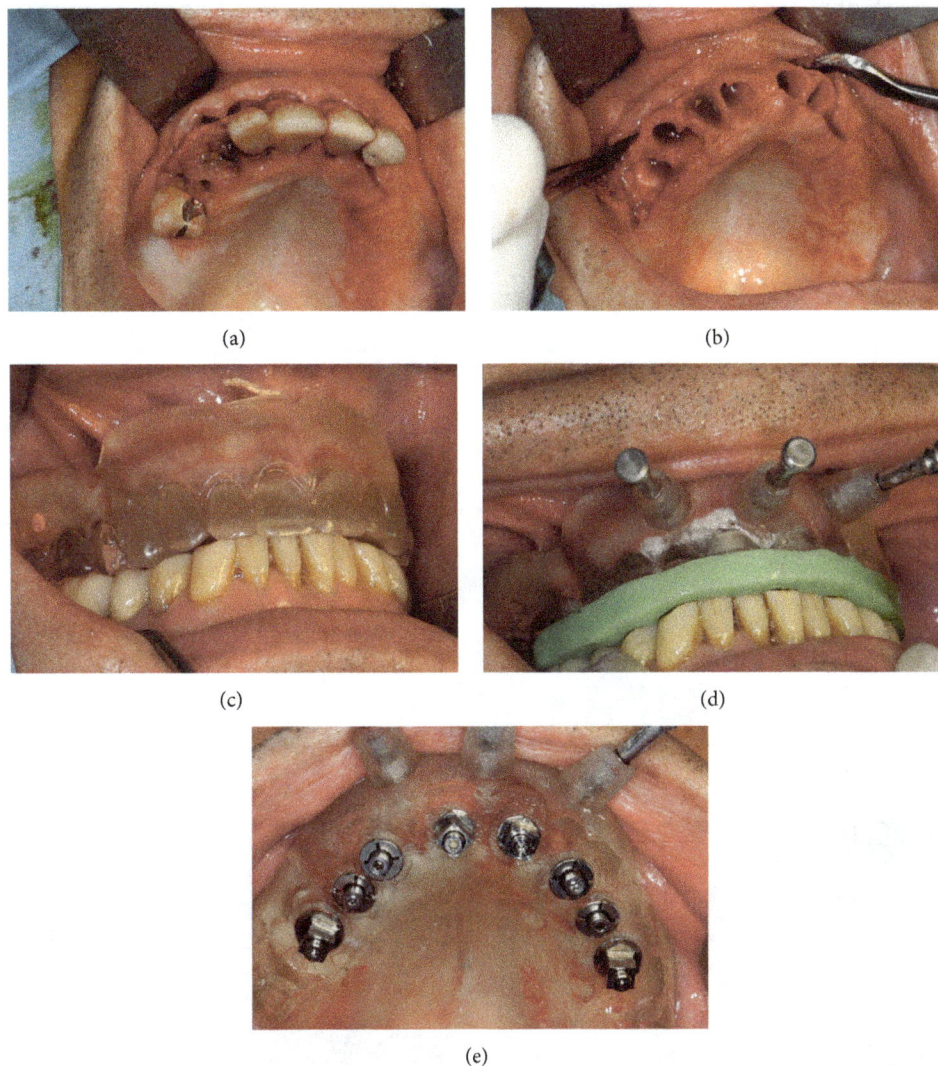

FIGURE 5: ((a) and (b)) Extraction of the 6 remaining teeth. (c) Blanching of the mucosa in a homogeneous way proves the correct positioning of the conventional surgical guide. (d) The stereolithographic surgical guide can thus be correctly placed via a lab-made occlusal index (using the articulator) and then stabilized with 3 transfixation screws. (e) Eight implants have been inserted according to the NobelGuide procedure.

when needed (Figure 6). The abutment screws were then tightened to 35 Ncm.

The subjects were enrolled in an implant maintenance program (Table 2) and a soft diet was instructed for 2 months. After 4 months, the prostheses were removed and the implants were individually tested for stability. If the implants were judged stable, the definitive fixed prosthesis was made as follows: two ceramic restorations (Procera Implant Bridge Zirconia, Nobel Biocare AB), seven metal-ceramic restorations, and fife hybrid prostheses (Figure 7).

2.6. Follow-Up. No subjects dropped out of this study. Subjects were examined at 1 week and at 1, 3, 6, and 12 months after the surgery. Examination included the assessment of prosthesis stability, peri-implant soft-tissue conditions, correct occlusion, and individual implant stability with the prosthesis removed at the 4-month follow-up.

To be classified as surviving, the implants were required to fulfill the following criteria: clinical stability, subject reported function without any discomfort, absence of suppuration, infection, or radiolucent areas around the implants.

Periapical radiographs (Figure 8) were made at implant insertion and then at 6-month intervals. The film was oriented with a conventional radiograph holder (Rinn XCP, Dentsply Rinn), manually positioned for an estimated orthogonal position of the film. An independent radiologist unaffiliated with the clinic interpreted the radiographs. The reference point for the reading was the implant platform. Marginal bone remodeling was calculated as the difference between readings at the examination and the baseline value at time of surgery. The radiographs were grouped as follows: implant insertion, 6 months, 1-year follow-up, 1-year and half follow-up, and 2-year follow-up. Implant survival and bone resorption data were analyzed with descriptive statistics.

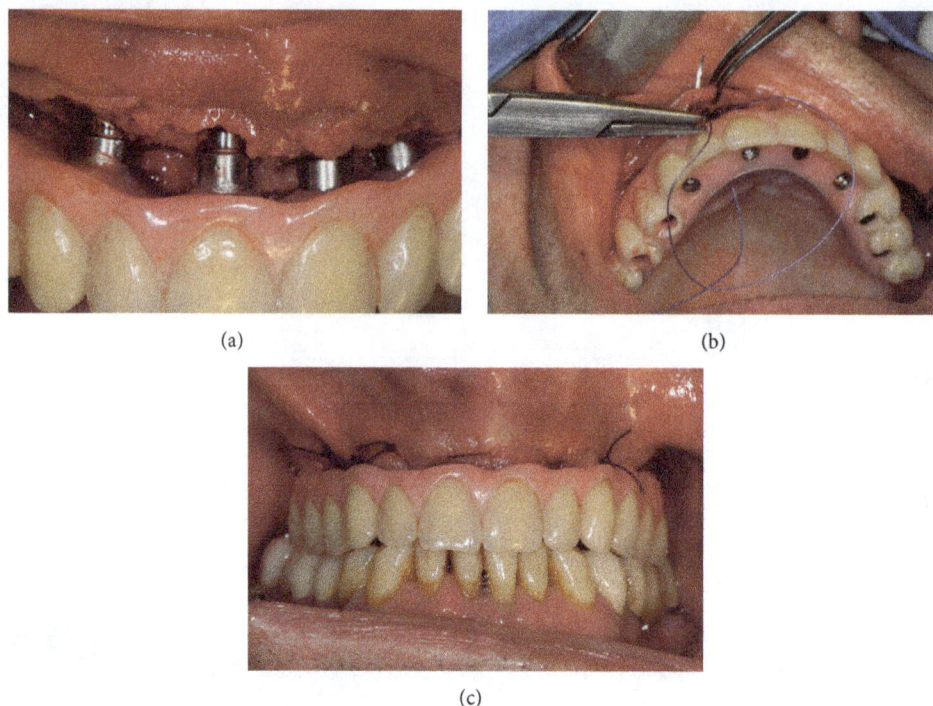

FIGURE 6: (a) Insertion of the restoration, in this protocol and because of the flap, the correct seating of the prosthesis can be checked visually. (b) The flap is sutured after the correct insertion of the restoration. (c) Final intraoral view.

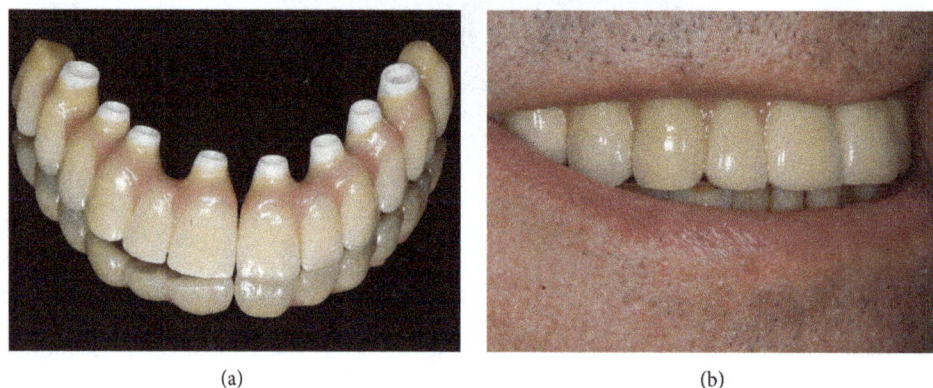

FIGURE 7: Final prosthesis. (a) Fixed ceramic one-piece prosthesis (Procera Implant Bridge Zirconia, Nobel Biocare AB). (b) Final extra oral view.

3. Results

Implant survival rates are presented in Table 3. The cumulative survival rate at 2 years was 97.97%. Sixty six implants have passed the 1- to 2-year follow-up. The mean follow-up time was 16.15 months.

Two implants in two different subjects were lost after 4 months at time of substituting the provisional restorations with the permanent ones: one implant in the first molar position in one heavy bruxing subject and the other in the second premolar position and that already was not stable at the time of placement. Both implants were reinserted and were not included in the statistical analysis. The prosthesis in these two subjects survived with the support of the remaining implants.

Twelve subjects experienced slight postoperative pain and two subjects experienced moderate or severe pain. Slight oedema was recorded for 11 subjects and moderate or severe oedema for the remaining three.

Three subjects experienced fracture of the transitional acrylic resin prostheses. One of them practically did not follow the instructions of soft food diet in the first few months. The handling of these problems necessitated the repair of the prostheses, adjustment of occlusion, and night guard fabrication. No further mechanical complications occurred.

The radiographic assessment of marginal bone level concerning the 66 implants available at the end of the 2-year follow-up period showed a mean marginal bone loss of approximately 0,9 mm.

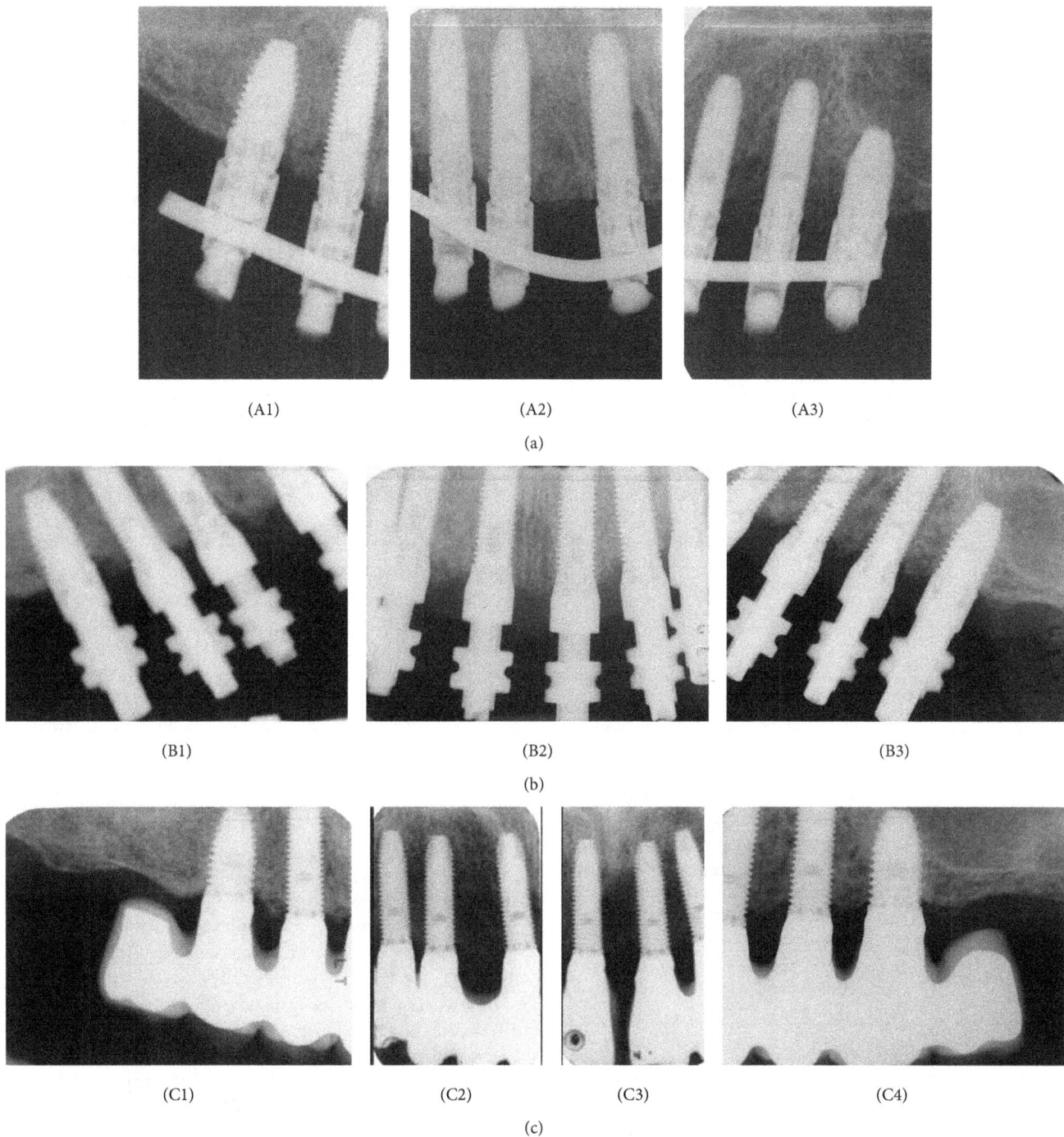

FIGURE 8: Radiographic examination: (A1), (A2), and (A3): postoperative radiographs. (B1), (B2), and (B3): at 6 months during the impression for the final restoration. (C1), (C2), (C3), and (C4): 18 months after the surgery.

4. Discussion

Immediate implant placement in fresh extraction sockets has been investigated in several clinical studies, showing clear scientific evidence that osseointegration may be successfully achieved [11, 15]. Later, the growing need for avoiding temporary removable prostheses after surgery led to considering immediate loading of implants inserted in fresh extraction sockets, even in the chronically infected alveolar bone [16]. However, the few studies available on immediate implants in postextraction sites supporting immediate full-arch rehabilitation show lack of homogeneity and comprehensive protocols [17].

The number of studies investigating the clinical and radiological outcome of guided implant placement seems to confirm the high predictability of 3D planning software and

TABLE 2: Postsurgical maintenance protocol.

Maintenance protocol	
Day of surgery (day 1)	Panoramic and periapical radiographs, explanation of maintenance procedures to the patient, application of chlorhexidine gel after surgery, evaluation of occlusion, and instructions to avoid prosthesis overload.
Day 10	Application of chlorhexidine gel, control of suppuration by finger pressure, removal of the sutures, evaluation of occlusion, instructions to avoid prosthesis overload, and evaluation for fracture or loosening of prosthetic components.
Month 1	Application of chlorhexidine gel, control of suppuration by finger pressure, tightening of the guided abutments at 35 Ncm, evaluation of occlusion, instructions to avoid prosthesis overload, and evaluation for fracture or loosening of prosthetic components.
Month 4	Panoramic and periapical radiographs, removal of prosthesis for cleaning and disinfecting, application of chlorhexidine gel, evaluation for inflammation/infection, evaluation of occlusion, instructions to avoid prosthesis overload, and evaluation for fracture or loosening of prosthetic components.
Month 6 or at definitive prosthesis placement	Panoramic and periapical radiographs, oral hygiene procedures every 3 months without removal of the prosthesis, evaluation of occlusion, and evaluation for inflammation/infection.
Month 12 and after	Panoramic and periapical radiographs, oral hygiene procedures every 6 months without removal of the prosthesis, and evaluation of occlusion, evaluation for inflammation/infection.
Problem-related visit	Removal of prosthesis for disinfection and cleaning and for testing implants for infections and stability.

TABLE 3: Life table of cumulative survival rate for implants.

	Number	Failures	Withdrawn	CSR %
Placement to 6 months	99	2	0	97.97%
6 to 12 months	93	0	0	97.97%
1 to 2 years	66	0	0	97.97%

indicate that immediate loading of oral implants yield acceptable to excellent results in full arch prosthetic restorations [14].

This preliminary study clearly demonstrates the high precision of transferring the virtual planning to the surgical field via the computer-aided technology even with extractions performed in the same surgical session. As in any extraction/implantation procedure, a judicious selection of the clinical case is essential for success. The presence of enough supra-alveolar bone is crucial for the primary stability of the fixture.

The benefits provided by computer-based planning seem to be superior with immediate implants cases in postextraction sites. Even without the use of the surgical template, there is a better match between the planned and the used implant when planning is done in a three-dimensional mode [18–20]. The preoperative choice of correct implant length and diameter can provide good primary stability through maximum filling of the extraction sockets and optimal engagement of the extra-apical alveolar bone. While no axial instability of any of the implants was observed, the insertion of some of the implants blocked at couples inferior to the recommended 35 Ncm. No adverse consequences were seen as these implants were connected to the others via a passive prosthesis. Knowing that primary stability measurements show significant correlations with different bone densities [21–23], the lesser density in the edentulous posterior regions could explain the encountered problems of stability, in opposition to the extraction sites where it was possible to engage in the nasal cortical bone.

Other benefits of guided implant planning and placement can be noted. (1) The remaining bone volume is used with more efficiency and predictability, (2) implant placement is made according to the prosthetic plan, and (3) the immediate cross-arch splinting of the freshly installed implant, another key factor for success [18, 19, 24–26], is easily obtained via the prefabricated prosthesis [27, 28].

The changes in marginal bone level were similar to those observed in the studies of Ganeles and Wismeijer in 2004 [24] and Glauser et al. in 2005 [25] on immediate loading and of Sanna et al. in 2007 on immediate loading and flapless surgery [26]. It can therefore be concluded that the applied protocol may improve the results of such prosthetic treatments renowned to be complex and unpredictable. It also offers a more adequate biomechanical environment for the implants, one that is "prosthetically driven."

However, the successful use of this approach requires advanced clinical experience, surgical judgment, and proper case selection. Further studies with larger sample size, including control groups (full-arch immediate implant rehabilitations with delayed healing or with the absence of extraction sockets), are necessary to confirm the suggested protocol.

5. Conclusion

Within the limitations of this study, combining a computed tomographic scan-derived surgical template to an immediate implant placement in postextraction sites together with immediate temporization and loading seems to be a predictable therapy, with high survival rate at 2-year period and valid functional and aesthetic results when applied in selected cases.

The applied protocol provides a safer procedure for both surgeon and patient and may become the gold standard for such treatments.

More clinical trials and follow-up studies are necessary before final conclusions can be drawn in relation to the long-term safety and efficacy of this proposed protocol.

Conflict of Interests

The authors declare that there is no conflict of interests regarding the publication of this paper.

References

[1] P. I. Brånemark, B. O. Hansson, R. Adell et al., "Osseointegrated implants in the treatment of the edentulous jaw. Experience from a 10-year period," *Scandinavian Journal of Plastic and Reconstructive Surgery*, vol. 16, pp. 1–132, 1977.

[2] D. Buser, H. P. Weber, U. Bragger, and C. Balsiger, "Tissue integration of one stage ITI implants: 3-year results of a longitudinal study with hollow-cylinder and hollow screw implants," *International Journal of Oral & Maxillofacial Implants*, vol. 6, no. 4, pp. 405–412, 1991.

[3] S. Szmukler-Moncler, H. Salama, Y. Reingewirtz, and J. H. Dubruille, "Timing of loading and effect of micromotion on bone-dental implant interface: review of experimental literature," *Journal of Biomedical Materials Research*, vol. 43, no. 2, pp. 192–203, 1998.

[4] L. Schropp, A. Wenzel, L. Kostopoulos, and T. Karring, "Bone healing and soft tissue contour changes following single-tooth extraction: a clinical and radiographic 12-month prospective study," *International Journal of Periodontics and Restorative Dentistry*, vol. 23, no. 4, pp. 313–323, 2003.

[5] G. Anneroth, K. G. Hedström, O. Kjellman, P.-Å. Köndell, and A. Nordenram, "Endosseus titanium implants in extraction sockets: an experimental study in monkeys," *International Journal of Oral Surgery*, vol. 14, no. 1, pp. 50–54, 1985.

[6] Y. H. Jo, P. K. Hobo, and S. Hobo, "Freestanding and multiunit immediate loading of the expandable implant: an up-to-40-month prospective survival study," *Journal of Prosthetic Dentistry*, vol. 85, no. 2, pp. 148–155, 2001.

[7] T. J. Balshi and G. J. Wolfinger, "Immediate loading of Brånemark implants in edentulous mandibles: a preliminary report," *Implant Dentistry*, vol. 6, no. 2, pp. 83–88, 1997.

[8] G. Chaushu, S. Chaushu, A. Tzohar, and D. Dayan, "Immediate loading of single tooth implants: immediate versus non immediate implantation. A clinical report," *International Journal of Oral and Maxillofacial Implants*, vol. 16, no. 2, pp. 267–272, 2001.

[9] L. F. Cooper, A. Rahman, J. Moriarty, N. Chaffee, and D. Sacco, "Immediate mandibular rehabilitation with endosseous implants: simultaneous extraction, implant placement and loading," *International Journal of Oral and Maxillofacial Implants*, vol. 17, no. 4, pp. 517–525, 2002.

[10] U. Grunder, "Immediate functional loading of immediate implants in edentulous arches: two year results," *International Journal of Periodontics and Restorative Dentistry*, vol. 21, no. 6, pp. 545–551, 2001.

[11] M. de Sanctis, F. Vignoletti, N. Discepoli, G. Zucchelli, and M. Sanz, "Immediate implants at fresh extraction sockets: bone healing in four different implant systems," *Journal of Clinical Periodontology*, vol. 36, no. 8, pp. 705–711, 2009.

[12] R. Villa and B. Rangert, "Early loading of interforaminal implants immediately installed after extraction of teeth presenting endodontic and periodontal lesions," *Clinical Implant Dentistry and Related Research*, vol. 7, no. 1, pp. S28–S35, 2005.

[13] S. F. Balshi, G. J. Wolfinger, and T. J. Balshi, "Surgical planning and prosthesis construction using computed tomography, CAD/CAM technology, and the internet for immediate loading of dental implants," *Journal of Esthetic and Restorative Dentistry*, vol. 18, no. 6, pp. 312–323, 2006.

[14] S. M. Meloni, G. de Riu, M. Pisano, and A. Tullio, "Full arch restoration with computer-assisted implant surgery and immediate loading in edentulous ridges with dental fresh extraction sockets. One year results of 10 consecutively treated patients: guided implant surgery and extraction sockets," *Journal of Maxillofacial and Oral Surgery*, vol. 12, no. 3, pp. 321–325, 2013.

[15] C. Blus, S. Szmukler-Moncler, P. Khoury, and G. Orrù, "Immediate implants placed in infected and noninfected sites after atraumatic tooth extraction and placement with ultrasonic bone surgery," *Clinical Implant Dentistry and Related Research*, vol. 17, supplement 1, pp. e287–e297, 2015.

[16] R. Villa and B. Rangert, "Immediate and early function of implants placed in extraction sockets of maxillary infected teeth: a pilot study," *Journal of Prosthetic Dentistry*, vol. 97, supplement, no. 6, pp. S96–S108, 2007.

[17] D. Peñarrocha-Oltra, U. Covani, M. Peñarrocha-Diago, and M. Peñarrocha-Diago, "Immediate loading with fixed full-arch prostheses in the maxilla: review of the literature," *Medicina Oral, Patología Oral y Cirugía Bucal*, vol. 19, no. 5, pp. e512–e517, 2014.

[18] R. Jacobs, A. Adriansens, K. Verstreken, P. Suetens, and D. van Steenberghe, "Predictability of a three-dimensional planning system for oral implant surgery," *Dentomaxillofacial Radiology*, vol. 28, no. 2, pp. 105–111, 1999.

[19] S. Szmukler-Moncler, H. Salama, Y. Reingewirtz, and J. H. Dubruille, "Timing of loading and effect of micromotion on bone-dental implant interface: review of experimental literature," *Journal of Biomedical Materials Research*, vol. 43, no. 2, pp. 192–203, 1998.

[20] O. Ozan, I. Turkyilmaz, A. E. Ersoy, E. A. McGlumphy, and S. F. Rosenstiel, "Clinical accuracy of 3 different types of computed tomography-derived stereolithographic surgical guides in implant placement," *Journal of Oral and Maxillofacial Surgery*, vol. 67, no. 2, pp. 394–401, 2009.

[21] L. Molly, "Bone density and primary stability in implant therapy," *Clinical Oral Implants Research*, vol. 17, supplement 2, pp. 124–135, 2006.

[22] N. Farré-Pagès, M. L. Augé-Castro, F. Alaejos-Algarra, J. Mareque-Bueno, E. Ferrés-Padró, and F. Hernández-Alfaro, "Relation between bone density and primary implant stability," *Medicina Oral, Patologia Oral y Cirugia Bucal*, vol. 16, no. 1, Article ID 16799, pp. e62–e67, 2011.

[23] H. G. Yoon, S. J. Heo, J. Y. Koak, S. K. Kim, and S. Y. Lee, "Effect of bone quality and implant surgical technique on implant stability quotient (ISQ) value," *Journal of Advanced Prosthodontics*, vol. 3, no. 1, pp. 10–15, 2011.

[24] J. Ganeles and D. Wismeijer, "Early and immediately restored and loaded dental implants for single-tooth and partial-arch applications," *International Journal of Oral and Maxillofacial Implants*, vol. 19, pp. 92–102, 2004.

[25] R. Glauser, P. Ruhstaller, S. Windisch et al., "Immediate occlusal loading of Brånemark System TiUnite implants placed predominantly in soft bone: 4-Year results of a prospective clinical

study," *Clinical Implant Dentistry and Related Research*, vol. 7, supplement 1, pp. S52–S59, 2005.

[26] A. M. Sanna, L. Molly, and D. van Steenberghe, "Immediately loaded CAD-CAM manufactured fixed complete dentures using flapless implant placement procedures: a cohort study of consecutive patients," *Journal of Prosthetic Dentistry*, vol. 97, no. 6, pp. 331–339, 2007.

[27] R. Crespi, P. Capparè, E. Gherlone, and G. E. Romanes, "Immediate occlusal loading of implants placed in fresh sockets after tooth extraction," *International Journal of Oral and Maxillofacial Implants*, vol. 22, no. 6, pp. 955–962, 2007.

[28] G. O. Gallucci, D. Morton, and H.-P. Weber, "Loading protocols for dental implants in edentulous patients," *The International Journal of Oral & Maxillofacial Implants*, vol. 24, pp. 132–146, 2009.

13

Soft Tissue Surgical Procedures for Optimizing Anterior Implant Esthetics

Andreas L. Ioannou,[1] **Georgios A. Kotsakis,**[1] **Michelle G. McHale,**[1] **Donald E. Lareau,**[1,2] **James E. Hinrichs,**[1] **and Georgios E. Romanos**[3]

[1] *Advanced Education Program in Periodontology, University of Minnesota, 515 Delaware Street SE, Minneapolis, MN 55455, USA*
[2] *Private Practice, Edina, MN 55435, USA*
[3] *Department of Periodontology, School of Dental Medicine, Stony Brook, NY 11794, USA*

Correspondence should be addressed to Georgios A. Kotsakis; geo.kotsakis@gmail.com

Academic Editor: Francesco Carinci

Implant dentistry has been established as a predictable treatment with excellent clinical success to replace missing or nonrestorable teeth. A successful esthetic implant reconstruction is predicated on two fundamental components: the reproduction of the natural tooth characteristics on the implant crown and the establishment of soft tissue housing that will simulate a healthy periodontium. In order for an implant to optimally rehabilitate esthetics, the peri-implant soft tissues must be preserved and/or augmented by means of periodontal surgical procedures. Clinicians who practice implant dentistry should strive to achieve an esthetically successful outcome beyond just osseointegration. Knowledge of a variety of available techniques and proper treatment planning enables the clinician to meet the ever-increasing esthetic demands as requested by patients. The purpose of this paper is to enhance the implant surgeon's rationale and techniques beyond that of simply placing a functional restoration in an edentulous site to a level whereby an implant-supported restoration is placed in reconstructed soft tissue, so the site is indiscernible from a natural tooth.

1. Introduction

Implant dentistry has been definitively established as a predictable treatment modality for replacing missing or nonrestorable teeth which yields excellent clinical success rates. During the last decade, the focus of implant research has shifted from the functional stability of the implant to its esthetic integration in the smile. The esthetics of implant restorations is dictated by two fundamental components: the reproduction of the natural tooth characteristics on the implant crown and the establishment of a soft tissue housing that will intimately embrace the crown. Therefore, the success of implant rehabilitation in the esthetic zone relies heavily on the preservation or the augmentation of peri-implant soft tissue by means of periodontal surgical procedures.

The aim of this paper is to enhance the implant surgeon's armamentarium with rationale and techniques that extend beyond the placement of a functional restoration in an edentulous site to the restoration of soft tissue harmony so that the implant-supported restoration is indiscernible from a natural tooth. This is especially important in areas of esthetic concern but not negligible in posterior sites where the added benefits of enhanced tissue contours cannot be overlooked.

2. Indications

It may not be an overstatement that every surgical implant procedure in the esthetic region constitutes an indication for soft tissue grafting. The inevitable alteration of the alveolar ridge dimensions that follows a tooth extraction often results in the placement of the implant in a site that has undergone a reduction in soft and hard tissue volume in comparison to its neighboring dentate sites [1–3]. This discrepancy is even more pronounced in single-implant sites where a concavity forms between the edentulous site and the root prominences of the neighboring dentition. Subepithelial connective tissue grafts (SCTG) or free gingival grafts (FGG) can be employed

Implants in the anterior maxilla: aesthetic challenges

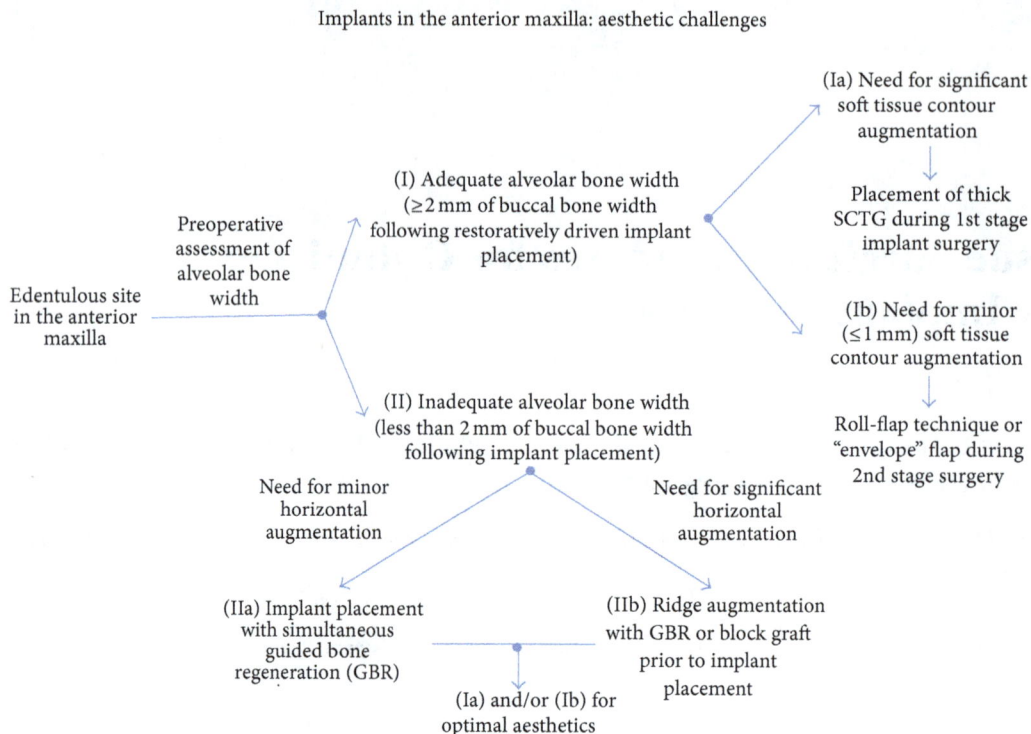

FIGURE 1: Implants in the anterior maxilla: a clinical decision-tree for overcoming aesthetic challenges.

in these cases to reconstruct the buccal dimensions of the site improving the tissue thickness. In addition, they create the illusion of root prominence and increase the width of the crestal peri-implant mucosa in order to provide an emergence profile for the restoration and enable the constructed site to closely resemble a natural tooth.

The long-term stability of pink esthetics around dental implant prostheses has been strongly correlated with adequate peri-implant soft tissue thickness, that is, a thick peri-implant biotype [4, 5]. When a thin biotype is diagnosed, a SCTG or a FGG can be used to prevent potential long-term recession of the facial mucosal margin or permeation of a gray color from the implant [6–8].

Factors that should be considered when evaluating the need for soft tissue grafting include the level of clinical attachment on adjacent teeth to support papillary height, the thickness of the coronal soft tissue margin to ensure a proper emergence profile, the thickness of labial soft tissue to simulate root eminence and prevent transillumination of underlying metallic structure, and the position of the mucogingival junction and amount of keratinized tissue so as to blend harmoniously with that of the adjacent teeth [9, 10] (Figure 1).

3. Contraindications and Limitations

General and specific limitations apply to the use of a soft tissue augmentation technique around dental implants. Certain medical conditions are considered general contraindications to surgical intervention. Collagen disorders, such as erosive

lichen planus and pemphigoid, may pose a risk to the viability of autogenous connective tissue grafts placed on a recipient bed that exhibits a pathologic healing response. There is no published evidence to either support or discourage the use of soft tissue grafting techniques in such cases.

Smoking is another relative contraindication. It is well established that a key determinant of soft tissue augmentation success is revascularization of the graft. Nicotine contained in cigarettes causes vasoconstriction to the surgical site, often resulting in necrosis of the graft [11]. This nicotine-associated vasoconstriction, in combination with lack of adherence of the fibroblasts [12] and alteration in immune response [13, 14], diminishes the likelihood for a successful outcome. Preoperative assessment should attempt to identify such at-risk patients whereby the clinician must inform the patients of the potential adverse effects associated with smoking. Local factors that may also limit patient selection include lack of adequate tissue thickness at the palatal donor site or restricted surgical access to intraoral donor sites such as the posterior of the hard palate or maxillary tuberosity.

4. Treatment Planning and Timing for Soft Tissue Grafting Procedures

A thorough 3-dimensional preoperative evaluation of the edentulous site is critical to properly planning an implant case that will result in an esthetic outcome. Two diagnostic variables that should be taken into account preoperatively are bone and soft tissue volumes [15]. Long-term stability of esthetics for an implant requires the implant to be surrounded by ~1.8–2.0 mm of vital bone [16]. Lack of adequate bone necessitates hard tissue grafting. Sites should also be evaluated for soft tissue profile. A discrepancy of soft tissue contours with adjacent teeth can be addressed with augmentation.

Soft tissue augmentation can be performed simultaneously with implant placement and/or during the second stage surgery, as will be described in the following technique section. There is no evidence in the literature to support any advantage of simultaneous soft tissue augmentation over augmentation during second stage surgery. Both treatment modalities have been shown to lead to better esthetics and increased soft tissue thickness [17]. Even though both techniques yield favorable esthetics, the earlier the intervention is performed, the more opportunities the clinician has to better control the final outcome. For instance, in a case where the residual ridge has undergone significant atrophy, the simultaneous soft tissue augmentation in conjunction with first stage surgery will allow sufficient healing time to properly assess the site during second stage surgery. Consequently, additional soft tissue augmentation can be performed simultaneously when uncovering the implant(s) in order to achieve a more ideal outcome.

Soft tissue grafting can also be utilized as a "rescue procedure" to manage esthetic complications associated with implants. Labial inclination of implants, buccal placement, or use of wide body contributes to a thin tissue biotype or thin buccal bone that may lead to recessions [18], permeation of gray from the implant structure through the tissue, and exposure of the titanium implant neck, all of which contribute to an inharmonious emergence profile of the implant-supported restoration and an ersatz appearance of the patient's smile [19, 20]. Additionally, soft tissue grafting following implant placement can be used to correct complications associated with soft tissue color mismatch to a level below clinical perception [21].

5. Free Gingival Graft

The use of autogenous FGG in mucogingival surgeries predates that of any other type of graft. FGGs are considered a reliable and efficacious approach for augmenting peri-implant soft tissue defects and are most often utilized to increase the amount of keratinized tissue around an implant. FGGs are the gold standard in cases when an increase in keratinized tissue is desired.

The most common donor site of a FGG is the highly keratinized hard palate. That being said, the color and shade of the augmented recipient site do not often blend naturally with the adjacent soft tissues. This produces a nonesthetic result, contradicting the initial purpose of the procedure. Even so, a FGG to increase the keratinized tissue is recommended for "rescue" procedures to cover exposed implant threads. In addition, a FGG can be used for patients with low smile lines, when extensive soft tissue augmentation is needed, or where the color of a FGG will not compromise the esthetic appearance of the implant site (Figure 2).

6. Subepithelial Connective Tissue Graft

SCTG procedures have been used successfully throughout the years for the management of recession and soft tissue defects around natural teeth and for augmenting alveolar ridge contours [22, 23]. Some may argue that the traditional approaches for connective tissue grafting do not fare well when one attempts to graft and achieve cover of a nonvital implant surface since the soft tissues around the implant do not respond in the same manner as a vital tooth. Nonetheless, many of these procedures can be translated directly to peri-implant soft tissue modification and esthetic optimization. When indicated and properly utilized, these surgical procedures can provide stable and significant gains in soft tissue volume and contour that can contribute to the successful esthetic management of implant sites (Figure 3).

7. Technique for Soft Tissue Grafting during 1st Stage Implant Surgery

Step 1: Treatment Planning. As in all surgical procedures, treatment planning is the cornerstone of success. Preoperative identification of potential soft and/or hard tissue deficiencies allows for the construction of an implant restoration that will closely mimic that of the natural dentogingival complex and blend with the existing dentition in a pleasing and esthetic fashion. A decision should be made preoperatively whether soft tissue augmentation alone will be adequate to develop the desired treatment outcome or if bone augmentation is also needed to achieve ideal implant position and soft tissue esthetics.

Step 2: Graft Harvesting. The three most common intraoral donor sites for harvesting connective tissue grafts are the tuberosity [24], the single incision-deep palatal [25], and the free gingival graft method-superficial palatal [26]. Donor tissue for FGGs is routinely harvested from the hard palate since this area provides an ample surface area of keratinized tissue. Nonetheless, relatively any intraoral site with adequate tissue thickness that displays keratinization, such as the keratinized epithelium apical to the gingival crest of the maxillary molars, may be utilized to procure a FGG. The amount and quality of soft tissue available for harvesting depend on donor site, that is, tuberosity versus palate. The tuberosity generally provides enough tissue to cover a single or two implant site(s), while adequate tissue can be obtained from the palate to cover an area two or three times wider than that of the tuberosity, depending on the incision design. The quality of the tissue harvested from the tuberosity is superior to that obtained from the palate since the tuberosity offers a graft composed of dense connective tissue, whereas the portion of the palatal connective tissue donor usually consists of adipose tissue. Tissue obtained from the tuberosity usually permits the harvesting of a significantly thicker graft than that obtained from the palate [27]. This broad piece of tuberosity can be longitudinally sectioned to increase the amount of donor tissue.

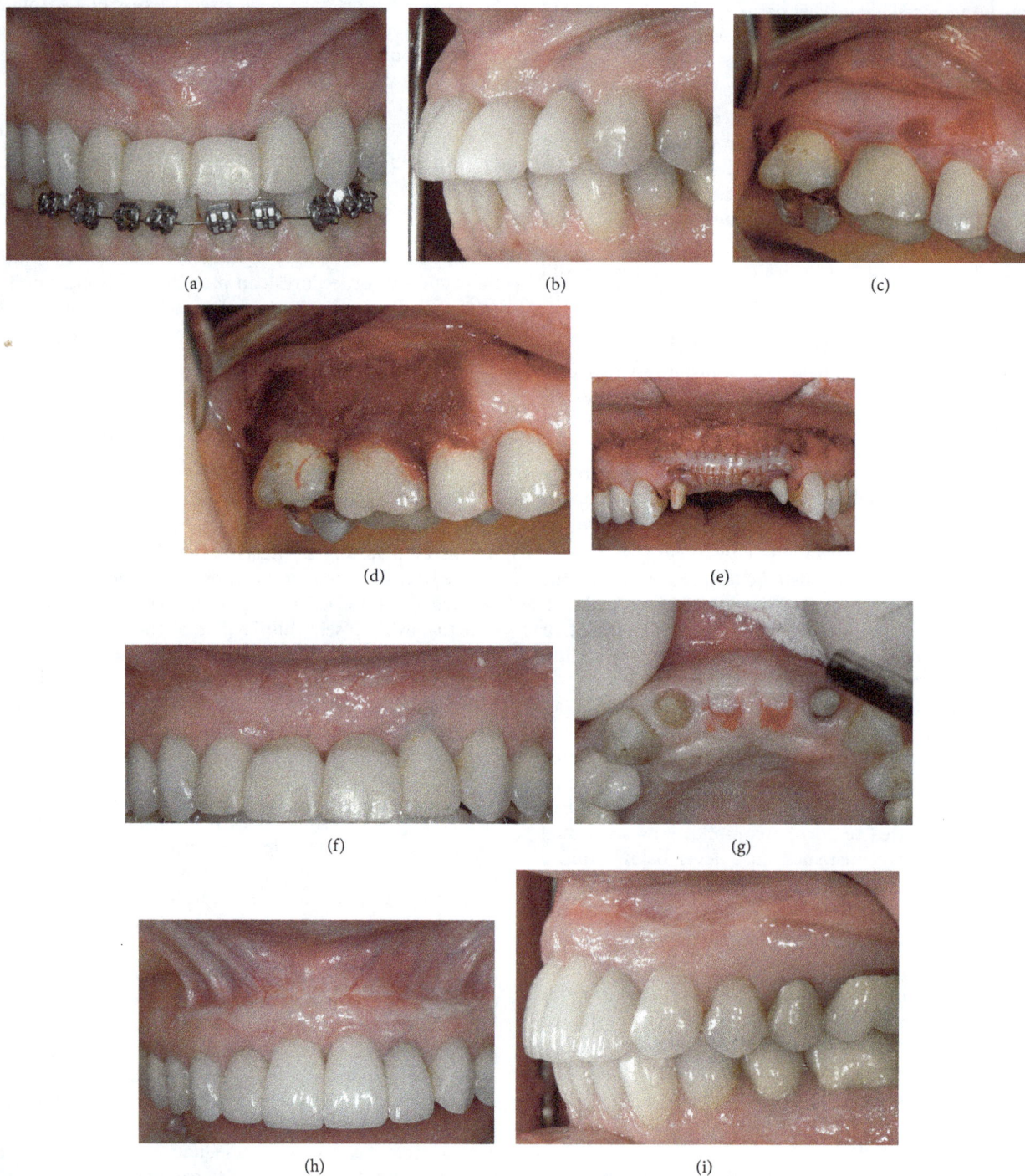

FIGURE 2: (a) Patient had previous bone grafting and numbers 8 and 9 implant placement. Note minimal keratinized attached gingiva over grafted area of numbers 8 and 9 due to coronal advancement of the flap. (b) Note the deficient soft tissue profile following placement of a provisional prosthesis with appropriate tooth emergence. (c) Donor site and graft procurement. (d) Collagen tape and cyanoacrylate to reduce discomfort over donor site. (e) Graft secured and well adapted to recipient bed with multiple sutures. (f) Recipient site following healing. Note the increase in height and thickness of the keratinized attached gingiva. (g) Numbers 8 and 9 implant sites prepared for second stage surgery. (h) Recipient site after numbers 8 and 9 implant restorations, showing stable keratinized attached gingiva. (i) Lateral view of recipient site. Note the thick buccal keratinized attached gingiva, establishing an esthetic emergence profile for the implant restorations.

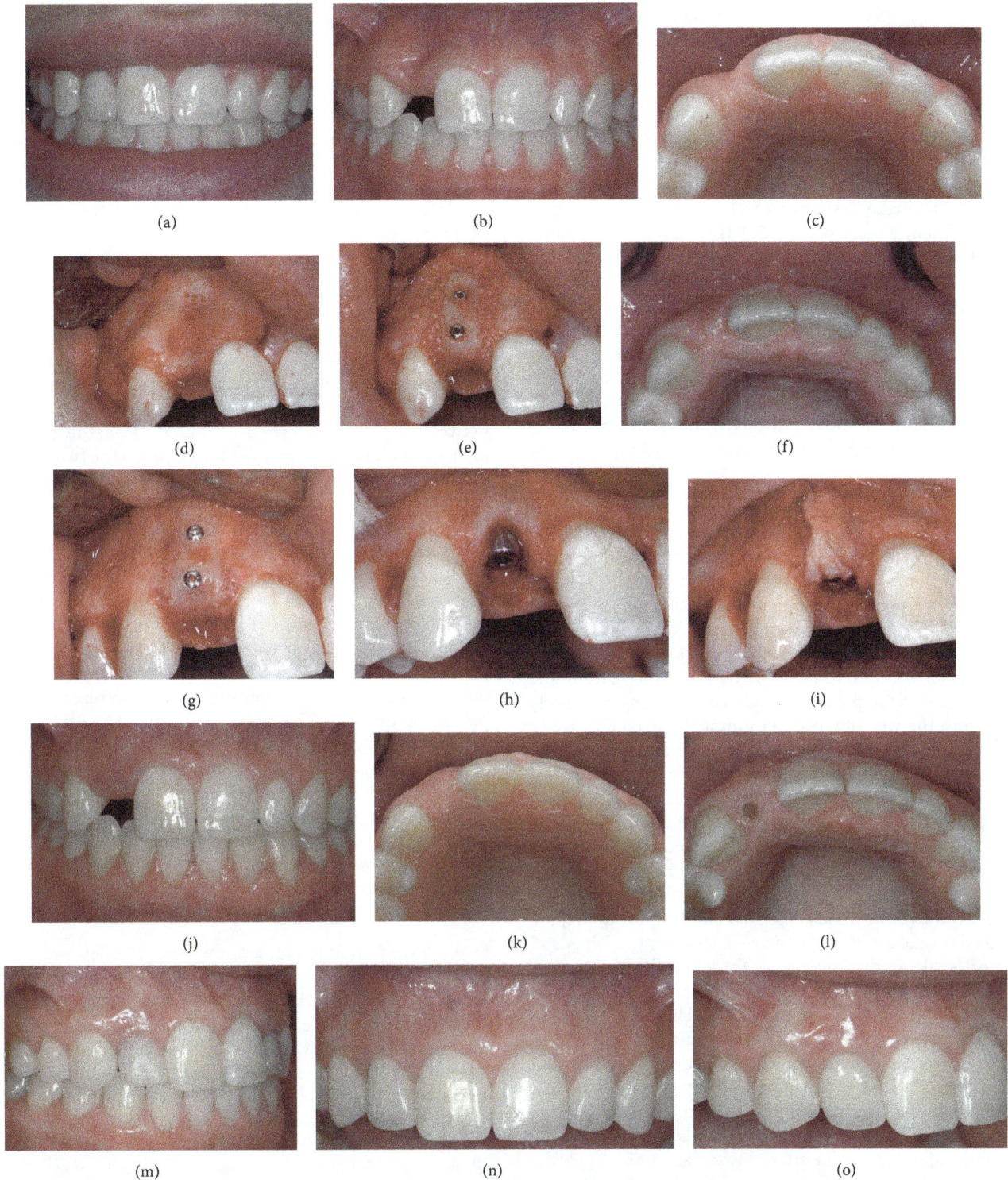

FIGURE 3: ((a), (b), and (c)) Patient presented for implant rehabilitation of number 7 lateral incisor. Not the high interdental smile line that poses an esthetic challenge. Following ridge resorption, a concavity consistent with a Seibert Class I defect is seen in the edentulous site. ((d), (e), and (f)) A block autograft was screwed in place to achieve horizontal ridge augmentation prior to implant placement. Particulated allograft was utilized to graft the area between the block and the recipient bed. Note the significant enhancement of the tissue profile postsurgically. ((g), (h), and (i)) At four months after grafting the site was reentered and an implant was placed in the ideal 3-dimensional position. A SCTG was utilized to replicate the root eminence and provide a natural emergence profile. ((j), (k), (l), and (m)) Postoperative healing view shows excellent tissue contours at the site. A customized healing abutment was selected to mold the tissues after 2nd stage surgery. Note the excellent positioning of the mucosal zenith at the time of provisionalization. ((n), (o)) Intraoral view of the final restorations in place. Crown lengthening was performed on the adjacent teeth to address the patient's overall esthetic demands. Note the excellent replication of gingival characteristics on the peri-implant mucosa and the natural appearance of the restoration as it emerges from the augmented hard on soft tissues at the site.

7.1. Harvesting from the Tuberosity. On the distal aspect of the tuberosity a single, crestal beveled incision is made from the mucogingival junction to the distofacial line angle of the most distal tooth. The incision is located on the buccal aspect of the ridge crest rather than midcrestal and connected to the distal surface of the most posterior tooth via a sulcular incision. Use of an Orban knife enhances the access to performing the sulcular incision. At this point, the palatal flap is raised until the distopalatal surface of the most distal tooth is exposed. Then, a new blade (15c) is used to meticulously dissect the connective tissue from the flap and the underlying periosteum. Tissue forceps and the suction tip should be delicately employed during procurement of the graft in order to minimize excessive trauma to the donor tissue and prevent inadvertent loss of the graft through the suction tip. Once the graft has been obtained, it is stored in saline to prevent dehydration while the recipient bed is prepared. The donor site flap is sutured closed at this time, preferably using 4-0 chromic gut and a continuous interlocking suturing technique.

7.2. Harvesting from Deep Palatal Tissue. If a deep palatal donor site is selected for harvesting the connective tissue graft, the donor site should be sounded to bone. This is performed to verify that the incision will not involve a periodontal pocket or bony dehiscence of a palatal root in order to avoid postoperative recession. A single, full-thickness horizontal incision is made at a right-angle to the alveolar bone of the palatal keratinized tissue approximately 3 mm from the free gingival margin of the maxillary teeth. This first incision extends from the mesial aspect of the palatal root of the maxillary first molar as far anteriorly as needed for the appropriate amount of donor tissue required. A second incision is made parallel to the underlying bone so that a thin split-thickness flap is created to separate the underlying connective tissue from the superficial flap. When the desired volume of SCTG has been identified, the blade is directed towards the bone at the edges of the graft so that the SCTG is free except for its periosteal attachment. A Woodson elevator is slid under the partial-thickness flap to separate the graft from the underlying bone. The procured graft is kept in saline-soaked gauzes until used. The palatal flap can be closed with either single interrupted sutures, sling sutures around the maxillary teeth, or a combination of the above. It is important that the clinician be familiar with the anatomy of the palate in order to minimize the risk of hemorrhage associated with traumatizing the major palatine artery during harvesting of the graft. The arterial vascular trunk is typically located ~12–17 mm from the CEJ of the posterior teeth in patients with an average or high palatal vault while the artery is usually within 7 mm of the CEJ in patients with a shallow palatal vault [28].

7.3. Harvesting from the Superficial Palatal Tissue. This technique is used for the harvesting of both the FGG and the SCTG. This technique utilizes a very similar method to that of a FGG to harvest the SCTG, with the only difference being that the epithelium is removed after harvesting. The rationale for using this technique is that sounding reveals a limited amount of connective tissue beneath the palatal mucosa. In contrast to the tuberosity area where connective tissue occupies the whole tissue volume underneath the epithelium, here a limited amount of connective tissue exists between the epithelium (superficial) and adipose tissue (deep). Consequently, use of the deep palatal harvest technique in patients with thin palatal mucosa as described before would not procure an adequate thickness/volume of graft after removal of the adipose tissue.

The superficial palatal harvest technique places a horizontal anterior/posterior incision 3 mm away from the maxillary teeth, as described in the deep palatal harvest technique, as a partial-thickness incision of only 1.5–2 mm in thickness and leaves the periosteum intact. A second anterior/posterior horizontal partial-thickness incision is traced parallel to the first incision at a position closer to the midline. The distance between these two incisions is based upon the estimated amount of tissue graft required for grafting. The two horizontal incisions are connected via anterior and posterior vertical partial-thickness incisions on the mesial and distal aspect of the graft. Either a sharpened gingivectomy knife (Kirkland knife) or a blade (15c) is utilized to separate the graft from the underlying tissue for an ideal thickness of 1.5 mm to 2 mm. Then the graft is placed on a moist, sterile surface whereby the superficial epithelium is removed by sharp dissection. Adipose tissue is removed from the periosteal side of the graft with the aid of a fresh blade or LaGrange scissors until the harvested graft consists of only connective tissue or/and epithelium. The tissue graft is used as a template to trim a collagen biomaterial in the proper dimensions to cover the donor site wound. After adequate hemostasis has been achieved at the denuded donor site by application of gauze with digital pressure for 5–10 minutes, the collagen biomaterial is placed over the wound and secured by the application of cyanoacrylate via pipette. Periodontal dressing may be utilized depending on the surgeon's preference to improve patient comfort.

Step 3: Preparation of the Recipient Site. The flap is designed to retain a band of keratinized mucosa on the buccal aspect of the flap whenever possible. Consequently, it may be advisable to place the initial incision slightly palatal rather than midcrestal. The crestal incision is extended as sulcular incisions onto the adjacent teeth or as papillae sparing vertical releasing incisions passing to the level of the mucogingival junction. The length of each incision depends on the individualized treatment plan. A full-thickness flap is raised to allow access for surgical placement of the implant(s). The successful incorporation of a tissue graft does not depend on the thickness of the incision since the combination of a tissue graft with either a full- or partial-thickness flap yields similar clinical results [29]. The recipient bed should be kept well-hydrated with frequent irrigation throughout the procedure.

In order to create a partial-thickness flap, the dissection should occur beyond the mucogingival junction, leaving a layer of approximately 2 to 3 mm of connective tissue and periosteum intact.

Step 4: Adaptation of the Soft Tissue Graft. Following placement of the implant(s), the procured graft is adapted to the area. The dimensions of the graft should be adequate to provide soft tissue bulk at the level of the neck of the implant to ensure an esthetic emergence profile for the restoration as well as simulate a root prominence for the missing tooth. The tissue graft should be trimmed to resemble a semicircular cone so that the apical aspect does not span to the proximal surfaces of adjacent teeth. Such excessive soft tissue will create a bulky visual effect rather than that resembling the natural gingival contours of adjacent teeth. There is no significant clinical difference in regard to the orientation of the SCTG during its placement into the recipient site. Based on studies on root coverage procedures, when the periosteal side of the graft opposes the flap rather than the recipient bed, the success of the outcome will not be compromised [30].

Step 5: Suturing at the Recipient Bed. After trimming the graft to the appropriate dimensions, the graft is secured in the recipient bed utilizing a palatal-locking suture technique. The suture needle initially penetrates the palatal keratinized tissue in a palatobuccal direction. The needle then passes through the mesial aspect of the graft employing a faciopalatal direction. The sequence is repeated for the distal portion of the graft, and as the needle exits the palatal flap a second time, a knot is placed on the palatal side. The apex of the graft is stabilized in the connective tissue at the base of the flap so that the graft is stretched and well adapted onto the recipient bed. It is emphasized that the graft should be uniformly adapted and well secured on the recipient bed to prevent disruption of plasmatic circulation and healing. The final adaptation should be verified with the aid of a periodontal probe. Pressure is applied with moist gauze for 5 minutes. The flap is closed with single interrupted sutures using a 4-0 or 5-0 suturing material. If passive closure cannot be achieved, then horizontal vestibular releasing incisions should be placed in the base of the labial flap with a fresh 15C blade until tension-free flap adaptation and closure can be accomplished.

8. Technique for Soft Tissue Grafting during 2nd Stage Implant Surgery

A broad variety of techniques have been proposed to augment the soft tissue profile of implants at second stage surgery. Ideally, second stage surgery should be a minimally invasive procedure whereby minor revisions in soft tissue architecture can be accomplished to create a natural emergence profile for the healing abutment and/or final restoration [31]. A rolled pedicle flap can be used to augment the connective tissue that covers the coronal portion of a submerged implant. Tissue sounding is utilized to locate the palatal shoulder of the cover screw followed by an arcing crestal incision around the palatal aspect of the cover screw. Papillae sparing mesial and distal vertical releasing incisions are placed, leaving the labial pedicle flap intact. A blade (15c) is used to deepithelize the superficial layer of the labial pedicle flap. The labial pedicle is elevated as a full-thickness mucoperiosteal flap and a Woodson elevator is used to create a small tunnel beneath the base of the labial pedicle. A horizontal mattress suture with absorbable suturing material (5-0 chromic gut or vicryl) is initially passed from the base of the tunnel horizontally through the coronal margin of the deepithelized pedicle flap and back through the base of the tunnel in order to invert the deepithelized pedicle beneath the labial marginal gingiva. A knot is tied to secure the rolled pedicle flap beneath the labial pouch and can be verified by slight blanching of the area. The patient is instructed to avoid mechanical trauma to the area for the next couple of weeks and to use only a chlorhexidine rinse while the deepithelized pedicle flap heals. As in all implant cases, the construction of a well-contoured restoration is critical to the maintenance of a desirable soft tissue profile and an acceptable esthetic outcome.

Other minimally invasive techniques for contour augmentation are also available. One such example is the use of a buccal "envelope" technique for sliding a connective tissue graft on the labial aspect of the implant, as was originally described by Raetzke for use around teeth with mucogingival defects [32]. In this technique, sharp dissection is employed to produce a partial-thickness "envelope" flap that extends beyond the mucogingival junction on the facial of the implant [33]. Subsequently, a SCTG is procured and slid in the buccal envelope at the implant site. Lastly, sling sutures are utilized to secure the graft and coronally advance the flap [33]. Eghbali et al. have shown that a mean increase of 0.8 mm of mucosal thickness can be achieved with the use of this technique, whose increase is stable for at least 9 months after surgery. Therefore this procedure could be also considered in cases where minor buccal contour enhancement is indicated [33].

9. Conclusions

Implant dentistry has been established as a predictable treatment modality with high clinical success rates. Esthetic considerations for implant restorations and the role of surgical procedures in the creation and maintenance of peri-implant soft tissue have been gaining interest over the years. Clinicians who practice implant dentistry should attain more than just implant osseointegration to achieve an esthetic, successful outcome. Knowledge of the variety of techniques available and proper planning enable clinicians to meet patients' increasing esthetic demands. However, the need for soft tissue augmentation procedures around dental implants in the anterior esthetic zone remains a controversial topic and lacks support from the literature. Long-term clinical trials are needed for better assessment of these surgical procedures.

Conflict of Interests

All of the authors declare that they have no conflict of interests regarding this paper.

References

[1] J. Pietrokovski and M. Massler, "Alveolar ridge resorption following tooth extraction," *The Journal of Prosthetic Dentistry*, vol. 17, no. 1, pp. 21–27, 1967.

[2] M. Farmer and I. Darby, "Ridge dimensional changes following single-tooth extraction in the aesthetic zone," *Clinical Oral Implants Research*, vol. 25, no. 2, pp. 272–277, 2014.

[3] L. Schropp, A. Wenzel, L. Kostopoulos, and T. Karring, "Bone healing and soft tissue contour changes following single-tooth extraction: a clinical and radiographic 12-month prospective study," *International Journal of Periodontics and Restorative Dentistry*, vol. 23, no. 4, pp. 313–323, 2003.

[4] N. C. Geurs, P. J. Vassilopoulos, and M. S. Reddy, "Soft tissue considerations in implant site development," *Oral and Maxillofacial Surgery Clinics of North America*, vol. 22, no. 3, pp. 387–405, 2010.

[5] J.-H. Fu, A. Lee, and H.-L. Wang, "Influence of tissue biotype on implant esthetics," *The International Journal of Oral & Maxillofacial Implants*, vol. 26, no. 3, pp. 499–508, 2011.

[6] J. Y. K. Kan, K. Rungcharassaeng, J. L. Lozada, and G. Zimmerman, "Facial gingival tissue stability following immediate placement and provisionalization of maxillary anterior single implants: a 2- to 8-year follow-up," *The International Journal of Oral and Maxillofacial Implants*, vol. 26, no. 1, pp. 179–187, 2011.

[7] Y.-T. Hsu, C.-H. Shieh, and H.-L. Wang, "Using soft tissue graft to prevent mid-facial mucosal recession following immediate implant placement," *Journal of the International Academy of Periodontology*, vol. 14, no. 3, pp. 76–82, 2012.

[8] J. Cosyn, N. Hooghe, and H. De Bruyn, "A systematic review on the frequency of advanced recession following single immediate implant treatment," *Journal of Clinical Periodontology*, vol. 39, no. 6, pp. 582–589, 2012.

[9] K. Nisapakultorn, S. Suphanantachat, O. Silkosessak, and S. Rattanamongkolgul, "Factors affecting soft tissue level around anterior maxillary single-tooth implants," *Clinical Oral Implants Research*, vol. 21, no. 6, pp. 662–670, 2010.

[10] H.-C. Lai, Z.-Y. Zhang, F. Wang, L.-F. Zhuang, X. Liu, and Y.-P. Pu, "Evaluation of soft-tissue alteration around implant-supported single-tooth restoration in the anterior maxilla: the pink esthetic score," *Clinical Oral Implants Research*, vol. 19, no. 6, pp. 560–564, 2008.

[11] D. A. Tipton and M. K. Dabbous, "Effects of nicotine on proliferation and extracellular matrix production of human gingival fibroblasts in vitro," *Journal of Periodontology*, vol. 66, no. 12, pp. 1056–1064, 1995.

[12] D. A. Tipton and M. K. Dabbous, "Effects of nicotine on proliferation and extracellular matrix production of human gingival fibroblasts in vitro.," *Journal of periodontology*, vol. 66, no. 12, pp. 1056–1064, 1995.

[13] W. S. Cheung and T. J. Griffin, "A comparative study of root coverage with connective tissue and platelet concentrate grafts: 8-month results," *Journal of Periodontology*, vol. 75, no. 12, pp. 1678–1687, 2004.

[14] A. P. Saadoun, "Current trends in gingival recession coverage. Part I. The tunnel connective tissue graft," *Practical Procedures & Aesthetic Dentistry*, vol. 18, no. 7, pp. 433–440, 2006.

[15] K. Phillips and J. C. Kois, "Aesthetic peri-implant site development. The restorative connection," *Dental Clinics of North America*, vol. 42, no. 1, pp. 57–70, 1998.

[16] J. R. Spray, C. G. Black, H. F. Morris, and S. Ochi, "The influence of bone thickness on facial marginal bone response: stage 1 placement through stage 2 uncovering," *Annals of Periodontology*, vol. 5, no. 1, pp. 119–128, 2000.

[17] M. Esposito, H. Maghaireh, M. G. Grusovin, I. Ziounas, and H. V. Worthington, "Soft tissue management for dental implants: what are the most effective techniques? A Cochrane systematic review," *European Journal of Oral Implantology*, vol. 5, no. 3, pp. 221–238, 2012.

[18] P. N. Small and D. P. Tarnow, "Gingival recession around implants: a 1-year longitudinal prospective study," *International Journal of Oral and Maxillofacial Implants*, vol. 15, no. 4, pp. 527–532, 2000.

[19] M. Al-Sabbagh, "Implants in the esthetic zone," *Dental Clinics of North America*, vol. 50, no. 3, pp. 391–407, 2006.

[20] P. V. Goldberg, F. L. Higginbottom, and T. G. Wilson Jr., "Periodontal considerations in restorative and implant therapy," *Periodontology 2000*, vol. 25, no. 1, pp. 100–109, 2001.

[21] O. Moses, Z. Artzi, A. Sculean et al., "Comparative study of two root coverage procedure: a 24-month follow-up multicenter study," *Journal of Periodontology*, vol. 77, no. 2, pp. 195–202, 2006.

[22] C. E. Nemcovsky, Z. Artzi, H. Tal, A. Kozlovsky, and O. Moses, "A multicenter comparative study of two root coverage procedures: coronally advanced flap with addition of enamel matrix proteins and subpedicle connective tissue graft," *Journal of Periodontology*, vol. 75, no. 4, pp. 600–607, 2004.

[23] A. Happe, M. Stimmelmayr, M. Schlee, and D. Rothamel, "Surgical management of peri-implant soft tissue color mismatch caused by shine-through effects of restorative materials: one-year follow-up," *The International Journal of Periodontics & Restorative Dentistry*, vol. 33, no. 1, pp. 81–88, 2013.

[24] A. Hirsch, U. Attal, E. Chai, J. Goultschin, B. D. Boyan, and Z. Schwartz, "Root coverage and pocket reduction as combined surgical procedures," *Journal of Periodontology*, vol. 72, no. 11, pp. 1572–1579, 2001.

[25] M. B. Hürzeler and D. Weng, "A single-incision technique to harvest subepithelial connective tissue grafts from the palate," *The International Journal of Periodontics and Restorative Dentistry*, vol. 19, no. 3, pp. 279–287, 1999.

[26] R. J. Harris, "A comparison of two techniques for obtaining a connective tissue graft from the palate," *International Journal of Periodontics and Restorative Dentistry*, vol. 17, no. 3, pp. 260–271, 1997.

[27] S. P. Studer, E. P. Allen, T. C. Rees, and A. Kouba, "The thickness of masticatory mucosa in the human hard palate and tuberosity as potential donor sites for ridge augmentation procedures," *Journal of Periodontology*, vol. 68, no. 2, pp. 145–151, 1997.

[28] G. M. Reiser, J. F. Bruno, P. E. Mahan, and L. H. Larkin, "The subepithelial connective tissue graft palatal donor site: anatomic considerations for surgeons," *International Journal of Periodontics and Restorative Dentistry*, vol. 16, no. 2, pp. 130–137, 1996.

[29] F. Mazzocco, L. Comuzzi, R. Stefani, Y. Milan, G. Favero, and E. Stellini, "Coronally advanced flap combined with a subepithelial connective tissue graft using full- or partial-thickness flap reflection," *Journal of Periodontology*, vol. 82, no. 11, pp. 1524–1529, 2011.

[30] A. Lafzi, R. M. Z. Farahani, N. Abolfazli, R. Amid, and A. Safaiyan, "Effect of connective tissue graft orientation on the root coverage outcomes of coronally advanced flap," *Clinical Oral Investigations*, vol. 11, no. 4, pp. 401–408, 2007.

[31] C. E. Nemcovsky and Z. Artzi, "Split palatal flap. II. A surgical approach for maxillary implant uncovering in cases with reduced keratinized tissue: technique and clinical results," *The International Journal of Periodontics and Restorative Dentistry*, vol. 19, no. 4, pp. 387–393, 1999.

[32] P. B. Raetzke, "Covering localized areas of root exposure employing the "envelope" technique," *Journal of Periodontology*, vol. 56, no. 7, pp. 397–402, 1985.

[33] A. Eghbali, H. de Bruyn, J. Cosyn, I. Kerckaert, and T. van Hoof, "Ultrasonic assessment of mucosal thickness around implants: validity, reproducibility, and stability of connective tissue grafts at the buccal aspect," *Clinical Implant Dentistry and Related Research*, 2014.

14

Protocol for Bone Augmentation with Simultaneous Early Implant Placement: A Retrospective Multicenter Clinical Study

Peter Fairbairn[1] and Minas Leventis[2]

[1]Department of Periodontology and Implant Dentistry, School of Dentistry, University of Detroit Mercy,
 2700 Martin Luther King Jr. Boulevard, Detroit, MI 48208, USA
[2]Department of Oral and Maxillofacial Surgery, Dental School, University of Athens, 2 Thivon Street, Goudi, 115 27 Athens, Greece

Correspondence should be addressed to Peter Fairbairn; peterdent66@aol.com

Academic Editor: Ali I. Abdalla

Purpose. To present a novel protocol for alveolar bone regeneration in parallel to early implant placement. *Methods.* 497 patients in need of extraction and early implant placement with simultaneous bone augmentation were treated in a period of 10 years. In all patients the same specific method was followed and grafting was performed utilizing *in situ* hardening fully resorbable alloplastic grafting materials consisting of β-tricalcium phosphate and calcium sulfate. The protocol involved atraumatic extraction, implant placement after 4 weeks with simultaneous bone augmentation, and loading of the implant 12 weeks after placement and grafting. Follow-up periods ranged from 6 months to 10 years (mean of 4 years). *Results.* A total of 601 postextraction sites were rehabilitated in 497 patients utilizing the novel protocol. Three implants failed before loading and three implants failed one year after loading, leaving an overall survival rate of 99.0%. *Conclusions.* This standardized protocol allows successful long-term functional results regarding alveolar bone regeneration and implant rehabilitation. The concept of placing the implant 4 weeks after extraction, augmenting the bone around the implant utilizing fully resorbable, biomechanically stable, alloplastic materials, and loading the implant at 12 weeks seems to offer advantages when compared with traditional treatment modalities.

1. Introduction

According to the Branemark original protocol, implant placement was carried out 6 to 8 months after tooth extraction followed by a 3- to 6-month stress-free osseointegration period resulting in a long overall treatment time [1]. In an attempt to shorten the time frame between extraction and prosthetic delivery and to reduce cost, patient discomfort, and the number of surgical interventions, the immediate placement of implants at the time of tooth extraction has been proposed [2]. Other potential advantages with immediate implants are that the amount of bone loss at the extraction site might be reduced and optimal soft tissue aesthetics may be achieved [3]. On the other hand, there are some disadvantages with immediate implants such as the enhanced risk of infection and the lack of soft tissue closure [4, 5]. In order to overcome these potential problems early placement of implants has been proposed [2]. In this technique the clinicians wait 2 to 8 weeks before placing the implant to achieve some soft tissue healing and decrease the risk of infections [5].

The short-term survival rate of implant placement appears similar between immediate, early, and late approaches. However, at present there is little data on the success of immediate and early placement compared to late placement [2, 3, 5]. A few reviews evaluating the efficacy of immediate or early implants have been published over the years, but so far evidence is inconclusive [4–11].

With immediate or early implants it is possible that one or more bony walls of the postextraction socket are either partly or completely missing due to the preexisting inflammatory processes or damaged as a complication of the tooth extraction procedure. As a result, a portion of the implants could remain exposed due to hard tissue defect. Sockets with dehiscence defects may lack the potential for complete bone regeneration, and the risk of long-term complications may be increased with immediate or early implants placed at these sites [5]. However, several reports have shown that bone regeneration may be achieved in defective sites adjacent to immediate or early implants using a variety of bone augmentation techniques, such as autogenous bone grafts, bone substitutes, and guided bone regeneration with resorbable or nonresorbable barriers [4]. However, there is no enough reliable evidence supporting or refuting the need for augmentation procedures in parallel to immediate or early implant placement or whether any of the augmentation techniques is superior to the others [4, 5, 12].

When regenerating lost alveolar bone with the use of grafting materials, an important concern is the presence of residual particles, which might interfere with normal healing and bone-to-implant contact. The quality of the regenerated bone around immediate or early implants might be critical in determining the long-term function and stability of dental implants and the peri-implant tissues [13]. Beta-tricalcium phosphate (β-TCP) has a compressive strength similar to that of cancellous bone and undergoes resorption over a 6–18-month period being completely replaced by newly formed vital bone [14–18]. However, few studies to date have evaluated the long-term outcome of using β-TCP as grafting material simultaneously with implant placement into extraction sites [14, 19].

It would be of great benefit to investigate if completely resorbable *in situ* hardening alloplastic grafting materials could be used, without the need of membrane coverage, during early implant placement in a successful and predictable way. The purpose of the present study was therefore to assess the long-term survival rate of implants early placed into defective sockets with simultaneous bone grafting with *in situ* hardening β-TCP, following a standardized protocol.

2. Patients and Methods

This study reports a series of 497 patients treated according to the novel protocol, from August 2004 to July 2014. Patients were referred for consultation and treatment of nonsalvageable teeth due to root fractures, advanced caries, trauma, periodontitis, or failed endodontic treatment. All patients were treated in 2 private implantology clinics by 2 different clinicians. In the present study, only cases with defective buccal bone wall and need for bone augmentation in parallel to early implant placement were included. Patients with intact 4-wall postextraction sockets, with uncontrolled diabetes, alcoholics, and drug abusers were excluded, but smokers were included. All patients signed a letter of consent for the use of the alloplastic bone graft substitutes and implant placement.

After thorough clinical examination, periapical radiographs were taken. In 48% of the cases where additional information was required, a CBCT was prescribed.

In all cases the same standardized methodology was followed: Firstly, after local anaesthesia, teeth were "atraumatically" extracted without raising a flap. Extractions were facilitated by the use of periotomes and gentle elevation. Attention was given not to damage the surrounding soft and hard tissues. In cases of multirooted teeth, teeth were sectioned and removed in pieces. After extraction, the sockets were thoroughly curetted and debrided of inflammatory

tissue, followed by rinsing with sterile saline. Postextraction sockets were allowed to heal by secondary intention.

After 4 weeks a site-specific full thickness flap was raised buccally using vertical releasing incisions, without including the papillae of the adjacent teeth. After flap elevation all granulation tissue was removed from the site and a tapered implant (Dio, Dio Co., Busan, Korea) was placed in the optimal position. After placing the cover screw, the site was augmented utilizing an *in situ* hardening resorbable alloplastic bone grafting material.

Fortoss Vital (Biocomposites, Staffordshire, UK) is a biphasic alloplastic bone graft consisting of β-TCP in a calcium sulfate (CS) matrix. This graft material has an increased negative isoelectric charge (Zeta Potential Charge [ZPC]) in an aqueous solution, which has been shown to upregulate the host response by attracting positively charged host bone morphogenetic proteins to the site. These in turn result in the increased presence of osteoblasts to the site for improved early bone regeneration. Fortoss Vital acts as a scaffold for bony proliferation as it is slowly resorbed by osteoclastic activity and substituted by living bone cells that grow directly in contact with the mineral. The product forms a simple to use, moldable cohesive paste that sets to form a hard, but resorbable, osteoconductive bone graft material.

Ethoss (Regenamed Ltd., London, UK) is a biphasic alloplastic grafting material consisting of β-TCP (65%) and CS (35%). When mixed with sterile saline, the material forms an easily handling moldable mass that hardens *in situ*.

No barrier membranes were used. The mucoperiosteal flap was repositioned and sutured without tension with resorbable 4-0 sutures (Vicryl, Ethicon, Johnson & Johnson, Somerville, NJ, USA). The sutures were removed after a 7-day healing period.

After 10 weeks a similar site-specific full-thickness flap was raised to access the cover screw. In 60% of the cases the stability of the implants was evaluated by resonance frequency analysis (Osstell ISQ, Gothenburg, Sweden). A healing abutment was placed and the flap was then sutured using 4-0 sutures (Vicryl Rapide, Ethicon, Johnson & Johnson, Somerville, NJ, USA). Lastly after allowing the soft tissue to mature for 2 weeks the final titanium abutment was placed and a cemented metal-ceramic restoration was fabricated.

3. Results

This retrospective study of 497 patients included 243 females (48.9%) and 254 males (51.1%) with mean age of 54.24 years (range 23 to 91). In total 601 implants were early placed in different locations according to the novel protocol, and, of the 601 sites, 471 (78.4%) were grafted with Fortoss Vital, and 130 (21.6%) were grafted with Ethoss. The implant distribution, in accordance with the grafting material used, is shown in Figures 1 and 2.

Of the 601 implants placed, 3 were lost before loading (2 grafted with Fortoss Vital and 1 with Ethoss) due to infection and granulation tissue development; and 3 implants (2 grafted with Fortoss Vital and 1 with Ethoss) were lost 1 year after loading, corresponding to an overall success rate of 99.0%.

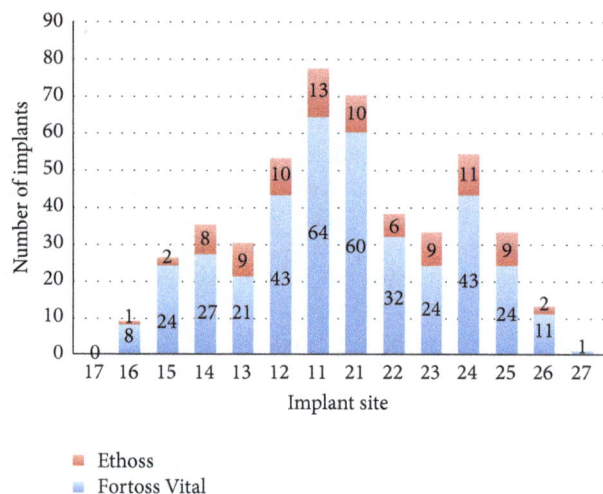

FIGURE 1: Implant distribution and grafting material used in maxilla.

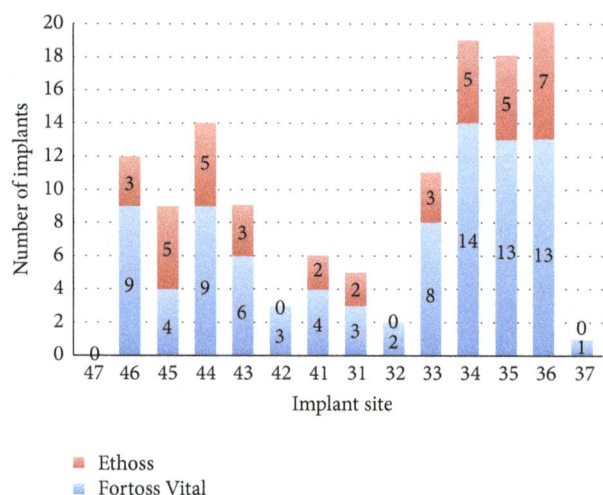

FIGURE 2: Implant distribution and grafting material used in mandible.

Apart from the 6 lost implants, none of the patients experienced postoperative complications.

At reentry, 10 weeks after implant placement and grafting, the sites were filled with newly formed bone. Remnants of the grafting materials could be identified, be embedded, and be in continuity with the newly formed bone. In many cases, the regenerated bone was completely or partially covering the implant cover screw. Out of the 595 successful cases only 5 (3 grafted with Fortoss Vital and 2 grafted with Ethoss) needed minor additional grafting buccally with the same material in order to cover still exposed cervical implant threads, without compromising the final result. At this time point all implants were firmly integrated and ISQ measurements, when available, showed high (70–84) values.

All successful cases were loaded with cemented crowns and the pleasing esthetic outcomes were noted.

Follow-up radiological examinations with periapical X-rays (follow-up periods ranged from 6 months to 10 years,

mean of 4 years) demonstrated stable peri-implant hard tissues.

Figures 3–6 show 4 cases treated according to the proposed protocol.

4. Discussion

This report proposes a protocol for early implant placement and simultaneous bone augmentation in sites with dehiscence-type bone defects.

A potential advantage with early implantation compared to immediate placement seems to be the decreased risk of infections and associated implant failures. The findings of the present study support this hypothesis as from the 601 placed implants 4 weeks after extraction only 3 (0.5%) were lost due to infection during the healing period. The overall success rate in this study was 99.0%, higher than the success rate reported in the literature with regard to survival percentages ranging from 95% to 97.5% [7, 8, 20–24].

Although there is currently too little evidence to draw definitive conclusions [5], the literature suggests that the placement of dental implants at an early timing after tooth extraction may also offer advantages in terms of soft and hard tissue preservation, when compared with immediate or delayed protocols [7, 12, 20–26]. The survival rates presented in this case series study show stable functional outcomes in a follow-up period up to 10 years (mean of 4 years). In 595 cases the contour augmentation technique described in this protocol was able to regenerate the hard tissues around the implants, as observed at the 10-week postop reentry, and allow for long-term function and clinical survival of the implants.

The concept of bone augmentation with the use of xenogeneic bone graft and a resorbable barrier membrane in conjunction with early implant placement was carried out in several clinical studies with successful results [23, 24, 26, 27].

In contrast to the above augmentation protocols, in the present study a different rationale for bone augmentation in parallel with early implant placement was followed. In all cases the dehiscence-type bone defects were treated with resorbable biphasic alloplastic bone grafting materials composed of β-TCP and CS and no barrier membranes were used. Significant bone formation at the buccal aspect of the implants was demonstrated at reentry after 10 weeks and only in 0.8% of the cases additional grafting was needed in order to cover still exposed cervical implant threads. It seems that the biomechanical properties of the grafting materials used in this study fulfilled the main principles of successful bone regeneration of the alveolar bone, that is, exclusion of gingival tissue from the regenerating site and maintenance of a stable bacterial-free closed compartment [28]. The CS component of the grafting materials used is pyrogen-free and bacteriostatic, creating a nanoporous cell-occlusive membrane that prevents the early stage invasion of unwanted soft tissue cells and when mixed with other grafting materials enhances graft containment, making the mixture more stable and pressure resistant [29–31]. Adding CS to β-TCP produces an *in situ* hardening grafting material that binds directly to the host bone, maintains the space and shape of the grafted

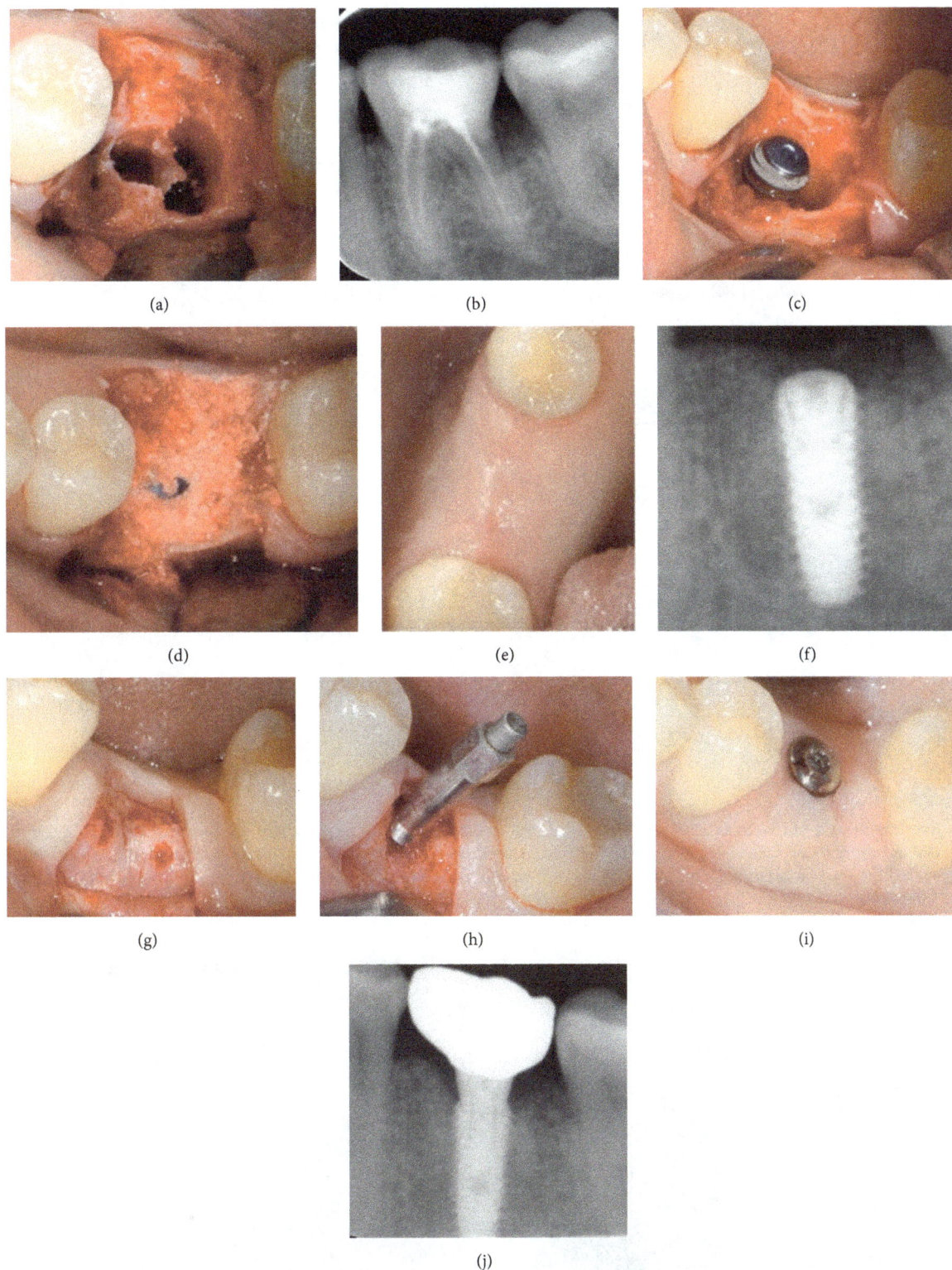

FIGURE 3: Case 1: a 47-year-old woman with crown and root fracture in the left mandibular first molar. (a) Clinical view of the site after thorough debridement of the socket. (b) Periapical X-ray of the nonrestorable tooth. (c) Implant placement at the correct 3D positioning. ISQ reading was 48. (d) Grafting with β-TCP/CS (Ethoss). (e) Clinical view after 10 weeks. (f) X-ray 10 weeks after implant placement and grafting showing the consolidation of the grafting material around the implant and new bone formation over the implant head and towards the adjacent interproximal heights of bone. (g) At reentry the site is filled with regenerated bone. Note the head of the implant covered by newly formed bone. (h) After removing the supernatant newly formed bone with a round burr implant stability is assessed (ISQ measurement: 78) revealing a significant increase through the 10-week healing period. (i) Maturation of the soft tissues 2 weeks after placement of the healing abutment. (j) X-ray 9 months after loading.

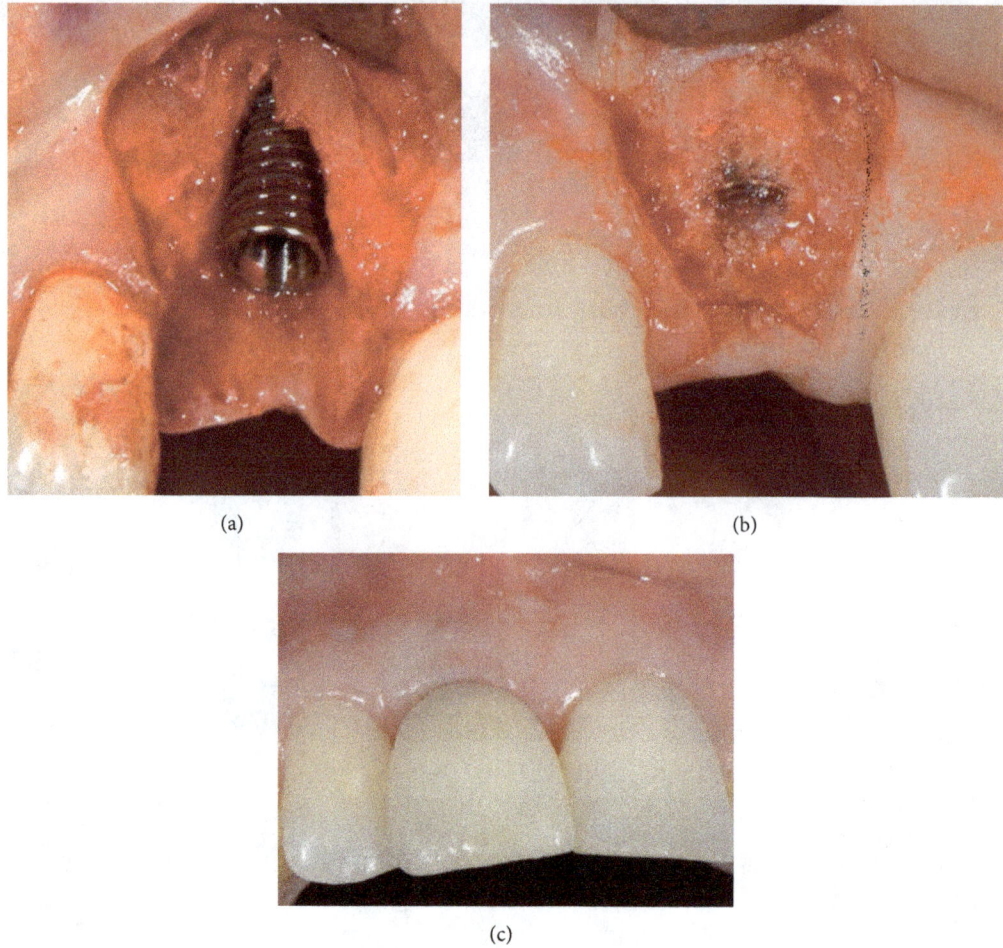

(a)

(b)

(c)

FIGURE 4: Case 2: a 28-year-old woman with root fracture in the maxillary right central incisor. (a) Implant placed at the optimum 3D positioning leaving a buccal dehiscence. (b) Reentry after 10 weeks revealing complete bone regeneration of the site. The head of the implant is partially covered by newly formed bone and the ridge is also significantly augmented laterally. ISQ reading was 75. (c) Six months after loading, excellent preservation of the buccal profile.

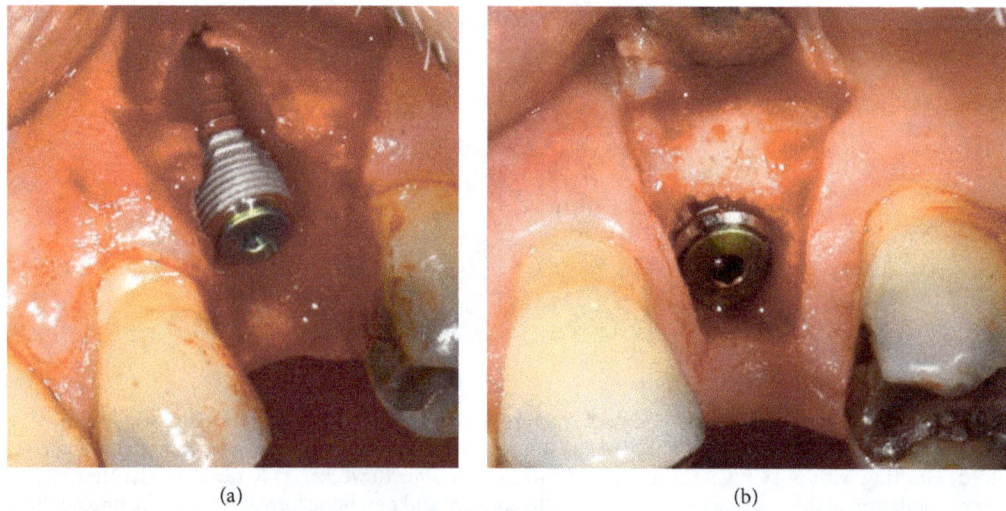

(a)

(b)

FIGURE 5: Case 3: a 62-year-old male with root fracture in the maxillary left second premolar. (a) Implant placed at the optimum 3D positioning with low initial stability, leaving a buccal dehiscence. (b) Reentry after 10 weeks showing excellent bone regeneration of the site. ISQ reading was 76.

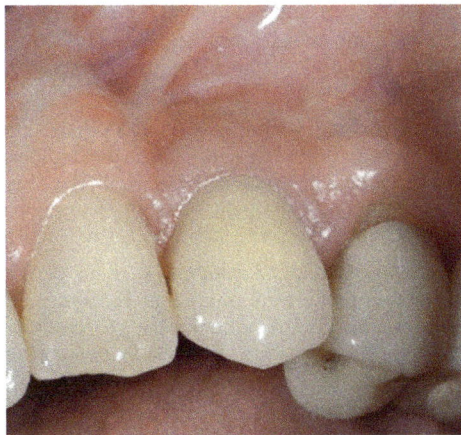

FIGURE 6: Seven-year follow-up clinical picture of a maxillary left canine case treated according to the protocol and grafted with Fortoss Vital.

site, and acts as a stable osteoconductive scaffold [32, 33]. The improved stability throughout the graft material seems to further improve the quality of the bone to be regenerated due to reduced micromotion of the material, which may lead to mesenchymal differentiation to fibroblasts instead of osteoblasts [34]. It is known that micromovements between bone and any implanted grafted material prevent bone formation, resulting in the development of fibrous tissue [35]. A possible problem with particulate grafts like deproteinized bovine bone mineral might be the lack of stability of the grafting material at the recipient site. In such cases a resorbable membrane is needed to cover and stabilize the particulate grafting material [36].

In the present study the β-TCP/CS bone grafts were covered only with the mucoperiosteal flap. The 4-week healing period after the extraction enabled the production of adequate newly formed keratinized tissue, achieving tension-free primary closure and maintenance throughout the healing and regeneration phases. The no need for a barrier membrane in the proposed protocol significantly reduced the surgical time and cost and may be attributed to enhanced bone regeneration as the periosteum was not isolated from the grafted site. Periosteum has been shown to play a pivotal role in bone graft incorporation, healing, and remodeling, as it contains multipotent mesenchymal stem cells that are capable of differentiating into bone and cartilage and provides a source of blood vessels and growth factors [37, 38].

The profound bone regeneration shown after 10 weeks in the present study may also be explained by the biological properties that characterize alloplastic materials used. It has been found that β-TCP when covered with vascularized periosteum enhances osteoconduction and osteoblastic activity while resorbing simultaneously with the formation of new bone. There is also ongoing important evidence that TCP possesses high osteoinductive potential [14, 39–42]. Moreover, experimental research has shown that the addition of the resorbable CS to the graft significantly accelerates osteogenesis and increases calcification and the quantity of new bone in a shorter period of time [33, 43]. It is also important that the most intensive osteogenic activity during

healing of extraction sites takes place between 4 and 8 weeks after extraction. Placement of the implant and the grafting material at 4 weeks after atraumatic extraction takes advantage of this enhanced host bone-healing environment [14, 44]. Also, it has been found that implant insertion increases bone metabolic activity at the site [45], further contributing to enhanced bone regeneration. Although a histological evaluation of the regenerated hard tissue was not performed in this study, it can be assumed that the bone defects around the implants have been repaired and finally filled with high quality vital bone free of residual graft particles.

There are concerns that bone grafting materials like β-TCP and CS that are fully resorbed in a short timeframe may contribute to site collapse [15, 16, 33, 42, 46]. Early loading of the implants after 12 weeks, as proposed in the present protocol, may further enhance the metabolic activity and trigger the remodelling of the regenerated labial bone [44]. Assuming that the newly formed hard tissue at the facial aspect of the implant is vital bone with no residual graft particles, it can be concluded that it adapted successfully to the transmitted occlusal forces according to Wolff's law, became stronger to resist to the type of loading, and thus maintained long-term the bone function [47, 48].

5. Conclusions

The results of this study suggest that this novel standardized protocol allows successful and predictable long-term successful functional outcomes regarding alveolar bone regeneration and implant rehabilitation. The concept of placing the implant 4 weeks after extraction, augmenting the bone around the implant utilizing only fully resorbable, biomechanical stable, alloplastic β-TCP/CS materials, and loading the implant at 12 weeks seems to offer advantages when compared with traditional treatment modalities. Additional studies are needed in order to confirm the present findings.

Conflict of Interests

The authors declare that there is no conflict of interests regarding the publication of this paper.

References

[1] P.-I. Branemark, "Osseointegration and its experimental background," The Journal of Prosthetic Dentistry, vol. 50, no. 3, pp. 399–410, 1983.

[2] R. U. Koh, I. Rudek, and H.-L. Wang, "Immediate implant placement: positives and negatives," Implant Dentistry, vol. 19, no. 2, pp. 98–108, 2010.

[3] J. Jofre, D. Valenzuela, P. Quintana, and C. Asenjo-Lobos, "Protocol for immediate implant replacement of infected teeth," Implant Dentistry, vol. 21, no. 4, pp. 287–294, 2012.

[4] S. T. Chen, T. G. Wilson Jr., and C. H. F. Hämmerle, "Immediate or early placement of implants following tooth extraction: review of biologic basis, clinical procedures, and outcomes," The International Journal of Oral & Maxillofacial Implants, vol. 19, no. 19, pp. 12–25, 2004.

[5] M. Esposito, M. G. Grusovin, I. P. Polyzos, P. Felice, and H. V. Worthington, "Timing of implant placement after tooth extraction: immediate, immediate-delayed or delayed implants? A Cochrane systematic review," *European Journal of Oral Implantology*, vol. 3, no. 3, pp. 189–205, 2010.

[6] P. A. Fugazzotto, "Treatment options following single-rooted tooth removal: a literature review and proposed hierarchy of treatment selection," *Journal of Periodontology*, vol. 76, no. 5, pp. 821–831, 2005.

[7] L. Schropp and F. Isidor, "Timing of implant placement relative to tooth extraction," *Journal of Oral Rehabilitation*, vol. 35, supplement 1, pp. 33–43, 2008.

[8] D. Rieder, J. Eggert, T. Krafft, H.-P. Weber, M. G. Wichmann, and S. M. Heckmann, "Impact of placement and restoration timing on single-implant esthetic outcome—a randomized clinical trial," *Clinical Oral Implants Research*, 2014.

[9] S. T. Chen and D. Buser, "Esthetic outcomes following immediate and early implant placement in the anterior maxilla—a systematic review," *The International Journal of Oral & Maxillofacial Implants*, vol. 29, supplement, pp. 186–215, 2014.

[10] K. L. Knoernschild, "Early survival of single-tooth implants in the esthetic zone may be predictable despite timing of implant placement or loading," *Journal of Evidence-Based Dental Practice*, vol. 10, no. 1, pp. 52–55, 2010.

[11] M. Hof, B. Pommer, H. Ambros, P. Jesch, S. Vogl, and W. Zechner, "Does timing of implant placement affect implant therapy outcome in the aesthetic zone? A clinical, radiological, aesthetic, and patient-based evaluation," *Clinical Implant Dentistry and Related Research*, 2014.

[12] L. Schropp, L. Kostopoulos, and A. Wenzel, "Bone healing following immediate versus delayed placement of titanium implants into extraction sockets: a prospective clinical study," *The International Journal of Oral & Maxillofacial Implants*, vol. 18, no. 2, pp. 189–199, 2003.

[13] H.-L. Chan, G.-H. Lin, J.-H. Fu, and H.-L. Wang, "Alterations in bone quality after socket preservation with grafting materials: a systematic review," *The International Journal of Oral & Maxillofacial Implants*, vol. 28, no. 3, pp. 710–720, 2013.

[14] N. Harel, O. Moses, A. Palti, and Z. Ormianer, "Long-term results of implants immediately placed into extraction sockets grafted with β-tricalcium phosphate: a retrospective study," *Journal of Oral and Maxillofacial Surgery*, vol. 71, no. 2, pp. e63–e68, 2013.

[15] A. Palti and T. Hoch, "A concept for the treatment of various dental bone defects," *Implant Dentistry*, vol. 11, no. 1, pp. 73–78, 2002.

[16] Z. Artzi, M. Weinreb, N. Givol et al., "Biomaterial resorption rate and healing site morphology of inorganic bovine bone and beta-tricalcium phosphate in the canine: a 24-month longitudinal histologic study and morphometric analysis," *The International Journal of Oral & Maxillofacial Implants*, vol. 19, no. 3, pp. 357–368, 2004.

[17] P. Trisi, W. Rao, A. Rebaudi, and P. Fiore, "Histologic effect of pure-phase beta-tricalcium phosphate on bone regeneration in human artificial jawbone defects," *International Journal of Periodontics and Restorative Dentistry*, vol. 23, no. 1, pp. 69–78, 2003.

[18] P. N. Nair, H.-U. Luder, F. A. Maspero, J. H. Fischer, and J. Schug, "Biocompatibility of b-tricalcium phosphate root replicas in porcine tooth extraction sockets—a correlative histological, ultrastructural, and X-ray microanalytical pilot study," *Journal of Biomaterials Applications*, vol. 20, no. 4, pp. 307–324, 2006.

[19] Z. Ormianer, A. Palti, and A. Shifman, "Survival of immediately loaded dental implants in deficient alveolar bone sites augmented with β-tricalcium phosphate," *Implant Dentistry*, vol. 15, no. 4, pp. 395–403, 2006.

[20] L. Schropp, F. Isidor, L. Kostopoulos, and A. Wenzel, "Interproximal papilla levels following early versus delayed placement of single-tooth implants: a controlled clinical trial," *The International Journal of Oral & Maxillofacial Implants*, vol. 20, no. 5, pp. 753–761, 2005.

[21] L. Schropp, A. Wenzel, L. Kostopoulos, and T. Karring, "Bone healing and soft tissue contour changes following single-tooth extraction: a clinical and radiographic 12-month prospective study," *International Journal of Periodontics and Restorative Dentistry*, vol. 23, no. 4, pp. 313–323, 2003.

[22] L. Schropp, L. Kostopoulos, A. Wenzel, and F. Isidor, "Clinical and radiographic performance of delayed–immediate single–tooth implant placement associated with peri–implant bone defects. A 2–year prospective, controlled, randomized follow–up report," *Journal of Clinical Periodontology*, vol. 32, no. 5, pp. 480–487, 2005.

[23] C. E. Nemcovsky, Z. Artzi, O. Moses, and I. Geernter, "Healing of dehiscence defects at delayed-immediate implant sites primarily closed by a rotated palatal flap following extraction," *The International Journal of Oral & Maxillofacial Implants*, vol. 15, no. 4, pp. 550–558, 2000.

[24] C. E. Nemcovsky and Z. Artzi, "Comparative study of buccal dehiscence defects in immediate, delayed, and late maxillary implant placement with collagen membranes: clinical healing between placement and second-stage surgery," *Journal of Periodontology*, vol. 73, no. 7, pp. 754–761, 2002.

[25] I. Sanz, M. Garcia-Gargallo, D. Herrera, C. Martin, E. Figuero, and M. Sanz, "Surgical protocols for early implant placement in post-extraction sockets: a systematic review," *Clinical Oral Implants Research*, vol. 23, no. 5, pp. 67–79, 2012.

[26] D. Buser, V. Chappuis, U. Kuchler et al., "Long-term stability of early implant placement with contour augmentation," *Journal of Dental Research*, vol. 92, no. 12, supplement, pp. 176S–182S, 2013.

[27] D. Buser, V. Chappuis, M. M. Bornstein, J.-G. Wittneben, M. Frei, and U. C. Belser, "Long-term stability of contour augmentation with early implant placement following single tooth extraction in the esthetic zone: a prospective, cross-sectional study in 41 patients with a 5-to 9-year follow-up," *Journal of Periodontology*, vol. 84, no. 11, pp. 1517–1527, 2013.

[28] O. Moses, S. Pitaru, Z. Artzi, and C. E. Nemcovsky, "Healing of dehiscence-type defects in implants placed together with different barrier membranes: a comparative clinical study," *Clinical Oral Implants Research*, vol. 16, no. 2, pp. 210–219, 2005.

[29] E. Eleftheriadis, M. D. Leventis, K. I. Tosios et al., "Osteogenic activity of β-tricalcium phosphate in a hydroxyl sulphate matrix and demineralized bone matrix: a histological study in rabbit mandible," *Journal of Oral Science*, vol. 52, no. 3, pp. 377–384, 2010.

[30] R. A. Horowitz, M. D. Rohrer, H. S. Prasad, N. Tovar, and Z. Mazor, "Enhancing extraction socket therapy with a biphasic calcium sulfate," *Compendium of Continuing Education in Dentistry*, vol. 33, no. 6, pp. 420–428, 2012.

[31] R. Smeets, A. Kolk, M. Gerressen et al., "A new biphasic osteoinductive calcium composite material with a negative Zeta potential for bone augmentation," *Head & Face Medicine*, vol. 5, no. 1, article 13, 2009.

[32] L. Podaropoulos, A. A. Veis, S. Papadimitriou, C. Alexandridis, and D. Kalyvas, "Bone regeneration using β-tricalcium

phosphate in a calcium sulfate matrix," *The Journal of Oral Implantology*, vol. 35, no. 1, pp. 28–36, 2009.

[33] K. A. Al Ruhaimi, "Effect of adding resorbable calcium sulfate to grafting materials on early bone regeneration in osseous defects in rabbits," *International Journal of Oral and Maxillofacial Implants*, vol. 15, no. 6, pp. 859–864, 2000.

[34] R. Dimitriou, G. I. Mataliotakis, G. M. Calori, and P. V. Giannoudis, "The role of barrier membranes for guided bone regeneration and restoration of large bone defects: current experimental and clinical evidence," *BMC Medicine*, vol. 10, no. 1, article 81, 2012.

[35] D. Buser, C. Dahlin, and R. K. Schenk, *Guided Bone Regeneration in Implant Dentistry*, Quintessence Publishing, London, UK, 1995.

[36] Y. Amano, M. Ota, K. Sekiguchi, Y. Shibukawa, and S. Yamada, "Evaluation of a poly-l-lactic acid membrane and membrane fixing pin for guided tissue regeneration on bone defects in dogs," *Oral Surgery, Oral Medicine, Oral Pathology, Oral Radiology, and Endodontics*, vol. 97, no. 2, pp. 155–163, 2004.

[37] A. Elshahat, N. Inoue, G. Marti, I. Safe, P. Manson, and C. Vanderkolk, "Guided bone regeneration at the donor site of iliac bone grafts for future use as autogenous grafts," *Plastic and Reconstructive Surgery*, vol. 116, no. 4, pp. 1068–1075, 2005.

[38] X. Zhang, H. A. Awad, R. J. O'Keefe, R. E. Guldberg, and E. M. Schwarz, "A perspective: engineering periosteum for structural bone graft healing," *Clinical Orthopaedics and Related Research*, vol. 466, no. 8, pp. 1777–1787, 2008.

[39] M. Saito, H. Shimizu, M. Beppu, and M. Takagi, "The role of β-tricalcium phosphate in vascularized periosteum," *Journal of Orthopaedic Science*, vol. 5, no. 3, pp. 275–282, 2000.

[40] H. Yuan, H. Fernandes, P. Habibovic et al., "Osteoinductive ceramics as a synthetic alternative to autologous bone grafting," *Proceedings of the National Academy of Sciences of the United States of America*, vol. 107, no. 31, pp. 13614–13619, 2010.

[41] A. M. C. Barradas, H. Yuan, C. A. van Blitterswijk, and P. Habibovic, "Osteoinductive biomaterials: current knowledge of properties, experimental models and biological mechanisms," *European Cells & Materials*, vol. 21, pp. 407–429, 2011.

[42] R. J. Miron, A. Sculean, Y. Shuang et al., "Osteoinductive potential of a novel biphasic calcium phosphate bone graft in comparison with autographs, xenografts, and DFDBA," *Clinical Oral Implants Research*, 2015.

[43] R. A. Horowitz, M. D. Leventis, M. D. Rohrer, and H. S. Prasad, "Bone grafting: history, rationale, and selection of materials and techniques," *Compendium of Continuing Education in Dentistry*, vol. 35, no. 4, supplement, pp. 1–6, 2014.

[44] C. I. Evian, E. S. Rosenberg, J. G. Coslet, and H. Corn, "The osteogenic activity of bone removed from healing extraction sockets in humans," *Journal of Periodontology*, vol. 53, no. 2, pp. 81–85, 1982.

[45] H. Sasaki, S. Koyama, M. Yokoyama, K. Yamaguchi, M. Itoh, and K. Sasaki, "Bone metabolic activity around dental implants under loading observed using bone scintigraphy," *The International Journal of Oral & Maxillofacial Implants*, vol. 23, no. 5, pp. 827–834, 2008.

[46] M. D. Leventis, P. Fairbairn, I. Dontas et al., "Biological response to β-tricalcium phosphate/calcium sulfate synthetic graft material: an experimental study," *Implant Dentistry*, vol. 23, no. 1, pp. 37–43, 2014.

[47] J. B. Brunski, D. A. Puleo, and A. Nanci, "Biomaterials and biomechanics of oral and maxillofacial implants: current status and future developments," *The International Journal of Oral & Maxillofacial Implants*, vol. 15, no. 1, pp. 15–46, 2000.

[48] J. Duyck and K. Vandamme, "The effect of loading on peri–implant bone: a critical review of the literature," *Journal of Oral Rehabilitation*, vol. 41, no. 10, pp. 783–794, 2014.

15

Evaluation of Static Friction of Polycrystalline Ceramic Brackets after Conditioning with Different Powers of Er:YAG Laser

Valiollah Arash,[1,2] **Saeed Javanmard,**[1,2] **Zeinab Eftekhari,**[1,2]
Manouchehr Rahmati-Kamel,[1,2] **and Mohammad Bahadoram**[3]

[1]*Department of Orthodontics, Faculty of Dentistry, Babol University of Medical Sciences, Babol, Iran*
[2]*Dental Materials Research Center, Babol University of Medical Sciences, Babol, Iran*
[3]*Medical Student Research Committee & Social Determinant of Health Research Center,*
 Ahvaz Jundishapur University of Medical Sciences, Ahvaz, Iran

Correspondence should be addressed to Zeinab Eftekhari; eftekhari_z83@yahoo.com

Academic Editor: Spiros Zinelis

This research aimed to reduce the friction between the wire and brackets by Er:YAG laser. To measure the friction between the wires and brackets in 0° and 10° of wire angulations, 40 polycrystalline ceramic brackets (Hubit, South Korea) were divided into 8 study groups and irradiated by 100, 200, and 300 mj/s of Er:YAG laser power. Two groups of brackets were not irradiated. The friction between the wires and brackets was measured with universal testing machine (SANTAM) with a segment of .019 × .025 SS wire pulled out of the slot of bracket. ANOVA and t-test were used for analyzing the results. To evaluate the effect of the laser on surface morphology of the bracket, SEM evaluations were carried out. The mean frictional resistances between the brackets and wires with 0° of angulation by increasing the laser power decreased compared with control group, but, in 10° of angulation, the friction increased regardless of the laser power and was comparable to the friction of nonirradiated brackets. Furthermore, with each laser power, frictional resistance of brackets in 10° of angulation was significantly higher than 0° of angulation. These results were explained by SEM images too.

1. Introduction

In the mid-1980s the first brackets made of monocrystalline ceramic (Sappire) and polycrystalline ceramic were marketed [1]. These brackets had many advantages compared with other esthetic appliances, including higher strength, more resistance to wear and deformation, more color stability, biocompatibility, and, above all, better appearance that is most demanded by patients during treatment nowadays. Ceramic brackets have some disadvantages, too, such as enamel wear, brittleness, difficulty debonding, and high coefficient of friction, which result in more resistance to sliding of wire in the slot [2].

It has been shown that, under all test circumstances, ceramic brackets have more frictional resistance compared with metal brackets because of their higher surface roughness. This concept is well ascertained by comparing these two brackets under a scanning electron microscope [3].

During orthodontic movement more over 60% of the force applied to teeth may disappear due to frictional resistance of ceramic brackets [4]. Higher frictional resistance increases the orthodontic force needed to move the teeth [5].

Reinforcing ceramic brackets with SS, improvement of manufacturing process of ceramic brackets, insertion of bumps on the floor of the slot of brackets, and so forth have been tried to reduce different problems of these brackets, including friction, strength, and force control [2, 4, 6–8]. However, investigations have shown inefficacy of some of these methods [4, 9].

Few researches have been carried out in orthodontics on the reduction of frictional resistance of ceramic brackets by laser. Abdallah et al. reported that glazing In-Ceram Alumina dental ceramics with high power settings of CO_2 laser and high energy density of excimer (XeCl) laser can improve the surface hardness and smoothness of ceramic surfaces [10]. Kara et al. and Dilber et al. reported that application of

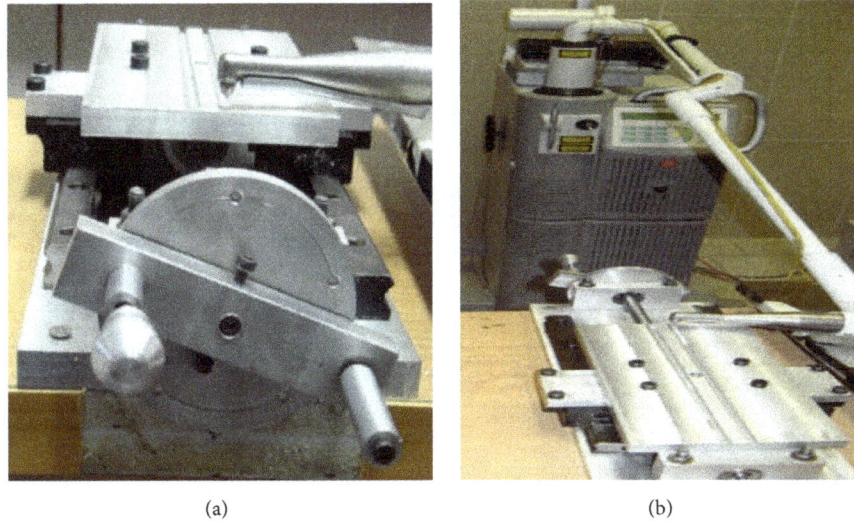

(a) (b)

FIGURE 1: The table was designed to keep the laser sample distance, laser speed, and angle of laser ray constant. The brackets were placed on a slot propped on the table. The laser handpiece-bracket distance was 1 mm for all the samples.

Er:YAG and Nd:YAG lasers changed the surface roughness of ceramic blocks used in their study [11, 12]. Considering the results of these studies, this study aimed to reduce the friction between the wire and brackets by different powers of Er:YAG laser to improve surface characteristics of ceramic brackets.

2. Materials and Methods

In this experimental study 40 polycrystalline ceramic brackets (Hubit, South Korea) and 40 pieces of .019 × .025-inch stainless steel wire (Orthotechnology, USA) were used to measure the friction between the wires and brackets in 0° and 10° of wire-bracket angulations. The brackets were randomly divided into 8 study groups, each group including 5 brackets; 6 groups were irradiated with 100, 200, and 300 mj/s of Er:YAG laser with wavelength 2940 at room temperature. Therefore, for each power setting and in each wire-bracket angulation, 5 brackets were used. Two groups of 5 brackets in 0° and 10° served as controls for friction test and were not irradiated. The brackets were placed on a designed table under a fixed laser handpiece. The table was aimed at keeping the laser sample distance, laser speed, and angle of laser ray constant. The handpiece light fiber diameter was 0.9 mm, so the table was designed so that a screw could move the table 0.9 mm in each turn and move the bracket with it at the same distance (Figure 1). Bracket irradiation was carried out for 20 seconds on each 0.9 mm of bracket surface from a distance of 1 mm from the brackets to apply the maximum power of the laser.

2.1. Evaluation of Bracket Surface.
The effect of the laser on the surface morphology of the brackets was evaluated under a scanning electron microscope (model KYKY-EM3200).

2.2. Friction Test.
To measure the friction between the wire and bracket, a universal testing machine (SANTAM) (Sahand

TABLE 1

Power of Er:YAG laser irradiated to samples (mj/s)	Average of frictional force between wire and bracket (N)
0	2.59 ± 0.74
100	1.66 ± 0.31
200	1.05 ± 0.56
300	0.59 ± 0.25

Company, Iran) was used. Straight line static traction test was carried out by this machine to simulate sliding of wire in the bracket. At one end of the machine there was an aluminum device that was attached to a 50 N load cell; this device included two plates. The brackets were bonded to the lower stable plate; then artificial saliva was sprayed on them. The wire was attached to the upper plate and then engaged in the bracket by elastomeric ligation. The upper end of the wire was attached to the upper plate; the wire was pulled out of the slot of the bracket with 50 N load cell at a rate 1 mm/min (Figure 2).

To place the brackets on the plate at 0° of angulation, the slots of the brackets were aligned precisely parallel to the edge of the plate by a conveyor (the edges of the plate were perpendicular to each other). To place the brackets on the plate at 10° of angulation, a line was drawn with 10° of angulation to the edge of the plate and the brackets were attached to the plate so that their slots were parallel to the line. The data were analyzed with ANOVA and t-test using SPSS 20.

3. Results

Table 1 and Figure 3 show the results of friction test between the wires placed at 0° of angulation and brackets irradiated with different laser powers.

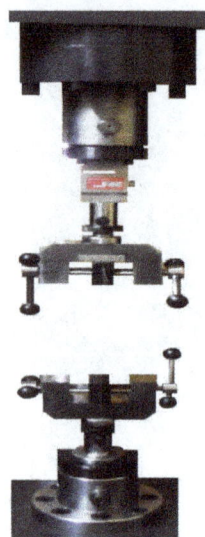

FIGURE 2: Schematic of universal testing machine. To measure the friction between the wire and bracket, a universal testing machine (SANTAM) (Sahand Company, Iran) was used. Straight line static traction test was carried out by this machine to simulate sliding of wire in the bracket. At one end of the machine there was an aluminum device that was attached to a 50 N load cell; this machine included two plates. The brackets were bonded to the lower stable plate. The wire was attached to the upper plate and then engaged in the bracket by elastomeric ligation; the wire was pulled out of the slot of the bracket with 50 N load cell at a rate 1 mm/min.

TABLE 2

Power of Er:YAG Laser irradiated to samples (mj/s)	Average of frictional force between the wire and bracket (N)
0	3.97 ± 0.75
100	2.97 ± 1.02
200	2.9 ± 1.66
300	3.8 ± 1.18

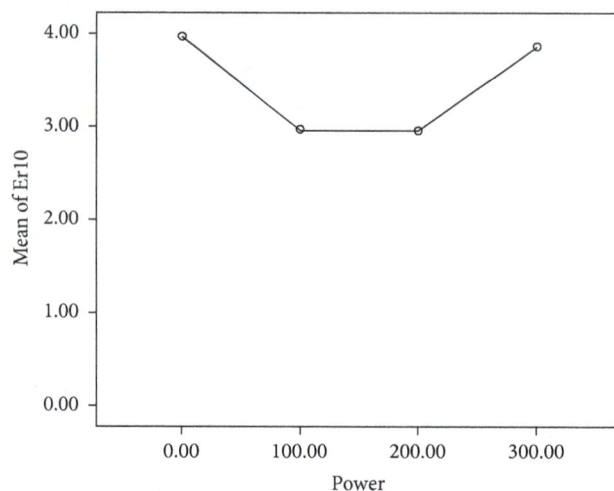

FIGURE 4: This diagram shows the changes in frictional forces (N) between the wire and bracket at 10° of angulation of wire with an increase in the laser power (mj/s).

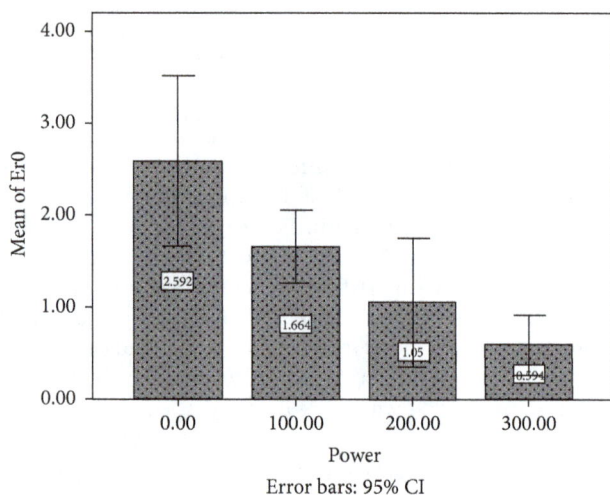

FIGURE 3: This diagram shows the changes in frictional force (N) between the wire and bracket at 0° of angulation with an increase in laser power (mj/s). Frictional resistance decreased with an increase in Er:YAG laser power ($P = 0.000$).

As shown in Figure 3, irradiation of brackets with 100 mj/s laser power and an increase in the power to 300 mj/s resulted in a significant decrease in frictional resistance compared with the control group ($P = 0.000$).

The differences between the frictional resistance of samples irradiated with 100 mj/s and 200 mj/s were not significant ($P = 0.264$). In addition, there were no significant differences

in the frictional resistance between samples irradiated with 200 mj/s and 300 mj/s ($P = 0.508$). However, the differences between the frictional resistance of the samples irradiated with 100 mj/s and 300 mj/s laser power were significant ($P = 0.020$).

Table 2 and Figure 4 show the results of friction test between the wires placed with 10° of angulation and brackets irradiated with different laser powers.

The changes in frictional resistance between the bracket and wire with an increase in the power of Er:YAG laser was not statistically significant ($P = 0.397$).

As shown in the diagram, irradiation of the brackets with 100 mj/s laser and an increase in the power to 300 mj/s did not result in statistically significant changes in frictional resistance compared with the control group.

The differences between the frictional resistance of the samples irradiated with 100 mj/s and 200 mj/s ($P = 1.000$); 200 mj/s and 300 mj/s ($P = 0.642$); 100 mj/s and 300 mj/s ($P = 0.649$) were not significant.

Table 3 shows the comparisons between the results of friction test between the wires placed at 10° of angulation and 0° of angulation and brackets irradiated with different laser powers. As shown in Table 3, with each laser power, the frictional resistance at 10° of angulation was statistically higher than frictional resistance at 0° of angulation with all laser powers.

TABLE 3

Power of Er:YAG laser beams used (mj/s)	Means of frictional forces between the wire at 0° of angulation and the bracket (N)	Means of frictional forces between the wire at 10° of angulation and the bracket (N)	P value
0	2.59 ± 0.74	3.97 ± 0.75	0.020
100	1.66 ± 0.31	2.97 ± 1.02	0.026
200	1.05 ± 0.56	2.9 ± 1.66	0.041
300	0.59 ± 0.25	3.8 ± 1.18	0.000

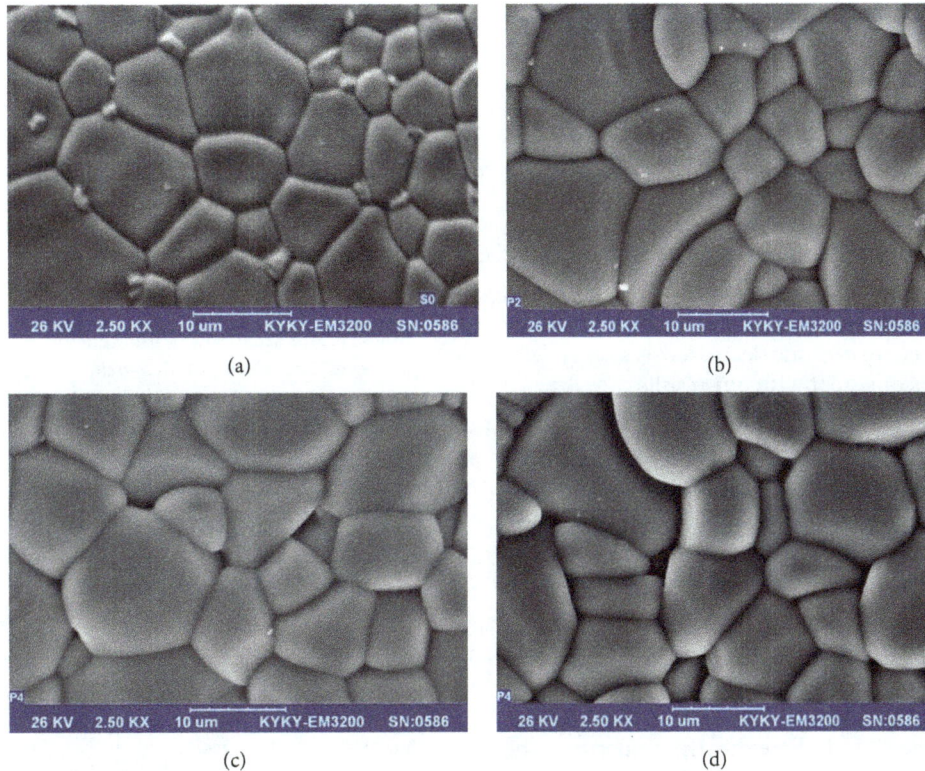

(a)

(b)

(c)

(d)

FIGURE 5: SEM images of brackets irradiated with 0, 100, 200, and 300 mj/s laser powers.

4. Discussion

Friction control is a major challenge in orthodontic treatment since a part of the applied force is dissipated to overcome friction [13]. In this study we aimed to reduce the frictional force between ceramic brackets and wires by irradiation of Er:YAG laser beams on ceramic brackets. When we have adequate temperature and time for atomic displacement on the surface the sharp angles of grains tend to become rounding (atomic displacement is the process of movement of atoms from rough and bumpy regions to depressed regions) [14].

As seen in Figure 5, by increasing the laser intensity, the temperature increases and more intergranular melting and grain contraction happen; the result is rounded angles of grains. Of course for more accurate evaluation of surface morphology to determine the relation between friction and surface changes, atomic force microscope (AFM) imaging is needed.

On the other hand, there was no significant difference between frictional resistance of brackets irradiated with different laser powers and wires placed in 10° of angulation, which might be attributed to more impressive effect of binding (deflection of wire against the corners of bracket) compared with surface friction in producing frictional resistance when the wire is placed with an angle in the bracket. As the angle between the wires and brackets in all the samples of this group was the same regardless of the laser power and the angle between the wire and bracket determines the binding rate, the frictional resistances between these brackets were not significantly different from each other. Therefore when binding of wire against the corners of brackets occurs the surface friction between the wire and the floor of the slot does not represent frictional resistance [15]. This can also explain the higher frictional resistance of samples irradiated with each laser power with 10° angle of wire in the bracket compared with 0° angle.

Jones and Amoah compared the static frictional resistance of ceramic brackets with a conventional slot (Allure), a glazed slot (Mystique), and a metal slot insert (Clarity) in three different simulated binding angulations (0°, 5°, and 10°) for each type of bracket. They concluded that brackets with glazed slot demonstrated low frictional resistance at 0° of angulation (without binding) and their friction was comparable to a metal slot in a ceramic bracket; however, by increasing angulations from 5 to 10 degrees frictional resistance increased so that the bracket behaved more like a conventional polycrystalline ceramic bracket [16]. The results of this study, especially about the prominent effect of binding on frictional resistance, are consistent with our results.

Abdallah et al. reported that glazing In-Ceram Alumina dental ceramics with high power settings of CO_2 laser and high energy density of excimer (XeCl) laser improved the surface hardness and smoothness of ceramic surfaces without affecting their internal structures [10]. Also Folwaczny et al. reported a significant reduction in roughness of dental ceramic surfaces under 308 nm excimer laser irradiation [17]. Zum Gahr et al. treated the surface of alumina with two procedures, followed by melting the surface with 200 W CO_2 laser; friction coefficient of ceramic decreased as a result [18]. These results are also consistent with our results.

Since frictional force is caused by several factors, which are usually correlated and dependent, these factors can also influence and create undesirable behavior in the frictional force values. Moreover, it is difficult to compare studies because of different methodologies; these variables can be considered influencing factors in data registers. Intraoral variables such as saliva, plaque, acquired pellicle, corrosion, chewing, bone density, tooth number, anatomic configuration, root surface area, and occlusion were not evaluated in this study, but they can influence frictional force values. In vitro studies do not correspond to what really happens during dental movement, and, therefore, the reader must be careful when evaluating the results from this research. The friction magnitude recorded is substantially different from the applied forces in clinical orthodontic movement. The values recorded should be used to compare the effects of different factors rather than to quantify in vivo friction.

5. Conclusion

By increasing the power of laser beams applied to the brackets, the friction between the wire and bracket at 0° of angulation decreased; but, at 10° of angulation, the friction increased regardless of the laser power and was comparable to the friction of nonirradiated brackets.

Conflict of Interests

The authors declare that there is no conflict of interests regarding the publication of this paper.

Acknowledgments

This study is a part of Saeed Javanmard's Ph.D. theses of orthodontics, which were supervised by the Department of Orthodontics & Craniofacial Orthopedics of Babol University of Medical Science. The authors would like to thank the Babol University of Medical Sciences for the laboratory technicians for their collaboration in measurement of the samples and also the financial support was provided by Ahvaz Jundishapur University of Medical Sciences, Ahvaz, Iran.

References

[1] A. K. Jena, R. Duggal, and A. K. Mehrotra, "Physical properties and clinical characteristics of ceramic brackets: a comprehensive review," *Trends in Biomaterials and Artificial Organs*, vol. 20, no. 2, pp. 123–138, 2007.

[2] J. S. Russell, "Current products and practice: aesthetic orthodontic brackets," *Journal of Orthodontics*, vol. 32, no. 2, pp. 146–163, 2005.

[3] D. H. Pratten, K. Popli, N. Germane, and J. C. Gunsolley, "Frictional resistance of ceramic and stainless steel orthodontic brackets," *American Journal of Orthodontics and Dentofacial Orthopedics*, vol. 98, no. 5, pp. 398–403, 1990.

[4] A. P. Guerrero, O. G. Filho, O. Tanaka, E. S. Camargo, and S. Vieira, "Evaluation of frictional forces between ceramic brackets and archwires of different alloys compared with metal brackets," *Brazilian Oral Research*, vol. 24, no. 1, pp. 40–45, 2010.

[5] A. P. Samant, S. P. Harimkar, and N. B. Dahotre, "The laser surface modification of advanced ceramics: a modeling approach," *JOM*, vol. 59, no. 8, pp. 35–38, 2007.

[6] R. P. Kusy and J. Q. Whitley, "esistances of metal-lined ceramic brackets versus conventional stainless steel brackets and development of 3-D frictional maps," *Angle Orthodontist*, vol. 71, no. 5, pp. 364–374, 2001.

[7] R. P. Kusy, "Orthodontic biomaterials: from the past to the present," *Angle Orthodontist*, vol. 72, no. 6, pp. 501–512, 2002.

[8] G. A. Thorstenson and R. P. Kusy, "Resistance to sliding of orthodontic brackets with bumps in the slot floors and walls: effects of second-order angulation," *Dental Materials*, vol. 20, no. 9, pp. 881–892, 2004.

[9] R. P. Kusy and J. Q. Whitley, "Friction between different wire-bracket configurations and materials," *Seminars in Orthodontics*, vol. 3, no. 3, pp. 166–177, 1997.

[10] R. M. Abdallah, I. M. Hammouda, M. Kamal, and O. B. Abouelatta, "Evaluation of hardness surface morphology and structure of laser irradiated ceramics," *Journal of Ovonic Research*, vol. 6, no. 5, pp. 227–238, 2010.

[11] H. B. Kara, E. Dilber, O. Koc, A. N. Ozturk, and M. Bulbul, "Effect of different surface treatments on roughness of IPS Empress 2 ceramic," *Lasers in Medical Science*, vol. 27, no. 2, pp. 267–272, 2012.

[12] E. Dilber, T. Yavuz, H. B. Kara, and A. N. Ozturk, "Comparison of the effects of surface treatments on roughness of two ceramic systems," *Photomedicine and Laser Surgery*, vol. 30, no. 6, pp. 308–314, 2012.

[13] S. Arango, A. Peláez-Vargas, and C. García, "Coating and surface treatment on orthodontic metallic materials," *Coatings*, vol. 3, no. 1, pp. 1–15, 2013.

[14] ASM International and Handbook Committee, *Powder Metal Technologies and Applications: ASM Handbook*, chapter 7, ASM International, Geauga County, Ohio, USA, 2nd edition, 1998.

[15] W. R. Proffit, "Mechanical principles in orthodontic force control," in *Contemporary Orthodontics*, chapter 9, pp. 330–332, Mosby Elsevier, St. Louis, Mo, USA, 5th edition, 2013.

[16] S. P. Jones and K. G. Amoah, "Static frictional resistances of polycrystalline ceramic brackets with conventional slots, glazed slots and metal slot inserts," *Australian orthodontic journal*, vol. 23, no. 1, pp. 36–40, 2007.

[17] M. Folwaczny, T. Liesenhoff, N. Lehn, and H. H. Horch, "Bactericidal action of 308 nm excimer-laser radiation: an in vitro investigation," *Journal of Endodontics*, vol. 24, no. 12, pp. 781–785, 1998.

[18] K.-H. Zum Gahr and J. Schneider, "Surface modification of ceramics for improved tribological properties," *Ceramics International*, vol. 26, no. 4, pp. 363–370, 2000.

16

Various Techniques to Increase Keratinized Tissue for Implant Supported Overdentures: Retrospective Case Series

Ahmed Elkhaweldi,[1] Carmen Rincon Soler,[2] Rodrigo Cayarga,[2] Takanori Suzuki,[1] and Zev Kaufman[1]

[1]*Department of Periodontology and Implant Dentistry, New York University College of Dentistry, 345 East 24th Street, New York City, NY 10010, USA*
[2]*Universidad Francisco Marroquín, 01010 Guatemala City, Guatemala*

Correspondence should be addressed to Ahmed Elkhaweldi; akh4243@gmail.com

Academic Editor: Sang-Choon Cho

Purpose. The purpose of this retrospective case series is to describe and compare different surgical techniques that can be utilized to augment the keratinized soft tissue around implant-supported overdentures. *Materials and Methods.* The data set was extracted as deidentified information from the routine treatment of patients at the Ashman Department of Periodontology and Implant Dentistry at New York University College of Dentistry. Eight edentulous patients were selected to be included in this study. Patients were treated for lack of keratinized tissue prior to implant placement, during the second stage surgery, and after delivery of the final prosthesis. *Results.* All 8 patients in this study were wearing a complete maxillary and/or mandibular denture for at least a year before the time of the surgery. One of the following surgical techniques was utilized to increase the amount of keratinized tissue: apically positioned flap (APF), pedicle graft (PG), connective tissue graft (CTG), or free gingival graft (FGG). *Conclusions.* The amount of keratinized tissue should be taken into consideration when planning for implant-supported overdentures. The apical repositioning flap is an effective approach to increase the width of keratinized tissue prior to the implant placement.

1. Introduction

Dental implant-supported overdentures have been documented to be a predictable and successful option to treat edentulous patients [1, 2]. Currently, with the evolution of implant surfaces, osseointegration of implants is less of a challenge [3]. However, the stability and health of the peri-implant soft tissue is necessary for the success and the long-term maintenance of dental implants [4]. Two millimeters wide band of keratinized tissue has been considered clinically desirable to provide a soft tissue seal around natural teeth [5]. However, controversy still remains over the necessity for a band of keratinized tissue around dental implants [6–9]. The role of dental plaque in the etiology of peri-implant diseases is well documented in the literature [10, 11]. The absence of periodontal ligament, supracrestal fibers attachment around dental implants may make peri-implant tissue more susceptible to an inflammatory process caused by plaque accumulation [12].

Several studies have reported increased gingival and plaque index scores, mucosal recession, and marginal bone resorption in areas around implants with less than 2 mm of keratinized tissue [4, 8, 13–16]. Conversely, some authors have claimed that, with adequate plaque control, peri-implant tissues can be maintained in a healthy state with a minimum amount of keratinized tissue [6–9].

However, patient discomfort has been reported to be associated with insufficient keratinized tissue in implant-supported overdentures [17]. In many cases, performing oral hygiene was reported to be painful as a result to the absence of the keratinized tissue surrounding the implant. Moreover, discomfort has been related to mechanical irritation due to the mobility of the nonkeratinized tissue under function [17, 18].

In 1999, Kaptein et al. investigated the peri-implant tissue health of loaded implants. There was a significantly higher gingival index and probing depth in overdenture versus fixed prosthesis cases [18]. It has been reported that implants supporting overdentures had more risk for bone loss, based on poorer peri-implant tissue health [18]. Adibrad et al. investigated the association between the width of the keratinized tissue and the health status of the soft tissue around implants supporting overdentures. They concluded that the absence of adequate keratinized tissue was associated with a higher plaque accumulation, gingival inflammation, bleeding on probing, and mucosal recession [17].

To date, there are a limited number of studies that discuss peri-implant tissue health and the presence of keratinized tissue around implants supporting overdentures [17–19]. These studies conclude that the presence of keratinized tissue around implant-supported overdentures is a factor effecting bone maintenance and soft tissue health around those implants [17, 18].

Various surgical procedures have been developed to preserve and/or reconstruct keratinized tissue around dental implants [20–24]. These techniques, including apically positioned flaps, pedicle grafts, free gingival grafts, and connective tissue grafts, can be performed prior to implant placement, during the second stage surgery or after delivery of the final prosthesis. Allogenic and xenogenic soft tissue grafts have also been used as other options for increasing peri-implant keratinized tissue [24–27].

The purpose of this retrospective case series was to describe and compare different surgical techniques that can be utilized to augment the keratinized soft tissue around dental implant-supported overdentures.

2. Materials and Methods

Clinical data in this study was obtained from implant database (ID). This data set was extracted as deidentified information from the routine treatment of patients at the Ashman Department of Periodontology and Implant Dentistry at New York University College of Dentistry. The ID was certified by the Office of Quality Assurance at NYUCD. This study is in compliance with the Health Insurance Portability and Accountability Act (HIPAA) requirements.

2.1. Study Subjects. Eight edentulous cases were selected from the ID to be included in this retrospective study. Patients were treated for lack of keratinized tissue prior to implant placement, during the second stage surgery or after delivery of the prosthesis. The population consisted of 2 females and 6 males, with a mean age of 65 years (range: 54 to 83). In 7 out of 8, the augmentation procedure was performed in the mandible.

2.2. Inclusion Criteria

(1) Patients who underwent implant surgery and were restored with a maxillary and/or mandibular implant-supported overdenture.

(2) Patients wearing a maxillary and/or mandibular implant-supported overdenture.

(3) Clinical symptoms of discomfort or difficulty to perform oral hygiene due to insufficient keratinized

tissue around implant-supported overdentures. Insufficient was defined as <2 mm of keratinized gingiva.

(4) Patients who underwent a surgical procedure to increase keratinized tissue around implant-supported overdentures.

2.3. Exclusion Criteria

(1) Presence of systemic diseases that influence bone or soft tissue metabolism.

(2) Smoking habit of more than a pack a day, and unwillingness to stop.

(3) Radiotherapy to head/neck region in the past 12 months prior to surgery.

(4) Chemotherapy in the past 12 months prior to surgery.

(5) Unwillingness to commit to a long-term maintenance program after treatment.

2.4. Description of the Protocol

(1) Preoperative measurement of the width of keratinized tissue, in the area of the planned implants, or around already placed implants, measured in millimeters using a periodontal probe from the free soft tissue margin to the mucogingival junction. All the measurements were performed by the same investigator.

(2) Antibiotic premedication: 2 g Amoxicillin 1 hour prior to surgery or 600 mg Clindamycin in case of penicillin allergy.

(3) Infiltrative local anesthesia using Lidocaine HCl 2% containing epinephrine 1:100,000 or Carbocaine 3% without epinephrine in cases where a vasoconstrictor was contraindicated.

(4) One of the following techniques was utilized to increase the amount of keratinized tissue: apically positioned flap, pedicle graft, connective tissue graft, or free gingival graft. The technique was selected depending on the time the surgery was performed and operator preferences (Table 1).

(5) Postsurgically, the patient was instructed to not wear their prosthesis for 3 weeks.

(6) Postoperative antibiotics (Amoxicillin 500 mg tid or Clindamycin 150 mg qid) and analgesics (Ibuprophen 600 mg q 4–6 hrs) were prescribed for a week.

(7) Postoperative care instructions were given, including use of Clorhexidine gluconate 0.12% rinses 3 times a day and soft diet, for two weeks.

(8) Postoperative measurement of the width of keratinized tissue taken 1 month and 3 months after the surgery, using a periodontal probe and measured from the free gingival margin to the mucogingival junction in the area where the preoperative measurement was taken and where the surgical technique was performed. Photos of the surgical procedure were used to duplicate the area of measurement.

TABLE 1: Gain in keratinized tissue three months after surgical procedure.

Case	Gender	Age	Site	KT initial (mm)	KT final (mm)	Increase KT (mm)	Time of surgery	Technique
1	Male	65	#22	3	8	5	Prior to implant placement	APF
			#27	4	9	5		
2	Male	72	#22	0-1	4	3-4	2nd stage	APF
			#27	1-2	5	3-4		
3	Female	54	#22	1	4	3	2nd stage	APF
4	Male	59	#22	1	4	3	2nd stage	APF
			#27	0-1	3	2-3		
5	Male	61	#22	1	3	2	2nd stage	PG
			#27	1	4	3		
6	Male	60	#11	1	4	3	After	FGG
			#13	1	3	2		
7	Female	65	#22	1	2-3	1-2	After	CTG
			#27	1	2-3	1-2		
8	Male	83	#22	0-1	0-1	0	After	CTG
			#27	0-1	0-1	0		

3. Results and Discussion

Over time, clinicians have used different surgical techniques to increase the width of keratinized tissue around natural teeth. These techniques have also been applied around implant-supported restorations. Each of these techniques has advantages and limitations. Understanding these techniques would help the clinician to decide which one to use in specific circumstances. In this study, fifteen sites in eight patients were treated to increase the amount of keratinized tissue. All 8 patients in this study were wearing a complete maxillary and/or mandibular denture for at least a year before the time of the surgery. One of the following surgical techniques was utilized to increase the amount of keratinized tissue: apically positioned flap (APF), pedicle graft (PG), connective tissue graft (CTG), or free gingival graft (FGG). In seven out of the eight cases, the surgery was performed in the mandible. The augmentation procedure was performed on three cases with the implants already restored with the final prosthesis. Four cases had the procedure done as part of the second stage implant surgery. However, in one case the augmentation utilized before the implants were placed.

When planning for implant-supported overdentures, a preoperative assessment of the amount of keratinized tissue is an important step. When necessary, augmentation of keratinized mucosa should be done prior to implant placement. In case 1, an apically positioned flap was performed one month before the stage 1 surgery to allow adequate soft tissue closure (Figure 1). The initial measurement of the band of keratinized tissue in sites #22 and #27 was 3 and 4 mm, respectively. A single horizontal beveled incision was made into the attached gingiva (Figure 1(b)). The mesiodistal extension of the incision was made from #21 to #28, making it possible to elevate a partial thickness flap which was apically repositioned by suturing the flap to the periosteum with Vicryl 4.0 (Polyglactin 910) (Figure 1(c)). As a result of this procedure, a 5 mm increase in the width of keratinized tissue was obtained at both sites (Figure 1(d)). When a surgery to increase the width of keratinized tissue is performed during implant placement, the incision should be designed to maintain the amount of keratinized tissue. This incision design will allow the implant to be surrounded by at least 2 mm of keratinized tissue all around.

A second stage surgery is a good opportunity to increase the width of keratinized tissue (Figures 2(a), 2(b), 2(c), and 2(d)). This approach was utilized in cases 2, 3, and 4. In three patients, an apically repositioned flap was used as described in case 1, which resulted in a mean increase in the width of keratinized tissue of 3.1 mm. Case 5 was also treated as part of the second stage surgery utilizing pedicle flap with a mean increase of 2.8 mm. The pedicle flap technique is an approach similar to an apically repositioned flap and should be used when there is adequate keratinized tissue adjacent to the implant. A beveled horizontal incision of approximately 6 mm was made distal to the implant, with a small vertical incision at the distal end part of the first incision. A partial thickness flap was then elevated and the pedicle flap sutured apically (Figures 3(a), 3(b), and 3(c)).

In some cases, a lack of keratinized tissue is evident after the insertion of the final prosthesis, causing discomfort and restricting oral hygiene performance. Moreover, since implant-supported overdentures are a removable prosthesis, patients often experience pain when taking the overdenture on and off. In this retrospective case series, three patients had surgery to increase the amount of keratinized tissue around 6 implants supporting overdentures, either by utilizing free gingival grafts or connective tissue grafts. The selection was based on the anatomy of the palate. Preference was giving to connective tissue graft when the patient had high vault palate, which allows harvesting a good amount tissue and reduces the risk of endangering the greater palatine artery. In case 6, an autogenous free gingival graft was harvested from the palatal premolar area, around #12, 13, and then sutured to the periosteal recipient bed of #11 and #13 (Figures 4(a), 4(b), and 4(c)). After healing and maturation of the soft tissue

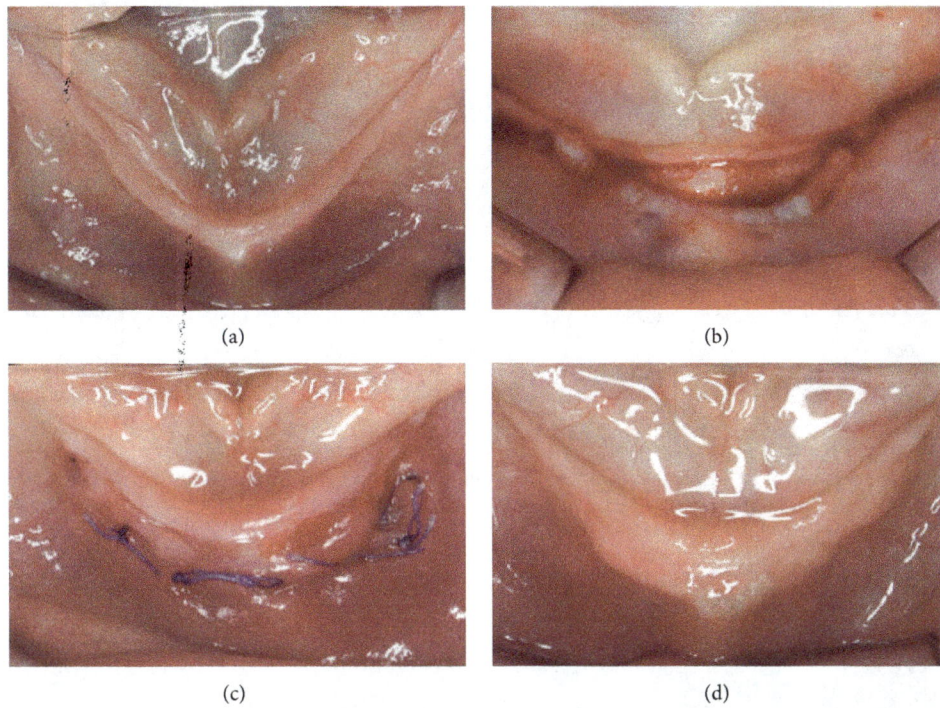

FIGURE 1: (a) Initial clinical appearance of the mandibular ridge with 3-4 mm of keratinized tissue. (b) Crestal horizontal beveled incision made. (c) The flap sutured apically with Vicryl 4.0 to the periosteum. (d) Final result 3 months after the surgery showed 5 mm increase in the width of keratinized tissue.

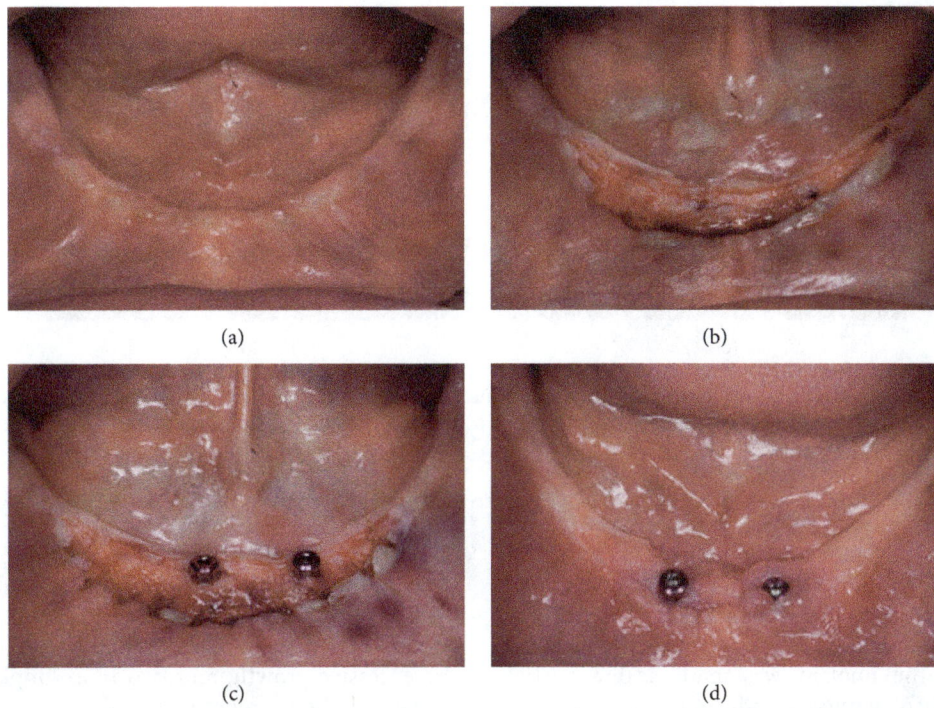

FIGURE 2: (a) Presurgical appearance of mandibular ridge with 0-1 mm of keratinized tissue. (b) Partial thickness flap reflection. (c) Apical suturing of the flap to the periosteum using Chromic Gut 4.0. (d) Final result after the surgery showed a 2-3 mm increase in keratinized tissue.

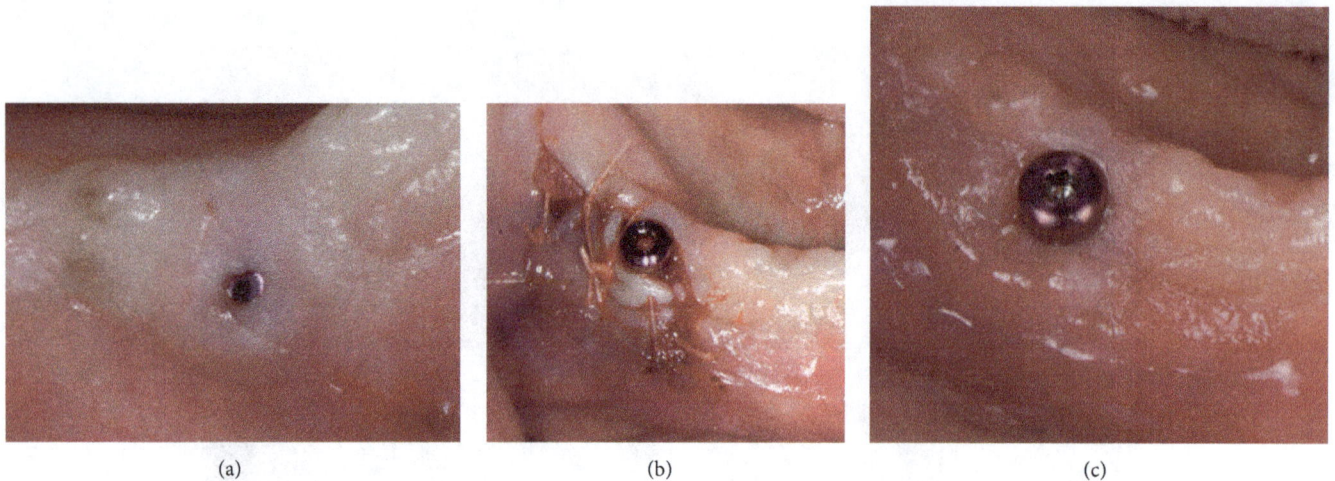

FIGURE 3: (a) Presurgical appearance of an implant supporting overdenture, 1 mm keratinized tissue. (b) Pedicle graft elevated and suture buccally. (c) Final result with 3 mm gain of keratinized tissue.

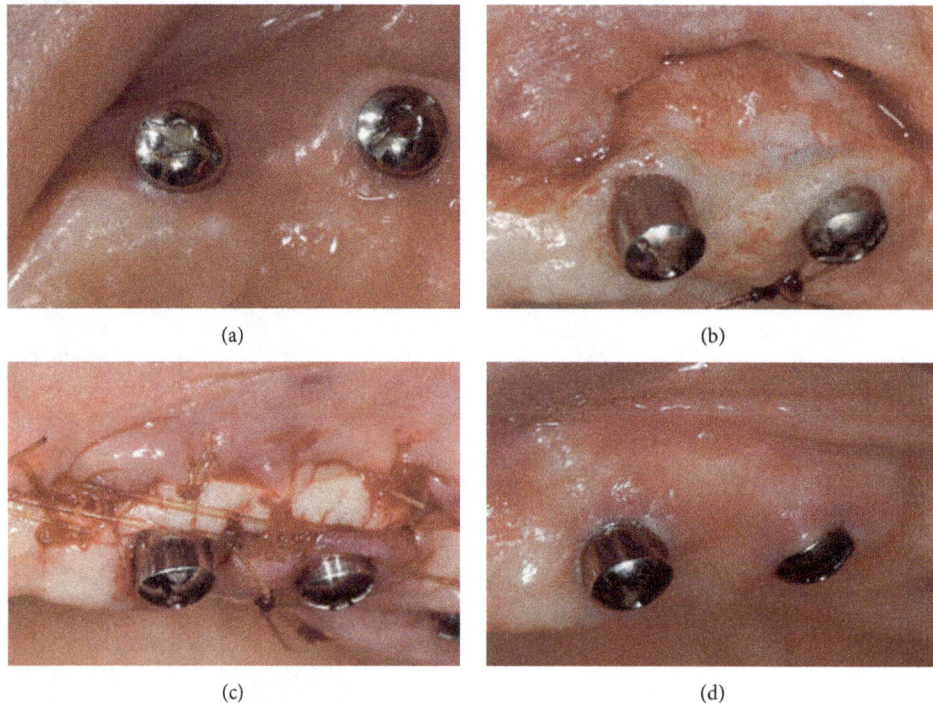

FIGURE 4: (a) Presurgical appearance of two implants with 1 mm of buccal keratinized tissue. (b) Partial thickness flap on the recipient bed prepared for the FGG. (c) Interrupted and horizontal mattress sutures to stabilize the FGG obtained from the palate. (d) Three-month follow-up showing an increase of 2-3 mm of keratinized tissue.

an increase of 3 and 2 mm was obtained, respectively, (Figure 4(d)). Cases 7 and 8 were treated with connective tissue grafts harvested from the premolar area of the palate. At the same time, the recipient site was prepared; a vertical incision mesial to the implant was made and a partial thickness flap was then elevated, creating a tunnel where the connective tissue graft was inserted and sutured. One of them (case 7) resulted in no increase of keratinized tissue as a result of significant decrease of the vestibular depth following the excessive amount of alveolar bone resorption. In case

8, the healing was accompanied with nonkeratinized soft tissue growth over the implant which made it very difficult both to perform oral hygiene and to insert the overdenture. A customized healing abutment was designed to control the excessive growth, and two more implants were placed, converting the overdenture prosthesis.

Each of the soft tissue augmentation techniques has advantages and limitations. The apically repositioned flap is a relatively simple procedure that provides a good esthetic outcome, as the newly formed tissue is indistinguishable from the surrounding mucosa. Moreover, shorter operative time and low morbidity is involved [20]. The main limitation of this technique is the need for at least 0.5 mm millimeters of keratinized tissue preoperatively. In cases where less than 0.5 mm of keratinized tissue is present preoperatively, autogenous free gingival grafts present an effective option. Free gingival grafts have been proven to be successful and predictable. However, these also present disadvantages. They involve two surgical sites with the consequent morbidity in both areas. Moreover, discrepancies in color and texture with the surrounding mucosa oftentimes result in a compromised esthetic outcome [24]. When using these techniques, some percentage of shrinkage should be expected. After one year, it has been reported that in the case of a free gingival graft, shrinkage of 38 to 45% occurs in relation to the thickness of the graft [28]. This shrinkage is even greater in cases where acellular dermal allografts are used [24]. Connective tissue graft was utilized in two cases. Although the augmentation was not successful in one case, this technique can still be an option to augment the keratinized tissue around implants restorations. There was average of 1.5 mm increase in the width of the keratinized tissue. Zucchelli et al. reported a similar result for CTG around single implant restoration. However, the author believes that the stability of the graft is very important for this technique to be successful. Pedicle Graft was utilized in one case as part of second stage surgery. This technique was less invasive and resulted in up to 3 mm increase in the keratinized tissue. This technique can be very useful in unilateral single implant cases where only small areas of narrow keratinized tissue need to be augmented [29].

4. Conclusions

The amount of keratinized tissue should be taken into consideration when planning for implant-supported overdentures. When the initial amount is considered insufficient, surgical augmentation procedures should be performed. An apical repositioning flap is an effective approach to increase the width of keratinized tissue prior to the implant placement if 0.5 mm of keratinized tissue was preoperatively available. During the second stage surgery, lingualized incision designs and pedicle grafts are a less invasive alternative to increase a limited zone of keratinized mucosa. Although free gingival graft or connective tissue graft could also be utilized but around implants, they can impose some challenges to the clinician during the surgery or throughout the healing. When patients experience discomfort after insertion of the final prosthesis due to a lack of keratinized mucosa, free gingival or connective tissue grafts are a feasible alternative. In some cases, a change of design of the prosthesis could be performed, placing more implants and converting from overdenture to a fixed restoration.

Conflict of Interests

The authors declare that there is no conflict of interests regarding the publication of this paper.

References

[1] T. Jemt, J. Chai, J. Harnett et al., "A 5-year prospective multicenter follow-up report on overdentures supported by osseointegrated implants," *International Journal of Oral and Maxillofacial Implants*, vol. 11, no. 3, pp. 291–298, 1996.

[2] N. J. Attard and G. A. Zarb, "Long-term treatment outcomes in edentulous patients with implant overdentures: the Toronto study," *The International Journal of Prosthodontics*, vol. 17, no. 4, pp. 425–433, 2004.

[3] A. Wennerberg and T. Albrektsson, "On implant surfaces: a review of current knowledge and opinions," *The International Journal of Oral & Maxillofacial Implants*, vol. 25, no. 1, pp. 63–74, 2010.

[4] B.-S. Kim, Y.-K. Kim, P.-Y. Yun et al., "Evaluation of peri-implant tissue response according to the presence of keratinized mucosa," *Oral Surgery, Oral Medicine, Oral Pathology, Oral Radiology, and Endodontology*, vol. 107, no. 3, pp. e24–e28, 2009.

[5] N. P. Lang and H. Löe, "The relationship between the width of keratinized gingiva and gingival health," *Journal of Periodontology*, vol. 43, no. 10, pp. 623–627, 1972.

[6] J. L. Wennström, F. Bengazi, and U. Lekholm, "The influence of the masticatory mucosa on the peri-implant soft tissue condition," *Clinical Oral Implants Research*, vol. 5, no. 1, pp. 1–8, 1994.

[7] J. L. Wennström and J. Derks, "Is there a need for keratinized mucosa around implants to maintain health and tissue stability?" *Clinical Oral Implants Research*, vol. 23, no. 6, pp. 136–146, 2012.

[8] D. M. Chung, T.-J. Oh, J. L. Shotwell, C. E. Misch, and H.-L. Wang, "Significance of keratinized mucosa in maintenance of dental implants with different surfaces," *Journal of Periodontology*, vol. 77, no. 8, pp. 1410–1420, 2006.

[9] F. Bengazi, J. L. Wennström, and U. Lekholm, "Recession of the soft tissue margin at oral implants: a 2-year longitudinal prospective study," *Clinical Oral Implants Research*, vol. 7, no. 2, pp. 303–310, 1996.

[10] Å. Leonhardt, S. Renvert, and G. Dahlén, "Microbial findings at failing implants," *Clinical Oral Implants Research*, vol. 10, no. 5, pp. 339–345, 1999.

[11] E. Romeo, M. Ghisolfi, and D. Carmagnola, "Peri-implant diseases. A systematic review of the literature," *Minerva Stomatologica*, vol. 53, no. 5, pp. 215–230, 2004.

[12] T. Berglundh and J. Lindhe, "Dimension of the periimplant mucosa. Biological width revisited," *Journal of Clinical Periodontology*, vol. 23, no. 10, pp. 971–973, 1996.

[13] D. Boynueğri, S. K. Nemli, and Y. A. Kasko, "Significance of keratinized mucosa around dental implants: a prospective comparative study," *Clinical Oral Implants Research*, vol. 24, no. 8, pp. 928–933, 2013.

[14] A. R. Schrott, M. Jimenez, J.-W. Hwang, J. Fiorellini, and H.-P. Weber, "Five-year evaluation of the influence of keratinized mucosa on peri-implant soft-tissue health and stability around implants supporting full-arch mandibular fixed prostheses," *Clinical Oral Implants Research*, vol. 20, no. 10, pp. 1170–1177, 2009.

[15] A. Bouri Jr., N. Bissada, M. S. Al-Zahrani, F. Faddoul, and I. Nouneh, "Width of keratinized gingiva and the health status of the supporting tissues around dental implants," *International Journal of Oral and Maxillofacial Implants*, vol. 23, no. 2, pp. 323–326, 2008.

[16] L. Gobbato, G. Avila-Ortiz, K. Sohrabi, C.-W. Wang, and N. Karimbux, "The effect of keratinized mucosa width on peri-implant health: a systematic review," *The International Journal of Oral & Maxillofacial Implants*, vol. 28, no. 6, pp. 1536–1545, 2013.

[17] M. Adibrad, M. Shahabuei, and M. Sahabi, "Significance of the width of keratinized mucosa on the health status of the supporting tissue around implants supporting overdentures," *Journal of Oral Implantology*, vol. 35, no. 5, pp. 232–237, 2009.

[18] M. L. A. Kaptein, G. L. De Lange, and P. A. Blijdorp, "Peri-implant tissue health in reconstructed atrophic maxillae—report of 88 patients and 470 implants," *Journal of Oral Rehabilitation*, vol. 26, no. 6, pp. 464–474, 1999.

[19] R. Mericske-Stern, T. Steinlin Schaffner, P. Marti, and A. H. Geering, "Peri-implant mucosal aspects of ITI implants supporting overdentures. A five-year longitudinal study," *Clinical Oral Implants Research*, vol. 5, no. 1, pp. 9–18, 1994.

[20] J. Carnio and P. M. Camargo, "The modified apically repositioned flap to increase the dimensions of attached gingiva: the single incision technique for multiple adjacent teeth," *The International Journal of Periodontics & Restorative Dentistry*, vol. 26, no. 3, pp. 265–269, 2006.

[21] G. Wiesner, M. Esposito, H. Worthington, and M. Schlee, "Connective tissue grafts for thickening peri-implant tissues at implant placement. One-year results from an explanatory split-mouth randomised controlled clinical trial," *European Journal of Oral Implantology*, vol. 3, no. 1, pp. 27–35, 2010.

[22] C. E. Nemcovsky and O. Moses, "Rotated palatal flap. A surgical approach to increase keratinized tissue width in maxillary implant uncovering: technique and clinical evaluation," *The International Journal of Periodontics and Restorative Dentistry*, vol. 22, no. 6, pp. 607–612, 2002.

[23] F. Cairo, U. Pagliaro, and M. Nieri, "Soft tissue management at implant sites," *Journal of Clinical Periodontology*, vol. 35, no. 8, pp. 163–167, 2008.

[24] J.-J. Yan, A. Y.-M. Tsai, M.-Y. Wong, and L.-T. Hou, "Comparison of acellular dermal graft and palatal autograft in the reconstruction of keratinized gingiva around dental implants: a case report," *International Journal of Periodontics and Restorative Dentistry*, vol. 26, no. 3, pp. 287–292, 2006.

[25] M. Sanz, R. Lorenzo, J. J. Aranda, C. Martin, and M. Orsini, "Clinical evaluation of a new *collagen matrix* (Mucograft prototype) to enhance the width of keratinized tissue in patients with fixed prosthetic restorations: a randomized prospective clinical trial," *Journal of Clinical Periodontology*, vol. 36, no. 10, pp. 868–876, 2009.

[26] K.-H. Lee, B.-O. Kim, and H.-S. Jang, "Clinical evaluation of a collagen matrix to enhance the width of keratinized gingiva around dental implants," *Journal of Periodontal & Implant Science*, vol. 40, no. 2, pp. 96–101, 2010.

[27] J.-B. Park, "Increasing the width of keratinized mucosa around endosseous implant using acellular dermal matrix allograft," *Implant Dentistry*, vol. 15, no. 3, pp. 275–281, 2006.

[28] W. Mormann, F. Schaer, and A. R. Firestone, "The relationship between success of free gingival grafts and transplant thickness. Revascularization and shrinkage: a one year clinical study," *Journal of Periodontology*, vol. 52, no. 2, pp. 74–80, 1981.

[29] G. Zucchelli, C. Mazzotti, I. Mounssif, M. Mele, M. Stefanini, and L. Montebugnoli, "A novel surgical-prosthetic approach for soft tissue dehiscence coverage around single implant," *Clinical Oral Implants Research*, vol. 24, no. 9, pp. 957–962, 2013.

17

In Vitro Ability of a Novel Nanohydroxyapatite Oral Rinse to Occlude Dentine Tubules

Robert G. Hill,[1] Xiaohui Chen,[1,2] and David G. Gillam[3]

[1]*Dental Physical Sciences, Barts and The London School of Medicine and Dentistry, Queen Mary University of London (QMUL), London E1 4NS, UK*
[2]*School of Dentistry, The University of Manchester, Manchester M13 9PL, UK*
[3]*Centre for Adult Oral Health, Barts and The London School of Medicine and Dentistry, Queen Mary University of London (QMUL), London E1 2AD, UK*

Correspondence should be addressed to David G. Gillam; d.g.gillam@qmul.ac.uk

Academic Editor: Patricia Pereira

Objectives. The aim of the study was to investigate the ability of a novel nanohydroxyapatite (nHA) desensitizing oral rinse to occlude dentine tubules compared to selected commercially available desensitizing oral rinses. *Methods.* 25 caries-free extracted molars were sectioned into 1 mm thick dentine discs. The dentine discs ($n = 25$) were etched with 6% citric acid for 2 minutes and rinsed with distilled water, prior to a 30-second application of test and control oral rinses. Evaluation was by (1) Scanning Electron Microscopy (SEM) of the dentine surface and (2) fluid flow measurements through a dentine disc. *Results.* Most of the oral rinses failed to adequately cover the dentine surface apart from the nHa oral rinse. However the hydroxyapatite, 1.4% potassium oxalate, and arginine/PVM/MA copolymer oral rinses, appeared to be relatively more effective than the nHA test and negative control rinses (potassium nitrate) in relation to a reduction in fluid flow measurements. *Conclusions.* Although the novel nHA oral rinse demonstrated the ability to occlude the dentine tubules and reduce the fluid flow measurements, some of the other oral rinses appeared to demonstrate a statistically significant reduction in fluid flow through the dentine disc, in particular the arginine/PVM/MA copolymer oral rinse.

1. Introduction

Dentine hypersensitivity (DH) is a clinical problem that may impact on the quality of life of individuals who may experience discomfort when eating and drinking hot and cold food and drink during their day to day activities [1]. Currently there is no recognized ideal desensitizing product (over-the-counter [toothpaste or mouthwash] or dentist [professionally] applied) that provides both fast acting and long lasting protection against the pain associated with DH [2]. This concern has subsequently led to the development of novel substances or reformulation of existing technologies for example, bioactive glasses (Novamin) and hydroxyapatite/nanohydroxyapatite/nanocarbonate apatite crystal toothpastes (HAP) [3–7], Colgate Sensitive Pro-Relief toothpastes and oral rinses [8–11], and a 1.4% potassium oxalate oral rinse (LISTERINE Advanced Defence Sensitive) [12–15]. Currently toothpastes, gels, and oral rinses are designed to reduce or relieve pain arising from DH based on either their (1) tubular occluding or (2) nerve desensitization properties. Recently a number of novel nanohydroxyapatite toothpastes and oral rinses (nHAs) have been developed for home use (over-the-counter [OTC]) and these products may be an attractive alternative to the traditional desensitizing toothpastes and oral rinses for treating DH [16, 17]. The aim of the present study therefore was to investigate the ability of a novel nanohydroxyapatite desensitizing oral rinse to occlude dentine tubules and reduce fluid flow in comparison with other selected commercially available desensitizing oral rinses.

2. Materials and Methods

25 caries-free extracted maxillary and mandibular molars were obtained from the tooth bank at the Royal London

Dental Hospital, London, UK. The *in vitro* occlusion of the dentine tubules was investigated using the dentine disc model [18]. The teeth were sectioned mesiodistally into discs approximately 1 mm thick using an internal edge annular diamond blade (Microslice annular blade, Ultratec, USA) mounted on the Microslice 2 saw (Malvern Instruments Ltd., UK) and halved (test and control sections). The dentine discs (*n* = 25) were etched with 6% citric acid for 2 minutes and rinsed with distilled water for 30 seconds, prior to the application of the test and control oral rinses. Each disc was divided into a control and test section by masking half the disk prior to application of the selected oral rinses for 30 seconds (*n* = 5 samples per group). Evaluation of the tubule occluding ability of the test and control oral rinses was by (1) Scanning Electron Microscopy (SEM) of the dentine surface and (2) measurement of the fluid flow (hydraulic conductance) through the dentine disc before and after 30 seconds of rinsing of the test and control oral rinses. One disc from each of the test and control oral rinses was used in the hydraulic conduction aspect of the study; each disc was subjected to 5 evaluations.

2.1. Materials. Five oral rinses, namely, two Hydroxyapatite based nHA (UltraDEX Recalcifying & Whitening, Periproducts Ltd., UK) and zinc substituted HA (BioRepairMicroRepair BioRepair/ACDOCO) oral rinses, potassium oxalate (1.4%) (LISTERINE Advanced Defence Sensitive, Johnson and Johnson Inc., New Brunswick, New Jersey, USA), arginine and PVM/MA copolymer oral rinse (Colgate Sensitive Pro-Relief, Colgate-Palmolive, UK), and a negative control oral rinse containing potassium nitrate (Sensodyne Pronamel Daily Mouthwash, GSK Consumer HealthCare, Weybridge, UK), were evaluated. The nHA powder used for the novel hydroxyapatite oral rinse (UltraDEX Recalcifying & Whitening) was also supplied separately by Periproducts Ltd., UK. A commercial high purity sintered hydroxyapatite powder (Captal R) was obtained from Plasma Biotal Ltd. (Matlock, Derbyshire, UK) as a reference. The remaining test and negative control formulations were obtained commercially.

Tubule occlusion was assessed as described above using Scanning Electron Microscopy (SEM) and by measuring the fluid flow (hydraulic conductance [Lp]) through the dentine discs using a modified Pashley hydraulic conductance model [19, 20].

2.1.1. Evaluation of the Dentine Specimens by Tubule Occlusion (Scanning Electron Microscopy [SEM]). The methodology used for preparation follow those described by Gillam et al. [21]. Half the dentine disc section was masked and the remaining half treated with the oral rinse/mouthwash for 30 seconds and then rinsed in distilled water for a further 30 s (dilution factor 1 : 2). The samples were then dried and gold coated prior to SEM examination.

2.1.2. Effectiveness of Tubule Occlusion Using Hydraulic Conductance (Fluid Flow) Measurements. The use of hydraulic conductance evaluation in order to assess the dentine fluid flow has been established by Pashley and coworkers [19, 20]

TABLE 1: Fluid flow reduction measurements for the test and control oral rinses (*n* = 5).

Oral rinse	Mean FFR (%)	SD (%)
UltraDEX Recalcifying & Whitening	40.3	9.6
BioRepair MicroRepair	48.7	15.9
LISTERINE Advanced Defence Sensitive	41.7	14.2
Colgate Sensitive Pro-Relief	66.9	6.6
Sensodyne Pronamel Daily Mouthwash	24	9.3

and is a useful *in vitro* method recognized by the American Dental Association (ADA) to evaluate both desensitizing toothpastes and oral rinses that work via a dentine occlusion mechanism. Fluid flow can be measured using a Pashley cell hydrodynamic flow device [19, 20]. The tests were performed on 1 mm thick dentine discs cut from the mid coronal section of human molars. The dentine discs (*n* = 5; one per test and control group) were then etched using 6% citric acid for 2 minutes to remove the smear layer and open the tubules. The disc was then mounted in the Pashley cell and the fluid flow measured over time.

2.2. Analysis of the Fluid Flow Measurements. The differences between the flow rates between the test and control oral rinses were analysed by Student *t*-test. Mean and Standard deviations of the test and control oral rinses were also assessed.

3. Results

3.1. Scanning Electron Microscopy (SEM) of the Effects of the Test and Control Oral Rinses on Tubule Occlusion. Figures 1–5 show the SEMs of the dentine discs before and after treatment with the test and control oral rinses. When treated with the nHA oral rinse for 30 seconds a number of the dentine tubules were occluded by the HA particles as observed in Figure 1. The HA particles appear to cover the dentine surface of the dentine disc as well as penetrate into the dentine tubules. The zinc substituted HA oral rinse (BioRepair MicroRepair Mouthwash) (Figure 2) however provided a less dense particle coverage and occlusion of the dentine tubules compared to the nHA oral rinse (Figure 1); this may have been as a consequence of the much lower HA concentration in this oral rinse. In comparison, the other oral rinse formulations do not appear to demonstrate any clear evidence of occlusion of the dentine surface compared with the etched control (before treatment) (Figures 3–5).

3.2. Hydraulic Conductance Fluid Flow Measurements. The fluid flow reduction (FFR) results for the desensitizing oral rinses were recorded in Table 1. Student *t*-tests ($p < 0.05$) were used to analyze the data from the results.

4. Discussion

There have been concerns previously expressed in the literature that the current strategies for treating DH may not

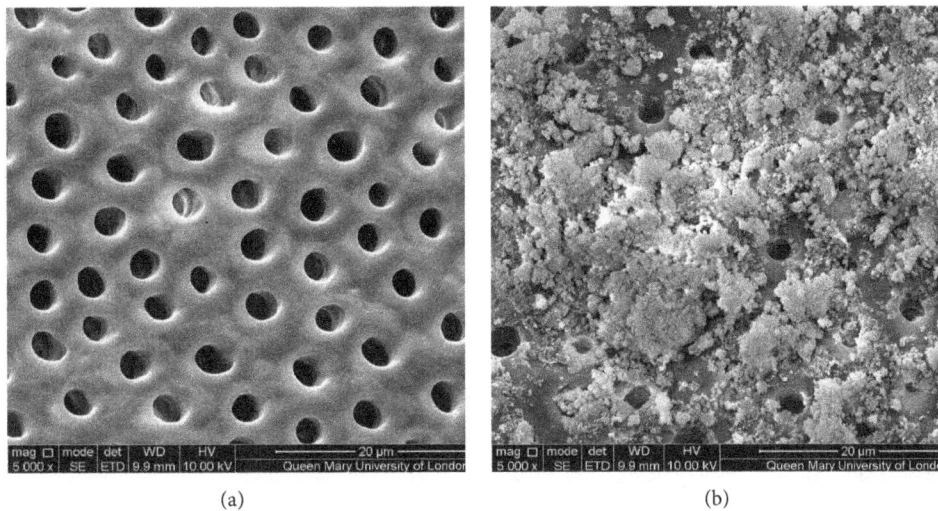

FIGURE 1: SEM images of dentine tubules treated with nHA oral rinse (UltraDEX HA Recalcifying oral rinse), before treatment (a) and after treatment (b).

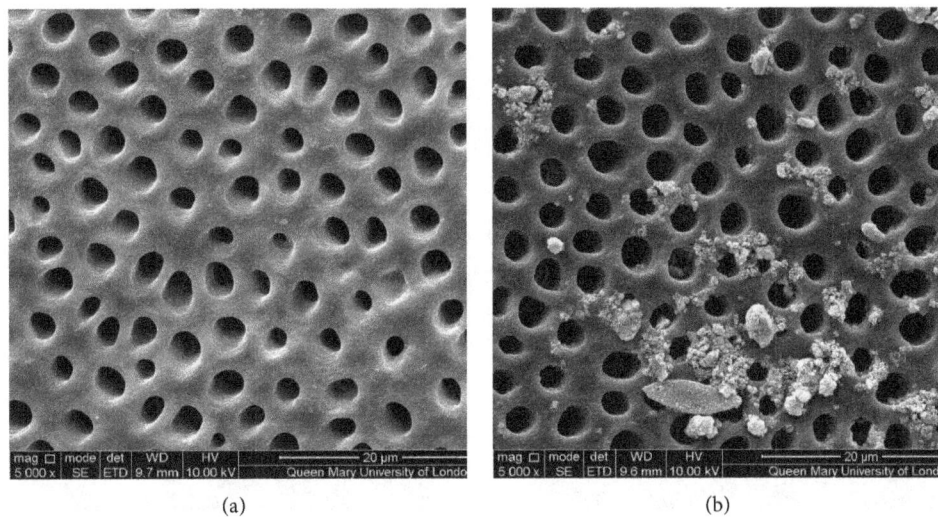

FIGURE 2: SEM images of dentine tubules treated with a zinc substituted HA oral rinse (Biorepair MicroRepair Mouthwash), before treatment (a) and after treatment (b).

provide a lasting solution to the problem of both tooth surface loss and pain associated with DH [2]. According to Gillam [15] a number of novel substances or reformulation of previously described technologies have been reintroduced into the consumer market, for example, bioactive glasses (Novamin) and hydroxyapatite/nanohydroxyapatite/ nanocarbonate apatite crystal toothpastes (HAP) [3–7], Colgate ProArgin toothpastes and oral rinses [8–11], and a 1.4% potassium oxalate mouth rinse (LISTERINE Advanced Defence Sensitive) [13, 14]. More recently a novel nanohydroxyapatite formulation (UltraDEX Recalcifying & Whitening toothpaste and oral rinse) has been developed [16, 17]. According to Hill et al. [16, 17] the advantages of using hydroxyapatite in a toothpaste and oral rinse formulation would be that as a natural component of tooth and bone, the HA component has the ability to be incorporated into

the tooth structure [16]. For the purposes of evaluating this new desensitizing formulation, the Investigators used a dentine disc methodology to determine the effectiveness of a number of commercially available oral rinses in reducing fluid flow through tubular occlusion. The zinc substituted HA was included to compare the effectiveness of a commercially available oral rinse: both the arginine and PVM/MA copolymer and 1.4% potassium oxalate oral rinses have been reported to be effective in reducing DH and were used as positive controls [10, 11, 13, 14] and the potassium nitrate oral rinse was included as a negative control as its mode of action is generally considered to be by nerve desensitization rather than by tubular occlusion. In order to test the potential ability of a desensitizing product prior to clinical evaluation, in vitro and/or in situ studies are often conducted in order to determine a possible mode of action of the product. One of

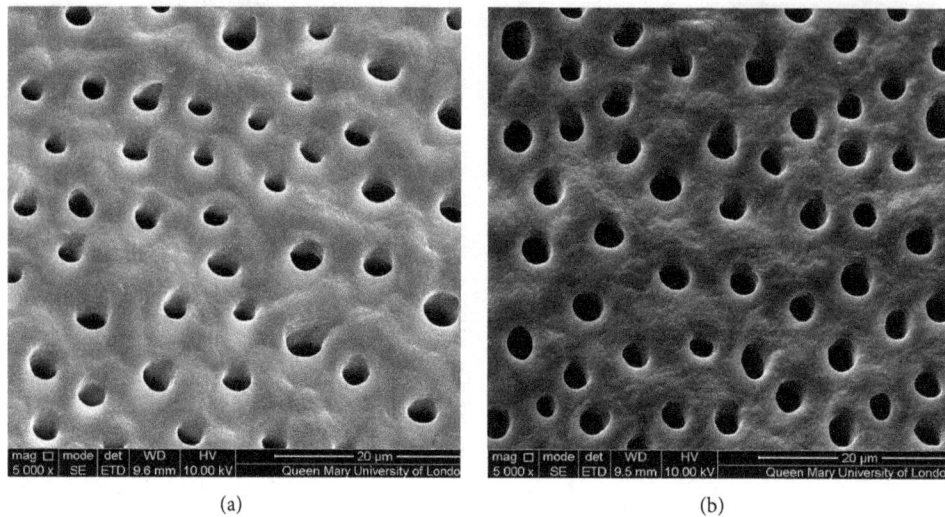

(a)   (b)

FIGURE 3: SEM images of dentine tubules treated with arginine and PVM/MA copolymer oral rinse (Colgate Sensitive Pro-Relief Mouthwash), before treatment (a) and after treatment (b).

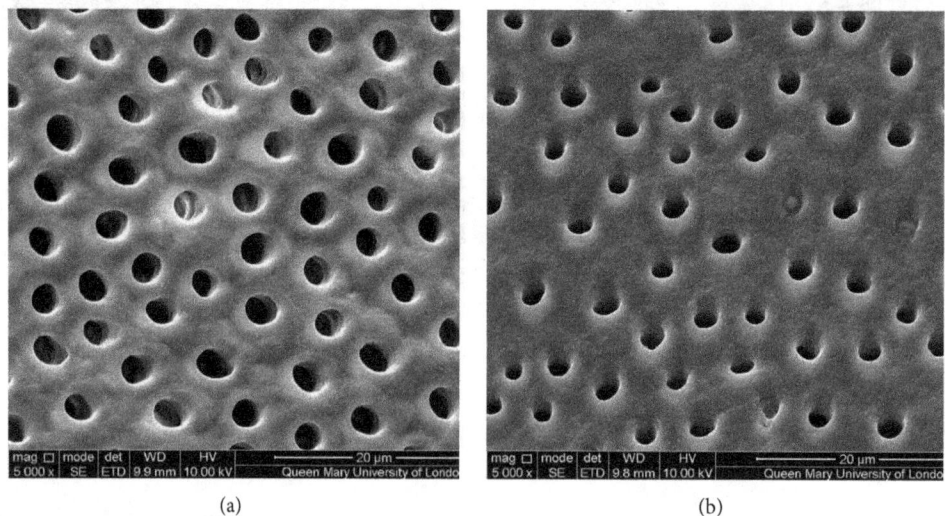

(a)   (b)

FIGURE 4: SEM images of dentine tubules treated with a 1.4% potassium oxalate oral rinse (LISTERINE Advanced Defence Sensitive Mouthwash), before treatment (a) and after treatment (b).

the problems however when conducting *in vitro* evaluation outside the oral environment is that it is very difficult to completely mimic the dynamics and interaction of saliva, and so forth. For example, most *in vitro* studies will evaluate the surface deposit of a particular formulation using Tris buffer, artificial saliva, and so forth, when brushing or rinsing with a test or control formulation, and will report on the ability of these products to occlude the dentine tubule. However it may be possible that this observation alone may be ineffective in identifying any potential of effectiveness in the oral environment when a particular formulation interacts with the saliva over time. Furthermore reporting on the surface precipitation or deposit alone without evaluating the hydraulic conductance measurements following the application of a

particular desensitizing product may also be misleading. According to the principles underpinning the hydrodynamic theory fluid flow through dentine is inversely proportional to 1/radius^4 and therefore relatively small reductions in the functional radius of the tubule diameter will have a significant effect on fluid flow. In the present study it was observed that not all of the test and control formulations covered the dentine surface (Figures 1–5) although it was evident from the fluid flow measurements (Table 1) that a degree of tubular occlusion must have occurred occurred below the dentine surface in order to have an effect on this change. One of the criticisms of the present study, however, would be that no investigation was undertaken to determine whether there was a degree of subsurface occlusion that would account for this

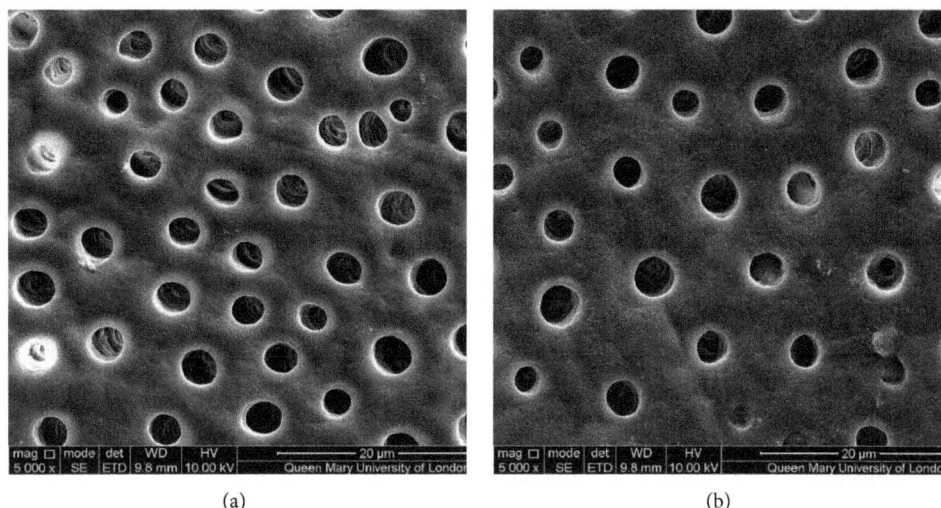

(a)   (b)

FIGURE 5: SEM images of dentine tubules treated with a potassium nitrate oral rinse (Sensodyne Pronamel Daily Mouthwash), before treatment (a) and after treatment (b).

observation. This particular phenomenon has been reported in the published literature for potassium oxalate previously used for in-office applications to treat DH [22–24].

The results from the SEM analysis of the test and control oral rinses provided a wide variation in the manner and extent of the surface precipitate (Figures 1–5). For example, the novel nHA and zinc substituted HA demonstrated varying degrees of surface coverage whereas potassium nitrate formulation failed to demonstrate any surface deposition which may be explained as indicated above that the recognized mode of action is through reducing nerve desensitization rather than by tubule occlusion. Both the arginine and PVM/MA copolymer and 1.4% potassium oxalate oral rinses also failed to show any surface deposit although as previously described it is more likely that there was subsurface precipitation within the dentine tubules which may explain why these two formulations demonstrated reductions in the fluid flow measurements (Table 1).

All the oral rinses investigated in the present study to some degree resulted in a fluid flow reduction (Table 1). For example, the arginine and PVM/MA copolymer oral rinse (66.9%) was the most effective in reducing FFR values compared to the 1.4% potassium oxalate (41.7%), nHa (40.3%)/zinc substituted HA (48.7%), respectively. It was apparent from these results that the arginine and PVM/MA copolymer oral rinse was statistically significant compared to the new nHA ($p = 0.0002$) and the 1.4% potassium oxalate ($p = 0.0036$) oral rinses, respectively, although there were no statistically significant differences between the new nHA/zinc substituted HA 1.4% potassium oxalate oral rinses. The negative control formulation (potassium nitrate) resulted in the least reduction in FFR values (24%) and all the other oral rinses demonstrated statistically significant differences in FFR in relation to the negative control (arginine and PVM/MA copolymer oral rinse ($p = 0.0000$), 1.4% potassium oxalate (0.0051), zinc substituted HA ($p = 0.0087$), and nHA ($p = 0.0098$)), respectively. This observation is perhaps not

surprising given that its primary mode of action does not involve a tubule occlusion mechanism. There does, however appear to be a limited correlation between the observed tubule occlusion observed by SEM and the measured FFR values and this is as a result of the SEM methodology used in the present study being more appropriate for the physical deposition of the particles rather than the differences in the mode of action for the other tested oral rinses. Furthermore the variations within the dentine disc particularly with the differences in the FFR values (Table 1) are primarily due to the anatomical variations (in terms of tubule size and tubule orientation) within the dentine disc itself which may complicate obtaining an ideal surface to evaluate these products. In the present study one dentine disc was evaluated for each oral rinse ($n = 5$) when assessing the FFR values in order to limit the variation in testing between different dentine discs. This may have accounted for the differences between the published values in the literature.

For example, Sharma et al. [14] investigated the composition used in the 1.4% potassium oxalate formulation and reported that the oral rinse demonstrated a 55% reduction in FFR values following three treatment applications and an approximately 100% reduction after 12 treatment applications. The 55% reduction compares reasonably with the 42% FFR reduction reported for one treatment in the present study. Mello et al. [11] investigated the hydraulic conductance of a prototype oral rinse similar to the arginine and PVM/MA copolymer oral rinse formulation. These investigators used a very different procedure from that used in the present study and included two treatments of 10 minutes which appeared excessive for an oral rinse application and reported a 59% reduction in FFR values. This percentage reduction is reasonably comparable to the 67% reduction demonstrated for the arginine and PVM/MA copolymer oral rinse in the present study following one treatment application.

Eliades et al. [13] used 12 treatment applications when investigating the tubule occluding properties of an arginine and PVM/MA copolymer oral rinse using back scattered SEM; there was however no significant evidence of tubule occlusion reported either on the dentine surface or in the subsurface of the dentine section. These investigators also investigated the 1.4% potassium oxalate formulation and in contrast to Sharma et al. [14] study there was little evidence of tubule occlusion at the surface, but there was, however, evidence of crystals in the tubules beneath the dentine surface as well as a degree of tubule occlusion which is consistent with the evidence reported in the literature [22–24].

A criticism of both the existing studies and the present study was the use of sections of mid coronal dentine for the studies of tubule occlusion and hydraulic conductance. For example, clinically DH is diagnosed on the buccal (facial) surfaces of the cervical region of the tooth where the dentine tubule size is generally considered to be smaller in diameter and has a different orientation from the tubules in the mid coronal region of dentine. Furthermore acid etching of the dentine surface prior to treatment not only removes the smear layer and opens up the tubules but also makes the openings to the tubules more funnel shaped in nature that may aid particles and liquids entering the tubules. Root dentine taken from the cervical region of the tooth would therefore be a more appropriate model than mid coronal sections; however, as indicated above there is greater variability in terms of tubule orientation of the root dentine compared to mid coronal dentine. A further problem as observed in the studies using the dentine disc model was the difficulty in reproducing the hydraulic conductance measurements. One possible method of reducing this variation in scatter would be to measure the flow rate prior to and after the application of the oral rinse using the same disc as indicated above, although the variation in scatter may be still evident as reported in the present study.

5. Conclusions

Although the new nanohydroxyapatite (nHA) demonstrated the ability to both occlude the dentine tubules and reduce the fluid flow values, nevertheless some of the other oral rinses appeared to demonstrate a statistically significant reduction in fluid flow through the dentine disc, in particular the arginine and PVM/MA copolymer oral rinse compared to the other test and control rinses.

Conflict of Interests

The authors have received financial support for conducting the laboratory research on behalf of Periproducts Ltd., Middlesex, UK.

References

[1] D. G. Gillam, "Current diagnosis of dentin hypersensitivity in the dental office: an overview," *Clinical Oral Investigations*, vol. 17, supplement 1, pp. 21–29, 2013.

[2] D. Gillam, R. Chesters, D. Attrill et al., "Dentine hypersensitivity—guidelines for the management of a common oral health problem," *Dental Update*, vol. 40, no. 7, pp. 514–524, 2013.

[3] L. Rimondini, B. Palazzo, M. Iafisco et al., "The remineralizing effect of carbonate-hydroxyapatite nanocrystals on dentine," *Materials Science Forum*, vol. 539–543, no. 1, pp. 602–605, 2007.

[4] G. Orsini, M. Procaccini, L. Manzoli, F. Giuliodori, A. Lorenzini, and A. Putignano, "A double-blind randomized-controlled trial comparing the desensitizing efficacy of a new dentifrice containing carbonate/hydroxyapatite nanocrystals and a sodium fluoride/potassium nitrate dentifrice," *Journal of Clinical Periodontology*, vol. 37, no. 6, pp. 510–517, 2010.

[5] P. Tschoppe, D. L. Zandim, P. Martus, and A. M. Kielbassa, "Enamel and dentine remineralization by nano-hydroxyapatite toothpastes," *Journal of Dentistry*, vol. 39, no. 6, pp. 430–437, 2011.

[6] Z. Wang, T. Jiang, S. Sauro et al., "The dentine remineralization activity of a desensitizing bioactive glass-containing toothpaste: an in vitro study," *Australian Dental Journal*, vol. 56, no. 4, pp. 372–381, 2011.

[7] P. Yuan, X. Shen, J. Liu et al., "Effects of dentifrice containing hydroxyapatite on dentinal tubule occlusion and aqueous hexavalent chromium cations sorption: a preliminary study," *PLoS ONE*, vol. 7, no. 12, Article ID e45283, 2012.

[8] D. Cummins, "The efficacy of a new dentifrice containing 8.0% arginine, calcium carbonate, and 1450 ppm fluoride in delivering instant and lasting relief of dentin hypersensitivity," *Journal of Clinical Dentistry*, vol. 20, no. 4, pp. 109–114, 2009.

[9] R. Docimo, L. Montesani, P. Maturo et al., "Comparing the efficacy in reducing dentin hypersensitivity of a new toothpaste containing 8.0% arginine, calcium carbonate, and 1450 ppm fluoride to a benchmark commercial desensitizing toothpaste containing 2% potassium ion: an eight-week clinical study in Rome, Italy," *The Journal of Clinical Dentistry*, vol. 20, no. 4, pp. 137–143, 2009.

[10] S. V. Mello, E. Arvanitidou, M. A. Stranick, R. Santana, Y. Kutes, and B. Huey, "Mode of action studies of a new desensitizing mouthwash containing 0.8% arginine, PVM/MA copolymer, pyrophosphates, and 0.05% sodium fluoride," *Journal of Dentistry*, vol. 41, supplement 1, pp. S12–S19, 2013.

[11] S. V. Mello, E. Arvanitidou, and M. Vandeven, "The development of a new desensitising mouthwash containing arginine, PVM/MA copolymer, pyrophosphates, and sodium fluoride—a hydraulic conductance study," *Journal of Dentistry*, vol. 41, supplement 1, pp. S20–S25, 2013.

[12] D. G. Gillam, J. Y. Tang, N. J. Mordan, and H. N. Newman, "The effects of a novel Bioglass dentifrice on dentine sensitivity: a scanning electron microscopy investigation," *Journal of Oral Rehabilitation*, vol. 29, no. 4, pp. 305–313, 2002.

[13] G. Eliades, M. Mantzourani, R. Labella, B. Mutti, and D. Sharma, "Interactions of dentine desensitisers with human dentine: morphology and composition," *Journal of Dentistry*, vol. 41, supplement 4, pp. S28–S39, 2013.

[14] D. Sharma, C. X. Hong, and P. S. Heipp, "A novel potassium oxalate-containing tooth-desensitising mouthrinse: a comparative in vitro study," *Journal of Dentistry*, vol. 41, supplement 4, pp. S18–S27, 2013.

[15] D. G. Gillam, "Chapter 5: treatment approaches for dentin hypersensitivity," in *Clinician's Guide to the Diagnosis and management of Tooth Sensitivity*, S. Taha and B. H. Clarkson, Eds., pp. 51–79, Springer, Berlin, Germany, 2014.

[16] R. Hill, D. Gillam, and N. Karpukhina, "Tubular occluding properties of a novel biomimetic hydroxyapatite toothpaste,"

in *Proceedings of the IADR/PER Pan-European Region Meeting*, Poster Presentation (Abstract no. 640), Helsinki, Finland, September 2012.

[17] R. G. Hill, A. J. Collings, I. Baynes, and D. G. Gillam, "Multi-component oral care composition," Patent 3 WO/2013/117913, Periproducts, 2013.

[18] N. J. Mordan, P. M. Barber, and D. G. Gillam, "The dentine disc. A review of its applicability as a model for the in vitro testing of dentine hypersensitivity," *Journal of Oral Rehabilitation*, vol. 24, no. 2, pp. 148–156, 1997.

[19] J. D. Greenhill and D. H. Pashley, "The effects of desensitizing agents on the hydraulic conductance of human dentin in vitro," *Journal of Dental Research*, vol. 60, no. 3, pp. 686–698, 1981.

[20] D. H. Pashley, J. A. O'Meara, E. E. Kepler, S. E. Galloway, S. M. Thompson, and F. P. Stewart, "Dentin permeability. Effects of desensitizing dentifrices in vitro," *Journal of Periodontology*, vol. 55, no. 9, pp. 522–525, 1984.

[21] D. G. Gillam, N. J. Mordan, and H. N. Newman, "The Dentin Disc surface: a plausible model for dentin physiology and dentin sensitivity evaluation," *Advances in Dental Research*, vol. 11, no. 4, pp. 487–501, 1997.

[22] D. H. Pashley and S. E. Galloway, "The effects of oxalate treatment on the smear layer of ground surfaces of human dentine," *Archives of Oral Biology*, vol. 30, no. 10, pp. 731–737, 1985.

[23] D. H. Pashley, R. M. Carvalho, J. C. Pereira, R. Villanueva, and F. R. Tay, "The use of oxalate to reduce dentin permeability under adhesive restorations," *American Journal of Dentistry*, vol. 14, no. 2, pp. 89–94, 2001.

[24] D. G. Gillam, N. J. Mordan, A. D. Sinodinou, J. Y. Tang, J. C. Knowles, and I. R. Gibson, "The effects of oxalate-containing products on the exposed dentine surface: an SEM investigation," *Journal of Oral Rehabilitation*, vol. 28, no. 11, pp. 1037–1044, 2001.

18

Knowledge of Future Dental Practitioners towards Oral Cancer: Exploratory Findings from a Public University in Malaysia

Akshaya Srikanth Bhagavathula,[1] Nazrin Bin Zakaria,[2] and Shazia Qasim Jamshed[2]

[1]*Department of Clinical Pharmacy, University of Gondar, College of Medicine and Health Sciences, School of Pharmacy, Gondar, Ethiopia*
[2]*Department of Pharmacy Practice, Kulliyyah of Pharmacy, International Islamic University Malaysia, Kuantan, Pahang, Malaysia*

Correspondence should be addressed to Akshaya Srikanth Bhagavathula; akshaypharmd@gmail.com

Academic Editor: Gilberto Sammartino

Objective. To assess knowledge and awareness of oral cancer in the early identification of risk factors among undergraduate dental students. *Methods.* A total of 162 undergraduate (third, fourth, and fifth year) dental students at International Islamic University, Malaysia, were approached to participate in the study, and those who agreed were administered. A 9-item pretested questionnaire contains questions on oral examination, oral cancer risk factors, and requests for further information. Descriptive statistics were conducted using chi-square testing. *Results.* The response rate of the study was 70.3% (114/162), with 26 (22.8%) males and 88 (77.2%) females. All undergraduate dental students were familiar with examining the oral mucosa of their patients and most were likely to advise patients about the risk factors for developing oral cancer (98.2%). Nearly one-third (32.4%) of students reported examining patients with oral lesions as early signs for oral cancer ($P < 0.001$) and nearly 70% agreed that they did not have sufficient knowledge regarding the prevention and detection of oral cancer ($P < 0.001$). In addition, more than 95.6% agreed that there is a need for additional information/teaching regarding oral cancer. Further, 61.3% and 14.1% identified tobacco smoking and drinking alcohol as major risk factors for developing oral cancer. *Conclusion.* This study demonstrated lack of awareness about risk factors among undergraduate dental students regarding oral cancer. Reinforcing awareness and enhancing the benefits of early detection on prevention of oral cancer should be done through training and/or educational intervention.

1. Introduction

The incidence of oral cancer especially squamous cell carcinoma accounts for nearly 2.4% of all cancers [1]. Due to significant number of oral cancer cases raising rapidly in the developing regions this is found to be the sixth most common cancer worldwide [2]. Life style habits such as heavy smoking and alcoholism are the important risk factors for developing oral cancer that increases at least three- to fifteenfold especially in females and young people [3]. In addition, marijuana, chewing beetle-leaf, human papilloma virus, ultraviolet radiations, iron deficiency anemia, candida infections, immunosuppression, and deletion or mutation of tumor suppressor genes are some of the other causes of oral cancer [4].

Lack of public awareness regarding oral health and low intake of fruits and vegetables, older age, and poor oral

hygiene are some of the implications for oral cancer [2]. Majority of the oral cancer was detected at late stages (III and IV) and early diagnosis is important to increase patient survivability and to delay its prognosis [5]. In 2011, World Health Organization (WHO) reported the incidence of oral cancer deaths in Malaysia to about 1.5% of the total deaths, with age adjusted death rate of 7.72 per 100,000 populations [6]. Malaysia ranked 14 in the world with annual oral cancer deaths of 1,587 [7].

Increasing the public awareness and early diagnosis can significantly improve oral cancer surveillance and prevent the delaying factors. To achieve these, it is important to have sufficient knowledge and awareness among dentists for detection and early diagnosis. Initiatives were undertaken by University of Malaya to increase the oral cancer awareness in Malaysia such as Malaysian Oral Cancer Research Initiative (MOCRI)

TABLE 1: Age and sex distribution of dental student respondents.

Number of students approached		Student participants (%)	Male	Female
Total	162	114 (70.3)	26 (22.8%)	88 (77.2%)
Fifth year	52	37 (32.5)	12 (10.5%)	25 (21.9%)
Fourth year	40	32 (28.1)	6 (5.2%)	26 (22.8%)
Third year	70	45 (39.5)	8 (7%)	37 (32.4%)
Participants age	Mean	Standard deviation	Median	IQR*	Wilcoxon rank-sum test
	24.36	7.127	24	1	$P < 0.001$

*IQR: interquartile range.

and Oral Cancer Research & Coordinating Centre (OCRCC) [8]. These publicity initiatives are crucial to improve the oral cancer awareness among general public and health professionals in Malaysia. In addition, general dental practitioner's role is decisive in identifying the oral mucosal changes that may lead to oral cancer. Assessing the knowledge of dental students paves the way towards understanding their level of awareness in the early detection and prevention of oral cancer. To the best of our knowledge, previous researches on dental students' knowledge and awareness were conducted in the University of Malaya (UM) and Universiti Sains Malaysia (USM) [9, 10]. Since there is a paucity of information regarding oral cancer awareness in undergraduate dental students in different other regions of Malaysia, therefore it is pertinent to assess these characteristics in senior dental students (third, fourth, and fifth year) at International Islamic University, Kuantan, Pahang, Malaysia. The aim of the current research was to assess the knowledge and awareness of oral cancer towards early identification of risk factors among undergraduate dental students.

2. Methodology

This is a descriptive cross-sectional study to assess the oral cancer knowledge and awareness of senior undergraduate dental students using a survey questionnaire, adopted by Carter and Ogden [11] and Brzak et al. [12]. Ethical permission to conduct the study was obtained from the respective Deans, International Islamic University, Malaysia. The study was conducted via face-to-face interview at International Islamic University Malaysia during the period of February to March, 2015. Verbal consent was obtained from each participant prior to administration of study questionnaire.

2.1. Sampling Technique. Sample size was determined using 95% confidence interval, with an accuracy of 60% for the total dental students being 300 studying in International Islamic University given a confidence interval of 5.5; the recommended sample size is 155 or more. A systemic random sampling technique was used to select senior dental students which includes third, fourth, and fifth years.

In general, as included in the curriculum, dental students receive information regarding oral cancer during their oral pathology and oral medicine sessions in their first and second year as well as oral examination during their clinical sessions.

Students of both gender studying third-, fourth-, and fifth-year dentistry were included in the study. Students who failed to meet the above criteria were excluded.

A 9-item pretested questionnaire was employed after explaining the purpose of the study and verbal consent was obtained from each study participant. The questionnaire constitutes 7 close-ended (yes/no) questions such as (1) oral mucosal examination (2 items), (2) advising current and future patients regarding risk factors for oral cancer, (3) opportunity to examine oral lesions, (4) knowledge regarding prevention and detection of oral cancer, (5) point of referral selection, and (6) desire for further information or teaching regarding oral cancer. Two open-ended questionnaires were asked to identify the risk factors for development of oral cancer and encouraged to select at least three to four options out of 10 options. In addition, interest of preferences for obtaining oral cancer information (1 out of 3 options).

Statistical analysis was performed using SPSS version 21 (SPSS Inc., Chicago, IL, USA). Descriptive data were analysed using frequencies and percentages. The Wilcoxon rank-sum test and chi-square were used to identify the difference between groups. The level of significance was set at $P < 0.05$.

3. Results

A total of 162 students were approached, and 114 questionnaires were returned with an overall response rate of 70.3%. Eighty-eight were females and twenty-six were males with a mean age (standard deviation) of 24.36 (7.12). Sex distribution with the number of respondents per year of course was shown in Table 1.

4. Knowledge about Oral Cancer

When asked about the examination of oral mucosa of the patients, all the students answered "yes" during their clinical training. Of those who examine the oral mucosa routinely, a high majority of the students (97.3%) would not examine the oral mucosa of the patient with high risk of developing oral cancer. Significantly, 67.5% of the students did not get opportunity to examine the oral lesions ($\chi^2 = 15.892$, df = 2, and $P = 0.000$) (Table 2). More than ninety percent of the participants preferred to refer patients with oral lesion as a point of care to dental specialties rather than doctors. However, significantly, two-thirds (65.7%) of students felt that

TABLE 2: Level of knowledge of participants on oral cancer.

Variables	Dental students (%)			Total 114 (%)	Stat. cal. value
	Fifth year (%)	Fourth year (%)	Third year (%)		
Do you examine patients' oral mucosa routinely?					—
Yes	37 (32.4)	32 (28.0)	45 (39.4)	114 (100%)	
No	0	0	0	0 (0.0)	
Do you screen the oral mucosa if the patients are in high risk of categories?					$\chi^2 = 2.358$, DF = 2, $P = 0.308$
Yes	2 (1.7)	1 (0.8)	0	3 (2.6)	
No	35 (30.7)	31 (27.2)	45 (39.4)	111 (97.3)	
When you have graduated will you advise patients about the risk factors for oral cancer?					$\chi^2 = 0.822$, DF = 2, $P = 0.663$
Yes	36 (31.5)	32 (28.0)	44 (38.6)	112 (98.2)	
No	1 (0.8)	0	1 (0.8)	2 (1.7)	
Have you had the opportunity to examine patients with oral lesions?					$\chi^2 = 15.892$, DF = 2, $\boldsymbol{P = 0.000^*}$
Yes	13 (11.4)	18 (15.7)	6 (5.2)	37 (32.4)	
No	24 (21.0)	14 (12.2)	39 (34.2)	77 (67.5)	
Do you think a patient should go to a doctor or dentist if he/she has an oral lesions?					$\chi^2 = 2.107$, DF = 2, $P = 0.349$
Doctor	5 (4.3)	3 (2.6)	2 (1.7)	10 (8.7)	
Dentist	32 (28.0)	29 (25.4)	43 (37.7)	104 (91.2)	
Do you feel that you have sufficient knowledge concerning prevention and detection of oral cancer?					$\chi^2 = 28.598$, DF = 2, $\boldsymbol{P = 0.000^*}$
Yes	23 (20.1)	13 (11.4)	3 (2.6)	39 (34.2)	
No	14 (12.2)	19 (16.6)	42 (36.8)	75 (65.7)	
Would you like more information or teaching on oral cancer?					$\chi^2 = 4.055$, DF = 2, $P = 0.132$
Yes	35 (30.7)	29 (25.4)	45 (39.4)	109 (95.6)	
No	2 (1.7)	3 (2.6)	0	5 (4.3)	

*Significant at $P < 0.05$ were bold.

they did not have sufficient knowledge about prevention and early detection of oral cancer. This was much higher observed in third-year student participants (42/45) than others ($\chi^2 = 28.598$, df = 2, and $P = 0.000$). Of note, most of the study participants (95.6%) requested further information regarding oral cancer prevention and early detection, with more than fifty percent preferred to obtain in the form of information package (52.6%), twenty-eight percent through seminars, and nearly twenty percent as lectures (Figure 1).

5. Risk Factors for Oral Cancer

A majority of the dental students (93%) identified a number of different risk factors for oral cancer were shown in Figure 2.

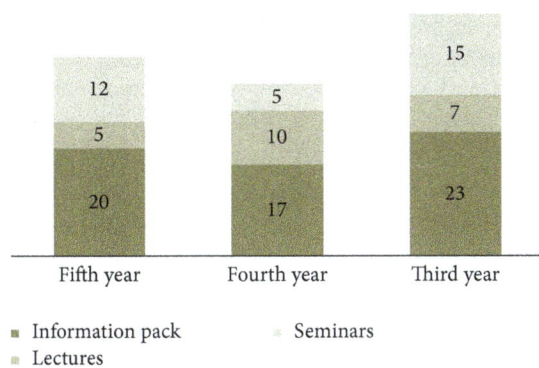

FIGURE 1: Students preferences for obtaining further information about oral cancer.

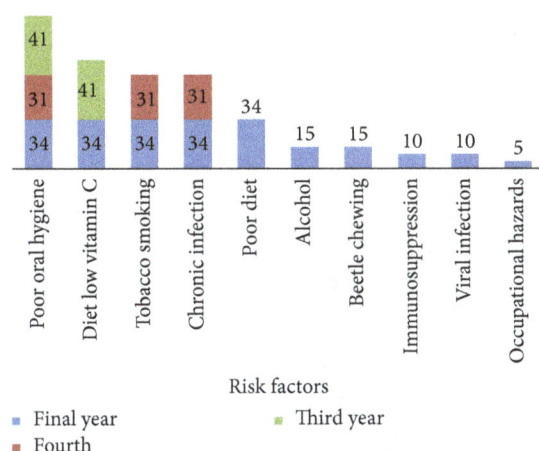

FIGURE 2: Dental students identifying risk factors for oral cancer ($N = 106$).

All the participants identified poor oral hygiene as a major risk factor, whereas 70.7% identified diet with low vitamin c levels as a risk factor for oral cancer. In addition, tobacco smoking and chronic infections were correctly reported by 61.3%. Only 14.5% of the participants identified alcohol and chewing beetle leaves as a risk factors. However, other oral cancer risk factors such as immunosuppression, viral infections, and occupational hazards were poorly reported by the final year students, and none of the other students identified these as a risk factors.

6. Discussion

Squamous cell carcinoma accounts for 90% of oral cancer and it is a general practice of the dental students to examine the patients' oral mucosa. Providing opportunity to examine and early detection can reduce the morbidity of oral cancer especially in high risk patients. It is the prime responsibility of the dental schools to provide sufficient knowledge to students for early diagnose in asymptomatic patients and prevent prevalent oral diseases. Hence, this study was carried out to determine the level of knowledge and awareness of oral cancer among dental students at International Islamic University, Selangor, Malaysia.

The response rate of the current study was 70.3% which is much lower than the studies conducted on dental students in Croatia (95%) [12], India (90.6%) [13], Iran (88%) [1], and Brazil (75.1%) [14] but fairly higher than the similar studies conducted in other specialties [15]. Although the response rate was low, a comparable number of students from different academic years participated in the study.

6.1. Level of Knowledge. In the present study, all the student participants routinely carried out oral mucosal examination of patients. Further, it was identified that a large majority of the students had an opportunity to examine patients with oral lesions. But unfortunately, a high majority of these students claimed that they failed to screen the high risk patient groups, which implies the gaps in their knowledge regarding oral cancer risk factors. Poor knowledge is directly related to lack of awareness, and emphasis should be taken to provide more opportunities engaging undergraduates to take oral health histories and examine oral lesions in patients during clinical attachments that should be undertaken. It is arguable that majority of the oral cancer patients are asymptomatic and identifying the changes in their cancerous and precancerous lesions in the oral cavity would help them to apply their critical knowledge into practice, importantly needed in high prevalent countries like Malaysia. For such reasons, Ogden et al. [1] claimed to implement work-based assessments to know these gaps and specific test for oral cancer within the curriculum prior to dental students graduation.

Regarding referral pattern for oral cancer, more than ninety percent felt that it is the dentist's responsibility to diagnose the oral malignancies. These results are encouraging as they demonstrate the recognition of dentistry, and it is their responsibility of dentists to diagnose and evaluate oral cancer. These results were consistent with other studies conducted by Ogden and Mahboobi [1], Awan et al. [9], Carter and Ogden [11], and Fotedar et al. [13] but contradict with study by Brzak et al. [12] where majority of the undergraduate dental students chose to refer oral cancer patients to a plastic surgeon specialist. A recent meta-analysis concluded that diagnosis delay is a potential risk factor for developing advanced stage oral cancer [16].

In our study, the majority reported that they would advise their patients about oral cancer and associated risk factors after graduation. These findings were similar to the previous study performed in Malaysia [9], UK [10], and Croatia [12]. It is crucial role of dentists to take a strong responsibility to offer advice to the patients on high-risk habits like cessation of smoking cigarettes [17] and self-examination of oral mucosa to improve the oral hygiene. These counseling techniques also enhance early detection of oral mucosal changes in the oral cavity [9].

Approximately, seventy percent felt that they are have insufficient knowledge ($P < 0.001$) with regard to prevention and early detection of oral cancer. These numbers are higher in those who were in third year (36.8%). In McCready et al.'s study [15] 77% of dental students from second year and fourth year reported that they were poorly informed regarding oral cancer, whereas in Carter and Ogden's study [11] 93% of the final-year medical students also reported the same. A well-designed institutional-based clinical training by incorporating different dental specialties such as oral medicine, dental oncology, and oral and maxillofacial surgery to improve the knowledge about oral cancer is highly recommended to increase the students confidence. However, almost all the students requesting further information regarding oral cancer which is similarly identified in studies by Awan et al [9], Brzak et al [12], and McCready et al [15] where more than 90% of the students requested to receive more information regarding oral cancer. Further, majority of the students are interested in receiving further information in the form of information package which is also most preferred in other studies [1, 9, 10, 12]. Seoane et al. [18] study assessing the oral cancer prevention and clinical attitude among Spanish dentists highlighted that providing continuous education through scientific newsletters and journals can provide positive preventive attitude in oral cancer.

6.2. Risk Factors for Development of Oral Cancer. In our study, 106 out of 114 participants identified the risk factors for oral cancer. Of these, all the students felt poor oral hygiene as the single most important risk factor. Only sixty percent of students identified tobacco smoking as a risk factor for development of oral cancer. Although previous studies revealed that smoking tobacco and alcohol consumption increase the incidence of oral cancer, these were unidentified by our third-year dental students. These findings were contradictory with other studies in the literatures, which show that around 90% of the dental and medical students identified tobacco smoking as an important risk factor 12,58 [1, 9, 10, 12–14, 17, 19]. However, alarmingly, none of the third and fourth years identified alcohol, beetle-chewing, and immunosuppression as a risk factor. Thus the knowledge on risk factors was poor in both third and fourth years and also very minimal in final-year dental students. There was trend towards better identification of risk factors which was observed with progression of their academic years, which is similarly noticed in other studies [9, 11, 14]. All these findings identified different knowledge gaps in identification of risk factors among dental students, and there is a need of educational intervention by implementing training or workshop particularly focusing on oral cancer.

7. Study Limitations

We used a prevalidated questionnaire which is used in other surveys assessing oral cancer knowledge [9, 11] on dental students to reduce selection bias. Further, recent research identified that nearly 20–30% of the oropharyngeal squamous cell cancer did not have traditional risk factors of smoking and cancer [20] which may be falsely interpreted in the light of respondents' knowledge.

The study has some limitations that should be taken into consideration. The study was conducted on senior dental students in a single institution in Malaysia and may not be generalized to other regions. In addition, the data presented here is self-reported, and some of the respondents may provide extreme responses than others, due to the motivations and beliefs of the participants, and might be subjected to recall bias. However, we believed that the participants were honest to provide appropriate responses conducted in a single institution, and national level multifaceted studies are further needed to assess dental students' knowledge about oral cancer.

8. Conclusion

This study showed knowledge gaps about oral cancer among undergraduate dental students. Lack of awareness about the risk factors initiates the need based educational interventions among future dental practitioners regarding early detection and prevention of oral cancer in Malaysia.

Conflict of Interests

The authors declare that there is no conflict of interests regarding the publication of this paper.

References

[1] G. R. Ogden and N. Mahboobi, "Oral cancer awareness among undergraduate dental students in Iran," *Journal of Cancer Education*, vol. 26, no. 2, pp. 380–385, 2011.

[2] R. S. Kulkarni, D. P. Arun, R. Rai, S. V. Kanth, V. Sargaiyan, and S. Kandasamy, "Awareness and practice concerning oral cancer among Ayurveda and Homeopathy practitioners in Davangere District: a speciality-wise analysis," *Journal of Natural Science, Biology and Medicine*, vol. 6, no. 1, pp. 116–119, 2015.

[3] J. P. Shah, N. W. Johnson, and J. G. Batsakis, *Oral Cancer*, Martin Dunitz, London, UK, 1st edition, 2003.

[4] Y. Hassona, C. Scully, M. Abu Ghosh, Z. Khoury, S. Jarrar, and F. Sawair, "Mouth cancer awareness and beliefs among dental patients," *International Dental Journal*, vol. 65, no. 1, pp. 15–21, 2015.

[5] I. Gómez, S. Warnakulasuriya, P. I. Varela-Centelles et al., "Is early diagnosis of oral cancer a feasible objective? Who is to blame for diagnostic delay?" *Oral Diseases*, vol. 16, no. 4, pp. 333–342, 2010.

[6] World Health Organization, "Oral health," Fact Sheet 318, 2012, http://www.who.int/mediacentre/factsheets/fs318/en/.

[7] A. Jemal, F. Bray, M. M. Center, J. Ferlay, E. Ward, and D. Forman, "Global cancer statistics," *CA: A Cancer Journal for Clinicians*, vol. 61, no. 2, pp. 69–90, 2011.

[8] R. B. Zain, V. Athirajan, W. M. N. Ghani et al., "An oral cancer biobank initiative: a platform for multidisciplinary research in a developing country," *Cell and Tissue Banking*, vol. 14, no. 1, pp. 45–52, 2013.

[9] K. H. Awan, T. W. Khang, T. K. Yee, and R. B. Zain, "Assessing oral cancer knowledge and awareness among Malaysian dental and medical students," *Journal of Cancer Research and Therapeutics*, vol. 10, no. 4, pp. 903–907, 2014.

[10] M. Sitheeque, Z. Ahmad, and R. Saini, "Awareness of oral cancer and precancer among final year medical and dental students of UniversitiSains Malaysia (USM), Malaysia," *Archives of Orofacial Sciences*, vol. 9, no. 2, pp. 53–64, 2014.

[11] L. M. Carter and G. R. Ogden, "Oral cancer awareness of undergraduate medical and dental students," *BMC Medical Education*, vol. 7, article 44, 2007.

[12] B. L. Brzak, I. Canjuga, M. Baričević, and M. Mravak-Stipetić, "Dental students' awareness of oral cancer," *Acta Stomatologica Croatica*, vol. 46, no. 1, pp. 50–58, 2012.

[13] S. Fotedar, V. Fotedar, K. Manchanda, A. Sarkar, N. Sood, and V. Bhardwaj, "Knowledge, attitude and practices about oral cancers among dental students in H.P Government Dental College, Shimla-Himachal Pradesh," *South Asian Journal of Cancer*, vol. 4, no. 2, pp. 65–67, 2015.

[14] T. R. C. Soares, M. E. A. Carvalho, L. S. S. Pinto, C. A. Falcao, F. T. C. Matos, and T. C. Santos, "Oral cancer knowledge and awareness among dental students," *Brazilian Journal of Oral Sciences*, vol. 13, no. 1, pp. 28–33, 2014.

[15] Z. R. McCready, P. Kanjirath, and B. C. Jham, "Oral cancer knowledge, behavior, and attitude among osteopathic medical students," *Journal of Cancer Education*, vol. 30, pp. 231–236, 2015.

[16] J. Seoane, P. Alvarez-Novoa, I. Gomez et al., "Early oral cancer diagnosis: the Aarhus statement perspective. A systematic review and meta-analysis," *Head & Neck*, 2015.

[17] T. Hanioka, M. Ojima, Y. Kawaguchi, Y. Hirata, H. Ogawa, and Y. Mochizuki, "Tobacco interventions by dentists and dental hygienists," *Japanese Dental Science Review*, vol. 49, no. 1, pp. 47–56, 2013.

[18] J. Seoane, P. Varela-Centelles, I. Tomás, J. Seoane-Romero, P. Diz, and B. Takkouche, "Continuing education in oral cancer prevention for dentists in Spain," *Journal of Dental Education*, vol. 76, no. 9, pp. 1234–1240, 2012.

[19] O. G. Uti and A. A. Fashina, "Oral cancer education in dental schools: knowledge and experience of Nigerian undergraduate students," *Journal of Dental Education*, vol. 70, no. 6, pp. 676–680, 2006.

[20] A. Panwar, R. Batra, W. M. Lydiatt, and A. K. Ganti, "Human papilloma virus positive oropharyngeal squamous cell carcinoma: a growing epidemic," *Cancer Treatment Reviews*, vol. 40, no. 2, pp. 215–219, 2014.

19

Cone-Beam Computed Tomographic Assessment of Mandibular Condylar Position in Patients with Temporomandibular Joint Dysfunction and in Healthy Subjects

Maryam Paknahad,[1,2] **Shoaleh Shahidi,**[1] **Shiva Iranpour,**[1]
Sabah Mirhadi,[1] **and Majid Paknahad**[3]

[1]*Oral Radiology Department, Dental School, Shiraz University of Medical Sciences, Shiraz 7145613466, Iran*
[2]*Prevention of Oral and Dental Disease Research Center, Dental School, Shiraz University of Medical Sciences,*
Shiraz 7145613466, Iran
[3]*Radiology Department, Medical School, Shiraz University of Medical Sciences, Shiraz 7145613466, Iran*

Correspondence should be addressed to Maryam Paknahad; paknahadmaryam@yahoo.com

Academic Editor: Francesco Mangano

Statement of the Problem. The clinical significance of condyle-fossa relationships in the temporomandibular joint is a matter of controversy. Different studies have evaluated whether the position of the condyle is a predictor of the presence of temporomandibular disorder. *Purpose.* The purpose of the present study was to investigate the condylar position according to gender in patients with temporomandibular disorder (TMD) and healthy controls using cone-beam computed tomography. *Materials and Methods.* CBCT of sixty temporomandibular joints in thirty patients with TMD and sixty joints of thirty subjects without TMJ disorder was evaluated in this study. The condylar position was assessed on the CBCT images. The data were analyzed using Pearson chi-square test. *Results.* No statistically significant differences were found regarding the condylar position between symptomatic and asymptomatic groups. Posterior condylar position was more frequently observed in women and anterior condylar position was more prevalent in men in the symptomatic group. However, no significant differences in condylar position were found in asymptomatic subjects according to gender. *Conclusion.* This study showed no apparent association between condylar positioning and clinical findings in TMD patients.

1. Introduction

The temporomandibular joint (TMJ) is one of the most complex joints in the body which is located between the mandibular condyle and the temporal bone [1, 2]. The radiographic joint space is a radiolucent area between the mandibular condyle and the temporal bone [3]. Joint space measurements were introduced by Ricketts to describe condylar position [4]. The condylar position can be determined by the relative dimensions of the radiographic joint spaces between the glenoid fossa and the mandibular condyle [3].

The clinical significance of condyle-fossa relationships in the temporomandibular joint is a matter of controversy [5]. Some studies have suggested an association between

eccentric condylar position and temporomandibular disorder (TMD) [6–9]. These studies have suggested therapeutic procedures to optimize the condylar position in some patients [6, 10, 11]. However, other studies failed to demonstrate significant association between the condylar positioning and the incidence of TMD [12, 13].

Various radiographic methods have been used in previous studies to determine condylar position such as plain film radiography, conventional tomography, computed tomography, cone-beam tomography, and magnetic resonance imaging [5, 14–18]. Cone-beam computed tomography (CBCT) is the modality of choice for the assessment of temporomandibular osseous structures [19]. In the present study, the observers have used CBCT to study condylar positioning.

The aim of the present study was to investigate the condylar position according to gender in patients with TMD and healthy controls using CBCT.

2. Materials and Methods

This study was carried out at the Department of Maxillofacial Radiology at Shiraz Dental University in Shiraz, Iran. An expert radiologist examined the participants and divided them into two groups including symptomatic group and asymptomatic group. The symptomatic group consisted of 30 patients (20 females and 10 males) aged 20 to 42 years (mean 33/4 years) with clinical signs and symptoms of TMD such as joint pain, muscle pain, mouth-opening limitation, joint noise (click or crepitation), and nonharmonic movements of the joint who were referred to the Department of Maxillofacial Radiology for the treatment of TMDs and required CBCT for more investigation. The asymptomatic group consisted of 30 adults (18 females and 12 males) who had no temporomandibular symptoms and no history of occlusal equilibration or masticatory disorders referred to our department for reasons other than TMJ problems. The age of the patients in the control group ranged from 15 to 34 years (mean 24 years). In the control group, the patients who had any evidence of TMD in clinical or radiological examination were excluded from the present study. In both groups, the exclusion criteria were the presence of any congenital abnormalities and/or any systemic disease which could affect joint morphology such as rheumatoid arthritis.

All the participants took part voluntarily in this study and the written consent forms were taken from each of them after being informed about the nature of the study in detail. The study was approved by the local Ethical Committee of Shiraz Dental School.

2.1. CBCT of the TMJ. The CBCT scans of bilateral TMJs were performed by a NewTom VGi (QR Srl, Italy) with a field of view 15 cm × 15 cm. The exposure factors were 120 kv, 5 mA, and exposure time of 5 seconds. The subjects were standing and biting their teeth into maximum intercuspal position. Their heads were positioned with the Frankfurt plane parallel to the floor.

2.2. Condylar Position Assessment. The axial view, in which the condylar process had the widest mediolateral diameter, was chosen as the reference view for secondary reconstruction. On this selected axial view, a line parallel to the long axis of the condylar process was drawn and lateral slices were reconstructed with 0.5 mm slice interval and 0.5 mm thickness (Figure 1(a)). On the central sagittal section, an expert maxillofacial radiologist measured the values of the narrowest posterior (P) and anterior (A) joint space accurately using NewTom NNT analysis software (Figure 1(b)). Condylar position was expressed by the following formula according to the method of Pullinger and Hollender [20]:

$$\text{condylar ratio} = \frac{P - A}{P + A} \times 100. \qquad (1)$$

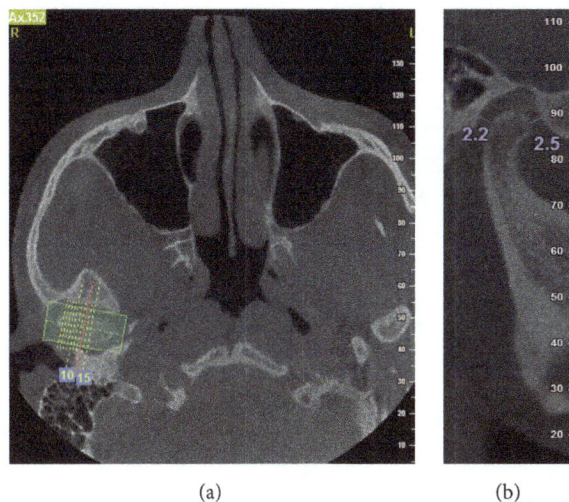

(a) (b)

FIGURE 1: Linear measurement of anterior (A) and posterior (P) subjective closest joint spaces in a sample patient. (a) Axial view; (b) sagittal view.

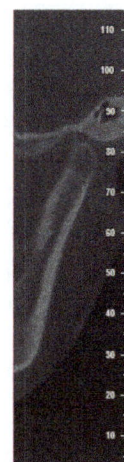

FIGURE 2: Posterior condylar position in a sample patient in the symptomatic group.

The position of the condyle was considered concentric if the ratio was within ±12%. If the ratio was smaller than −12%, the condylar position was considered posterior and if the ratio was greater than +12%, the condyle was considered in an anterior position (Figures 2 and 3).

2.3. Statistical Analysis. All data were analyzed with the SPSS program (SPSS 15.0, IBM, Chicago, IL, USA). The statistical analysis was performed using Pearson chi-square test to compare the condylar positions between two groups at the significance level of 0.05. To assess the significance of any errors during measurement, all images were revaluated over one-week interval. The mean difference between the first and second measurement was analyzed using paired t-test. The level for significance was set at $P < 0.05$.

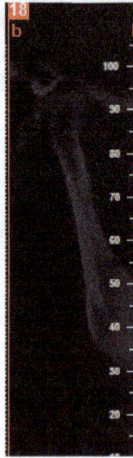

FIGURE 3: Anterior condylar position in a sample patient in the symptomatic group.

3. Results

There were no significant differences between dual measurements. The means of these two measurement values were used to minimize the error in identifying the reference points.

In the asymptomatic group, the frequency of posterior position was 25%, concentric position 38.5%, and anterior position 36.7%. In the symptomatic objects the incidence of posterior condylar position was 38.3%, concentric position 36.7%, and anterior position 35% (Table 1). There was no significant difference between the symptomatic and the asymptomatic groups for condylar position (P value = 0.22). Distribution of the condylar position in the symptomatic and asymptomatic groups according to gender is summarized in Table 2. No significant differences in condylar position between men and women were found in the asymptomatic subjects (P value = 0.757). The condylar position in the symptomatic group was significantly different in men and women (P value < 0.05) (Table 2). Posterior condylar position is significantly more prevalent in women (50%) and anterior condylar position more prevalent in men (55%).

4. Discussion

The clinical significance of condyle-fossa relationships in the temporomandibular joint is a matter of controversy [5]. Some studies have suggested eccentric condylar position is associated with temporomandibular disorder [6–9]. The aim of this study was to evaluate the condylar position according to gender in patients with TMD and healthy controls using CBCT.

Different radiographic techniques including conventional radiography [15], conventional tomography [18], computed tomography [1], MRI [14, 16, 17], and cone-beam computed tomography [5, 14, 21] have been used to study the condylar position in the glenoid fossa and the articular eminence morphology. Previously conventional radiography, especially transcranial radiography, has been used to assess condylar position and morphology [7]. However, transcranial

TABLE 1: Distribution of condyle position in the symptomatic and asymptomatic group.

| Group | Condylar position | | | P value |
	Posterior	Concentric	Anterior	
Asymptomatic	15 (25.0%)	23 (38.3%)	22 (36.7%)	0.22
Symptomatic	23 (38.3%)	16 (26.7%)	16 (26.7%)	

radiographs only represent the lateral third of the condyle. Therefore the reliability of these radiographs or assessing condylar position is questioned. Some researchers used conventional tomography to evaluate condylar position in the glenoid fossa [20]. However because slice thickness is large ranging between 1.0 and 3.0 mm, it does not represent the margins of joint structure as clearly as CT and CBCT [22].

The recently developed CBCT represents the joint structures with high accuracy which produces submillimeter spatial resolution as high as or even superior to spiral CT [23, 24]. Kobayashi et al. reported that the measurement error in CBCT was significantly less than spiral CT [24]. The bony component can be visualized in 3 planes without any superimposition, distortion, or magnification [25, 26]. CBCT has the advantage of reduced radiation dose and shorter scanning time compared with CT [27]. Therefore, CBCT has been used in the present study.

In studies that used transcranial radiographs actually the most lateral part of the joint is evaluated. Rammelsberg et al. selected three tomograms including central, 3 mm more lateral, and 3 mm more medial and measured data in tomograms [28]. Ikeda and Kawamura evaluated joint spaces on the central cuts of joints within 3.5 mm range medially and laterally to the central cut in CBCT [29]. They found that landmark identification outside this range was default because of the glenoid fossa anatomy. They also suggested that there were not significant differences in the joint spaces in this section [29]. Therefore we only considered the central slice of sagittal section of condyles in order to simplify analyzing the data.

There is a controversy over the clinical significance of condylar position [5]. Many studies have reported nonconcentric condylar position in association with disk displacement [14, 17], osteoarthritic changes [5], remodeling of the articular eminence and the condyle [30], and predisposition to arthrosis [31]. Nonconcentric condylar positioning is seen in one-third to one-half of asymptomatic volunteers [3]. On the other hand, concentric positioning in patients with TMD has high prevalence [32]. Aggressive condylar repositioning therapies are frequently performed to reestablish the mandibular condyle in an optimal position [6, 10]. However, according to the present study, condylar eccentricity is not a sufficient evidence for diagnosis of TMD and besides the evaluation of TMJ clinical symptoms and assessment of condylar eccentricity, additional investigations are required before a therapeutic change is performed.

Some studies represented no significant association between condylar positioning and clinical findings [12, 33, 34]. However, many studies showed significant difference in

TABLE 2: The condylar position in the symptomatic and asymptomatic groups according to gender.

Group	Sex	Condylar position			P value
		Posterior	Concentric	Anterior	
Asymptomatic	Female	10 (27.8%)	14 (38.9%)	12 (33.3%)	0.757
	Male	5 (20.8%)	9 (37.5%)	10 (41.7%)	
Symptomatic	Female	20 (50%)	10 (25%)	10 (25%)	0.020*
	Male	3 (15%)	6 (30%)	11 (55%)	

*A P value less than 0.05 was considered statistically significant.

the condylar positions in patients with TMD and asymptomatic subjects [27, 35]. Cho and Jung found concentric condylar position was more common in the asymptomatic group and posterior condylar position was more frequent in the symptomatic group [5]. Paknahad and Shahidi reported posteriorly seated condyles in patients with severe TMD and anteriorly and concentric seated condyles in patients with mild to moderate TMD [36]. Lelis et al. evaluated the condyle-mandibular fossa relationship in young individuals with intact dentitions and compared it to that between individuals with and without symptoms of temporomandibular disorder using CBCT [37]. They concluded that the presence or absence of temporomandibular disorder was not correlated with the condyle position in the temporomandibular joint which was similar to our findings.

In some previous studies asymptomatic groups represented more posterior condylar position in women and more anterior positions in men [20, 38]. Madsen found in the transcranial radiographs of asymptomatic adults that women and men were more likely to present posterior and anterior condylar positioning, respectively [39]. However in the present study, no significant difference in condylar position was found between men and women in asymptomatic subjects. Similarly some previous studies found no significant sex difference in condylar position joint spaces in normal joints [35, 40]. Ikeda and Kawamura found no significant sex difference in joint spaces, using CBCT in symptom-free subjects [29].

On the other hand in the symptomatic group posterior condylar position in women and anterior position in men were noticed. Some authors have reported an association between posterior condylar positioning and internal derangement [14, 16]. Higher incidence of posterior condylar position in women may be the etiological factor for preponderance of TMD and disk instability in women.

In this study the subjects who had history of occlusal therapy, prosthodontics treatment, and any systemic disorders such as rheumatoid arthritis were not included because these factors could affect the condylar morphology and position.

The present study did not demonstrate any significant differences in condylar position between symptomatic and asymptomatic groups. However several different factors such as radiographic technique used, accuracy of clinical examination, sample size, and the method of condylar position measurement can influence the results. Therefore, further investigations for assessing the correlation between temporomandibular disorder and condylar position are necessary.

Conflict of Interests

The authors declare that there is no conflict of interests regarding the publication of this paper.

Acknowledgments

The authors thank the Vice-Chancellery of Shiraz University of Medical Sciences for supporting this research. The authors would like to thank Dr. Sh. Hamedani (DDS, M.S.) for his suggestions and English writing assistance in the paper. The authors also thank Dr. M. Vosoughi of the Center for Research, of the School of Dentistry, for statistical analysis.

References

[1] C.-K. Wu, J.-T. Hsu, Y.-W. Shen, J.-H. Chen, W.-C. Shen, and L.-J. Fuh, "Assessments of inclinations of the mandibular fossa by computed tomography in an Asian population," Clinical Oral Investigations, vol. 16, no. 2, pp. 443–450, 2012.

[2] P. M. Som and H. D. Curtin, Head and Neck Imaging, Elsevier Health Sciences, 5th edition, 2011.

[3] S. C. White and M. J. Pharoah, Oral Radiology: Principles and Interpretation, Elsevier Health Sciences, 6th edition, 2009.

[4] R. M. Ricketts, "Variations of the temporomandibular joint as revealed by cephalometric laminagraphy," American Journal of Orthodontics, vol. 36, no. 12, pp. 877–898, 1950.

[5] B.-H. Cho and Y.-H. Jung, "Osteoarthritic changes and condylar positioning of the temporomandibular joint in Korean children and adolescents," Imaging Science in Dentistry, vol. 42, no. 3, pp. 169–174, 2012.

[6] L. A. Weinberg, "An evaluation of occlusal factors in TMJ dysfunction-pain syndrome," The Journal of Prosthetic Dentistry, vol. 41, no. 2, pp. 198–208, 1979.

[7] L. A. Weinberg, "Correlation of temporomandibular dysfunction with radiographic findings," The Journal of Prosthetic Dentistry, vol. 28, no. 5, pp. 519–539, 1972.

[8] D. D. Blaschke, W. K. Solberg, and B. Sanders, "Arthorgraphy of the temporomandibular joint: review of current status," The Journal of the American Dental Association, vol. 100, no. 3, pp. 388–395, 1980.

[9] W. B. Farrar and W. L. McCarthy Jr., "Conventional radiography compared with arthrography in internal derangements of the temporomandibular joint," The Journal of Prosthetic Dentistry, vol. 50, no. 4, pp. 585–586, 1983.

[10] F. Mongini, "Combined method to determine the therapeutic position for occlusal rehabilitation," *The Journal of Prosthetic Dentistry*, vol. 47, no. 4, pp. 434–439, 1982.

[11] L. A. Weinberg, "Definitive prosthodontic therapy for TMJ patients. Part I: Anterior and posterior condylar displacement," *The Journal of Prosthetic Dentistry*, vol. 50, no. 4, pp. 544–557, 1983.

[12] E. G. Herbosa, K. S. Rotskoff, B. F. Ramos, and H. S. Ambrookian, "Condylar position in superior maxillary repositioning and its effect on the temporomandibular joint," *Journal of Oral and Maxillofacial Surgery*, vol. 48, no. 7, pp. 690–696, 1990.

[13] F. O'Ryan and B. N. Epker, "Surgical orthodontics and the temporomandibular joint. I. Superior repositioning of the maxilla," *American Journal of Orthodontics*, vol. 83, no. 5, pp. 408–417, 1983.

[14] K. Ikeda and A. Kawamura, "Disc displacement and changes in condylar position," *Dentomaxillofacial Radiology*, vol. 42, no. 3, Article ID 84227642, 2013.

[15] A. V. Menezes, S. M. de Almeida, F. N. Bóscolo, F. Haiter-Neto, G. M. B. Ambrosano, and F. R. Manzi, "Comparison of transcranial radiograph and magnetic resonance imaging in the evaluation of mandibular condyle position," *Dentomaxillofacial Radiology*, vol. 37, no. 5, pp. 293–299, 2008.

[16] L. Incesu, N. Taşkaya-Yilmaz, M. Oğütcen-Toller, and E. Uzun, "Relationship of condylar position to disc position and morphology," *European Journal of Radiology*, vol. 51, no. 3, pp. 269–273, 2004.

[17] H. Kurita, A. Ohtsuka, H. Kobayashi, and K. Kurashina, "A study of the relationship between the position of the condylar head and displacement of the temporomandibular joint disk," *Dentomaxillofacial Radiology*, vol. 30, no. 3, pp. 162–165, 2001.

[18] P. W. Major, R. D. Kinniburgh, B. Nebbe, N. G. Prasad, and K. E. Glover, "Tomographic assessment of temporomandibular joint osseous articular surface contour and spatial relationships associated with disc displacement and disc length," *American Journal of Orthodontics and Dentofacial Orthopedics*, vol. 121, no. 2, pp. 152–161, 2002.

[19] M. L. Hilgers, W. C. Scarfe, J. P. Scheetz, and A. G. Farman, "Accuracy of linear temporomandibular joint measurements with cone beam computed tomography and digital cephalometric radiography," *American Journal of Orthodontics and Dentofacial Orthopedics*, vol. 128, no. 6, pp. 803–811, 2005.

[20] A. G. Pullinger, L. Hollender, W. K. Solberg, and A. Petersson, "A tomographic study of mandibular condyle position in an asymptomatic population," *The Journal of Prosthetic Dentistry*, vol. 53, no. 5, pp. 706–713, 1985.

[21] S. Shahidi, M. Vojdani, and M. Paknahad, "Correlation between articular eminence steepness measured with cone-beam computed tomography and clinical dysfunction index in patients with temporomandibular joint dysfunction," *Oral Surgery, Oral Medicine, Oral Pathology and Oral Radiology*, vol. 116, no. 1, pp. 91–97, 2013.

[22] K. Ikeda, A. Kawamura, and R. Ikeda, "Assessment of optimal condylar position in the coronal and axial planes with limited cone-beam computed tomography," *Journal of Prosthodontics*, vol. 20, no. 6, pp. 432–438, 2011.

[23] A. Nakajima, G. T. Sameshima, Y. Arai, Y. Homme, N. Shimizu, and H. Dougherty Sr., "Two- and three-dimensional orthodontic imaging using limited cone beam-computed tomography," *Angle Orthodontist*, vol. 75, no. 6, pp. 895–903, 2005.

[24] K. Kobayashi, S. Shimoda, Y. Nakagawa, and A. Yamamoto, "Accuracy in measurement of distance using limited cone-beam computerized tomography," *International Journal of Oral & Maxillofacial Implants*, vol. 19, no. 2, pp. 228–231, 2004.

[25] M. A. Sümbüllü, F. Çağlayan, H. M. Akgü, and A. B. Yilmaz, "Radiological examination of the articular eminence morphology using cone beam CT," *Dentomaxillofacial Radiology*, vol. 41, no. 3, pp. 234–240, 2012.

[26] Z. T. Librizzi, A. S. Tadinada, J. V. Valiyaparambil, A. G. Lurie, and S. M. Mallya, "Cone-beam computed tomography to detect erosions of the temporomandibular joint: effect of field of view and voxel size on diagnostic efficacy and effective dose," *American Journal of Orthodontics and Dentofacial Orthopedics*, vol. 140, no. 1, pp. e25–e30, 2011.

[27] O. B. Honey, W. C. Scarfe, M. J. Hilgers et al., "Accuracy of cone-beam computed tomography imaging of the temporomandibular joint: comparisons with panoramic radiology and linear tomography," *American Journal of Orthodontics and Dentofacial Orthopedics*, vol. 132, no. 4, pp. 429–438, 2007.

[28] P. Rammelsberg, L. Jäger, and J.-M. Pho Duc, "Magnetic resonance imaging-based joint space measurements in temporomandibular joints with disk displacements and in controls," *Oral Surgery, Oral Medicine, Oral Pathology, Oral Radiology, and Endodontics*, vol. 90, no. 2, pp. 240–248, 2000.

[29] K. Ikeda and A. Kawamura, "Assessment of optimal condylar position with limited cone-beam computed tomography," *American Journal of Orthodontics and Dentofacial Orthopedics*, vol. 135, no. 4, pp. 495–501, 2009.

[30] R. P. Scapino, "Histopathology associated with malposition of the human temporomandibular joint disc," *Oral Surgery, Oral Medicine, Oral Pathology*, vol. 55, no. 4, pp. 382–397, 1983.

[31] P.-L. Westesson and M. Rohlin, "Internal derangement related to osteoarthrosis in temporomandibular joint autopsy specimens," *Oral Surgery, Oral Medicine, Oral Pathology*, vol. 57, no. 1, pp. 17–22, 1984.

[32] M. A. Markovic and H. M. Rosenberg, "Tomographic evaluation of 100 patients with temporomandibular joint symptoms," *Oral Surgery, Oral Medicine, Oral Pathology*, vol. 42, no. 6, pp. 838–846, 1976.

[33] J. W. Brand, J. G. Whinery Jr., Q. N. Anderson, and K. M. Keenan, "Condylar position as a predictor of temporomandibular joint internal derangement," *Oral Surgery, Oral Medicine, Oral Pathology*, vol. 67, no. 4, pp. 469–476, 1989.

[34] S. R. Alexander, R. N. Moore, and L. M. DuBois, "Mandibular condyle position: comparison of articulator mountings and magnetic resonance imaging," *American Journal of Orthodontics & Dentofacial Orthopedics*, vol. 104, no. 3, pp. 230–239, 1993.

[35] H. Bonilla-Aragon, R. H. Tallents, R. W. Katzberg, S. Kyrkanides, and M. E. Moss, "Condyle position as a predictor of temporomandibular joint internal derangement," *The Journal of Prosthetic Dentistry*, vol. 82, no. 2, pp. 205–208, 1999.

[36] M. Paknahad and S. Shahidi, "Association between mandibular condylar position and clinical dysfunction index," *Journal of Cranio-Maxillofacial Surgery*, vol. 43, no. 4, pp. 432–436, 2015.

[37] É. R. Lelis, J. C. Guimarães Henriques, M. Tavares, M. R. de Mendonça, A. J. Fernandes Neto, and G. d. Almeida, "Cone-beam tomography assessment of the condylar position in asymptomatic and symptomatic young individuals," *The Journal of Prosthetic Dentistry*, vol. 114, no. 3, pp. 420–425, 2015.

[38] C. E. Rieder and J. T. Martinoff, "Comparison of the multiphasic dysfunction profile with lateral transcranial radiographs," *The Journal of Prosthetic Dentistry*, vol. 52, no. 4, pp. 572–580, 1984.

[39] B. Madsen, "Normal variations in anatomy, condylar movements, and arthrosis frequency of the temporomandibular joints," *Acta Radiologica*, vol. 4, no. 3, pp. 273–288, 1966.

[40] E. L. Christiansen, T. T. Chan, J. R. Thompson, A. N. Hasso, D. B. Hinshaw Jr., and S. Kopp, "Computed tomography of the normal temporomandibular joint," *European Journal of Oral Sciences*, vol. 95, no. 6, pp. 499–509, 1987.

20

Challenges Faced in Engaging American Indian Mothers in an Early Childhood Caries Preventive Trial

Tamanna Tiwari, Judith Albino, and Terrence S. Batliner

Centers for American Indian and Alaska Native Health, Colorado School of Public Health, University of Colorado Anschutz Medical Campus, Aurora, CO 80045, USA

Correspondence should be addressed to Tamanna Tiwari; tamanna.tiwari@ucdenver.edu

Academic Editor: Najla Dar-Odeh

Objective. This study explores the challenges faced by the research implementation team in engaging new mothers in a community oral health prevention intervention in an American Indian (AI) reservation community. *Methods*. Qualitative methods in the form of in-depth interviews were used in the study. Qualitative data were collected from research staff workers at a field site, who were involved in the implementation of a culturally tailored, randomized controlled trial of a behavioral intervention utilizing Motivational Interviewing (MI). *Results*. Several challenges were described by the field staff in engaging new mothers, including low priority placed on oral health, lack of knowledge, and distractions that reduced their ability to engage in learning about oral health of their child. Other difficulties faced in engaging the mothers and the AI community at large were distrust related to racial differences and physical and environmental barriers including poor road conditions, lack of transportation and communication, and remoteness of data collection sites. The field staff developed and applied many strategies, including conducting home visits, applying new communication strategies, and interacting with the community at various venues. *Conclusion*. Prevention interventions for ECC need to target AI mothers. Strategies developed by the field staff were successful for engaging mothers in the study.

1. Introduction

Mothers play an important role in determining the oral health of their children. Maternal oral health knowledge, behaviors and beliefs such as feeding practices, oral hygiene maintenance for the child, failure to access professional dental care, and the beliefs that a child is not susceptible to caries or that primary teeth are not important are associated with early childhood caries (ECC) [1]. These maternal beliefs and oral health practices appear to place a child at greater risk of developing dental caries [1]. Also, mothers' oral health status is a strong predictor of the oral health status of their children [2].

ECC is a multifactorial disease involving biological, microbial, and behavioral factors [3] and the three etiological factors must simultaneously be present for initiation and progression of the disease. There is strong evidence that *S. mutans* and lactobacilli are the primary agents involved in the development of caries in both children and adults [4]. Studies using genetic/molecular techniques have shown that the source of the *S. mutans* infection in children is, predominantly although not exclusively, attributed to vertical transmission from the mothers [5]. High levels of *S. mutans* andlactobacilli in the mother's mouth contribute to maternal transfer as do maternal dietary habits and poor oral hygiene [6]. Maternal behaviors such as tasting the infant's food and sharing utensils can transmit bacteria from the mother to the child [6].

Maternal psychosocial factors, including stress, oral health beliefs, fatalistic attitudes, and cultural factors, are associated with ECC and with dental health services utilization [1, 7–9]. Other characteristics such as maternal oral health literacy, self-efficacy, and ethnic and cultural-specific beliefs about oral health can be contributing factors to ECC [9, 10]. Because a child's oral health is largely dependent on maternal biological and psychosocial factors, ECC becomes a women's health issue, making it imperative to engage mothers in behavior change methods beginning at a child's birth, or even prenatally.

American Indian (AI) children have the highest rate of ECC of any population group within the United States [11]. American Indian mothers living on reservations often are disproportionately burdened with the social disadvantages associated with unemployment, low levels of education, and poverty [12]. These environmental factors may contribute to maternal psychological distress and, along with other factors such as low self-efficacy, social support, and inadequate preventive health services, can place AI children at still higher risk of ECC. Our data have demonstrated that AI parents who do not adhere to recommended oral health behaviors also report more chronic distress than others [13]. They also had poor oral health knowledge and demonstrated external locus of control, suggesting little confidence in their ability to influence their children's oral health [13]. In fact, the oral health of these AI children was significantly worse than that of children whose parents had greater oral health knowledge and more positive attitudes [14]. These data suggested that working to improve maternal behavior, knowledge, and attitudes might lead to improved oral health in AI children.

An oral health prevention trial for behavior change using Motivational Interviewing (MI) in AI mothers is underway in a Northern Plains tribal region. We speculated that when mothers learn more about oral health during MI sessions and engaged in supportive discussions about the importance of oral health practices and appropriate action steps, they will be better able to formulate oral health care goals for their children and develop the confidence and motivation needed for behavior change. However, several challenges were faced by investigators and research field staff in recruiting and engaging these mothers in the study. This paper describes the challenges and barriers faced by the field staff for an oral health prevention trial as they worked to engage AI mothers living in rural and remote locations. We also discuss the strategies developed as these staff worked to overcome the challenges they faced.

2. Materials and Methods

In 2008, the Center for Native Oral Health Research at the University of Colorado Anschutz Medical Center was funded by the National Institute for Dental and Craniofacial Research (U54DE019259) to conduct a randomized controlled trial to determine whether a behavioral intervention using MI with AI new mothers will achieve a greater reduction of caries experience in children younger than three years than would enhanced community services alone [15]. Six hundred mothers and their newborns were enrolled and randomized to one of two groups over two years, with a period of follow-up lasting until the child's third birthday. The trial has been approved by the Tribal Research Review Board and the Colorado Multiple Institutional Review Board.

This study was a qualitative evaluation of the challenges faced by the field staff in engaging AI mothers in the prevention trial; as such, it falls under the purview of quality assurance and management of data collection for the trial and is not subject to IRB review, other than what is required for the clinical trial. The authors created a semistructured interview guide and conducted in-depth interviews, lasting 40–50 minutes each, with the five field staff members, who carried out the intervention. All interviews were digitally recorded and later transcribed. Verbal consent was obtained from the staff members who participated in the interviews, and participation was voluntary. Staff members were requested not to identify other staff members or themselves during the interviews to maintain confidentiality. All digital recordings are stored on a secure server. Following standard qualitative analysis procedures [16, 17], all the transcripts were coded. After initial coding was completed, codes were iteratively refined as various themes and subthemes emerged as shown as follows.

Challenges. They include the following.

Engaging the mothers:

low priority,
lack of knowledge,
distractions.

Balancing potential conflicts between research policy and cultural norms.

Not being American Indian.

No gender based challenges.

Barriers. They include the following.

Physical and environmental barriers:

poor road conditions,
lack of transportation and communication,
remoteness of data collection sites.

Strategies. They include the following.

Research implementation which is a teamwork.

Conducting home visits.

New communication methods.

Interacting with the community at various venues.

Culturally sensitive strategies.

3. Result and Discussion

3.1. Results. Three major themes and several subthemes emerged from the transcripts as shown above. The field staff described several challenges they faced in implementing the research, particularly those related to engaging new mothers in the study and the MI intervention. The staff pointed out that some mothers living on the reservation placed low priority on the oral health of their children, thus making it difficult to recruit them into the study. Reflecting on the fact that AI families living on the reservation often have to deal with unemployment, food insecurity, and problems related to inadequate housing and transportation, they expressed empathy and understanding that oral health often was not the highest priority for some of these mothers.

3.2. Comments of the Staff. Staff comment:

> *Mothers deal with so many things here, they want to participate in something like this, they want the best for their children but it is almost impossible.*

The field staff described that AI mothers had relatively little knowledge about oral health; for instance, they often did not have knowledge about the importance of primary teeth or about the causes of dental caries. Moreover, the main source of their knowledge was their mothers and extended family.

Staff comment:

> *I think my biggest challenge is ignorance; they just do not know. And the other challenge is to get them to think differently than their mothers and grandmothers.*

Pointing out that many study visits are done in the participants' homes, staff noted that the mothers often were distracted by older children or by household chores and could not always fully engage with the staff who were there for an MI session or for conducting the dental assessment for the child.

Staff comment:

> *The main challenge that I face in engaging new mothers is distractions, mainly their other older kids who want attention.*

Though all the staff are from the community, some of them are not American Indian, and this sometimes makes it difficult to create trust and thereby makes the job of recruiting mothers more difficult.

Staff comment:

> *I think it is also different for me because I am a Caucasian person, I am not from here and for me it is different to come in here, I am the outcast here, I am the different person here.*

All the field staff members are women, and they indicated that they have not faced any gender based challenges or barriers in engaging the mothers in the study. In fact, they said that being a woman was helpful in building rapport with the study participants. They believed that participants felt safer and more comfortable inviting women into their homes and sharing their stories with them.

Staff comment:

> *I always get positive responses from mothers as I am a mom too. I think mothers are more attentive to other women.*

The staff described some physical and environmental barriers they encountered that prevented them from being more productive in improving participant engagement in the study. They spoke about the vastness and remoteness of the reservation, poor road conditions, inclement weather, and poor communication methods—all of which could be overwhelming and delay the process of reaching out to study participants. They thought that not reaching the participants at a given time could send the wrong signals related to their role in helping new mothers in reaching oral health goals for their child.

Staff comments:

> *I guess the number one difficulty is that everything is so spread out and so far away. You have to have a vehicle to survive around here.*

> *Just access, whether we are going to them or they (study participants) are coming to us. Anytime it rains or snows it reduces our ability to reach to them as the roads are muddy.*

Despite all the challenges they have faced, the staff have developed innovative ways to engage the mothers and the AI community at large in this oral health prevention trial. They informed us in the interviews that they are using new communication strategies such as Facebook and sending postcards to interact and engage new mother on the reservation.

Staff comment:

> *People have no phone, no car, but they have Facebook 24/7.*

They said they interact with the mothers at various community events, health clinics, and after-school programs for the children. This has not only provided ways to gain the trust of the community and the study participants but also increased their interest in oral health in general. They said they try to be culturally sensitive and are adapting to the local culture.

Staff comment:

> *When I call them I talk to them as if they are my friends on an everyday basis rather than clients or a participant in the study.*

3.3. Discussion. Results from this qualitative assessment reveal a number of difficulties of engaging AI mothers in an oral health intervention for their children, even though AI children have the highest need for such preventive interventions. One of the challenges is to prioritize the child's oral health for AI mothers and to increase their acceptance of such interventions. Though there are many physical and environmental barriers in reaching out to these mothers, the most salient challenge is to get them interested in the prevention of oral disease and then to help them develop an understanding of oral health issues and the steps they can take to prevent oral disease in their children. The use of Motivational Interviewing (MI) in this trial is helping to prioritize the oral health of children for the participating mothers and the families. MI is complementary to the cultural values of AI/AN people; it emphasizes listening, learning, and respect, and it creates space to include spirituality and religious practices, all of which are essential to engage and elicit behavior change in AI mothers [15]. Previous studies have recommended including oral health in anticipatory guidance during prenatal visits for indigenous women and using community-based promotion initiatives to emphasize the importance of oral health for pregnant women and their infants, which might help to prioritize oral health in all indigenous children since birth [18].

Data from this study and the previous work reported in the research literature have shown that maternal physical and psychosocial health and oral health knowledge are associated with oral health in their children, or with oral health behavior on behalf of their children. For example, mother's self-efficacy is strongly associated with frequency of brushing child's teeth [5]. A number of false beliefs have been found, including the idea that primary teeth are not important because they fall out and the child will get a "second chance" with the permanent teeth [19]. We also have found that, in AI populations, oral health decisions for children often are made by multiple members of the family, and some of those family members may discourage preventive oral health practices and support accessing dental care only when there is a serious problem.

Research staff in the study are overcoming the barriers of conducting research in remote and rural settings and developing successful strategies to engage new mother in oral health interventions by gaining trust of the community and being sensitive to local norms. These include conducting home visits, applying new communication strategies (Facebook), and interacting with the community at various venues. By providing flexibility to accommodate the work and childcare schedules of the study participants, conducting home visits, and participating in community events and pow wows, the field staff not only have gained the trust of the participants and the community but also have been able to spread awareness about oral health in general. Involving the AI communities as active members of research and adapting engagement approaches according to community or tribal feedback are some of the successful strategies reported in the literature [20, 21].

These approaches were welcomed by the mothers and the AI community more generally and suggest that interacting with mothers, who are the main gatekeepers for a child's oral health, targeting behavior change in them, and building capacity at the family and community level could reduce ECC in AI children. Future oral health prevention interventions can utilize these tested strategies and approaches to successfully engage mothers and increase oral health awareness for the family at large.

4. Conclusion

Clearly, the prevention of ECC needs to target AI mothers; improving their oral health knowledge and decision making capacity could bring about family-level and community-level changes in preventing ECC.

Disclaimer

The content is solely the responsibility of the authors and does not necessarily represent the official views of the National Institutes of Health.

Conflict of Interests

The authors declare that there is no conflict of interests regarding the publication of this paper.

Acknowledgments

The grant support for this project is National Institute of Health-National Institute of Dental and Craniofacial Research (NIH-NIDCR) Award no. 1U54DE019259. The authors thank their staff, Erin Swyers, Tracy Zacher, Rocky Dubray, Leslie Skinner, Terri Rattler, and Margaret Beardmore, their community partners, and the study participants, without whom this work would not be possible.

References

[1] W. Kim Seow, "Environmental, maternal, and child factors which contribute to early childhood caries: a unifying conceptual model," *International Journal of Paediatric Dentistry*, vol. 22, no. 3, pp. 157–168, 2012.

[2] B. A. Dye, C. M. Vargas, J. J. Lee, L. Magder, and N. Tinanoff, "Assessing the relationship between children's oral health status and that of their mothers," *The Journal of the American Dental Association*, vol. 142, no. 2, pp. 173–183, 2011.

[3] P. W. Caufield, G. R. Cutter, and A. P. Dasanayake, "Initial acquisition of mutans streptococci by infants: evidence for a discrete window of infectivity," *Journal of Dental Research*, vol. 72, no. 1, pp. 37–45, 1993.

[4] J. M. Tanzer, J. Livingston, and A. M. Thompson, "The microbiology of primary dental caries in humans," *Journal of Dental Education*, vol. 65, no. 10, pp. 1028–1037, 2001.

[5] R. Harris, A. D. Nicoll, P. M. Adair, and C. M. Pine, "Risk factors for dental caries in young children: a systematic review of the literature," *Community Dental Health*, vol. 21, no. 1, pp. 71–85, 2004.

[6] M. G. Gussy, E. G. Waters, O. Walsh, and N. M. Kilpatrick, "Early childhood caries: current evidence for aetiology and prevention," *Journal of Paediatrics and Child Health*, vol. 42, no. 1-2, pp. 37–43, 2006.

[7] T. L. Finlayson, K. Siefert, A. I. Ismail, and W. Sohn, "Psychosocial factors and early childhood caries among low-income African-American children in Detroit," *Community Dentistry and Oral Epidemiology*, vol. 35, no. 6, pp. 439–448, 2007.

[8] A. J. Casanova-Rosado, C. E. Medina-Solís, J. F. Casanova-Rosado, A. A. Vallejos-Sánchez, G. Maupomé, and L. Ávila-Burgos, "Dental caries and associated factors in Mexican schoolchildren aged 6-13 years," *Acta Odontologica Scandinavica*, vol. 63, no. 4, pp. 245–251, 2005.

[9] R. B. Quiñonez, M. A. Keels, W. F. Vann Jr., F. T. McIver, K. Heller, and J. K. Whitt, "Early childhood caries: analysis of psychosocial and biological factors in a high-risk population," *Caries Research*, vol. 35, no. 5, pp. 376–383, 2001.

[10] A. I. Ismail, S. Lim, W. Sohn, and J. M. Willem, "Determinants of early childhood caries in low-income African American young children," *Pediatric Dentistry*, vol. 30, no. 4, pp. 289–296, 2008.

[11] K. R. Phipps, T. L. Ricks, M. C. Manz, and P. Blahut, "Prevalence and severity of dental caries among American Indian and Alaska Native preschool children," *Journal of Public Health Dentistry*, vol. 72, no. 3, pp. 208–215, 2012.

[12] U.S. Department of Health and Human Services. United States, *Facts on Indian Health Disparities*, Indian Health Service, Rockville, Md, USA, 2006, http://www.ihs.gov/newsroom/factsheets/disparities/.

[13] T. Tiwari, D. O. Quissell, W. G. Henderson et al., "Factors associated with oral health status in American Indian children," *Journal of Racial and Ethnic Health Disparities*, vol. 1, no. 3, pp. 148–156, 2014.

[14] J. Albino, T. Tiwari, W. G. Henderson et al., "Learning from caries-free children in a high-caries American Indian population," *Journal of Public Health Dentistry*, vol. 74, no. 4, pp. 293–300, 2014.

[15] T. Batliner, K. A. Fehringer, T. Tiwari et al., "Motivational interviewing with American Indian mothers to prevent early childhood caries: study design and methodology of a randomized control trial," *Trials*, vol. 15, no. 1, article 125, 2014.

[16] H. R. Bernard, *Research Methods in Anthropology: Qualitative and Quantitative Approaches*, vol. 4, AltaMira Press, Lanham, Md, USA, 2005.

[17] M. B. Miles and A. M. Huberman, *Qualitative Data Analysis: An Expanded Sourcebook*, vol. 2, Sage Publications, Thousand Oaks, Calif, USA, 1994.

[18] American Academy of Pediatrics, "Early childhood caries in indigenous communities," *Pediatrics*, vol. 127, no. 6, pp. 1190–1198, 2011.

[19] I. V. Hilton, S. Stephen, J. C. Barker, and J. A. Weintraub, "Cultural factors and children's oral health care: a qualitative study of carers of young children," *Community Dentistry and Oral Epidemiology*, vol. 35, no. 6, pp. 429–438, 2007.

[20] T. Tiwari, A. Casciello, S. A. Gansky et al., "Recruitment for health disparities preventive intervention trials: the early childhood caries collaborating centers," *Preventing Chronic Disease*, vol. 11, Article ID 140140, 2014.

[21] S. M. Davis and R. Reid, "Practicing participatory research in American Indian communities," *The American Journal of Clinical Nutrition*, vol. 69, no. 4, supplement, pp. 755S–759S, 1999.

21

Evaluation of Extraradicular Diffusion of Hydrogen Peroxide during Intracoronal Bleaching Using Different Bleaching Agents

Mohammad E. Rokaya,[1] Khaled Beshr,[2] Abeer Hashem Mahram,[2,3] Samah Samir Pedir,[2] and Kusai Baroudi[4]

[1] *Department of Endodontics, Faculty of Dentistry, Al-Azhar University, Assiut, Egypt*
[2] *Department of Restorative Dental Sciences, Al-Farabi Colleges, Riyadh, Saudi Arabia*
[3] *Department of Endodontics, Faculty of Dentistry, Ain Shams University, Cairo, Egypt*
[4] *Department of Preventive Dental Sciences, Al-Farabi Colleges, Riyadh, Saudi Arabia*

Correspondence should be addressed to Kusai Baroudi; d_kusai@yahoo.co.uk

Academic Editor: Patricia Pereira

Objectives. Extra radicular diffusion of hydrogen peroxide associated with intracoronal teeth bleaching was evaluated. *Methods*. 108 intact single rooted extracted mandibular first premolars teeth were selected. The teeth were instrumented with WaveOne system and obturated with gutta percha and divided into four groups ($n = 27$) according to the bleaching materials used. Each main group was divided into three subgroups ($n = 9$) according to the time of extra radicular hydrogen peroxide diffusion measurements at 1, 7, and 14 days: group 1 (35% hydrogen peroxide), group 2 (35% carbamide peroxide), group 3 (sodium perborate-30% hydrogen peroxide mixture), and group 4 (sodium perborate-water mixture). Four cemental dentinal defects were prepared just below the CEJ on each root surface. The amount of hydrogen peroxide that leached out was evaluated after 1, 7, and 14 days by spectrophotometer analysis. The results were analyzed using the ANOVA and Tukey's test. *Results*. Group 1 showed highest extra radicular diffusion, followed by group 3 and group 2, while group 4 showed the lowest mean extra radicular diffusion. *Conclusion*. Carbamide peroxide and sodium perborate-water mixture are the most suitable bleaching materials used for internal bleaching due to their low extra radicular diffusion of hydrogen peroxide.

1. Introduction

In modern society, greater emphasis is being placed on the cosmetic appearance of teeth [1]. Tooth discoloration is an aesthetic problem that may require treatment based on bleaching [2]. The causes of tooth discoloration are varied and complex but are usually classified as being either intrinsic or extrinsic in nature [3].

The main intrinsic factors are pulp hemorrhage, decomposition of pulp, bacteria and their products, tetracycline, pulp necrosis, intracanal medicaments, some endodontic filling materials, and metallic restorations, With the dissemination of blood components into the dentinal tubules caused by pulp extirpation or traumatically induced internal pulp bleeding, blood vessels are broken, promoting blood overflow into the pulp chamber [4]. Bleaching is considered as

a procedure, which involves lightening the color of a tooth through application of a chemical agent to oxidize the organic pigmentation in the tooth [5].

Correct diagnosis of the cause of tooth discolouration is important, as shade changes as a result of different etiologies may require different treatment strategies. Thus, teeth with healthy pulps may be bleached by the home technique, termed night guard vital bleaching, or vital tooth bleaching, in-office techniques, or an association of both. Root filled teeth may be treated by the walking bleach technique, thermocatalytic technique, or an association of techniques [6].

Inside outside bleaching at home using carbamide peroxide in bleaching gel is safe but there are chances of collection of debris and contamination in the open pulp chamber when tray is not in mouth. In-office laser bleaching is a dentist controlled bleaching and is safe but may cost the patient quite a bit and one needs to buy specific equipment for the same. Walking bleach procedure, on the other hand, can be undertaken in remotest places also as no special equipment is required and material cost is also minimal [7].

The walking bleach technique involves the application of a bleaching agent to the dentine of the pulp chamber between dental visits. A mixture of sodium perborate and distilled water has been extensively used as an effective agent for intracoronal bleaching. In order to enhance bleaching efficacy, 30% hydrogen peroxide (HP) was suggested as a substitute for water. A concentrated hydrogen peroxide (25–35%) is efficient for bleaching teeth with or without vital pulp. Another bleaching agent, 35–37% carbamide peroxide (CP), has emerged as a popular and effective agent for both in-office and intracoronal bleaching techniques [8]. One of the most important properties of a bleaching agent is its ability to allow penetration of the bleaching agent through the dentinal permeability; the deeper the penetration is, the more the pigment that causes chromatic alteration of the dental tissue can be reversed by the oxidation reaction [9].

However, laboratory studies have demonstrated that intracoronal hydrogen peroxide can diffuse through the root, and this diffusion is greater in the presence of cemental root defects. Animal studies have confirmed the association of intracoronal bleaching with cervical root resorption. There is speculation that diffusion of hydrogen ions from intracoronal bleaching agents may provide an acidic environment that is optimal for osteoclastic activity and bone resorption, resulting in external cervical root resorption over time [10].

Since dentinal tubules are oriented incisally, placing a protective base material at the lower level of the CEJ could reduce the leakage of hydrogen peroxide to the periodontal tissues. Deferent protective base materials have been compared. No significant differences were found between them [11].

This study aimed to compare by spectrophotometer analysis using potassium permanganate the extraradicular diffusion of hydrogen peroxide associated with intracoronal teeth bleaching by Opalescence Endo 35%, Opalescence PF 35%, sodium perborate with 30% hydrogen peroxide mixture, and sodium perborate with water mixture.

2. Materials and Methods

108 freshly extracted human single root canals (mandibular first premolars) for orthodontic reasons from patient less than 21 years old were collected with no sign of cracks or structural anomalies. A prior patient's consent was given to use their extracted teeth to conduct the study. Approval of Al-Azhar University Faculty of Oral and Dental Medicine, Egypt (under number 282/2009), was also obtained. The selected teeth were then immersed in 5.25% sodium hypochlorite for one hour to dissolve organic debris that was present on the external surface of the roots. Subsequently, they were cleaned with an ultrasonic scaler (satelec, Acteon, France) to remove calculus, discarding teeth with previous root canal treatment, internal resorption, and external resorption, localized or

diffuse calcifications. The selected teeth were stored in normal saline at room temperature until the time of use.

A standardized access cavity was made using a carbide bur loaded in a high speed handpiece. Each root canal orifice was enlarged using Gates-Glidden bur numbers 3 and 4 to enlarge root canals of the same size using 5.25% NaOCl solution for irrigation. The pulp tissues were removed with a barbed broach (Dentsply Maillefer, Ballaigues, Switzerland). Working length (WL) was determined by inserting a size 10 K-file (Dentsply Maillefer, Ballaigues, Switzerland) which was passively introduced into the canal until the tip was seen to exit at the major foramen. The real length of the canal was recorded and the working length calculated by subtracting 1 mm from this measurement.

The preparation was performed with a single rotary file, the WaveOne (Dentsply Maillefer, Ballaigues, Switzerland), and the preprogrammed motor (X-Smart Plus, Dentsply Maillefer, Ballaigues, Switzerland), using a specific movement of reciprocation: 170°CCW and 50°CW at a speed equivalent to 350 rpm.

Root canals were initially shaped with WaveOne primary reciprocating file (25/08) in the presence of 5.25% NaOCl as irrigant. The primary WaveOne file was used gently in a reciprocating, slow in- and out-pecking motion with short 2-3 mm amplitude strokes, to passively advance until it does not easily progress anymore. The shaping step was repeated until the coronal two-thirds of the canal has been prepared. The working length and canal patency were confirmed and then the primary file is carried to the full working length in one or more passes.

A larger WaveOne file 40/08 was carried to working length to fully shape and finish the preparation. The finished shape is confirmed in which the apical flutes of the file are loaded with dentin and a gauging 40/02 hand file is snugged at length. The apical foramen of each root was sealed with wax during instrumentation to prevent irrigating solutions from passing through the apical foramen. During instrumentation, the canals were irrigated with 2 mL of 5.25% NaOCl solution using a plastic syringe with 30-gauge closed-end needle (Hawe Max-I-probe, Hawe Neos, Bioggio, Switzerland). The needle was inserted within 1 to 2 mm of the working length. Then the root canals were dried by size 40/08 WaveOne paper point. Root canals are obturated with size 40/08 WaveOne gutta-percha using ProRoot Endo Sealer (Dentsply Maillefer, Ballaigues, Switzerland).

To simulate standardized breaks in the cemental covering, four cemental dentinal defects were prepared just below the CEJ on each root surface, mesial, distal, buccal, and lingual aspects [10]. The hemispherical defects (diameter 1.0 mm, depth 0.5 mm) were created using a round diamond bur (diameter 1.0 mm) in a high speed handpiece. The smear layer created in the defects was removed with 15% EDTA and then thoroughly washed with distilled water. The apical two-thirds of the root surface was coated with a double layer of a nail varnish to seal potential superficial defects as in Figure 1.

2.1. Specimen's Grouping. The prepared specimens were then divided randomly into four groups ($n = 27$) according to the beaching materials used. Each main group was subdivided

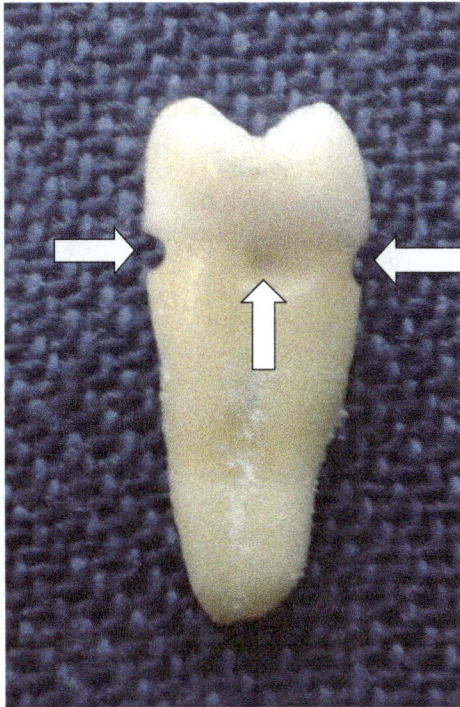

FIGURE 1: A photograph showing simulated defects below CEJ.

FIGURE 2: A schematic diagram showing KMnO$_4$ having a standard spectrum (absorbance 0.871 A) at wavelength 525 nm.

into three subgroups (n = 9) according to the time of extraradicular hydrogen peroxide diffusion measurements at 1, 7, and 14 days.

2.1.1. Group 1 (Opalescence Endo 35%). Opalescence Endo (Ultradent Products, South Jordan, UT, USA) is a 35% hydrogen peroxide specially formulated gel for the "walking" bleach technique (pH 5).

2.1.2. Group 2 (Opalescence PF 35%). Opalescence PF 35% (Ultradent Products, South Jordan, UT, USA) is 35% carbamide peroxide, 0.5% potassium nitrate, and 0.11% weight to weight (1100 ppm) fluoride ion. It is clear, high-viscosity, and sticky (pH 6.5).

2.1.3. Group 3 (Sodium Perborate-30% Hydrogen Peroxide Mixture). There is a mixture of sodium perborate (Degussa, Hanau, Germany) and 30% hydrogen peroxide (in the ratio, 1 g of powder : 0.5 mL of liquid) (pH 7.1).

2.1.4. Group 4 (Sodium Perborate-Water Mixture). There is a mixture of sodium perborate (Degussa, Hanau, Germany) and distilled water (in the ratio, 1 g of powder: 0.5 mL of distilled water) (pH 9.7).

2.2. Bleaching Procedure. The root filling in the coronal pulp chamber was removed to 2 mm below the facial cementoenamel junction. A barrier placement of 2 mm layer of glass-ionomer cement (Ketac-Molar, 3 M ESPE, St. Paul, MN, USA) was placed over the gutta-percha [12]. A pellet of cotton was placed in the chamber; it was sealed temporarily with Cavit

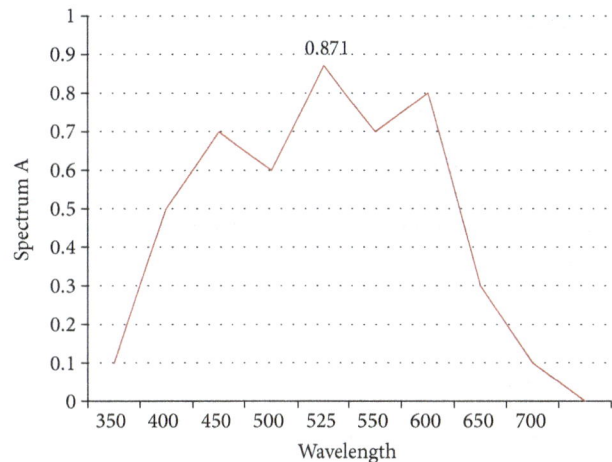

(3 M ESPE, St. Paul, MN, USA). After 24 hours, the temporary filling and the cotton pellet were removed completely.

The walls of the access cavity were cleaned of any residue using a small carbide bur followed by thorough rinsing with 2 mL of 5.25% NaOCl. The bleaching material of each group was placed in the pulp chamber and the access cavity of each specimen sealed temporarily with Cavit.

Each tooth was suspended in a plastic vial of 3 mL distilled water using laboratory sealing film Parafilm (Parafilm M, Neenah, WI, USA). The sealing film was cut to fit each tooth at the level of the CEJ and stabilized with sticky wax to achieve a tight seal and stored in an incubator at 37°C and 100% relative humidity during 14 days of bleaching; the bleaching materials were changed at 7 days, and the amount of hydrogen peroxide that leached out into the distilled water was evaluated after 1, 7, and 14 days.

3. Extraradicular Hydrogen Peroxide Diffusion Measurement

In this study we used titration method of permanganate and hydrogen peroxide according to the following equation [13]

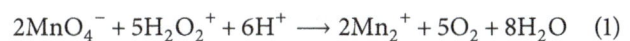

$$2MnO_4^- + 5H_2O_2^+ + 6H^+ \longrightarrow 2Mn_2^+ + 5O_2 + 8H_2O \quad (1)$$

The pink color of permanganate would be changed when reacted with peroxides; the color disappears according to the concentration of peroxide. The reaction is fast and does not need time or temperature for progression. The amount of radicular peroxide was measured using the UV-visible spectrophotometer (SpectraMax 1601, Molecular Devices Corp., Sunnyvale, CA, USA) at a wavelength of 480 nm (at room temperature), utilizing the potassium permanganate (KMnO$_4$) as peroxide indicator (redox reaction) and (KMnO$_4$) having a standard spectrum (absorbance 0.871 A) at wavelength 525 nm (Figure 2).

4. Results

4.1. After 1 Day. Group 1 (Opalescence Endo 35%) showed the statistically significantly highest extraradicular diffusion (0.168 ± 0.049) $P < 0.05$. There was no statistically significant difference between Group 2 (Opalescence PF 35%), Group 3 (sodium perborate-30% hydrogen peroxide mixture), and Group 4 (sodium perborate-water mixture) which showed the statistically significantly lowest mean extraradicular diffusion (Groups 2 and 4 showed no extraradicular diffusion).

4.2. After 7 Days. Group 1 (Opalescence Endo 35%) showed highest extraradicular diffusion (0.482 ± 0.051). This was followed by Group 3 (sodium perborate-30% hydrogen peroxide mixture (0.375 ± 0.049)) and Group 2 (Opalescence PF 35% (0.210 ± 0.125)) while Group 4 (sodium perborate-water mixture) showed the lowest mean extraradicular diffusion (0.141 ± 0.040). Statistically there was no statistically significant difference between Group 1 and Group 3 while there was statistically significant difference between the other tested groups. Meanwhile there was no statistically significant difference between Groups 2 and 4.

4.3. After 14 Days. Group 1 (Opalescence Endo 35%) showed highest extraradicular diffusion (0.865 ± 0.061). This was followed by Group 3 (sodium perborate-30% hydrogen peroxide mixture (0.743 ± 0.060)) and Group 2 (Opalescence PF 35% (0.430 ± 0.30)) while Group 4 (sodium perborate-water mixture) showed the lowest mean extraradicular diffusion (0.315 ± 0.046). Statistically there was no statistically significant difference between Group 1 and Group 3 while there was statistically significant difference between the other tested groups. Meanwhile there was no statistically significant difference between Groups 2 and 4.

4.4. On the Other Hand. All bleaching material used in this study recorded statistically significant increase in mean extraradicular diffusion after 7 and 14 days (Table 1).

5. Discussion

The current study employed the use of four different bleaching agents with intracoronal teeth bleaching and they are 35% hydrogen peroxide (Opalescence Endo), 35% carbamide peroxide (Opalescence PF 35%), sodium perborate with 30% hydrogen peroxide mixture, and sodium perborate with water mixture.

This study has been done to investigate the effect of these four bleaching agents on extraradicular hydrogen peroxide diffusion after one and seven days and fourteen days by potassium permanganate ($KMnO_4$) as peroxide indicator. Understanding the chemistry of the active ingredient of the bleaching agent would be useful.

Hydrogen peroxide (H_2O_2) is the main whitening agent employed. It is a thermally unstable free radical with a low molecular weight, which penetrates the enamel and dentin through diffusion. Complex molecules of organic pigments in the tissues are broken down into simpler hydrophilic molecules through an oxidation reduction reaction by the action of perhydroxyl ions originating from the degradation of H_2O_2. These simpler molecules are easily removed from the dental tissue when being in contact with water, thereby providing the desired whitening effect [14, 15].

Carbamide peroxide ($CH_4N_2O \cdot H_2O_2$) decomposes to 1/3 hydrogen peroxide and 2/3 urea [16]. The urea can theoretically be further decomposed to carbon dioxide and ammonia, which elevates the pH to facilitate the bleaching procedure further. This can be explained by the fact that, in a basic solution, lower activation energy is required for the formation of free radicals from hydrogen peroxide, and the reaction rate is higher [17].

Sodium perborate is an oxidizing agent available as a powder. It is stable when being dry; however, in the presence of acid, warm air, or water, it breaks down to form sodium metaborate, hydrogen peroxide, and nascent oxygen. Sodium perborate is easier to control and safer than concentrated hydrogen peroxide solutions [18].

This study compared extraradicular hydrogen peroxide diffusion of various bleaching agents after one and seven days and fourteen days. Previous studies of peroxide penetration have utilized different time periods [11, 19].

In the present study, single rooted mandibular premolars extracted for orthodontic reasons from patients below 21 years were used. They were selected because of the availability of such teeth and most reported cases of cervical root resorption associated with intracoronal bleaching were in young patients. It is probable that the wide and patent dentinal tubules in young teeth would favor ionic diffusion of the bleaching agent through dentine [10].

The walking bleach technique requires a sound coronal seal around the access cavity after application of bleaching paste in the chamber. It can be achieved with GIC, resin composite, or compomer to ensure its effectiveness and to avoid leakage of bleaching agent into the oral cavity. In addition, a good seal also prevents recontamination of the dentin with microorganisms and reduces the risk of renewed staining [18].

In the present study, although the teeth were not totally immersed in the distilled water, the access openings were protected in order to prevent the leakage of bleaching agents through this area. Thus, the diffusion of the bleaching material occurred only through the cervical dentin tubules, exposed by CJE defects. It is important to emphasize the difficulty to obtain teeth with similar CJE characteristics, which lead some researchers to create artificial defects along the external cervical area to standardize the diffusion of bleaching agents [20].

In this study, a 2 mm layer of glass-ionomer cement was applied over the canal filling due to its effectiveness in preventing penetration of 30% hydrogen peroxide solution into the root canal. Thus, the use of this material as a base during bleaching presents the additional advantage that it can be left in place after bleaching and can serve as a base for the final restoration [12].

The result of this study showed that after 1 day, Group 1 (*Opalescence Endo 35%*) showed the statistically significantly highest extraradicular diffusion $P < 0.05$. There was no statistically significant difference between group 2 (Opalescence

TABLE 1: The means, standard deviation (SD) values, and results of ANOVA and Tukey's test for comparison of extraradicular diffusion between four groups.

Time	Group 1 (Opalescence Endo 35%)		Group 2 (Opalescence PF 35%)		Group 3 (sodium perborate-30% hydrogen peroxide mixture)		Group 4 (sodium perborate-water mixture)		P value
	Mean	S.D	Mean	S.D	Mean	S.D	Mean	S.D	
1 day	0.168^c	0.049	0^d	0	0.068^d	0.021	0^d	0	* < 0.001
7 days	0.482^b	0.051	0.210^c	0.125	0.375^b	0.049	0.141^c	0.040	
14 days	0.865^a	0.061	0.430^b	0.030	0.743^a	0.060	0.315^b	0.046	

*Significant at $P \leq 0.05$; means with different letters are statistically significantly different according to Tukey's test.

PF 35%), group 3 (sodium perborate-30% hydrogen peroxide mixture), and group 4 (sodium perborate-water mixture) after 7 and 14 days. Group 1 showed highest extraradicular diffusion, followed by group 3 and group 2, while group 4 showed the lowest mean extraradicular diffusion.

The probable reasons for the results obtained in the present study could be [21] as follows. (a) As 35% carbamide peroxide decomposes on contact with moisture to yield approximately only 12% hydrogen peroxide. (b) It could be because of the fact that carbamide peroxide does not diffuse through dentine as fast as hydrogen peroxide. (c) With the rise in pH aided by the resultant ammonia from the carbamide peroxide, the deionization of the hydrogen peroxide is facilitated. Therefore, little unreacted hydrogen peroxide is left to diffuse through the root dentin into the extraradicular environment. These results were in agreement with that of Gökay et al. [22] who stated that higher peroxide penetration occurred with the 30% HP-SP mixture than with the CP bleaching gels, and the 37% CP group also promoted greater peroxide penetration than the other CP groups ($P < 0.05$). There was no statistically significant difference between 10% and 17% CP groups ($P > 0.05$). Lee et al. [10] stated that carbamide peroxide had very low levels of extraradicular diffusion of HP. Shivanna and Gupta [21] concluded that radicular peroxide penetration from carbamide peroxide gels is less than sodium perborate-hydrogen peroxide mixture, therefore carrying less risk of postbleaching external root resorption.

Heithersay analyzed cervical resorption cases and reported that 24.1% were caused by orthodontic treatment, 15.1% by dental trauma, 5.1% by surgery (e.g., transplantation or periodontal surgery), and 3.9% by intracoronal bleaching. A combination of internal bleaching with one of the other causes is responsible for 13.6% of cervical resorption cases. The combination of bleaching and history of trauma is the most important predisposing factor for cervical resorption [23].

6. Conclusion

Carbamide peroxide and sodium perborate-water mixture are the most suitable bleaching materials used for internal bleaching due to its low extraradicular diffusion of hydrogen peroxide.

Conflict of Interests

The authors declare that there is no conflict of interests regarding the publication of this paper.

References

[1] W. C. de Souza-Zaroni, E. B. Lopes, J. C. Ciccone-Nogueira, and R. C. S. P. Silva, "Clinical comparison between the bleaching efficacy of 37% peroxide carbamide gel mixed with sodium perborate with established intracoronal bleaching agent," *Oral Surgery, Oral Medicine, Oral Pathology, Oral Radiology, and Endodontology*, vol. 107, no. 2, pp. e43–e47, 2009.

[2] J. Kaneko, S. Inoue, S. Kawakami, and H. Sano, "Bleaching effect of sodium percarbonate on discolored pulpless teeth in vitro," *Journal of Endodontics*, vol. 26, no. 1, pp. 25–28, 2000.

[3] M. Addy, J. Moran, R. Newcombe, and P. Warren, "The comparative tea staining potential of phenolic, chlorhexidine and anti-adhesive mouthrinses," *Journal of Clinical Periodontology*, vol. 22, no. 12, pp. 923–928, 1995.

[4] M. C. Valera, C. H. R. Camargo, C. A. T. Carvalho, L. D. de Oliveira, S. E. A. Camargo, and C. M. Rodrigues, "Effectiveness of carbamide peroxide and sodium perborate in non-vital discolored teeth," *Journal of Applied Oral Science*, vol. 17, no. 3, pp. 254–261, 2009.

[5] A. Feiz, B. Barekatain, S. Khalesi, N. Khalighinejad, H. Badrian, and E. J. Swift, "Effect of several bleaching agents on teeth stained with a resin-based sealer," *International Endodontic Journal*, vol. 47, no. 1, pp. 3–9, 2014.

[6] K. C. K. Yui, J. R. Rodrigues, M. N. G. Mancini, I. Balducci, and S. E. P. Gonçalves, "Ex vivo evaluation of the effectiveness of bleaching agents on the shade alteration of blood-stained teeth," *International Endodontic Journal*, vol. 41, no. 6, pp. 485–492, 2008.

[7] R. Anuradha and G. Manisha, "Walking bleach-still relevant; a review with—a case report," *Indian Journal of Dental Sciences*, vol. 1, pp. 32–37, 2009.

[8] V. Cavalli, M. S. Shinohara, W. Ambrose, F. M. Malafaia, P. N. R. Pereira, and M. Giannini, "Influence of intracoronal bleaching agents on the ultimate strength and ultrastructure morphology of dentine," *International Endodontic Journal*, vol. 42, no. 7, pp. 568–575, 2009.

[9] L. D. Carrasco, I. C. Fröner, S. A. M. Corona, and J. D. Pécora, "Effect of internal bleaching agents on dentinal permeability of non-vital teeth: quantitative assessment," *Dental Traumatology*, vol. 19, no. 2, pp. 85–89, 2003.

[10] G. P. Lee, M. Y. Lee, S. O. Y. Lum, R. S. C. Poh, and K.-C. Lim, "Extraradicular diffusion of hydrogen peroxide and pH changes associated with intracoronal bleaching of discoloured teeth using different bleaching agents," *International Endodontic Journal*, vol. 37, no. 7, pp. 500–506, 2004.

[11] T. Lambrianidis, A. Kapalas, and M. Mazinis, "Effect of calcium hydroxide as a supplementary barrier in the radicular penetration of hydrogen peroxide during intracoronal bleaching in vitro," *International Endodontic Journal*, vol. 35, no. 12, pp. 985–990, 2002.

[12] I. Rotstein, D. Zyskind, I. Lewinstein, and N. Bamberger, "Effect of different protective base materials on hydrogen peroxide leakage during intracoronal bleaching in vitro," *Journal of Endodontics*, vol. 18, no. 3, pp. 114–117, 1992.

[13] L. Campanella, R. Roversi, M. P. Sammartino, and M. Tomassetti, "Hydrogen peroxide determination in pharmaceutical formulations and cosmetics using a new catalase biosensor," *Journal of Pharmaceutical and Biomedical Analysis*, vol. 18, no. 1-2, pp. 105–116, 1998.

[14] M. Pinto, C. H. de Godoy, C. Bortoletto et al., "Tooth whitening with hydrogen peroxide in adolescents: study protocol for a randomized controlled trial," *Trials*, vol. 15, article 395, 2014.

[15] M. M. Pinto, S. K. Bussadori, A. C. Guedes-Pinto, M. A. Rego, and P. Eberson, "Esthetic alternative for fluorosis blemishes with the usage of a dual bleaching system based on hydrogen peroxide at 35%," *Journal of Clinical Pediatric Dentistry*, vol. 28, pp. 143–146, 2004.

[16] A. Baltzer and V. Kaufmann-Jinoian, "Shading of ceramic crowns using digital tooth shade matching devices," *International Journal of Computerized Dentistry*, vol. 8, no. 2, pp. 129–152, 2005.

[17] G. S. Heithersay, S. W. Dahlstrom, and P. D. Marin, "Incidence of invasive cervical resorption in bleached root-filled teeth," *Australian Dental Journal*, vol. 39, no. 2, pp. 82–87, 1994.

[18] G. Plotino, L. Buono, N. M. Grande, C. H. Pameijer, and F. Somma, "Nonvital tooth bleaching: a review of the literature and clinical procedures," *Journal of Endodontics*, vol. 34, no. 4, pp. 394–407, 2008.

[19] A. R. Benetti, M. C. Valera, M. N. G. Mancini, C. B. Miranda, and I. Balducci, "In vitro penetration of bleaching agents into the pulp chamber," *International Endodontic Journal*, vol. 37, no. 2, pp. 120–124, 2004.

[20] I. Rotstein, Y. Torek, and R. Misgav, "Effect of cementum defects on radicular penetration of 30% H_2O_2 during intracoronal bleaching," *Journal of Endodontics*, vol. 17, no. 5, pp. 230–233, 1991.

[21] V. Shivanna and K. Gupta, "A spectrophotometric analysis of radicular peroxide penetration after intracoronal bleaching using different concentrations of carbamide peroxide gels," *Endodontology*, vol. 24, pp. 99–103, 2012.

[22] O. Gökay, F. Ziraman, A. Ç. Asal, and O. M. Saka, "Radicular peroxide penetration from carbamide peroxide gels during intracoronal bleaching," *International Endodontic Journal*, vol. 41, no. 7, pp. 556–560, 2008.

[23] G. S. Heithersay, "Invasive cervical resorption following trauma," *Australian Endodontic Journal*, vol. 25, no. 2, pp. 79–85, 1999.

22

A Comparative Evaluation of Static Frictional Resistance Using Various Methods of Ligation at Different Time Intervals: An In Vitro Study

Amanpreet Singh Natt, Amandeep Kaur Sekhon, Sudhir Munjal, Rohit Duggal, Anup Holla, Prahlad Gupta, Piyush Gandhi, and Sahil Sarin

Dasmesh Institute of Research and Dental Sciences, Faridkot, Punjab, India

Correspondence should be addressed to Amanpreet Singh Natt; dramanpreetnatt@gmail.com

Academic Editor: Carlos A. Munoz-Viveros

Aim. To compare and evaluate the static frictional resistance offered by the four different types of ligation methods in both dry and wet conditions and at different durations when immersed in artificial saliva. *Material and Methods.* Alastik Easy to Tie modules, Super Slick Mini Stix elastomeric modules, Power "O" modules, and $0.009''$ Stainless Steel ligatures were used to compare the static friction using maxillary canine and premolar Preadjusted Edgewise brackets with $0.022'' \times 0.028''$ slot and $0.019'' \times 0.025''$ stainless steel wires. *Results.* The mean frictional resistance for Alastik modules was the lowest and that of Stainless Steel ligatures was found to be highest among the four groups compared and the difference among the four groups was statistically significant ($P < 0.005$). The mean static frictional resistance in all groups under dry conditions was lower than that under wet conditions. No statistical significant differences were found when the groups were compared at different time periods of immersion in artificial saliva. *Conclusion.* This study concludes that the Alastik modules showed the lowest mean static frictional forces compared to any other ligation method, though no significant difference was found for different time periods of immersion in the artificial saliva.

1. Introduction

The success of the straight wire appliance depends on the ability of orthodontic arch wire to slide freely through brackets and tube. During orthodontic tooth movement with sliding mechanics, a frictional force generated at the bracket/arch wire interface tends to impede the desired movement [1]. In clinical terms, the force applied must overcome this unknown frictional component and achieve the desired tooth movement.

Friction is an important factor in all forms of sliding mechanics such as space closure and canine retraction into an extraction site and in leveling and alignment where the wire must slide through the brackets and tubes. The nature of friction in orthodontics is multifactorial, derived from a multitude of both mechanical and biological factors. The method of ligation is an important contributor to the frictional force generated at the bracket/archwire interface. The new super

slick modules introduced by TP Orthodontics and Alastik modules introduced by 3M Unitek claim to reduce friction more than other ligation methods [2]. Magnitude of friction depends upon the amount of normal force pushing the two surfaces together which is decided by the method of ligation, the surface roughness, and the nature of materials from which the surfaces are made [3].

The dissipation of the orthodontic force due to resistance to sliding may vary from 12% to 60%. On the other hand, an excessive increase in orthodontic force to overcome frictional resistance of the anterior teeth may produce increased posterior anchorage loss [4]. Baker et al. [5] using an artificial saliva substitute stated that 15 to 19% reduction in friction was seen in wet state, while some of the other studies [6, 7] showed that the coefficient of friction in the wet state is increased. Saliva could have lubricous as well as adhesive behavior, depending on which archwire bracket combination was under consideration.

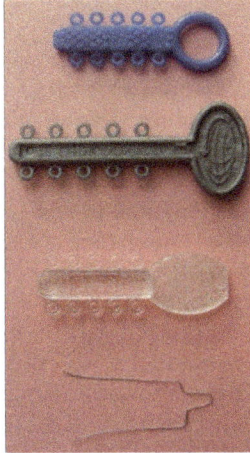

FIGURE 1: Four types of ligation materials used in the study.

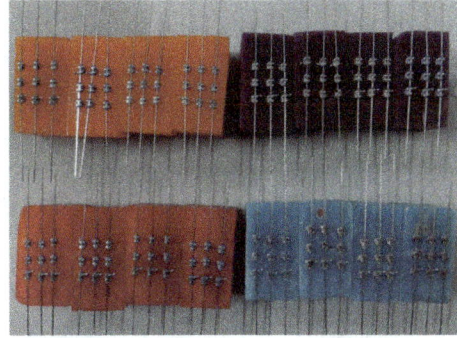

FIGURE 2: All custom made assemblies with different color coding of acrylic blocks.

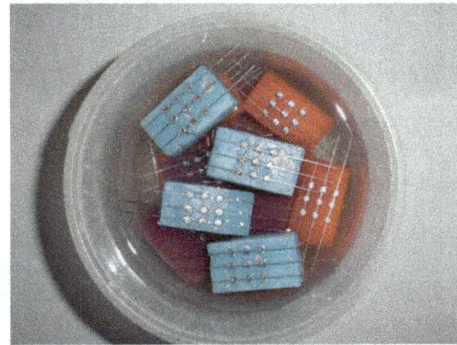

FIGURE 3: Custom made assemblies immersed in artificial saliva.

So the aim of the present in vitro study was to compare and evaluate the frictional resistance offered by the Alastik Easy to Tie modules, Super Slick Mini Stix elastomeric modules, Power "O" modules, and 0.009″ Stainless Steel ligatures for free sliding of stainless steel arch wires in stainless steel bracket slot in both dry and wet conditions.

2. Materials and Methods

The setup included the maxillary right canine and premolar Preadjusted Edgewise brackets with 0.022″ × 0.028″ slot and was of Roth Prescription (Ormco Corporation, Orange, CA). 0.019″× 0.025″ stainless steel wires (Libral Traders, New Delhi, India) of 5 cm length were used to test friction during sliding movement in the bracket slots. In order to test the friction in wet state, the artificial saliva was prepared at Rajiv Academy of Pharmacy, Mathura, as described by Fusayama Meyer [8].

Four types of ligation materials (Figure 1) used in the present study for ligating the wire to the bracket slots are mentioned as follows:

(a) GROUP I: Alastik Easy to Tie modules (3M Unitek, Minnesota, USA),

(b) GROUP II: Super Slick Mini Stix modules (TP Orthodontic, LaPorte, Indiana, USA),

(c) GROUP III: Power "O" modules (Ormco Corporation, Orange, CA),

(d) GROUP IV: Stainless Steel ligature, 0.009″ (Libral Traders, New Delhi, India).

3. Sample

156 stainless steel right maxillary canine and premolar PAE brackets (39 brackets for each group) were used. Sample size consisted of 5 bracket-wire-ligation assemblies, each assembly consisting of 3 bracket-wire-ligation setups for each of the four groups tested (Figure 2). Each assembly was soaked in artificial saliva for 1 hour, 24 hours, 15 days, and

1 month before the test run and one sample was tested in dry condition (Figure 3). The acrylic blocks of different groups were color coded as per time intervals as described in the following:

immediate (dry): white color;

1 hour: blue color;

24 hours: orange color;

15 days: violent color;

1 month: red color.

As 3 test readings were taken in each group for a particular time period, a total of sixty test runs were performed on the universal testing machine.

4. Methodology

A custom-made assembly was fabricated which consisted of acrylic block (2″ × 4″) prepared in a metal housing of the same dimensions (Figure 4). Once set, the acrylic block was removed and three sets of brackets-arch wire-ligation setup were bonded onto the acrylic block using an instant adhesive (Fevi Kwik, Pidilite Industries Ltd., Mumbai, India). Three right maxillary PAE brackets (canine, 1st premolar, and 2nd premolar) were bonded at 8 mm intervals and 5 cm long stainless steel straight length 0.019″ × 0.025″ wire was secured with the desired mode for ligation. This wire dimension was chosen because it is the recommended size for

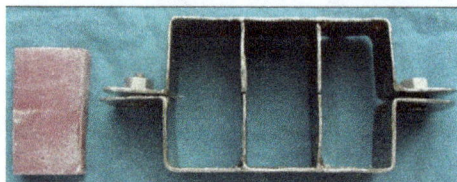

FIGURE 4: Metal housing in which acrylic block is fabricated ($2'' \times 4''$).

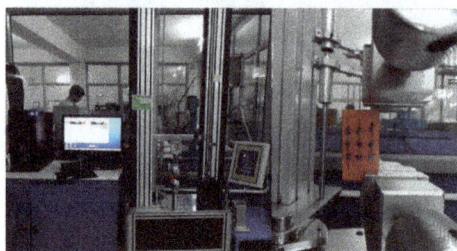

FIGURE 5: Custom made assembly mounted on the machine; test wire is being pulled in upward direction (universal testing machine, Blue Star, model number HZ 1004).

sliding mechanics with $0.022''$ slot brackets which were used in the present study.

The wires were secured to test brackets with the elastomeric modules and the preformed ligatures (prepared with ligature forming plier) using artery forceps. The Stainless Steel ligatures were fully tied with the wire. The static friction between bracket and arch wire was measured with a universal testing machine (Blue Star Testing Service, India, Figure 5), with a crosshead speed of 20 mm/min as done by Hain et al. [2, 11] and Chimenti et al. [10]. The lower end of the assembly was attached to the lower crosshead of the testing machine. The wire was pulled in a vertical direction by the upper crosshead of the machine (Figure 5) till the 5 mm span of the wire was completely pulled out through the brackets. The force to overcome resistance to initiate movement of the wire was measured. This maximum frictional force at initial movement was taken to represent the peak static frictional resistance.

Values for peak static frictional forces (in grams) were recorded for each test run, from the electronic monitor display in the universal testing machine (Blue Star, model number HZ 1004) for each assembly.

5. Statistical Analysis

All the statistical tests were carried out with the SPSS software (IBM, Version 17, USA) using ANOVA and post hoc Tukey's test. Analysis of variance (ANOVA) was used to determine the variance in between the different groups with different ligation methods. A post hoc Tukey's test was then done to compare each type of ligation with respect to the others in each group and at different time periods. The power of the study was kept at .80 and the error of the study is 5%.

6. Results

Table 1 shows the mean static frictional resistance values with the standard deviations in each of the four groups at different time intervals, which were calculated using the one-way analysis of variance (ANOVA). It was seen that the mean static frictional resistance in all groups was lower in dry conditions sample as compared to wet conditions in all the time intervals. There were no statistical significant differences among four groups at the different time periods of immersion in the artificial saliva.

The mean static frictional resistance for Group I (Alastik modules) was the lowest and that of Group IV (Stainless Steel ligatures) was the highest among the four groups compared in wet conditions and the difference in the frictional resistance offered by the four groups was statistically significant ($P < 0.005$). Thus these results showed clear differences between the frictional resistance values generated with the different ligation methods.

A post hoc Tukey's test revealed that the Alastik and Super Slick modules showed statistically significant differences from the other ligation methods. The Alastik modules lowered the frictional resistance to an even greater extent than the Super Slick modules, Power "O" modules, and Stainless Steel ligatures. The coated Super Slick modules showed significantly lowered frictional resistance than the Power "O" modules and Stainless Steel ligatures. Table 2 showed that the significant differences were found in the friction values between the immediate and 24-hour time periods in case of Group I (Alastik modules). The Group II (Super Slick modules) showed that no significant difference was seen in the different time periods of immersion. Table 3 showed the significant difference in the frictional values between the immediate and 1-month time periods in case of Group III (Power "O" modules). These statics showed significant differences for immediate sample in all groups except in Group II (Super Slick modules) and Group III (Power "O" modules) which showed a nonsignificant difference in values.

The bar diagram in Figure 6 shows the mean static friction with standard deviations between the groups at different time periods using ANOVA test and the bar diagram in Figure 7 depicts the mean static friction with standard deviations within the groups at different time periods.

7. Discussion

Many factors are involved within the bracket-arch wire-ligature system, which could influence the development of friction during sliding mechanics. This study was designed with the aim of standardizing as many of these factors as possible, so that the effects of different types of ligation methods could be objectively determined. Static friction was studied rather than the kinetic friction, since orthodontic tooth movement consists of a series of tipping and uprighting movements [4]. It is to be remembered that force required for overcoming static friction is greater than the force needed to sustain uniform sliding motion.

The results of this study showed that the 45° angulated Alastik Easy to Tie modules produced the lowest mean static

TABLE 1: Comparison of mean static friction between different groups (ANOVA test).

	Time	Mean	Standard deviation	F-ratio	P value	NS/S
	Immediate (dry)	270.00	50.00000			
	1 hour	370.00	36.05551			
GP I	24 hours	336.67	32.14550	3.497	**0.049**	**S**
	15 days	340.00	45.82576			
	1 month	400.00	55.67764			
	Immediate (dry)	443.33	30.55050			
	1 hour	450.00	52.91503			
GP II	24 hours	420.00	79.37254	2.060	0.161	NS
	15 days	476.67	32.14550			
	1 month	533.33	51.31601			
	Immediate (dry)	526.67	30.55050			
	1 hour	686.67	65.06407			
GP III	24 hours	780.00	141.06736	4.488	**0.025**	**S**
	15 days	690.00	26.45751			
	1 month	710.00	30.55050			
	Immediate (dry)	646.67	45.09250			
	1 hour	743.33	65.06407			
GP IV	24 hours	843.33	159.47832	2.605	0.100	NS
	15 days	780.00	26.45751			
	1 month	863.33	55.67764			

TABLE 2: Post hoc Tukey's test for Group I (Alastik).

Time	Immediate (dry)	1 hour	24 hours	15 days	1 month
Immediate (dry)	—	NS	**S**	NS	NS
1 hour	NS	—	NS	NS	NS
24 hours	**S**	NS	—	NS	NS
15 days	NS	NS	NS	—	NS
1 month	NS	NS	NS	NS	—

S: significant difference ($P < 0.05$); NS: nonsignificant difference.

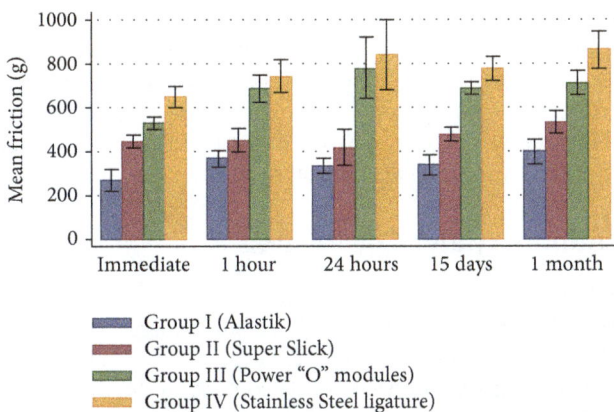

FIGURE 6: The bar diagram showing the mean static friction with standard deviations between the groups at different time periods (ANOVA test).

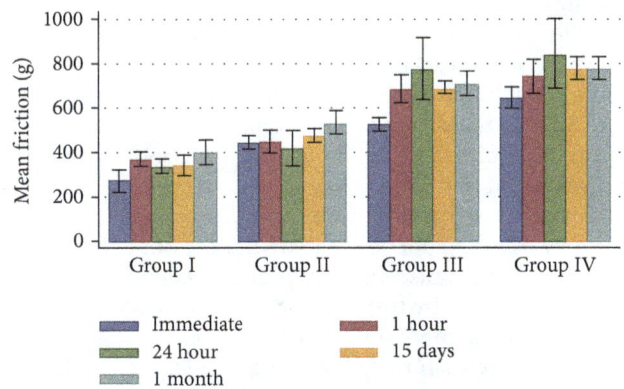

FIGURE 7: The bar diagram showing the mean static friction with standard deviations within the groups at different time periods (ANOVA test).

friction. This result compares favourably with the results of Khambay et al. [9, 13] and Arun and Vaz [14] who found that

Alastik Easy to Tie modules had the lowest mean frictional forces. A possible explanation could be that the bend in the module may prevent the entire module from contacting

TABLE 3: Post hoc Tukey's test for Group III (Power "O" modules).

Time	Immediate (dry)	1 hour	24 hours	15 days	1 month
Immediate (dry)	—	NS	NS	NS	**S**
1 hour	NS	—	NS	NS	NS
24 hours	NS	NS	—	NS	NS
15 days	NS	NS	NS	—	NS
1 month	**S**	NS	NS	NS	—

S: significant difference ($P < 0.05$); NS: nonsignificant difference.

the wire. Even though the Alastik module seats the wire firmly into the bracket slot, the incomplete contact between the module and the wire may allow easier sliding [9], but the results of this study were in contrast to the study by Hain et al. [11] who found that Super Slick Mini Stix modules had lower mean frictional values than Alastik modules.

The results of present study also revealed that the Super Slick Mini Stix modules also exhibited lower mean frictional forces than the Power "O" modules and Stainless Steel ligatures but higher than the Alastik modules. This compares favourably with the studies of Griffith et al. [1], Khambay et al. [9, 13], and Arun and Vaz [14]. But the results are in contrast with the study of Hain et al. [2, 11] who found that Super Slick Mini Stix modules have low frictional values compared to Alastik modules. This was attributed to the presence of highly lubricious polymer coating, based on Metafasix technology, wherein a water insoluble coating has been covalently bonded to the ligatures, E-chains, and separators causing a slippery surface when moistened reducing the friction as much by 70% as claimed by the manufacturer. Preangulated Alastik modules showed lower mean frictional force when compared with the Super Slick modules, though the difference was statistically not significant, implying that both the elastomeric ligatures were equally efficient in reducing frictional resistance when compared with Power "O" modules and Stainless Steel ligatures.

When comparing the results of Power "O" modules, it showed lower mean frictional force than the stainless steel ligatures but higher than the Alastik modules and Super Slick Mini Stix modules. These results compare favourably with the results of Griffith et al. [1], Hain et al. [11], Gandini et al. [12], and Arun and Vaz [14] but are in contrast with the results of the Khambay et al. [9, 13] who showed that regular modules have low frictional forces compared to the Super Slick Mini Stix modules because these modules need to remove the saliva film as the wire translates beneath them during sliding.

It is seen that the Stainless Steel ligatures had higher mean frictional force than the Alastik, Super Slick Mini Stix, and Power "O" modules. These results are in contrast with the studies of Hain et al. [2] and Khambay et al. [9, 13] who showed the lowest mean frictional force by the stainless steel ligature compared to any other ligation method. A possible explanation for this might be that in our study we fully ligated the Stainless Steel ligature with the wire but Khambay et al. [9, 13] and Bazakidou et al. [15] gave seven full turns of Spencer-Wells clips/Mathieu ligature tying plier after the ligature was placed and was ready for tightening. Rajendran

et al. [8] in their study initially fully tightened the ligature and then unwound it by 3 turns, but we found that unwinding the ligature by 3 turns would make the ligature very loose. In the present study, the value of frictional resistance offered by the stainless steel ligature was high as it may have been tighter than that done in other studies.

The effect of lubrication is debatable and the increased or decreased frictional resistance cannot be attributed to the lubricant used with any certainty [16, 17]. This study indicates that, with all types of the ligation materials, the static friction was increased in the wet conditions relative to the dry conditions. The results compare favourably with the studies of Edwards et al. [18], Griffith et al. [1], Stannard et al. [7], and Thorstenson and Kusy [19]. It could be due to the fact that these modules have to remove the saliva film as the wire translates beneath them during sliding.

Though it is not possible to reproduce and standardize the exact oral environmental conditions that influence the friction clinically, an attempt has been made to test friction at different time periods immersed artificial saliva with different ligation methods. The study shows that the saliva immersion increased the friction in wet conditions as compared to the dry condition but no significant difference was seen in each group between different immersion periods.

Difficulty in comparing the results of this study with the previous studies of the different elastomeric modules could be due to the differences in the methodologies and Table 4 shows the comparison of methodologies between the present and the previous studies. However, more research is needed to enhance our understanding of different methods of ligation and its effects on various bracket systems.

8. Summary and Conclusions

(1) The Alastik Easy to Tie modules showed the lowest mean static frictional forces compared to any other ligation method. This finding could be attributed to the bend in the module which prevents the entire module contacting the wire.

(2) The Super Slick Mini Stix elastomeric modules showed lower mean static frictional forces than the Power "O" modules and Stainless Steel ligatures but higher than the Alastik Easy to Tie modules. Though there was no statistically significant difference between the two. This finding could be attributed to the surface characteristics of these modules.

(3) The Power "O" modules showed lower mean static frictional forces than the Stainless Steel ligatures but higher

TABLE 4: Comparison of mean static friction found in other studies quoted and results obtained in the present study. A comparative evaluation of static frictional resistance.

Author	Type of bracket-wire used in the study and method of ligature placement	Type of ligation	Dry or wet medium	Mean static friction	
Stannard et al. [7], 1986	Stainless steel or Teflon coated brackets with $0.017 \times 0.025''$ SS, TMA, NiTi, and Co-Cr wires Placement of ligature not mentioned	Stainless Steel ligatures	Both	*Dry* 739 g SS	*Wet* 855 g SS
Baker et al. [5], 1987	PAE SS Brackets with $0.018''$, $0.020''$, and $0.018 \times 0.025''$ SS wires Placement of ligature not mentioned	$0.010''$ polyurethane ligatures	Both	142 g in saliva 170 g in dry 166 g in glycerine	
Dowling et al., 1998	Standard twin and mini twin brackets with $0.018 \times 0.025''$ wire Placement of ligature with an Orthopli 018R forceps	Elastomeric modules round A-grey, B-clear, C-orange, D-fluoride impregnated, rectangular E-grey	Both	*Dry* A-1.05 N B-1.06 N C-0.91 N D-1.16 N E-1.46 N	*Wet* A-1.25 N B-0.80 N C-1.22 N D-1.07 N E- 1.15 N
Khambay et al. [9], 2005	Self-ligating Damon II and PAE SS brackets with 0.017×0.025 SS and TMA and $0.019 \times 0.025''$ SS and TMA Placement of ligature with straight shooter gun	Elastomeric modules-, purple, grey, Alastik or Super Slick, and $0.09''$ SS ligature	Wet	*$0.019 \times 0.025''$ bracket* SS ligature-0.45 N Alastik-0.50 N Purple-0.56 N Grey-0.84 N Super Slick-0.98 N	
Chimenti et al. [10], 2005	$0.022''$ PAE SS brackets with $0.019 \times 0.025''$ SS wire Placement of ligature not mentioned	Elastic modules (small, medium, large, clear lubricated, and grey lubricated)	Dry	Small modules: 533.16 g Medium modules: 508.80 g Large modules: 611.14 g Clear lubricated: 392.44 g Gray lubricated: 350.38 g	
Hain et al. [11], 2006	Victory, speed, and Damon II brackets with $0.019 \times 0.025''$ SS wire Placement of ligature not mentioned	Regular uncoated, Super Slick, conventional silver, Alastik, Sili-Ties	Wet	Regular uncoated: 2 N Super Slick: 0.96 N Conventional silver: 2.80 N Alastik: 1.87 N Sili-Ties: 1.81 N	
Gandini et al. [12], 2008	SmartClip and conventional SS bracket with $0.014''$ NiTi and $0.019 \times 0.025''$ SS wire Placement of ligature not mentioned	Conventional elastomeric ligature (CEL) and unconventional elastomeric ligature (UEL)	Dry	*$0.019 \times 0.025''$ SS* CEL-177.4 g UEL-1.2 g	
Present study, 2014	$0.022''$ PAE SS bracket with $0.019 \times 0.025''$ SS wire Placement of ligature with artery forceps	Grp. I: Alastik Easy to Tie Grp. II: Super Slick Mini Stix Grp. IIII: Power "O" modules Grp. IV: $0.009''$ Stainless Steel ligature	Both dry and wet mediums at different time intervals	*Dry* Grp. I: 270 g Grp. II: 443 g Grp. III: 526 g Grp. IV: 646 g	*Wet* Grp. I: 343 g Grp. II: 464 g Grp. III: 678 g Grp. IV: 775 g

than the Alastik Easy to Tie modules and Super Slick Mini Stix modules.

(4) The Stainless Steel ligatures showed the highest mean static frictional forces compared to any other ligation method. This finding could be attributed to the tight ligation by these ligatures with the wire.

(5) This study showed that, with all four types of the ligation methods, the static friction was increased in the wet conditions relative to the dry condition, though no significant difference was found for the static frictional resistance for different time periods of immersion in the artificial saliva.

Conflict of Interests

The authors declare that there is no conflict of interests regarding the publication of this paper.

References

[1] H. S. Griffth, M. Sherrif, and A. J. Ireland, "Resistance to sliding with three types of elastomeric modules," *American Journal of Orthodontics and Dentofacial Orthopedics*, vol. 127, pp. 670–675, 2005.

[2] M. Hain, A. Dhopatkar, and P. Rock, "The effect of ligation method on friction in sliding mechanics," *American Journal of Orthodontics and Dentofacial Orthopedics*, vol. 123, no. 4, pp. 416–422, 2003.

[3] R. Nanda, *Biomechanics in Clinical Orthodontics*, WB Saunders, Philadelphia, Pa, USA, 1st edition, 1997.

[4] D. Drescher, C. Bourauel, and H.-A. Schumacher, "Frictional forces between bracket and arch wire," *The American Journal of Orthodontics and Dentofacial Orthopedics*, vol. 96, no. 5, pp. 397–404, 1989.

[5] K. L. Baker, L. G. Nieberg, A. D. Weimer, and M. Hanna, "Frictional changes in force values caused by saliva substitution," *American Journal of Orthodontics and Dentofacial Orthopedics*, vol. 91, no. 4, pp. 316–320, 1987.

[6] R. P. Kusy, J. Q. Whitley, and M. J. Prewitt, "Comparison of the frictional coefficients for selected archwire-bracket slot combinations in the dry and wet states," *Angle Orthodontist*, vol. 61, no. 4, pp. 293–302, 1991.

[7] J. G. Stannard, J. M. Gau, and M. A. Hanna, "Comparative friction of orthodontic wires under dry and wet conditions," *The American Journal of Orthodontics*, vol. 89, no. 6, pp. 485–491, 1986.

[8] S. Rajendran, J. Paulraj, P. Rengan, J. Jeyasundari, and M. Manivannan, "Corrosion behaviour of metals in artificial saliva in presence of spirulina powder," *Journal of Dentistry and Oral Hygiene*, vol. 1, no. 1, pp. 1–8, 2009.

[9] B. Khambay, D. Millett, and S. McHugh, "Archwire seating forces produced by different ligation methods and their effect on frictional resistance," *European Journal of Orthodontics*, vol. 27, no. 3, pp. 302–308, 2005.

[10] C. Chimenti, L. Franchi, M. G. Di Giuseppe, and M. Lucci, "Friction of orthodontic elastomeric ligatures with different dimensions," *The Angle Orthodontist*, vol. 75, no. 3, pp. 421–425, 2005.

[11] M. Hain, A. Dhopatkar, and P. Rock, "A comparison of different ligation methods on friction," *American Journal of Orthodontics and Dentofacial Orthopedics*, vol. 130, no. 5, pp. 666–670, 2006.

[12] P. Gandini, L. Orsi, C. Bertoncini, S. Massironi, and L. Franchi, "In vitro frictional forces generated by three different ligation methods," *Angle Orthodontist*, vol. 78, no. 5, pp. 917–921, 2008.

[13] B. Khambay, D. Millett, and S. McHugh, "Evaluation of methods of archwire ligation on frictional resistance," *European Journal of Orthodontics*, vol. 26, no. 3, pp. 327–332, 2004.

[14] A. V. Arun and A. C. Vaz, "Frictional characteristics of the newer orthodontic elastomeric ligatures," *Indian Journal of Dental Research*, vol. 22, no. 1, pp. 95–99, 2011.

[15] E. Bazakidou, R. S. Nanda, M. G. Duncanson Jr., and P. Sinha, "Evaluation of frictional resistance in esthetic brackets," *American Journal of Orthodontics and Dentofacial Orthopedics*, vol. 112, no. 2, pp. 138–144, 1997.

[16] M. Tselepis, P. Brockhurst, and V. C. West, "The dynamic frictional resistance between orthodontic brackets and arch wires," *The American Journal of Orthodontics and Dentofacial Orthopedics*, vol. 106, no. 2, pp. 131–138, 1994.

[17] B. K. Rucker and R. P. Kusy, "Resistance to sliding of stainless steel multistranded archwires and comparison with single-stranded leveling wires," *The American Journal of Orthodontics and Dentofacial Orthopedics*, vol. 122, no. 1, pp. 73–83, 2002.

[18] G. D. Edwards, E. H. Davies, and S. P. Jones, "The ex vivo effect of ligation technique on the static frictional resistance of stainless steel brackets and archwires," *British Journal of Orthodontics*, vol. 22, no. 2, pp. 145–153, 1995.

[19] G. Thorstenson and R. Kusy, "Influence of stainless steel inserts on the resistance to sliding of esthetic brackets with second-order angulation in the dry and wet states," *Angle Orthodontist*, vol. 73, no. 2, pp. 167–175, 2003.

23

Malocclusion in Elementary School Children in Beirut: Severity and Related Social/Behavioral Factors

Antoine Hanna,[1] **Monique Chaaya,**[2] **Celine Moukarzel,**[3] **Khalil El Asmar,**[2] **Miran Jaffa,**[2] **and Joseph G. Ghafari**[1]

[1]*Division of Orthodontics and Dentofacial Orthopedics, Department of Otolaryngology/Head and Neck Surgery,*
 American University of Beirut Medical Center, Beirut, Lebanon
[2]*Department of Epidemiology and Population Health, Faculty of Health Sciences, American University of Beirut, Beirut, Lebanon*
[3]*Private Practice, Beirut, Lebanon*

Correspondence should be addressed to Monique Chaaya; mchaaya@aub.edu.lb

Academic Editor: James K. Hartsfield

Aim. To assess severity of malocclusion in Lebanese elementary school children and the relationship between components of malocclusion and sociodemographic and behavioral factors. *Methods.* Dental screening was performed on 655 school children aged 6–11 from 2 public (PB) and 5 private (PV) schools in Beirut. A calibrated examiner recorded occlusion, overjet, overbite, posterior crossbite, midline diastema, and crowding. Another examiner determined the DMFT (Decayed/Missing/Filled Teeth) score. A questionnaire filled by the parents provided data on sociodemographic and behavioral factors. Multinomial, binomial, and multiple linear regressions tested the association of these factors with occlusal indices. *Results.* Malocclusion was more severe in PB students. Age and sucking habit were associated with various components of malocclusion. Crowding was more prevalent among males and significantly associated with the DMFT score. Income and educational level were significantly higher ($P < 0.05$) in PV pupils and deleterious habits were more frequent in PB children. *Conclusions.* Children of lower socioeconomic background had more severe malocclusions and poorer general dental health. Compared to Western and WHO norms, the findings prompt health policy suggestions to improve dental care of particularly public school children through regular screenings in schools, prevention methods when applicable, and cost effective practices through public and private enabling agencies.

1. Introduction

Malocclusion is defined as any deviation from the norm of the arrangement of the teeth and occurs commonly among various populations [1, 2]. While considered nonlife threatening, malocclusion may cause altered functions (mastication, speech) and poor dentofacial esthetics that reduce the quality of life of affected subjects including social and functional limitations [3]. Malocclusion has also been associated with the development of periodontal disease, albeit not a direct etiology [4].

The assessment of malocclusion has not been uniform. Relatively subjective weights are assigned to the components of malocclusions in different rating systems [5], eventually leading to variable reporting of orthodontic treatment need.

The corresponding scoring indices have been used by governmental and insurance agencies to determine eligibility and/or amount of treatment coverage.

Prevalence of malocclusion in the deciduous (primary), intermediate, and permanent dentitions varied widely across studies and countries because of population differences (races/ethnicity), sample sizes, age range of the surveyed children, and methods of measurement [6–10]. Yet, fewer differences were found in classification of malocclusion because of more standardized norms of the relationship between maxillary and mandibular molars (molar occlusion) or the overjet (horizontal overbite) between upper and lower incisors. In general, these relations are well correlated [11].

In Western Studies (mainly American) spanning over 50 years, the majority of malocclusions in Caucasian children exhibit Class I malocclusion (nearly 75%), with closer to normal relations between the posterior teeth, followed by Class II malocclusion (tendency to increased overjet, nearly 20%), then Class III (anterior underbite-less than 5%) [2]. Surveys of Brazilian children indicated lower proportions but still a majority of Class I malocclusion and higher percentages of Class II and Class III problems [12, 13].

Fewer studies are available on prevalence of malocclusion in the Middle East and Northern Africa region, but the same pattern of malocclusion as in Western countries seemingly holds, although in varied proportions. The majority of malocclusions in Middle Eastern countries related to Class I in children, adolescents, or young adults, followed by Classes II and III [14–18]. In some studies the components of the malocclusion were further qualified [14, 16–18].

Although scarce, studies that have directly related malocclusion and its severity to social status indicated that children with relatively poor lifestyle have higher orthodontic treatment need compared to their counterparts with wealthier lifestyle [19, 20]. Social condition also can affect malocclusion indirectly. Underprivileged people are more exposed to risk factors that affect oral health: unhealthy diet, tobacco use, excessive consumption of alcohol, poor sanitation and polluted water, poor oral hygiene, and HIV infection [21]. Poor oral health leads to caries and early tooth loss, facilitating the development of malocclusion, hence greater need for orthodontic treatment [22, 23].

The available data on malocclusion in Lebanon only cover the age range of 9–15 years. Prevention of oral disease or dysmorphology is usually implemented at an earlier age, thus the importance of assessing the prevalence of malocclusion at younger ages (6–11 years). Relating malocclusion to social/behavioral factors in early childhood shall facilitate the prevention or decrease in severity of malocclusion, particularly in the presence of guidelines recommending intervention before the emergence of all permanent teeth (usually by age 12 years) [24].

Accordingly, our aim was to evaluate in prepubertal Lebanese students from presumably varied backgrounds, attending public and private schools, the prevalence of malocclusion and its relation to social and behavioral characteristics. Such information potentially helps public health workers to plan intervention programs and highlight the importance of early orthodontic screening.

2. Material and Methods

The investigation was a comparative cross-sectional study of elementary school children in grades 2 to 5, aged 6–11 years, attending public and private schools in Beirut, Lebanon. The data were collected through an oral examination and a questionnaire sent to parents or guardians. The Institutional Review Board of the American University of Beirut and the Ethics committees of all participating institutions approved the study along with the pertinent consent forms secured by the parents and the assent provided by children.

2.1. Sample Size Calculation. A sample size of 721 was determined through the *A Priori Sample Size Calculator for Multiple Regression* [25] with an anticipated effect size (f2) of 0.02, a statistical power level of 0.8, 7 predictors, and a probability level of 0.05. Accounting for probable missing data we inflated the sample size by 1.2; for nonresponse from the parents or the children we further inflated the size by 1.25, whereby we sought to approach a number of nearly 1000 children.

2.2. Participants. Access to public schools was possible through a local nongovernmental organization (NGO, "Ajialouna") in Beirut, dedicated to improve life standards through various projects such as school health, health education programs, orphan sponsorship and other commitments. From a total of 30 public schools, two schools were chosen based on a timetable provided by the NGO indicating the readiness of schools for the survey and prior consent from parents that cleared our conduct of oral examination on 530 children. However, only 325 (61.3%) of these students were recruited, because the parents of the remaining 205 children did not consent to participate in the survey. The findings of the oral examinations of these pupils were used only to determine potential differences with the consenting participants.

Private schools were selected based on location (Beirut and suburbs) and willingness to participate. From 12 contacted schools, five agreed to partake in the study, encompassing 1119 children from average to high socioeconomic status. The parents/guardians of 333 children (29.76%) agreed to enroll their child and answered the survey. Excluding 3 subjects with prior or current interceptive orthodontic treatment, the final number was 330. The comparatively low response rate was probably related to the prior dental screening at the start of the school year in some of the schools, or to a more regular follow-up by a private dentist. The total sample size of both private and public schools was 655.

2.3. Instruments. The components of the US National Health and Nutrition Estimates Survey (NHANES) malocclusion assessment model were used. They included spacing within the arch (crowding, midline diastema) and relations between maxillary and mandibular teeth in the 3 planes of space: sagittal (relations between anterior teeth: overjet or anterior crossbite; relationship between the first permanent molars (Class I, II, or III)), vertical (overbite or open bite), and transversal (posterior crossbite). The study deviated from the NHANES gauge in 2 aspects.

(1) A more complete description of the malocclusion was added by dividing the molar occlusion into 5 categories based on half-cusp deviation and recording the overbite not only in millimeters but also as percentage of overlap of the mandibular incisors by the maxillary incisors.

(2) The maxillary irregularity index was discarded because the sample age bracket (6–11 years) was lower than the NHANES range (8–11 years), precluding the examination of a large number of children with nonerupted maxillary lateral incisors. Given a high correlation between the maxillary and mandibular irregularity scores [2], the latter increasing more from

childhood to adulthood, we projected the mandibular score to properly represent the presence and severity of crowding. Additional findings worth reporting were noted separately (missing and supernumerary teeth, impeded eruption of teeth).

Outcome was classified into quantitative measurements (number of teeth in crossbite and percentage of overbite), nominal measurements (molar and canine occlusion), or an ordinal variable reflecting severity (crowding, overjet, and overbite).

The DMFT (Decayed/Missing/Filled Teeth) score and the plaque index (a measure of hygiene) were recorded for each child to be analyzed in a different paper.

The questionnaire addressed to parents included 41 questions in the following categories:

(a) sociodemographic background of child and parents (family status and educational background of the respondent, family monthly income, and child's birth order),

(b) general health status of the child (presence/absence of chronic disease, child's breathing mode, and smoking status of the mother during pregnancy),

(c) sucking habits of the child (digit or other object, duration, and intensity of sucking),

(d) feeding methods of the child (feeding mode of child during infancy, consumption of detrimental foods),

(e) oral health behaviors (brushing habits, visits to the dentist),

(f) perception of parents towards their child's oral health (malocclusion and decays).

2.4. Procedure. Calibration studies preceded the in-field examinations. The dental examination comprised two distinct parts: the collection of occlusal data (investigator AH); the determination of the DMFT and plaque scores (investigator CM). The dental instruments used were noninvasive mouth mirrors, probes, and periodontal probes (ZFA043#11, Co), available in disposable packages. The screenings were performed according to WHO standards [26].

A document was sent with the children to their parents, including all pertinent information regarding the study, the IRB-approved questionnaire, and consent form. When the child was found to require treatment, a note was sent to the parents or legal guardian(s). Essential information contacts of nearby specialized dental centers with reasonable treatment cost were provided to the parents when the child was not being followed up by a dentist.

2.5. Data Analysis. Frequency distributions for all variables helped assess variability and data regrouping. Outcome indicators were chosen to represent each plane of space: overjet, overbite, and posterior crossbite. Bivariate associations gauged how different malocclusion components vary relative to selected characteristics, through chi-square tests or independent sample t-tests between each dependent variable

and the study covariates, depending on the nature of the variables.

Multivariate analysis was performed using the generalized estimated equations (GEEs), to estimate coefficients and odds ratios by fitting regression models with continuous (overjet in mm) and binary (presence/absence of posterior crossbite) outcomes adjusted for clustering effect. As GEE does not model multinomial outcome variables, generalized linear models (GLM) were used to estimate relative risk ratios (RRR) by fitting multinomial logistic regression models for outcome variables having more than 2 categories (overjet severity, overbite severity, and irregularity score severity). Clustering effect was adjusted for in the variance-covariance matrix structure and robust standard errors were reported. The multinomial regression was used instead of the ordinal logistic regression because the proportional odds assumption did not hold.

All covariates statistically associated with outcome variables at the bivariate level of $P < 0.2$ were included in the multivariate analysis. For all parameters, 95% CI and two-sided P values were reported. Statistical significance was set at $P < 0.05$. All analyses were completed in Stata SE 10.1.

3. Results

3.1. Sociobehavioral Characteristics. Mean age was not significantly different between private schools [PV] (8.57 ± 1.31 yrs.) and public schools [PB] (8.49 ± 1.59 yrs.) children. The proportion of girls was slightly higher in PV (52.8%) than in PB (46.2%) schools, but the difference was not statistically significant.

Statistically significant differences were found between both groups for family income and educational level of parents, the higher levels detected among parents of PVS children (Table 1). Regarding behavioral factors, the proportion of children whose mothers smoked during pregnancy was nearly 3 times higher among PB (20.4%) compared to PV schools. Reported sucking habits were also higher for PB children (Table 2).

3.2. Dental Measures. To facilitate the communication of a large set of data, only malocclusion parameters (by type of school) with statistically significant differences between PB and PV children are displayed in Table 3. The largest proportions of PB and PV children had Class I (normal) occlusion. The type of occlusion classified by molar relations (Class I, II, or III) was not statistically significantly different between school groups; however, when occlusion was stratified based on overjet severity the differences were significant (Table 3). PB children had statistically significantly greater mean and higher percentage of OJ compared with PV children. Anterior crossbite (reverse overjet) was statistically significantly different between the groups in Class III malocclusions. Midline diastema was more prevalent in public compared to private schools.

Vertical measures (open bite, overbite) were not statistically significantly different between school groups; however, transverse abnormalities (posterior crossbite and midline

TABLE 1: Sociodemographic variables.

Characteristics	School type		P value
	Public (n = 325)	Private (n = 330)	
Age (years)	8.49 ± 1.59	8.57 ± 1.31	NS
	%	%	
Gender			
Males	52.8	46.2	NS
Females	47.2	53.8	
Family income (LL)			
<500,000	33.6	1.4	
500,000–999,999	49.4	14.2	0.000
1,000,000–3,000,000	15.1	57.6	
>3,000,000	2.1	26.4	
Education of informant			
Low (illiterate-primary -elementary)	45.4	7.7	
Average (secondary-intermediate)	44.1	20.0	0.000
High (college/university)	10.5	72.4	

TABLE 2: Health and behavioral characteristics of child and mother.

Characteristics	School type		P value
	Public (n = 325) %	Private (n = 330) %	
Chronic diseases			
Yes	13.4	9.1	NS
No	86.6	90.9	
Mouth breathing			
Yes	9.8	7.7	NS
No	90.2	92.3	
Sucking habits			
Yes	19.56	14.9	0.030
No	80.43	85.1	
Maternal smoking during pregnancy (cigarettes)	20.4	7.0	0.000
Feeding method			
Breast	53.3	31.0	
Bottle	22.7	24.2	NS
Both	24.0	44.8	

diastema) were more frequent in PB. The overall DMFT scored a mean of 7.30 ± 3.98 in PB children compared with a mean of 3.50 ± 3.41 in PV schools (P < 0.0001). The number of decayed teeth was significantly higher in PB compared to PV (P ≤ 0.0001) schools, with means of 5.67 ± 3.81 and 1.48 ± 2.19, respectively.

3.3. Associations among Variables

3.3.1. Bivariate Associations. Only statistically significant associations are displayed in Table 4. Overjet was statistically significantly associated with age (6-7 years when permanent incisors and first molars erupt, and 8–11 years prior and during the eruption of permanent canines and premolars) and DMFT score. DMFT scores were significantly higher in children with more severe overjet. Overbite was significantly associated with age and plaque index. A higher proportion of older children had severe overbite compared to younger ones. The mean plaque index was greater in subjects with deeper bite. The post hoc test showed that the statistically significant difference existed between the subjects with moderate and deep bite (P = 0.043). Children with sucking habits were almost twice more likely to have at least one tooth in posterior crossbite compared to those with no sucking habit. None of the occlusal variables were associated with the amount or severity of the irregularity index.

3.3.2. Multivariate Analysis. The clustering by school did not appear to have any effect on the regression outcome of the overjet, overbite, and irregularity index. However, for the posterior crossbite, age only became significant following adjustment for clustering.

Adjusting for gender, school type, educational level, sucking duration, DMFT score, and plaque index, the results

TABLE 3: Percentage distribution of malocclusion characteristics in public and private school children.

Measures	School type		P value*
	Public (n = 325)	Private (n = 330)	
Overjet (%)			
1-2 [ideal]	27.4	36.3	
3-4 [mild]	46.2	45.0	0.022
>4 [mod-sev]	26.4	18.7	
Mean OJ (mm)	3.71 ± 1.77	3.41 ± 1.7	0.032
Anterior crossbite (%)			
0 [mild]	5.23	0.9	
−1 to −2 [moderate]	5.5	6.6	0.008
−3 to −4 [severe]	0.3	0.9	
<−4 [extreme]	0.0	0.0	
Occlusion** (%)			
I	72.93	77.57	
II	23.69	16.96	0.002
III	3.38	5.45	
Midline diastema (>2 mm)	16.1	10.5	0.036

*Chi-square.
**Cl I, Cl II, and Cl III classified based on OJ (ideal: 1–4; >4: Cl II; reverse overjet: Cl III).

indicate that a subject older than 8 years is at higher risk to have a mild rather than an ideal overjet (RRR: 1.35; 95% CI: 1.04–1.28; Table 5). Children with higher plaque index were at a lower risk of having a severe overjet (RRR: 0.93; 95% CI: 0.88–0.98).

TABLE 4: Associations in percentage between components of malocclusion and other variables.

	Associations			P value
Overjet	1-2 [ideal]	3-4 [mild]	4< [mod-sev]	
Age				
(6-7)	38.6	41.9	19.5	0.033
(8–11)	28.2	48.0	23.8	
DMFT	4.79 ± 3.98	5.36 ± 4.24	6.18 ± 4.12	0.030
Overbite	0–2 [ideal]	3-4 [moderate]	5< [mod-sev]	
Age				
(6-7)	63.9	24.4	11.8	0.033
(8–11)	48.7	27.4	23.8	
Plaque index (PI)	1.27 ± 0.21	1.24 ± 0.16	1.30 ± 0.22	0.049
Posterior crossbite	Present	Not present		
Sucking habits				
Present	75.8	24.2		0.005
Not present	86.9	13.1		

When using the overjet as a continuous outcome and adjusting for the same covariates employed in the multi-nomial model, the regression model resulted in a positive correlation between age and overjet (β: 0.14; 95% CI: 0.046–0.249; Table 5). PV students were more likely to have a lower overjet than those attending public school (β: −0.10; 95% CI: −0.185; −0.026). Family income was positively associated with overjet, children of lower income families (<500,000 LL) exhibiting a greater likelihood for increased overjet.

Subjects 8–11 years of age were at a higher risk of having mild (RRR: 1.71; 95% CI: 1.21; 2.39) and moderate to severe (RRR: 2.23; 95% CI: 1.03; 4.83) overbite (Table 5). Also, children with increased sucking habit duration (RRR: 0.98; 95% CI: 0.97; 0.99) and higher DMFT score (RRR: 0.93; 95% CI: 0.86; 0.99) were at a lower risk of reporting moderate to severe overbite.

The odds of having posterior crossbite in 8–11-year old children and those with increased sucking habit duration were 1.29 (95% CI: 1.18; 1.39) and 1.01 (95% CI: 1.01; 1.18), respectively. Subjects with mouth breathing habit were more likely to have a mild irregularity index (RRR: 2.61; 95% CI: 1.99; 3.42). A higher risk of moderate to severe irregularity index was determined for male subjects (RRR: 1.69; 95% CI: 1.36; 2.1) and children with higher DMFT score (RRR: 1.04; 95% CI: 1.03; 1.06).

4. Discussion

This study addressed for the first time the magnitude and severity of malocclusion conditions in preadolescent Lebanese children, a comparison between public and private school children, and the association of social and behavioral factors with a wide range of malocclusion features.

4.1. Malocclusion. In addition to high malocclusion severity in all children, this study disclosed varying magnitudes of severity between the two school groups, depending on the

malocclusion variable. The most prevalent variable was the overjet, which occurred in at least 20% of children. However, the statistically significant difference between OJ in PB (3.71 ± 1.77 mm) and PV (3.41 ± 1.70 mm) arguably may not be clinically significant.

For a more universal perspective, we compared our findings with the published data from the NHANES III survey, carried out between 1988 and 1999 on nearly 7000 individuals from different racial/ethnic and age groups [2]. Malocclusion in the NHANES was stratified on the overjet. Our findings regarding molar occlusion are consistent with other studies of Caucasian children [12, 13]. When malocclusion was classified on overjet, more similarities were found with the literature [2, 27] but the occlusion in public school children was most similar to the NHANES III data (Figure 1). Less Class II malocclusion and more Class I occlusions were found in the private schools (77.57% Class I, 16.96% Class II) compared to both NHANES III (74.8% Class I, 22.5% Class I) and public school (72.93% Class I, 23.69% Class II) data.

In some patients, the relationship between maxillary and mandibular molars falls between the three classes of malocclusion. Accordingly, the overjet was used as a more practical but not perfect proxy in various studies [27, 28]. In our sample, more than 9 of 10 subjects with an overjet greater than 6 mm had a Class II molar relationship, a finding consistent with other studies [28].

In other aspects of malocclusion, the following comparisons emerge (Figure 1).

(a) The prevalence of overjet and overbite in the moderate to severe range is greater in the NHANES III survey than in the PV schools, but less than in the PB schools. This disparity may relate to the wider range or lack of differentiation of socioeconomic backgrounds in the US survey compared to the differentiated socioeconomic levels of the PV and PB children in this study.

TABLE 5: Multivariate analysis of associations between categories of malocclusion and other variables.

		Overjet*		
Variable	RRR	Robust SE	95% CI	*P* value
Mild				
Age (6-7 versus 8–11)	1.35	0.16	[1.067; 1.71]	0.013
Moderate to severe				
Plaque index	0.93	0.024	[0.888; 0.983]	0.009
		Overjet (continuous measurement)		
Variable	*β*	Semi-Robust SE	95% CI	*P* value
Age	1.15	0.051	[1.04; 1.28]	0.004
School type	0.9	0.04	[0.831; 0.974]	0.009
Family income**				
500,000–999,999	1.229	0.070	[1.07; 1.41]	0.003
1,000,000–3,000,000	1.328	0.044	[1.209; 1.447]	0.000
>3,000,000	1.205	0.123	[0.94; 1.535]	0.131
		Overbite*		
Variable	RRR	Robust SE	95% CI	*P* value
Mild				
Age (6-7 versus 8–11)	1.709	0.294	[1.21; 2.39]	0.002
Moderate to severe				
Age (6-7 versus 8–11)	2.238	0.880	[1.035; 4.83]	0.040
Sucking duration	0.983	0.004	[0.97; 0.992]	0.000
DMFT	0.930	0.033	[0.866; 0.999]	0.048
		Posterior crossbite		
Variable	OR	Semi-Robust SE	95% CI	*P* value
Age (6-7 versus 8–11)	1.29	0.041	[1.188; 1.39]	0.000
Sucking duration	1.014	0.001	[1.011; 1.185]	0.000
		Irregularity index*		
Variable	RRR	Robust SE	95% CI	*P* value
Mild				
Mouth breathing	2.612	0.362	[1.99; 3.428]	0.000
Moderate to severe				
Gender	1.692	0.189	[1.359; 2.1]	0.000
DMFT	1.049	0.0082	[1.033; 1.065]	0.000

*Ideal category as base outcome.
**<500.000 as base outcome.
β—slope of regression; OR: odds ratio; RRR: relative risk ratio.

(b) A higher prevalence of open bite, posterior crossbite, and crowding in Lebanese school children compared to the NHANES III. The difference might relate to the higher prevalence/severity of sucking habits in our sample.

(c) A lower irregularity index in the NHANES III than in both groups. The higher incidence in males is similar to the NHANES III, while being inconsistent with other studies in which no differences [1] or higher female prevalence [29, 30] was found.

The epidemiology of malocclusion is significant because of multilevel impacts.

(a) Personal image: malocclusion may influence self-concept. Our findings on crowding (OR: 5.359) and crossbite (OR: 6.153) were reported by other investigators as risk factors for "global self-concept" (includes six domain-specific scales: social, competence, affect, academic, family, and physical) [31].

(b) Individual health: Our observations on anterior crossbite [underbite] (OR = 4.016) and molar relationship (OR = 1.661) match other findings that disclosed these characteristics as risk indicators for speech and chewing capabilities, respectively [32].

(c) Quality of life in general: patients with severe malocclusion scored poorer oral health-related quality of life (OHRQoL) than patients with less critical treatment need [33]. Also, orthodontic intervention would enhance some aspects of OHRQoL. More specific to the age bracket we investigated (6–11 years), early orthodontic intervention is beneficial because

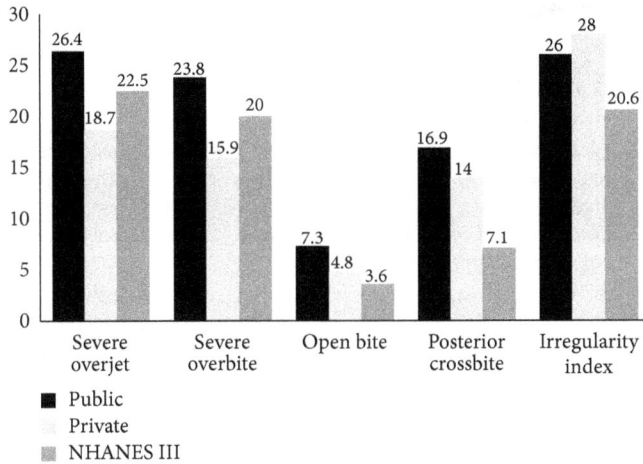

FIGURE 1: Percent distribution of students aged 8–11 by malocclusion characteristics and type of school (public and private) compared with the NHANES III findings.

younger children have high self-esteem and body-image and expect orthodontics to improve their lives [33].

4.2. Associations. Associations are listed in 2 categories, those first found in this study and those corroborated in other studies.

4.2.1. New/Different Findings

(a) Overbite was negatively associated with DMFT score. This finding might be partially explained by the association between mouth breathing (usually associated with open bite [34]) and increased risk of caries, through the reduction of the salivary flow that helps protect the teeth against decay [35].

(b) The multivariate analysis suggests that being in a private school is "protective" against increased overjet. The increased overjet might be linked to the environment in which the students live where some conditions (possibly higher rate of upper respiratory tract infections or pollution) enhance mouth breathing. Further research is needed to determine reasons for the differences.

4.2.2. Findings Supported in the Literature. Consider the following:

(a) correspondence of family income and education [36],

(b) more prevalent sucking habits in PB children, possibly reflecting the reported increase in sucking habits of children feeling insecure, lonely, or stressed [37],

(c) higher proportion (3-fold) of mothers of PB children who smoked during pregnancy, concurring with prior conclusions that smoking during pregnancy is negatively correlated with educational level and socioeconomic status [38, 39],

(d) the association between overbite and sucking duration [40, 41], possibly explained by the link of sucking habits with tongue thrust and abnormal swallowing pattern [42],

(e) positive associations between posterior crossbite and age and between crossbite and the presence (and duration) of a sucking habit [43],

(f) the association between irregularity of incisors and DMFT [44, 45]. More caries may develop because of inappropriate brushing of the crowded incisors,

(g) the association between mouth breathing and increased irregularity score of the mandibular incisor [46]. Focused investigation is needed for definitive explanation.

Because all investigated children were past the primary dentition, comparisons are not possible with reports of association between sucking habits and increased overjet in this dentition [47, 48]. However, it is plausible that the higher prevalence of severe OJ in public school children was related to higher prevalence and intensity of sucking duration at an earlier age.

4.3. Implications for School Health. The findings underscore the need to reduce social disparities in oral health among Lebanese city pupils. The inequality stems from living conditions and unequal access to proper dental awareness/education and care. Short- and long-term strategies are considered to remedy this problem.

4.3.1. Short-Term Recommendations. Regular annual dental screening is a public health service that should be generalized to all schools, not limited to mostly private and NGO-supported public schools, through the following:

(a) integrating orthodontic screening in the annual health evaluation, involving an orthodontist or trained dentist or dental hygienist, and basic screening tools. Several alternatives may be explored when funds are lacking: the assistance of civil NGO or charity organizations; volunteer dental examiners; coordination with orthodontic residency programs (possibly within a community service requirement for residency certification),

(b) the requirement by governmental health and educational agencies for all schools to institute an annual orthodontic/dental screening starting at age 7 years, the time recommended by the American Association of Orthodontists [24] or at least by the age of 8–8.5 years, the expected time for achieving the early mixed dentition,

(c) documentation by the pediatrician, during the child's regular medical screening, of mouth breathing and sucking habits, followed by referral for treatment of these habits. The prevalence/severity of certain aspects of malocclusion (posterior crossbite, irregularity index) would be decreased, oral health improved, awareness raised and potentially the screening protocol modified in pediatric residency.

4.3.2. Long-Term Recommendations. Current dental insurance schemes are limited in Lebanon particularly for orthodontic treatment. Affordable access to orthodontic care is facilitated by the presence of 4 postgraduate orthodontic programs in the Beirut area. In other countries, oral healthcare is provided through private dental insurance and poorly to moderately funded public programs. In Europe, particularly Scandinavian countries characterized by their universal healthcare coverage, severe malocclusion is treated free of charge until a certain age (usually 18 years) and at low cost thereafter [49].

Such schemes might not be cost effective in Lebanon before studies and pilot programs help weigh the viability of any insurance plan before implementation. Focus on prevention may be more effective in the initial phases. Interceptive orthodontic treatment in US Medicaid patients has been effective in reducing malocclusion severity; some subjects might not require additional comprehensive orthodontic treatment at later stages [50, 51].

4.4. Research Considerations. A number of parents of children in private schools refused to enlist their children in the study because they had their own dentist. The lower percentage of private school respondents possibly impacted the rate and severity of malocclusion between the school groups. The study did not include children from the more expensive private schools, presumably representing higher living standards and different lifestyles, thus possibly altering some findings with potentially more divergence between both types of schools investigated.

Self-reporting might have affected the accuracy or underestimated some variables because of recall bias or misinterpretation of the question. Both limitations might have been diminished or overcome if the investigators had a direct interview with the parents.

Long-term follow-up on the screened subjects should confirm the reported associations and explore new ones among the studied parameters.

5. Conclusions

Malocclusion was more severe in preadolescent school children from lower socioeconomic background, indicating social disparities in oral health. Some associations were found between malocclusion and societal/behavioral parameters (e.g., sucking habits, prevalent in public school children, with open bite and posterior crossbite; crowding among mandibular incisors with DMFT score [indicative of oral hygiene]). Except for a lower prevalence of overjet/overbite in private schools, Lebanese school children have more severe malocclusion components than American children.

Conflict of Interests

The authors declare that there is no conflict of interests regarding the publication of this paper.

References

[1] J. Kelly and C. Harvey, *An Assessment of the Teeth of Youths 12-17 Years*, DHEW Pub No. (HRA) 77-1644, National Center for Health Statistics, Washington, DC, USA, 1977.

[2] W. R. Proffit, H. W. Fields Jr., and L. J. Moray, "Prevalence of malocclusion and orthodontic treatment need in the United States: estimates from the NHANES III survey," *The International Journal of Adult Orthodontics & Orthognathic Surgery*, vol. 13, no. 2, pp. 97–106, 1998.

[3] B. W. Bresnahan, H. Asuman Kiyak, S. H. Masters, S. P. McGorray, A. Lincoln, and G. King, "Quality of life and economic burdens of malocclusion in U.S. patients enrolled in Medicaid," *The Journal of the American Dental Association*, vol. 141, no. 10, pp. 1202–1212, 2010.

[4] A.-M. Bollen, "Effects of malocclusions and orthodontics on periodontal health: evidence from a systematic review," *Journal of Dental Education*, vol. 72, no. 8, pp. 912–918, 2008.

[5] A. Bjork, A. Krebs, and B. Solow, "A method of epidemiological registration of malocclusion," *Acta Odontologica Scandinavica*, vol. 22, pp. 27–41, 1964.

[6] R. Grabowski, F. Stahl, M. Gaebel, and G. Kundt, "Relationship between occlusal findings and orofacial myofunctional status in primary and mixed dentition: part I: prevalence of Malocclusions," *Journal of Orofacial Orthopedics*, vol. 68, no. 1, pp. 26–37, 2007.

[7] F. Stahl and R. Grabowski, "Orthodontic findings in the deciduous and early mixed dentition—inferences for a preventive strategy," *Journal of Orofacial Orthopedics*, vol. 64, no. 6, pp. 401–416, 2003.

[8] F. J. Robke, "Effects of nursing bottle misuse on oral health: prevalence of caries, tooth malalignments and malocclusions in North-German preschool children," *Journal of Orofacial Orthopedics*, vol. 69, pp. 5–19, 2008.

[9] V. Dhar, A. Jain, T. E. van Dyke, and A. Kohli, "Prevalence of gingival diseases, malocclusion and fluorosis in school-going children of rural areas in Udaipur district," *Journal of Indian Society of Pedodontics and Preventive Dentistry*, vol. 25, no. 2, pp. 103–105, 2007.

[10] D. S. Rwakatema, P. M. Ng'ang'a, and A. M. Kemoli, "Prevalence of malocclusion among 12–15-year-olds in Moshi, Tanzania, using Bjork's criteria," *East African Medical Journal*, vol. 83, no. 7, pp. 372–379, 2006.

[11] J. Varrela, "Early developmental traits in Class II malocclusion," *Acta Odontologica Scandinavica*, vol. 56, no. 6, pp. 375–377, 1998.

[12] M. R. de Almeida, A. L. P. Pereira, R. R. de Almeida, R. R. de Almeida-Pedrin, and O. G. D. S. Filho, "Prevalence of malocclusion in children aged 7 to 12 years," *Dental Press Journal of Orthodontics*, vol. 16, no. 4, pp. 123–131, 2011.

[13] R. A. de Souza, M. B. B. D. A. Magnani, D. F. Nour, F. L. Romano, and M. R. Passos, "Prevalence of malocclusion in a Brazilian schoolchildren population and its relationship with early tooth loss," *Brazilian Journal of Oral Sciences*, vol. 7, no. 25, pp. 1566–1570, 2008.

[14] Z. A. Murshid, H. E. Amin, and A. M. Al-Nowaiser, "Distribution of certain types of occlusal anomalies among Saudi Arabian adolescents in Jeddah city," *Community Dental Health*, vol. 27, no. 4, pp. 238–241, 2010.

[15] F. Behbehani, J. Årtun, B. Al-Jame, and H. Kerosuo, "Prevalence and severity of malocclusion in adolescent Kuwaitis," *Medical Principles and Practice*, vol. 14, no. 6, pp. 390–395, 2005.

[16] E. S. J. Abu Alhaija, K. S. Al-Nimri, and S. N. Al-Khateeb, "Orthodontic treatment need and demand in 12–14-year-old north Jordanian school children," *European Journal of Orthodontics*, vol. 26, no. 3, pp. 261–263, 2004.

[17] A. Kassis, J. Bou Serhal, and N. Bassil Nassif, "Malocclusion in Lebanese orthodontic patients: an epidemiologic and analytic study," *International Arab Journal of Dentistry*, vol. 1, pp. 35–43, 2010.

[18] F. K. Saleh, "Prevalence of malocclusion in a sample of Lebanese schoolchildren: an epidemiological study," *Eastern Mediterranean Health Journal*, vol. 5, no. 2, pp. 337–343, 1999.

[19] A. A. Doğan, E. Sari, E. Uskun, and A. M. Şahin Sağlam, "Comparison of orthodontic treatment need by professionals and parents with different socio-demographic characteristics," *European Journal of Orthodontics*, vol. 32, no. 6, pp. 672–676, 2010.

[20] M. Mtaya, P. Brudvik, and A. N. Åstrøm, "Prevalence of malocclusion and its relationship with socio-demographic factors, dental caries, and oral hygiene in 12- to 14-year-old Tanzanian schoolchildren," *European Journal of Orthodontics*, vol. 31, no. 5, pp. 467–476, 2009.

[21] D. Gratrix and P. J. Holloway, "Factors of deprivation associated with dental caries in young children," *Community Dental Health*, vol. 11, no. 2, pp. 66–70, 1994.

[22] B. Melsen and S. Terp, "The influence of extractions caries cause on the development of malocclusion and need for orthodontic treatment," *Swedish Dental Journal*, vol. 15, pp. 163–169, 1982.

[23] P. Frazão and P. Capel Narvai, "Socio-environmental factors associated with dental occlusion in adolescents," *American Journal of Orthodontics and Dentofacial Orthopedics*, vol. 129, no. 6, pp. 809–816, 2006.

[24] American Association of Orthodontists, *Good Dental Health Starts Early 2011*, American Association of Orthodontists, St. Louis, Mo, USA, 2012, https://www.aaoinfo.org/.

[25] T. W. Beck, "The importance of a priori sample size estimation in strength and conditioning research," *Journal of Strength and Conditioning Research*, vol. 27, no. 8, pp. 2323–2337, 2013.

[26] World Health Organization, *Oral Health Surveys: Basic Methods*, World Health Organization, Geneva, Switzerland, 4th edition, 1997, http://apps.who.int/iris/.

[27] S. Zupančič, M. Pohar, F. Farčnik, and M. Ovsenik, "Overjet as a predictor of sagittal skeletal relationships," *European Journal of Orthodontics*, vol. 30, no. 3, pp. 269–273, 2008.

[28] P. M. Sinclair and R. M. Little, "Maturation of untreated normal occlusions," *American Journal of Orthodontics*, vol. 83, no. 2, pp. 114–123, 1983.

[29] S. E. Bishara, J. E. Treder, and J. R. Jakobsen, "Facial and dental changes in adulthood," *American Journal of Orthodontics and Dentofacial Orthopedics*, vol. 106, no. 2, pp. 175–186, 1994.

[30] L. Perillo, M. Esposito, A. Caprioglio, S. Attanasio, A. C. Santini, and M. Carotenuto, "Orthodontic treatment need for adolescents in the Campania region: the malocclusion impact on self-concept," *Patient Preference and Adherence*, vol. 8, pp. 353–359, 2014.

[31] S. H. D. C. S. Peres, S. Goya, K. L. Cortellazzi, G. M. B. Ambrosano, M. D. C. Meneghim, and A. C. Pereira, "Self-perception and malocclusion and their relation to oral appearance and function," *Ciencia e Saude Coletiva*, vol. 16, no. 10, pp. 4059–4066, 2011.

[32] H. A. Kiyak, "Does orthodontic treatment affect patients' quality of life?" *Journal of Dental Education*, vol. 72, no. 8, pp. 886–894, 2008.

[33] A. W. Tung and H. A. Kiyak, "Psychological influences on the timing of orthodontic treatment," *American Journal of Orthodontics and Dentofacial Orthopedics*, vol. 113, no. 1, pp. 29–39, 1998.

[34] B. Q. Souki, G. B. Pimenta, M. Q. Souki, L. P. Franco, H. M. G. Becker, and J. A. Pinto, "Prevalence of malocclusion among mouth breathing children: do expectations meet reality?" *International Journal of Pediatric Otorhinolaryngology*, vol. 73, no. 5, pp. 767–773, 2009.

[35] G. K. Stookey, "The effect of saliva on dental caries," *Journal of the American Dental Association*, vol. 139, no. 5, pp. 11–17, 2008.

[36] Y. Liu, Z. Li, and M. P. Walker, "Social disparities in dentition status among American adults," *International Dental Journal*, vol. 64, no. 1, pp. 52–57, 2014.

[37] R. A. van Norman, "Digit-sucking: a review of the literature, clinical observations and treatment recommendations," *The International Journal of Orofacial Myology*, vol. 23, pp. 14–34, 1997.

[38] R. Bachir and M. Chaaya, "Maternal smoking: determinants and associated morbidity in two areas in Lebanon," *Maternal and Child Health Journal*, vol. 12, no. 3, pp. 298–307, 2008.

[39] M. Chaaya, J. Awwad, O. M. R. Campbell, A. Sibai, and A. Kaddour, "Demographic and psychosocial profile of smoking among pregnant women in Lebanon: public health implications," *Maternal and Child Health Journal*, vol. 7, no. 3, pp. 179–186, 2003.

[40] E. Larsson, "Sucking, chewing, and feeding habits and the development of crossbite: a longitudinal study of girls from birth to 3 years of age," *Angle Orthodontist*, vol. 71, no. 2, pp. 116–119, 2001.

[41] J. J. Warren and S. E. Bishara, "Duration of nutritive and non-nutritive sucking behaviors and their effects on the dental arches in the primary dentition," *The American Journal of Orthodontics and Dentofacial Orthopedics*, vol. 121, no. 4, pp. 347–356, 2002.

[42] P. Cozza, T. Baccetti, L. Franchi, M. Mucedero, and A. Polimeni, "Sucking habits and facial hyperdivergency as risk factors for anterior open bite in the mixed dentition," *American Journal of Orthodontics and Dentofacial Orthopedics*, vol. 128, no. 4, pp. 517–519, 2005.

[43] S. Melink, M. V. Vagner, I. Hocevar-Boltezar, and M. Ovsenik, "Posterior crossbite in the deciduous dentition period, its relation with sucking habits, irregular orofacial functions, and otolaryngological findings," *American Journal of Orthodontics and Dentofacial Orthopedics*, vol. 138, no. 1, pp. 32–40, 2010.

[44] L. Szyszka-Sommerfeld and J. Buczkowska-Radlińska, "Influence of tooth crowding on the prevalence of dental caries. A literature review," *Annales Academiae Medicae Stetinensis*, vol. 56, no. 2, pp. 85–88, 2010.

[45] J. Buczkowska-Radlinska, L. Szyszka-Sommerfeld, and K. Wozniak, "Anterior tooth crowding and prevalence of dental caries in children in Szczecin, Poland," *Community Dental Health*, vol. 29, no. 2, pp. 168–172, 2012.

[46] B. Solow and L. Sonnesen, "Head posture and malocclusions," *European Journal of Orthodontics*, vol. 20, no. 6, pp. 685–693, 1998.

[47] O. Fukuta, R. L. Braham, K. Yokoi, and K. Kurosu, "Damage to the primary dentition resulting from thumb and finger (digit) sucking," *Journal of Dentistry for Children*, vol. 63, no. 6, pp. 403–407, 1996.

[48] S. M. Adair, M. Milano, and J. C. Dushku, "Evaluation of the effects of orthodontic pacifiers on the primary dentitions

of 24- to 59-month-old children: preliminary study," *Pediatric Dentistry*, vol. 14, no. 1, pp. 13–18, 1992.

[49] E. Capilouto, "The dentist's role in access to dental care by Medicaid recipients," *Journal of Dental Education*, vol. 52, no. 11, pp. 647–652, 1988.

[50] D. L. Patrick, R. S. Y. Lee, M. Nucci, D. Grembowski, C. Z. Jolles, and P. Milgrom, "Reducing oral health disparities: a focus on social and cultural determinants," *BMC Oral Health*, vol. 6, article S4, 2006.

[51] G. King, C. Spiekerman, G. Greenlee, and G. Huang, "Randomized clinical trial of interceptive and comprehensive orthodontics," *Journal of Dental Research*, vol. 91, no. 7, supplement, pp. 59S–64S, 2012.

24

Correlations between Perceived Oral Malodor Levels and Self-Reported Oral Complaints

Atsushi Kameyama,[1,2] **Kurumi Ishii,**[3] **Sachiyo Tomita,**[4] **Chihiro Tatsuta,**[3]
Toshiko Sugiyama,[2] **Yoichi Ishizuka,**[5] **Toshiyuki Takahashi,**[2] **and Masatake Tsunoda**[2]

[1]*Department of Endodontics and Clinical Cariology, Tokyo Dental College, Tokyo, Japan*
[2]*Division of General Dentistry, Tokyo Dental College Chiba Hospital, Chiba, Japan*
[3]*Tokyo Dental College School of Dental Hygiene, Chiba, Japan*
[4]*Department of Periodontology, Tokyo Dental College, Tokyo, Japan*
[5]*Department of Epidemiology and Public Health, Tokyo Dental College, Tokyo, Japan*

Correspondence should be addressed to Atsushi Kameyama; kameyama@tdc.ac.jp

Academic Editor: Manuel Lagravere

Objectives. Even though objective data indicating the absence of oral malodor are presented to patients, they may be skeptical about the results, possibly due to the presence of some discomfort in the oral cavity. The objective of this study was to investigate whether there is an association among self-perceptions of oral malodor, oral complaints, and the actual oral malodor test result. *Materials and Methods.* Questions concerning self-perceptions of oral malodor and subjective intraoral symptoms were extracted from a questionnaire on oral malodor completed by 363 subjects who visited the clinic for oral malodor of Tokyo Dental College Chiba Hospital and gave consent to this study. In addition, the association of self-perception of oral malodor with values obtained after organoleptic and OralChroma measurement was analyzed. *Results.* No correlation between 195 subjects (54%) who were judged "with oral malodor" (organoleptic score of ≥ 1) and 294 subjects (81.6%) who had a self-perceptions of oral malodor was observed. Self-perception of oral malodor was significantly correlated with tongue coating ($p = 0.002$) and a strange intraoral taste ($p = 0.016$). *Conclusions.* Subjects with a self-perception of oral malodor were not necessarily consistent with those actually having an oral malodor. In addition, it was suggested that patients became aware of oral malodor when they felt oral complaints.

1. Introduction

Increasing awareness of cleanliness by society in general has heightened interest in odor. Since one cannot sense oral malodor accurately by oneself, bad breath brings marked psychological discomfort and may interfere with social interactions [1]. Many people feel anxiety or distress regarding oral malodor, even though they may have no such oral malodor. They may believe they have oral malodor when they see someone touching his/her nose or grimacing during a conversation [2].

Even though a dentist judges the oral malodor level by smelling and informs patients that there is no oral malodor, it is difficult for them to accept it because the procedure is based on the examiner's subjectivity. Therefore, it is necessary to measure the actual oral malodor level by measuring major oral malodor-related volatile sulfur compounds (VSCs) contained in exhaled air, hydrogen sulfide (H_2S), methyl mercaptan (CH_3SH), and dimethyl sulfide (($CH_3)_2S$), and "objectively" inform patients of the actual oral malodor level [3]. Many pseudohalitosis patients are convinced and relieved when the examiner (dentists and dental hygienists) inform them that there is no need to worry about oral malodor by showing the VSC measurement results [3, 4].

On the other hand, some people visiting an outpatient clinic for oral malodor are skeptical even though these objective data are presented [5]. They may be diagnosed with "halitophobia" based on the classification reported by Murata et al. [6]. However, if they have some subjective intraoral symptoms (self-reported oral complaints), these may induce pseudohalitosis or real malodor. If so, their distress caused by oral malodor is not resolved unless oral complaints are resolved. Therefore, it is necessary to investigate whether there is an association between a self-perception of oral complaints and actual manifestation of oral malodor or number of complaints of pseudohalitosis.

To clarify the association between the presence or absence of oral complaints and actual oral malodor measurement results, it was necessary to investigate the association between various subjective intraoral symptoms and oral malodor parameters (VSCs) in subjects who initially visited the outpatient clinic for oral malodor of Tokyo Dental College Chiba Hospital. The following null hypotheses were set: (1) there is no correlation between self-perceptions of oral malodor and oral complaints and (2) there is no correlation between self-perception of oral malodor and oral malodor parameters.

2. Materials and Methods

2.1. Subjects. Of a total of 429 persons who visited the outpatient clinic for oral malodor at the Tokyo Dental College Chiba Hospital between January 2009 and December 2011, 363 (123 males and 240 females) gave written consent after an explanation of the objective of the study. Four of them were excluded because of data deficiency. This study was performed after approval by the Ethics Committee of Tokyo Dental College (protocol approval number 375).

2.2. Extraction of Responses to Questionnaire concerning Oral Malodor. All initial examinees completed to a self-administered questionnaire concerning oral malodor before examination of the oral cavity and the oral malodor test. Questions concerning the presence or absence of subjective oral malodor symptoms and related items (11 items in total) were extracted and adopted for this study as follows.

Questionnaire on Oral Malodor Responded to by Examinees of the Outpatient Clinic for Oral Malodor of Tokyo Dental College Chiba Hospital (List of Factors concerning Oral Complaints).

(1) Do you think you have bad breath?

(Yes/No/Unsure)

(2) Do your gums bleed during tooth brushing?

(Yes/No)

(3) Do your gums ooze out pus?

(Yes/No)

(4) Do you have a loose tooth/teeth?

(Yes/No)

(5) Do you grind your teeth while you are asleep?

(Yes/No)

(6) Does your mouth feel dry?

(Yes/No)

(7) Is your mouth viscous?

(Yes/No)

(8) Is your tongue frequently coated with deposits?

(Yes/No)

(9) Do you often remove tongue coating?

(Yes/No)

(10) Do you notice a bad taste in your mouth?

(Yes/No)

(11) Is there medicine you have to take regularly?

(Yes/No)

2.3. Evaluation of Oral Malodor Level. The oral malodor level was objectively evaluated by measuring the levels of 3 volatile sulfur compounds (VSCs) contained in intraoral gas using a portable gas chromatograph, OralChroma (FIS, Itami, Hyogo, Japan), and performing an organoleptic test.

To gather optimal test results, several precautions should be taken before the examinations: the patient should refrain from eating spicy foods, garlic, or onions the day before the examination. For at least 12 h before the consultation, the teeth should not be cleaned or rinsed, perfumes should be avoided, and, at least 6 h before the examination, the intake of food and liquids should be avoided. Smoking should be refrained from for at least 24 h before any examination [7].

To use breath odor at waking as the standard, measurement was performed between 9:30–11:30 a.m. [8]. The organoleptic test was performed employing 5-step grading: scores 0 = absence of odor, 1 = barely appreciable odor, 2 = moderate malodor, 3 = strong malodor, and 4 = severe malodor.

Prior to measurement using OralChroma, the patients were instructed to close their mouth and breathe through their nose for 30 seconds. A 1-mL disposable syringe (Top, Tokyo, Japan) was placed in the mouth through the lips and teeth, 1 mL of air in the mouth was aspirated, and 0.5 mL of this was immediately injected into OralChroma [9]. It was judged that oral malodor can be perceived when the H_2S level exceeds 600 ppb, the CH_3SH level exceeds 100 ppb, $(CH_3)_2S$ level exceeds 100 ppb [2, 10], or organoleptic level is 1–4.

2.4. Analysis. The associations between self-perception of oral malodor and each subjective intraoral symptom and oral malodor parameter were investigated using the Chi-square test ($p = 0.05$). When data involved only 20 or fewer subjects, Yates' correction was applied. The association between the parameters was analyzed using Spearman's rank-correlation coefficient test. Statistical analysis was performed using IBM SPSS statistics 18 for Windows (IBM Japan Inc., Tokyo, Japan).

TABLE 1: Correlation coefficients between the results of 4 parameters regarding oral malodor.

| | n | Spearman's correlation | | |
		CH_3SH	$(CH_3)_2S$	OT
H_2S				
<600 ppb	335	$r = 0.247$	$r = 0.449$	$r = 0.422$
≥600 ppb	24	$p < 0.001$	$p < 0.001$	$p < 0.001$
CH_3SH				
<100 ppb	165		$r = 0.294$	$r = 0.906$
≥100 ppb	194		$p < 0.001$	$p < 0.001$
$(CH_3)_2S$				
<100 ppb	305			$r = 0.472$
≥100 ppb	54			$p < 0.001$
OT				
Score 0	164			
Score 1	83			
Score 2	59			
Score 3	26			
Score 4	27			

OT: organoleptic test; n: number of subjects.
r: correlation coefficient.

TABLE 2: Relationships between self-perception of oral malodor and associated parameters.

| | Self-perceived oral malodor | | p value |
	(+) ($n = 294$)	(−) ($n = 65$)	
H_2S			
<600 ppb	22	2	0.311 NS
≥600 ppb	272	63	
CH_3SH			
<100 ppb	153	41	0.106 NS
≥100 ppb	141	24	
$(CH_3)_2S$			
<100 ppb	46	8	0.624 NS
≥100 ppb	248	57	
Organoleptic test			
Score 0	140	24	
Score 1	63	20	
Score 2	49	10	0.117 NS
Score 3	18	8	
Score 4	24	3	

NS: no significant difference (Chi-square test).

3. Results

3.1. Correlation between Oral Malodor Parameters. The associations among the 4 oral malodor parameters are shown in Table 1. Significant correlations were noted between the parameters of all combinations ($p < 0.001$). Particularly, a strong correlation was noted between the organoleptic test result and CH_3SH ($r = 0.906$, $p < 0.001$).

3.2. Association between Self-Perception of Oral Malodor and Oral Malodor Parameters. Only 9 (2.5%) of the 359 subjects responded that they were not aware of their own oral malodor, 294 subjects (81.9%) responded that they had self-perceived oral malodor, and 56 subjects (15.6%) stated that they did not know. The results of analysis of the association between self-perception of oral malodor and the results of VSC measurement using OralChroma and the organoleptic test are shown in Table 2. Subjects who chose "unsure" to the questions on self-perception of oral malodor were regarded as having no self-perception. No significant correlation with the presence or absence of self-perception of oral malodor was noted in any of H_2S, CH_3SH, $(CH_3)_2S$, or organoleptic test results.

3.3. Association between Self-Perception of Oral Malodor and Oral Complaints. The results of analysis of the association between self-perception of oral malodor and elements of oral complaints are shown in Table 3. No significant correlation was noted between the presence or absence of periodontal disease-associated intraoral symptoms and self-perception of oral malodor. In contrast, a significant correlation was noted between tongue coating and self-perception of oral malodor ($p = 0.002$). A significant correlation with a strange intraoral

taste was also observed ($p = 0.016$), but no significant correlation with intraoral viscosity was noted ($p = 0.067$).

The combinations of significantly correlated factors on analysis using Spearman's correction are shown in Table 4. Significant correlations were noted between oral dryness and intraoral viscosity, a strange taste, tongue coating, and frequent tongue brushing ($p < 0.05$). In addition, significant correlations were noted between intraoral viscosity and tongue coating and a strange intraoral taste ($p < 0.05$).

4. Discussion

The objective of this study was to clarify the association between the presence or absence of subjective intraoral symptoms and results of actual oral malodor measurement. The oral malodor level was judged based on the measurement of 3 VSCs, in addition to the organoleptic test. The organoleptic test is considered to be the gold-standard oral malodor test because whether oral malodor is perceived by human olfaction is important for the judgment of the presence or absence of oral malodor [11, 12]. However, tests employing human olfaction cannot be quantified because it is based on subjective judgment by the examiner (operator). Therefore, comparison of the test results between before and after treatment is difficult, and the test lacks persuasiveness as a material for explanation of the oral malodor level [3]. Therefore, to judge the oral malodor level, generally, the measurement of oral malodor-producing substances using an oral malodor-analyzing device is concomitantly employed in addition to the olfaction-based organoleptic test.

The organoleptic score is correlated with the levels of VSCs contained in intraoral gas determined using gas chromatography and a portable sulfide monitor. We also observed correlations among the 4 items: the H_2S, CH_3SH,

TABLE 3: Relationships between self-perception of oral malodor and oral complaints.

	Self-perceived oral malodor		p value
	(+)	(−)	
Bleeding from gum			
Yes	83	19	0.872 NS
No	211	46	
Pus from gum			
Yes	27	2	0.167 NS
No	267	63	
Tooth movement			
Yes	29	9	0.471 NS
No	265	56	
Grinding of teeth			
Yes	58	14	0.742 NS
No	236	51	
Mouth dryness*			
Yes	181	29	0.012
No	113	36	
Intraoral viscosity			
Yes	192	36	0.133 NS
No	102	29	
Tongue coating*			
Yes	200	31	0.002
No	94	34	
Frequent tongue brushing			
Yes	181	32	0.067 NS
No	113	33	
Strange taste*			
Yes	99	12	0.016
No	195	53	
Taking medicine			
Yes	141	27	0.348 NS
No	153	38	

*Significant difference (Chi-square test; $p < 0.05$).

TABLE 4: Correlated parameters analyzed by Spearman's correlation.

		r	p value
Bleeding from gum	Pus from gum	0.153	0.004
Tooth movement	Grinding of teeth	0.122	0.021
Mouth dryness	Intraoral viscosity	0.289	<0.001
	Tongue coating	0.199	<0.001
	Strange taste	0.197	<0.001
	Frequent tongue cleaning	0.108	0.040
Intraoral viscosity	Tongue coating	0.269	<0.001
	Strange taste	0.232	<0.001
Tongue coating	Frequent tongue cleaning	0.355	<0.001
	Strange taste	0.259	<0.001

and $(CH_3)_2S$ levels and organoleptic test result ($p < 0.001$). Particularly, the correlation between the organoleptic test

result and CH_3SH level was markedly stronger than those between the organoleptic test result and H_2S and $(CH_3)_2S$ levels ($r = 0.906$, $p < 0.001$). $(CH_3)_2S$ stimulates olfaction at 1/6 and 1/21,000 of the levels of H_2S and ammonia, respectively [13]. Accordingly, the strength of oral malodor is strongly correlated with the $(CH_3)_2S$ level [14].

Of the subjects who visited the outpatient clinic for oral malodor during the 3-year period, only 9 subjects (2.5%) felt that they had no oral malodor and more than 80% of the examinees felt that they had oral malodor. However, only 54.3% of them were judged as having some level of oral malodor on the organoleptic test, showing no correlation between their self-perception and the organoleptic test results ($r = 0.080$, $p = 0.128$). This finding suggests that persons who self-perceive oral malodor are not necessarily consistent with those who actually have it, and this finding was consistent with those of several reports [14, 15].

About 60% of the examinees felt oral dryness. A significant association was present between self-perception of oral malodor and oral dryness. Indeed, oral dryness due to reduced salivary flow is a cause of oral malodor [16], and the oral malodor level rises with a decrease in salivary flow [17]. On the other hand, feeling oral dryness was not significantly correlated in this study with the organoleptic test result, H_2S, or CH_3SH, suggesting that a feeling of oral dryness does not necessarily indicate the actual reduction of salivary flow [18].

A significant association was also noted between self-perceptions of oral malodor and frequent tongue coating. Tongue coating has been reported to be one of the typical factors of oral malodor [19, 20]. Amou et al. [21] visually evaluated the accumulation of tongue coating using Kojima's 5-step scoring criteria [22] and observed its correlations with the organoleptic score and CH_3SH level. Particularly, F. nucleatum and T. denticola contained in tongue coating have been reported to be closely involved in VSC production [23, 24]. Therefore, tongue cleaning is recommended to improve oral malodor [25–28]. A significant correlation was noted between tongue coating and frequent tongue brushing ($r = 0.355$, $p < 0.001$), possibly because patients know that tongue coating removal improves oral malodor. This was also demonstrated by the findings that frequent tongue brushing was inversely correlated with the organoleptic test result and CH_3SH level.

A feeling of oral dryness was also significantly correlated with subjective symptoms causing oral complaints, such as intraoral viscosity and a strange taste. Similarly, a significant correlation was noted between a feeling of oral dryness and tongue coating ($p < 0.001$). These findings suggest that persons who feel oral dryness tend to have some oral complaints, and tongue coating induced their anxiety regarding oral malodor. Based on these findings, first null hypotheses that there is no correlation between self-perception of oral malodor and oral complaints was rejected.

It was also determined that there is no association between self-perception of oral malodor and its actual presence. Thus, the second null hypothesis was accepted. This is because examinees/patients suspected having oral malodor even though it was not present when there was some oral complaints such as, for example, the feeling of oral dryness, tongue coating, and a strange intraoral taste. Particularly, when oral dryness is felt, the person becomes sensitive to intraoral viscosity and an unpleasant taste, aggravating the tendency. Pseudohalitosis patients, that is, persons who visit outpatient clinics for oral malodor although it is actually absent, do not necessarily self-perceive oral malodor simply due to mental stress. The study results therefore suggest that some forms of oral complaints induced self-perception of oral malodor. On interviews of halitosis patients in actual medical practice, it is necessary to sufficiently ask whether they have discomfort in the oral cavity, in addition to asking about anxiety and mental distress due to oral malodor. If this is the case, not only mental support but also instruction and treatment should be offered to improve such oral complaints.

5. Conclusions

Our study revealed that the subjects with a self-perception of oral malodor were not necessarily consistent with those actually having an oral malodor. In addition, it was suggested that patients became aware of oral malodor when they felt oral complaints.

Conflict of Interests

The authors declare that there is no conflict of interests regarding the publication of this paper.

Authors' Contribution

Drs. Atsushi Kameyama and Sachiyo Tomita designed and coordinated the study. Dr. Yoichi Ishizuka managed the statistical analysis. Dr. Toshiko Sugiyama, DH. Kurumi Ishii, and DH. Chihiro Tatsuta performed data analysis. Dr. Toshiyuki Takahashi and Dr. Masatake Tsunoda assisted in the conceptualization and planning of the paper preparation. All authors reviewed the paper critically for content and approved it for submission.

References

[1] M. Sanz, S. Roldán, and D. Herrera, "Fundamentals of breath malodour," *The Journal of Contemporary Dental Practice*, vol. 2, no. 4, pp. 1–17, 2001.

[2] S. Tomita, A. Kameyama, N. Watanabe et al., "Analysis of clinical data from a specialized clinic for oral malodor at the Tokyo Dental College Chiba Hospital, 2009–2011," *Nihon Shishubyo Gakkai Kaishi*, vol. 55, no. 1, pp. 15–23, 2013.

[3] C. M. L. Bollen and T. Beikler, "Halitosis: the multidisciplinary approach," *International Journal of Oral Science*, vol. 4, no. 2, pp. 55–63, 2012.

[4] R. Seemann, M. Bizhang, C. Djamchidi, A. Kage, and S. Nachnani, "The proportion of pseudo-halitosis patients in a multidisciplinary breath malodour consultation," *International Dental Journal*, vol. 56, no. 2, pp. 77–81, 2006.

[5] F. Romano, E. Pigella, N. Guzzi, and M. Aimetti, "Patients' self-assessment of oral malodour and its relationship with organoleptic scores and oral conditions," *International Journal of Dental Hygiene*, vol. 8, no. 1, pp. 41–46, 2010.

[6] T. Murata, T. Yamaga, T. Iida, H. Miyazaki, and K. Yaegaki, "Classification and examination of halitosis," *International Dental Journal*, vol. 52, no. 3, pp. 181–186, 2002.

[7] T. Zaitsu, M. Ueno, K. Shinada, F. A. Wright, and Y. Kawaguchi, "Social anxiety disorder in genuine halitosis patients," *Health and Quality of Life Outcomes*, vol. 9, article 94, 2011.

[8] D. Van Steenberghe, P. Avontroodt, W. Peeters et al., "Effect of different mouthrinses on morning breath," *Journal of Periodontology*, vol. 72, no. 9, pp. 1183–1191, 2001.

[9] S. Awano, Y. Takata, I. Soh et al., "Correlations between health status and OralChroma™-determined volatile sulfide levels in mouth air of the elderly," *Journal of Breath Research*, vol. 5, no. 4, Article ID 046007, 2011.

[10] T. Sugiyama, A. Kameyama, and M. Tsunoda, "Effect of initial periodontal therapy in patients with halitosis," *Journal of Japanese Academy of Malodor Syndrome*, vol. 1, pp. 23–27, 2010.

[11] R. Nalçaci and I. S. Sönmez, "Evaluation of oral malodor in children," *Oral Surgery, Oral Medicine, Oral Pathology, Oral Radiology, and Endodontology*, vol. 106, no. 3, pp. 384–388, 2008.

[12] B. U. Aylikci and H. Çolak, "Halitosis: from diagnosis to management," *Journal of Natural Science, Biology and Medicine*, vol. 4, no. 1, pp. 14–23, 2013.

[13] Y. Nagata and N. Takeuchi, "Measurement of odor threshold value by triangle odor bag method," *Bulletin of Japan Environmental Sanitation Center*, vol. 17, pp. 77–89, 1990.

[14] M. Rosenberg, A. Kozlovsky, I. Gelernter et al., "Self-estimation of oral malodor," *Journal of Dental Research*, vol. 74, no. 9, pp. 1577–1582, 1995.

[15] M. Rosenberg, A. Kozlovsky, Y. Wind, and E. Mindel, "Self-assessment of oral malodor 1 year following initial consultation," *Quintessence International*, vol. 30, no. 5, pp. 324–327, 1999.

[16] I. Kleinberg, M. S. Wolff, and D. M. Codipilly, "Role of saliva in oral dryness, oral feel and oral malodour," *International Dental Journal*, vol. 52, no. 3, pp. 236–240, 2002.

[17] S. Koshimune, S. Awano, K. Gohara, E. Kurihara, T. Ansai, and T. Takehara, "Low salivary flow and volatile sulfur compounds in mouth air," *Oral Surgery, Oral Medicine, Oral Pathology, Oral Radiology, and Endodontics*, vol. 96, no. 1, pp. 38–41, 2003.

[18] M. Bergdahl and J. Bergdahl, "Low unstimulated salivary flow and subjective oral dryness: association with medication, anxiety, depression, and stress," *Journal of Dental Research*, vol. 79, no. 9, pp. 1652–1658, 2000.

[19] H.-X. Lu, C. Tang, X. Chen, M. C. M. Wong, and W. Ye, "Characteristics of patients complaining of halitosis and factors associated with halitosis," *Oral Diseases*, vol. 20, no. 8, pp. 787–795, 2014.

[20] T. Kanehira, H. Hongo, J. Takehara et al., "A novel visual test for hydrogen sulfide on the tongue dorsum," *Open Journal of Stomatology*, vol. 02, no. 04, pp. 314–321, 2012.

[21] T. Amou, D. Hinode, M. Yoshioka, and D. Grenier, "Relationship between halitosis and periodontal disease—associated oral bacteria in tongue coatings," *International Journal of Dental Hygiene*, vol. 12, no. 2, pp. 145–151, 2014.

[22] K. Kojima, "Clinical studies on the coated tongue," *Japanese Journal of Oral & Maxillofacial Surgery*, vol. 31, no. 7, pp. 1659–1678, 1985.

[23] T. Yasukawa, M. Ohmori, and S. Sato, "The relationship between physiologic halitosis and periodontopathic bacteria of the tongue and gingival sulcus," *Odontology*, vol. 98, no. 1, pp. 44–51, 2010.

[24] R. Dinesh Kamaraj, S. B. Kara, and K. L. Vandana, "An evaluation of microbial profile in halitosis with tongue coating using PCR (polymerase chain reaction)—a clinical and microbiological study," *Journal of Clinical and Diagnostic Research*, vol. 8, no. 1, pp. 263–267, 2014.

[25] M. I. Van der Sleen, D. E. Slot, E. Van Trijffel, E. G. Winkel, and G. A. Van der Weijden, "Effectiveness of mechanical tongue cleaning on breath odour and tongue coating: a systematic review," *International Journal of Dental Hygiene*, vol. 8, no. 4, pp. 258–268, 2010.

[26] M. Quirynen, H. Zhao, and D. van Steenberghe, "Review of the treatment strategies for oral malodour," *Clinical Oral Investigations*, vol. 6, no. 1, pp. 1–10, 2002.

[27] D. Wilhelm, A. Himmelmann, C. Krause, and K. P. Wilhelm, "Short term clinical efficacy of new meridol halitosis tooth & tongue gel in combination with a tongue cleaner to reduce oral malodor," *The Journal of Clinical Dentistry*, vol. 24, no. 1, pp. 12–19, 2013.

[28] E. E. Aung, M. Ueno, T. Zaitsu, S. Furukawa, and Y. Kawaguchi, "Effectiveness of three oral hygiene regimens on oral malodor reduction: a randomized clinical trial," *Trials*, vol. 16, no. 1, article 31, 2015.

25

Comparing the Air Abrasion Cutting Efficacy of Dentine Using a Fluoride-Containing Bioactive Glass versus an Alumina Abrasive: An *In Vitro* Study

Melissa H. X. Tan, Robert G. Hill, and Paul Anderson

Centre for Oral Growth and Development, Barts and The London School of Medicine and Dentistry,
Unit of Dental Physical Sciences, Queen Mary University of London, Mile End Road, London E1 4NS, UK

Correspondence should be addressed to Robert G. Hill; r.hill@qmul.ac.uk

Academic Editor: Cornelis H. Pameijer

Air abrasion as a caries removal technique is less aggressive than conventional techniques and is compatible for use with adhesive restorative materials. Alumina, while being currently the most common abrasive used for cutting, has controversial health and safety issues and no remineralisation properties. The alternative, a bioactive glass, 45S5, has the advantage of promoting hard tissue remineralisation. However, 45S5 is slow as a cutting abrasive and lacks fluoride in its formulation. The aim of this study was to compare the cutting efficacy of dentine using a customised fluoride-containing bioactive glass Na0SR (38–80 μm) versus the conventional alumina abrasive (29 μm) in an air abrasion set-up. Fluoride was incorporated into Na0SR to enhance its remineralisation properties while strontium was included to increase its radiopacity. Powder outflow rate was recorded prior to the cutting tests. Principal air abrasion cutting tests were carried out on pristine ivory dentine. The abrasion depths were quantified and compared using X-ray microtomography. Na0SR was found to create deeper cavities than alumina ($p < 0.05$) despite its lower powder outflow rate and predictably reduced hardness. The sharper edges of the Na0SR glass particles might improve the cutting efficiency. In conclusion, Na0SR was more efficacious than alumina for air abrasion cutting of dentine.

1. Introduction

Broad Information on Topic. The conventional method of treatment for dental caries would be to remove carious tooth tissue, followed by replacement using a restorative material. The most common method of caries removal today is via the dental air rotor drill. Despite its widespread use, some associated problems include dentinal sensitivity after use, high-pitched noises during use, thermal stimulation of the pulp tissue, bone-conducted vibration, and pressure within the tooth structure [1]. Some other methods that have been explored include caries removal using hand excavation [2], chemical agents like Carisolv [3], and air abrasion [4]. As dentistry moves towards minimally invasive treatment [5–9] and tooth-coloured adhesive materials gain favour over amalgam, the importance of creating cavities with well-defined walls and retentive undercuts has diminished.

As a caries removal technique, air abrasion refers to a nonrotary method of abrading a surface using a stream of high-speed abrasive particles generated from compressed air [10]. It possesses an end-cutting mode of action [11, 12] and creates saucer-shaped cavities with indistinct walls and margins [13]. As compared to rotary drilling, air abrasion does not cause vibrational forces on the tooth due to the minute sizes of the particles that come into contact with it [14]. As such, it is more comfortable and creates less stress on the tooth structure [15]. Particularly in the dentine region close to the pulp, where careful caries removal using the slow speed handpiece often proves uncomfortable due to the vibrations produced, slow-cutting air abrasion becomes a viable option. The high velocity particles propelled by the air stream also translate into less exertion required by the operator [14].

Commercially, aluminium oxide abrasives are used for cutting tooth tissue using air abrasion. However, issues of indiscriminate cutting of sound tooth structure [15] coupled with controversial health and safety issues [16, 17] make it a less ideal material. An alternative material is bioactive glass, which was originally designed as a biocompatible bone replacement material [18]. A bioactive glass abrasive, Sylc, is also commercially available but indicated for the purpose of tooth polishing. Some work has also showed potential for Sylc to have selective cutting properties [19, 20]. However, its cutting time can take 2-3 times longer than alumina, making it clinically impractical [4, 21]. Neither alumina nor Sylc possesses fluoride in its composition yet there is evidence that remineralisation in dentine can be achieved [22] with locally available fluoride ions [23].

While carrying out research on a new composition of fluoride incorporated bioactive glass, Farooq et al. [24] found that the hardness of bioactive glass could be increased by reducing its sodium content. This variability in hardness was then postulated to be useful in producing bioactive glass air abrasives. Moreover, their research demonstrated apatite formation within their series of bioactive glasses when it was placed in Tris buffer solution for 6–24 hours whereas Sylc produced smaller peaks of apatite in the same time. This study aims to study a glass with a similar base composition to Farooq et al.'s [24] and compare its efficacy against alumina in air abrasion cutting of dentine.

Need for Study. Studying the behaviour of a new bioactive glass abrasive, Na0SR, within the field of air abrasion cutting is needed.

Focus of Paper. Determining the cutting efficacy of a customised fluoridated bioactive glass abrasive, Na0SR, against commercial alumina on dentine is the focus of the paper.

Null Hypothesis. Na0SR and alumina cut dentine equally well.

Hypothesis. Na0SR is not hard enough to cut dentine as efficiently as alumina.

Summary of Problem. Caries removal via rotary instruments is quick but aggressive. It not only removes sound tissue very quickly, but also creates mechanical stresses within the tooth structure. Caries removal via other methods, that is, hand excavation or the use of chemical agents, for example, Carisolv, has proven to be slow and inconsistent. While air abrasion cutting of carious dental tissue has been increasingly studied in recent years, alumina abrasives still indiscriminately cut sound structure and do not possess remineralisation properties. Bioglass abrasives on the other hand have been shown to promote hard tissue remineralisation yet they abrade at a slower rate. It can therefore be postulated that a fluoridated bioactive glass abrasive that possesses apatite-forming abilities would have an edge over the two abrasive types mentioned above.

2. Materials and Methods

2.1. Bioactive Glass Abrasive Fabrication. Bioactive glass Na0SR was produced in the in-house lab using the melt-quench technique using the composition shown in Table 1. To

TABLE 1: Composition of Na0SR by molecular weight percentage.

Na0SR composition	% by molecular weight
SiO_2	37%
P_2O_5	6.1%
SrO	53.9%
SrF_2	3%

produce glass of that molecular weight composition, 36.85 g of silicon dioxide, 14.35 g of phosphorus pentoxide, 131.89 g of strontium carbonate (all analytical grade products by Sigma-Aldrich, Gillingham, UK), and 6.25 g of strontium fluoride (Riedel-de Haën, Seelze, Germany) powder reagents (measured using weighing scale by Mettler PC 4400 Delta Range, Leicester, UK) were placed in a platinum crucible and heated in an electric furnace (Lenton, Derbyshire, UK) at 1540°C for 90 minutes. The viscous melted glass was then quenched by immediate pouring into a pail of deionised water at room temperature. The glass frit produced was immediately collected in a metal sieve and dried for at least 2 hours in a drying cabinet (LTE Scientific, Oldham, UK) at 65–80°C.

The dried glass frit was milled for 1 minute and 15 seconds using a milling machine (Gy-Ro Mill, Glen Creston, London, UK). This machine acts in a horizontal grinding motion and produces angular particles, ideal for air abrasion cutting. In order to select only abrasive particles between 38 and 80 microns in width, the ground powder was sieved using the Retsch VS 1000 sieve shaker (Retsch, Heidenheim, Germany) between two woven wire mesh analytical sieves (Endecotts Ltd., London, UK) of nominal apertures 38 and 80 microns for 30 minutes. The particle size distribution of the abrasives was visually examined under the Scanning Electron Microscope (SEM by Oxford Instruments, Abingdon, Oxfordshire, UK). Angular particles were observed but particles much smaller than 38 microns were noted to be present in masses. A second round of sieving was carried out for 30 minutes to remove the small particles.

Rubber balls were placed in the 80- and 38-micron sieves in the first and second rounds of sieving, respectively. This was to discourage particle adherence and to encourage particle flow through the sieves. A second round of examination under the SEM confirmed a more even size distribution of angular particles within the targeted range of 38 to 80 microns in width (Figure 1).

Eight batches of glass with the same composition were produced. To check for homogeneity among the batches, glass characterisation was performed for each batch. Differential Scanning Calorimetry (DSC) was carried out (DSC, Stanton Redcroft DSC1500, Rheometric Scientific, Epsom, UK) to map out the behaviour of the glass through thermal changes. 0.05 g (weighing scale by Balance Technology, Wanstead, London, UK) of each glass batch was analysed to determine the glass transition temperature (T_g). All eight batches of glass produced similar T_g values, which was indicative of the similarity in composition between them. The glass batches were also analysed using X-ray diffraction (XRD), a rapid analytical technique used for phase identification of a crystalline material. An amorphous material like glass

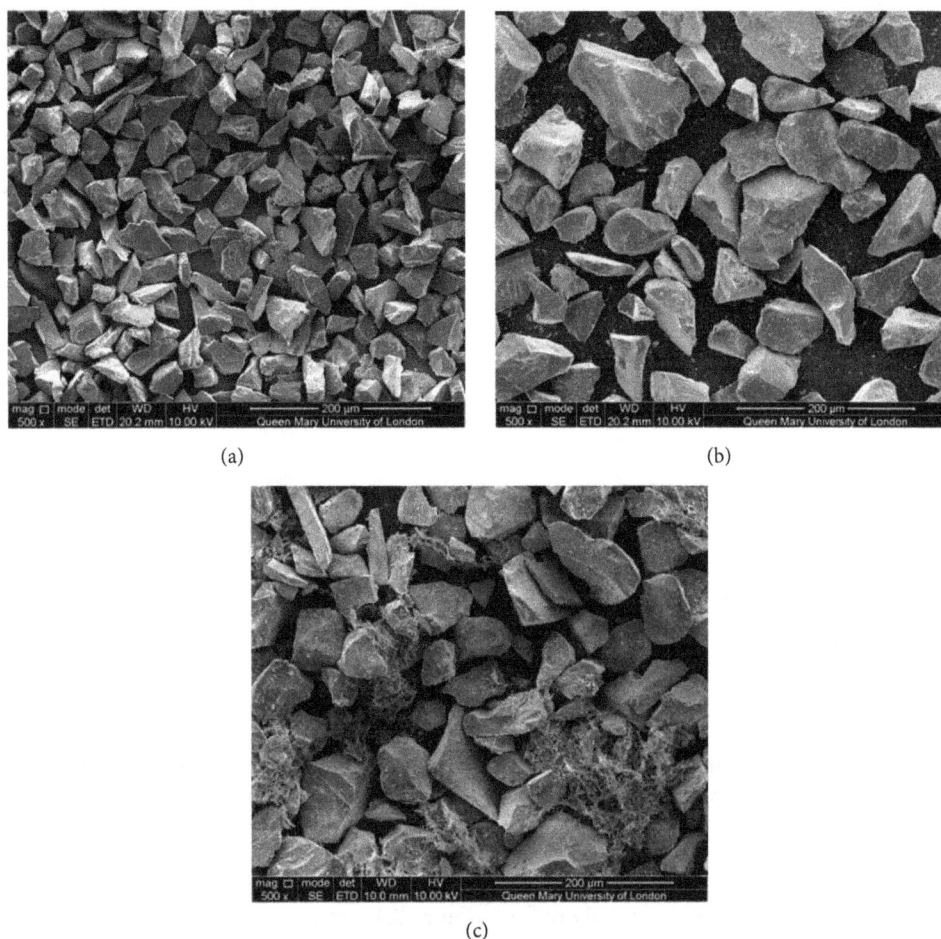

FIGURE 1: Scanning electron microscopy images of (a) alumina, adapted from Farooq et al. 2013 [24], (b) NaOSR, and (c) 45S5.

should not have any phases identified. XRD analyses revealed that all eight batches of glass were generally amorphous with the exception of one narrow peak of crystallisation, indicative of a small but insignificant percentage of crystalline nature present (Figure 2). All eight batches of glass were then combined into one.

2.2. Powder Flow Tests. This was carried out to determine the consistency of the powder output of both abrasives. It was also to ensure that the output flow was smooth with no clogging.

The design of the set-up as shown in Figure 3 was similar to the system described by Banerjee et al. [25]. A commercially available air abrasion unit that had undergone recent maintenance and calibration was used (Aquacut Quattro, Twin-Chamber Dental Air Abrasion and Air Polishing Unit, Velopex International, Harlesden, London, UK). This machine dispenses abrasives using a vibration mechanism. Its silicon carbide nozzle tip, 0.6 mm in diameter, was directed through an airtight opening into a container sealed at the base with a dry, porous cloth. This cloth enabled air to escape but trapped the abrasive particles in. As both abrasives were white in colour, a contrasting black paper was kept beneath the cloth to ensure no particle leakage. A sponge was placed in the centre of the container to absorb the highly pressurised

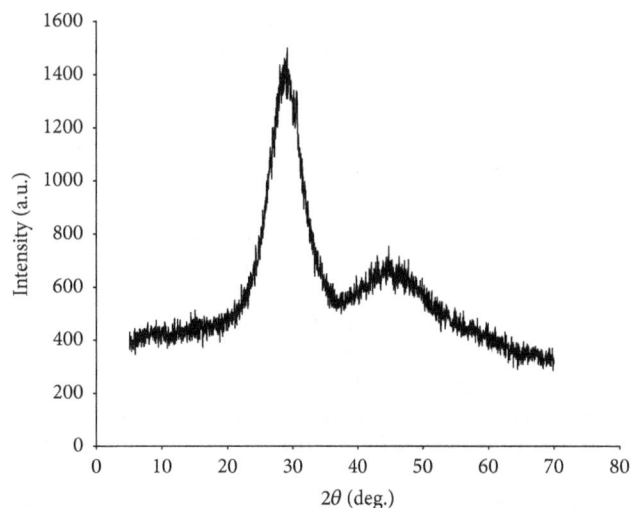

FIGURE 2: X-ray diffraction of one batch of NaOSR (#7) as an example.

air jet from the nozzle and avoid fenestration of the cloth. The powder flow tests were carried out dry at a pressure of 552 kPa

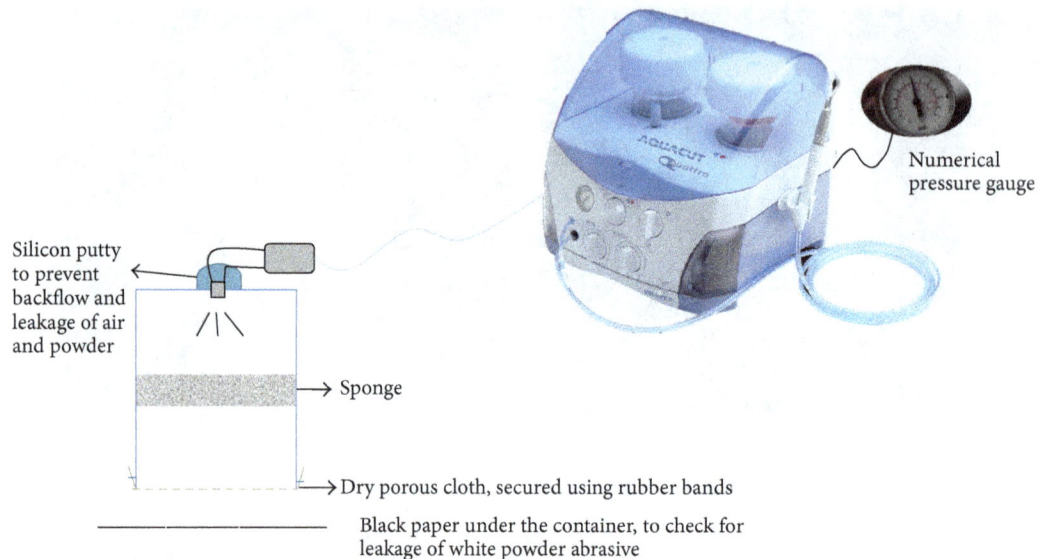

FIGURE 3: Air abrasion set-up of the abrasive powder outflow test.

(80 PSI), with the powder flow setting kept at 2. The reservoirs containing the abrasive powders were maintained to be one-quarter-filled to half-filled throughout the experiment. The weight of each container before and after each run lasting for 30 seconds was measured (weighing scale by Mettler PC 4400 Delta Range, Leicester, UK). Five rounds were carried out for each abrasive.

2.3. Samples Preparation. In order to reduce variation between samples, ivory dentine slabs were used instead of extracted teeth. Ivory was obtained by the airport customs and later gifted to the department for research purposes. All samples were prepared from the same piece of ivory, taking care to ensure that the working surfaces were from the same plane. 14 flat slabs of ivory dentine, with working surfaces measuring 5×5 mm and a depth of at least 5 mm, were prepared using an annular diamond blade (Microslice 2 Precision Slicing Machine by Malvern Instruments, Malvern, England) within the confines of a fume cupboard (Astec Monair Astec Microflow, Bioquell UK Ltd., Hampshire, UK). The outer lining of cementum was removed and the samples were mounted onto acrylic resin blocks (Meadway cold cure rapid repair powder and liquid, MR Dental Supplies Ltd., Surrey, England, UK) to obtain a stable base. Polishing of the working surfaces was achieved using rotating silicon carbide paper wheels in incremental grit sizes to obtain a smooth, flat surface. To prevent desiccation of the dentine samples, they were stored in a moist, airtight container.

2.4. Air Abrasion Cutting Tests. 14 samples of ivory dentine were used, with seven in each group of abrasives. Air abrasion tests were carried out using the same machine, Aquacut Quattro air abrasion machine (Velopex International, Harlesden, London, UK). It has a water spray feature coincident with and enveloping the particle stream. Two abrasive powders were compared, a commercial aluminium oxide abrasive (29 μm) (Velopex International, UK), and the lab-fabricated fluoridated bioactive glass abrasive NaOSR (38–80 μm). A 0.6 mm diameter nozzle tip was held stationary using a stand, at a distance of 1 mm and 90 degrees to the working surface of the dentine sample. The air abrasion was switched on for 10 seconds per round at a pressure of 552 kPa (80 PSI) and powder flow setting 2. Deionised water output was kept constant for this experiment. A rubber nozzle was used to funnel the water and the powder into a single stream. The nozzle was regularly checked to be centred and intact with no broken edges. The reservoirs holding the abrasives were kept between a quarter and half full throughout the experiment. Following each round of air abrasion treatment, a flush of deionised water over the working surface of each sample removed excess debris.

2.5. X-Ray Microtomography. Following the air abrasion procedure, the samples were scanned using X-ray micro-tomography on the MicroCT 40 Scanner (Scanco Medical, Switzerland). This is a nondestructive technique that characterises a material's microstructure in three dimensions at a micron level spatial resolution [26]. The specimen is mounted such that it can be stepped across a monochromatic beam and rotated about an axis normal to the beam. A detector measures the X-ray intensity and a line projection is calculated. A large number of line projections in multiple orientations can be collected to reconstruct a three-dimensional X-ray scan of the specimen [27].

An image of the plane through which the greatest cavity depth was observed for each sample was extracted from the three-dimensional scans using ImageJ program. Using a travelling microscope (Vickers Instruments, York, United

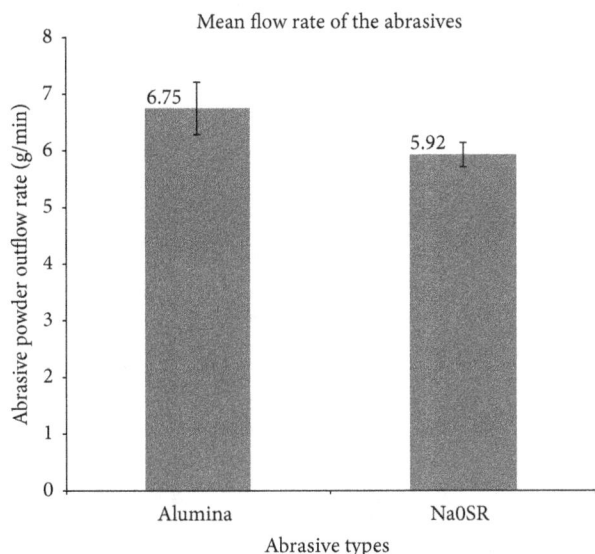

FIGURE 4: Comparison of mean flow rate between alumina and NaOSR abrasives.

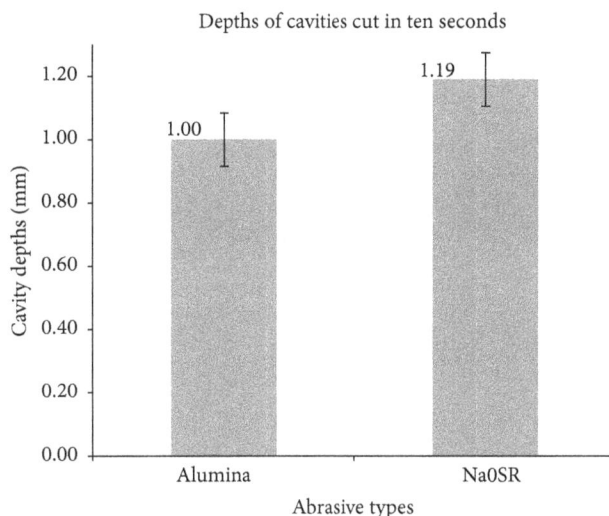

FIGURE 5: Comparison of cavity depths cut in 10 seconds between alumina and NaOSR abrasives.

Kingdom), physical measurements of the length of each slab as well as the diameter of the cavity were taken in the same plane as the extracted image. By calibrating the physical measurements with the length measurements on the image, the actual depths of the cavities were found.

3. Results

3.1. Powder Flow Tests (Figure 4). The mean weight of alumina abrasive output was 6.75 g/min ± 6.9%, whereas the mean weight of NaOSR abrasive output was 5.92 g/min ± 3.6%. Assuming normal distribution, the two-tailed t-test demonstrated that the mean powder output of alumina versus NaOSR was significantly different at the 95% confidence interval ($p = 0.023$).

3.2. Cavity Depths Cut Using Air Abrasion (Figure 5). The mean depth of cavity cut by alumina in ten seconds was 1.00 mm ± 8.4%, while NaOSR produced cavities of mean depth 1.19 mm ± 7.1%. Assuming normal distribution, the two-tailed t-test demonstrated that the mean cavity depths produced by NaOSR were nearly 0.2 mm deeper than alumina, significantly different at the 95% confidence interval ($p = 0.001$).

In conclusion, both the null hypothesis and hypothesis have been disproved. NaOSR abrasive was more efficacious at cutting dentine as compared to alumina despite its lower mean powder output.

4. Discussion

This study disproved the initial hypothesis. Instead of performing inferior to alumina in its cutting ability, the customised fluoridated bioactive glass abrasive NaOSR in this study produced significantly deeper cavities despite the lower powder outflow rate.

Bioactive glass is known to have a lower hardness as compared to alumina and it has also been consistently shown to cut at a slower rate than alumina [4, 19, 24]. Both Banerjee et al. [4] and Paolinelis et al. [19] used smaller particles of 45S5 Bioglass, 10–40 μm and 25–32 μm, respectively, similar in size to the alumina particles. The bioactive glass particles in this study were prepared as 38–80 μm, in comparison, larger than the 29 μm alumina particles used (Figure 1). It was modelled after the study by Farooq et al. [24], yet that study also demonstrated a lower cutting efficacy of bioactive glass. However, it might be useful to consider that the abrasives used in the study by Farooq et al. [24] appear to have multiple small particles within its distribution (observed from SEM images in the paper) and that might have affected the cutting ability or powder flow. The powder flow rate was not measured in that study.

The composition of NaOSR was adapted from Farooq et al. [24], which showed that the T_g values of the glass corresponded to the changes in sodium composition and hardness of the glass. As sodium levels decreased, hardness levels increased. The T_g values derived in this study corresponded to the T_g values of the 0% sodium glass in that study (Figure 6). Its Vickers hardness is therefore postulated to be similar and close to 6.65 GPa. As compared to alumina which has a known Knoop Hardness Value (KHV) of 2100 [28, 29], approximately equivalent to 19.86 GPa in Vickers hardness, NaOSR is substantially softer. Both particles of alumina and NaOSR were angular in shape. To explain the observed favourable cutting outcome of NaOSR, we can postulate that it may be due to the nature of broken glass. Glass is brittle and produces sharp edges when broken. This increased surface area of sharp cutting edges upon impact could be the reason behind more efficacious tooth structure abrasion despite its lower volume output per minute.

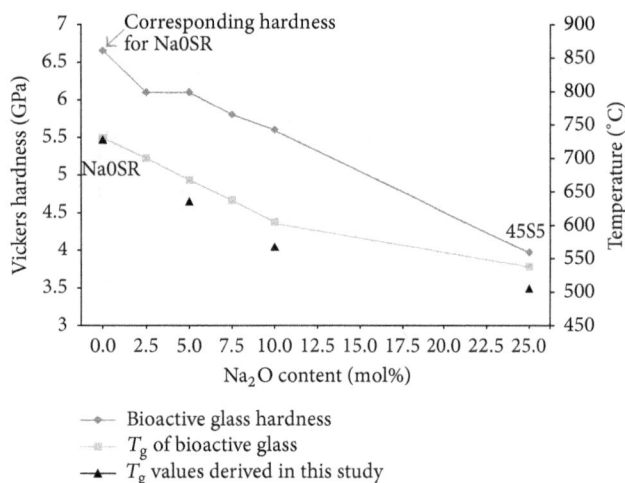

FIGURE 6: T_g and Vickers hardness values adapted from Farooq et al. 2013 [24], as comparison.

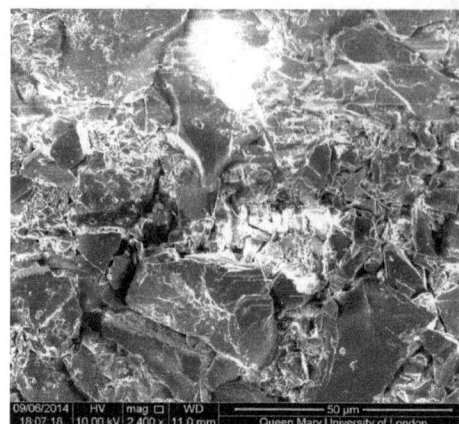

(a)

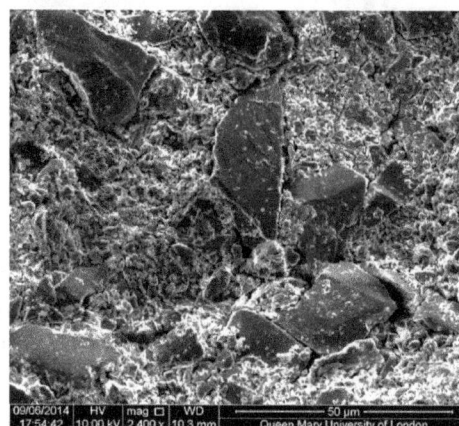

(b)

FIGURE 7: SEM image of the alumina (a) and NaOSR (b) remnant at the base of the cut cavities after air abrasion.

In the production of NaOSR, calcium was fully substituted by strontium from the zero-sodium composition in Farooq et al. [24] to increase the radiopacity of the abrasive for clearer XMT imaging. Due to the similarity in size and ionic charge of calcium and strontium, this substitution by molecular weight is not expected to change the structure [30, 31] or behaviour [32] of the glass. Farooq et al.'s [24] research demonstrated apatite formation within their series of bioactive glasses when it was placed in Tris buffer solution for 6–24 hours whereas Sylc produced smaller peaks of apatite within the same time frame. A comparison between the SEM images of the abrasives in their study and the SEM of NaOSR postoperatively (Figure 7) reveals the similarity of widespread small, broken down particles that would have an increased surface area for bioactivity to occur. Thus, NaOSR can be expected to behave in the same manner for apatite formation in Tris buffer solution.

The addition of fluorine, instead of substitution, ensured that the silicate network is not disrupted and the network connectivity remains unchanged [33]. Several studies have found that, by adding low amounts of fluorine to bioactive glass, fluorapatite is formed [34] and can be identified using MAS-NMR within six hours in Tris buffer [35]. This even occurs at a lower pH [36], which mimics an environment similar to an oral acid attack [37].

The important implication of this study is the emergence of an alternative abrasion cutting material, which not only has the ideal characteristics of being conservative and in line with minimally invasive dentistry, but also has likely remineralisation potential of hydroxyfluorapatite and uses a method with better patient acceptability due to its reduced vibrational forces, loud noises, and overall discomfort.

4.1. Limitations of Findings. The jet of water spray on each sample was insufficient to remove the layer of powder compacted onto the base of the cavity. This layer is visible to the naked eye in every sample. However, due to a limitation of the X-ray microtomography machine, this layer can be differentiated clearly in some images but not in others (Figure 8). This has led to a systematic error in the collection of results, where an underestimation of the cavity depths is carried out for all samples by measuring the depths to the top surface of the powder layer, instead of to the actual cavity depth. Leaving the layer of powder in situ has its potential benefit and risk. A potential benefit would be that it could potentially act as a nucleus of minerals for remineralisation to occur. The plausible risk on the other hand would be an interference with the strength of bond between the restorative material and the tooth structure. This would need to be further studied. An initial examination was carried out via SEM images on the appearance of the powder layer after the procedure. Alumina had formed a layer comprising particles with similar sizes whereas NaOSR had a few larger particles dispersed and embedded within a bed of fine particles (Figure 7).

A second limitation would be a lack of comparison to 45S5 Bioglass in this study. The original plan was to compare the cutting efficacy of NaOSR to both 45S5 Bioglass and alumina. This could not be carried out due to the poor, inconsistent flow rate of the commercial 45S5 Bioglass (Sylc©, Aquacut Quattro, Velopex International, Harlesden, London,

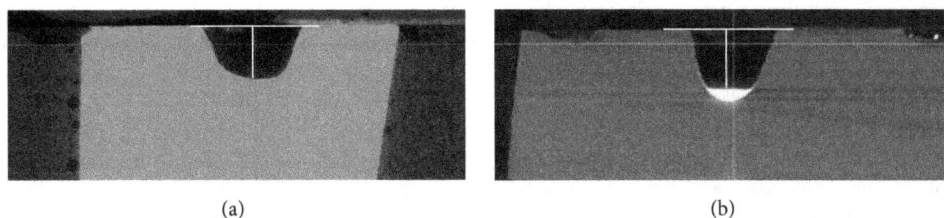

(a)   (b)

FIGURE 8: Samples of cavity cut by alumina ((a) with indistinguishable powder layer from dentine) and Na0SR ((b) with a very radiopaque powder layer due to the presence of strontium).

UK). Newly opened bottles of Sylc$^{©}$ were revealed to have multiple, interspersed regions of web-like structure, which led to its irregular flow (Figure 1(c)). These structures have been suggested to appear similar to octacalcium phosphate [38], a precursor of hydroxyapatite that forms when in contact with moisture. The advantage of Na0SR over 45S5 Bioglass that can be postulated through this observation is its reduced sensitivity and reactivity to environmental moisture, which would translate to a longer shelf life.

Future research that would advance the field of air abrasion cutting using bioactive glasses would be to test the cutting efficacy of Na0SR on carious dentine as compared to sound dentine. Selective cutting of carious dentine over sound structure can be examined using a series of fluoridated glass compositions with varying sodium content and hardness.

5. Conclusion

Na0SR, a fluoridated bioactive glass, performed significantly better than alumina at air abrasion cutting of dentine. This is despite having a significantly lower abrasive particle output. Both were calculated at the 95% confidence level. Na0SR can therefore be considered as a plausible abrasive substitute for alumina in air abrasion cutting as it performs as well and has the potential added benefit of promoting remineralisation and hydroxyfluorapatite formation.

Conflict of Interests

The authors hereby declare no potential conflict of interests with respect to the authorship and/or publication of this paper.

References

[1] A. Banerjee, E. A. M. Kidd, and T. F. Watson, "In vitro evaluation of five alternative methods of carious dentine excavation," *Caries Research*, vol. 34, no. 2, pp. 144–150, 2000.

[2] R. J. Smales and D. T. S. Fang, "In vitro effectiveness of hand excavation of caries with the ART technique," *Caries Research*, vol. 33, no. 6, pp. 437–440, 1999.

[3] M. Ahmed, G. R. Davis, and F. S. L. Wong, "X-ray microtomography study to validate the efficacies of caries removal in primary molars by hand excavation and chemo-mechanical technique," *Caries Research*, vol. 46, no. 6, pp. 561–567, 2012.

[4] A. Banerjee, I. D. Thompson, and T. F. Watson, "Minimally invasive caries removal using bio-active glass air-abrasion," *Journal of Dentistry*, vol. 39, no. 1, pp. 2–7, 2011.

[5] M. J. Tyas, K. J. Anusavice, J. E. Frencken, and G. J. Mount, "Minimal intervention dentistry—a review: FDI Commission Project 1-97," *International Dental Journal*, vol. 50, no. 1, pp. 1–12, 2000.

[6] S. O. Griffin, E. Oong, W. Kohn et al., "The effectiveness of sealants in managing caries lesions," *Journal of Dental Research*, vol. 87, no. 2, pp. 169–174, 2008.

[7] M. Dorri, A. Sheiham, and V. C. Marinho, "Atraumatic restorative treatment versus conventional restorative treatment for the management of dental caries," *Cochrane Database of Systematic Reviews*, 2009.

[8] N. P. T. Innes, D. J. P. Evans, and D. R. Stirrups, "Sealing caries in primary molars: randomized control trial, 5-year results," *Journal of Dental Research*, vol. 90, no. 12, pp. 1405–1410, 2011.

[9] D. Ricketts, T. Lamont, N. P. T. Innes, E. Kidd, and J. E. Clarkson, "Operative caries management in adults and children." *The Cochrane Database of Systematic Reviews*, no. 3, Article ID CD003808, 2013.

[10] V. S. Hegde and R. A. Khatavkar, "A new dimension to conservative dentistry: air abrasion," *Journal of Conservative Dentistry*, vol. 13, no. 1, pp. 4–8, 2010.

[11] A. Gabel, "Critical review of cutting instruments in cavity preparation: airbrasive technic," *International Dental Journal*, vol. 4, pp. 57–63, 1953.

[12] K. Laurell, W. Carpernter, and M. Beck, "Pulpal effects of airbrasion cavity preparation in dogs," *Journal of Dental Research*, vol. 72, p. 237, 1993.

[13] F. S. L. Wong, N. S. Willmott, and G. R. Davis, "Dentinal carious lesion in three dimensions," *International Journal of Paediatric Dentistry*, vol. 16, no. 6, pp. 419–423, 2006.

[14] R. B. Black, "Airbrasive: some fundamentals," *Journal of the American Dental Association*, vol. 41, no. 6, pp. 701–710, 1950.

[15] R. J. Cook, A. Azzopardi, I. D. Thompson, and T. F. Watson, "Real-time confocal imaging, during active air abrasion—substrate cutting," *Journal of Microscopy*, vol. 203, no. 2, pp. 199–207, 2001.

[16] G. Z. Wright, S. Hatibovic-Kofman, D. W. Millenaar, and I. Braverman, "The safety and efficacy of treatment with air abrasion technology," *International Journal of Paediatric Dentistry*, vol. 9, no. 2, pp. 133–140, 1999.

[17] E. Radziun, J. Dudkiewicz Wilczyńska, I. Ksiazek et al., "Assessment of the cytotoxicity of aluminium oxide nanoparticles on selected mammalian cells," *Toxicology in Vitro*, vol. 25, no. 8, pp. 1694–1700, 2011.

[18] L. L. Hench and A. E. Clark, *Adhesion to Bone*, CRC Press, Boca Raton, Fla, USA, 1982.

[19] G. Paolinelis, A. Banerjee, and T. F. Watson, "An in vitro investigation of the effect and retention of bioactive glass air-abrasive on sound and carious dentine," *Journal of Dentistry*, vol. 36, no. 3, pp. 214–218, 2008.

[20] A. Banerjee, H. Pabari, G. Paolinelis, I. D. Thompson, and T. F. Watson, "An in vitro evaluation of selective demineralised enamel removal using bio-active glass air abrasion," *Clinical Oral Investigations*, vol. 15, no. 6, pp. 895–900, 2011.

[21] H. Milly, R. S. Austin, I. Thompson, and A. Banerjee, "In vitro effect of air-abrasion operating parameters on dynamic cutting characteristics of alumina and bio-active glass powders," *Operative Dentistry*, vol. 39, no. 1, pp. 81–89, 2014.

[22] J. M. Ten Cate, "Remineralization of caries lesions extending into dentin," *Journal of Dental Research*, vol. 80, no. 5, pp. 1407–1411, 2001.

[23] J. D. B. Featherstone, "Prevention and reversal of dental caries: role of low level fluoride," *Community Dentistry and Oral Epidemiology*, vol. 27, no. 1, pp. 31–40, 1999.

[24] I. Farooq, M. Tylkowski, S. Müller, T. Janicki, D. S. Brauer, and R. G. Hill, "Influence of sodium content on the properties of bioactive glasses for use in air abrasion," *Biomedical Materials*, vol. 8, no. 6, Article ID 065008, 2013.

[25] A. Banerjee, M. Uddin, G. Paolinelis, and T. F. Watson, "An investigation of the effect of powder reservoir volume on the consistency of alumina powder flow rates in dental air-abrasion devices," *Journal of Dentistry*, vol. 36, no. 3, pp. 224–227, 2008.

[26] E. N. Landis and D. T. Keane, "X-ray microtomography," *Materials Characterization*, vol. 61, no. 12, pp. 1305–1316, 2010.

[27] X. J. Gao, J. C. Elliott, P. Anderson, and G. R. Davis, "Scanning microradiographic and microtomographic studies of remineralisation of subsurface enamel lesions," *Journal of the Chemical Society, Faraday Transactions*, vol. 89, no. 15, pp. 2907–2912, 1993.

[28] D. R. Lide, *CRC Handbook of Chemistry and Physics*, The Chemical Rubber, Boca Raton, Fla, USA, 74th edition, 1993.

[29] R. G. Craig, W. J. O'Brien, and J. M. Powers, *Dental Materials—Properties and Manipulation*, C.V. Mosby, St. Louis, Mo, USA, 1995.

[30] R. G. Hill, A. Stamboulis, R. V. Law, A. Clifford, M. R. Towler, and C. Crowley, "The influence of strontium substitution in fluorapatite glasses and glass-ceramics," *Journal of Non-Crystalline Solids*, vol. 336, no. 3, pp. 223–229, 2004.

[31] Y. C. Fredholm, N. Karpukhina, R. V. Law, and R. G. Hill, "Strontium containing bioactive glasses: glass structure and physical properties," *Journal of Non-Crystalline Solids*, vol. 356, no. 44–49, pp. 2546–2551, 2010.

[32] J. Du and Y. Xiang, "Effect of strontium substitution on the structure, ionic diffusion and dynamic properties of 45S5 Bioactive glasses," *Journal of Non-Crystalline Solids*, vol. 358, no. 8, pp. 1059–1071, 2012.

[33] D. S. Brauer, N. Karpukhina, R. V. Law, and R. G. Hill, "Structure of fluoride-containing bioactive glasses," *Journal of Materials Chemistry*, vol. 19, no. 31, pp. 5629–5636, 2009.

[34] D. S. Brauer, N. Karpukhina, M. D. O'Donnell, R. V. Law, and R. G. Hill, "Fluoride-containing bioactive glasses: effect of glass design and structure on degradation, pH and apatite formation in simulated body fluid," *Acta Biomaterialia*, vol. 6, no. 8, pp. 3275–3282, 2010.

[35] X. Chen, X. Chen, D. S. Brauer, R. M. Wilson, R. G. Hill, and N. Karpukhina, "Bioactivity of sodium free fluoride containing glasses and glass-ceramics," *Materials*, vol. 7, no. 8, pp. 5470–5487, 2014.

[36] M. Mneimne, R. G. Hill, A. J. Bushby, and D. S. Brauer, "High phosphate content significantly increases apatite formation of fluoride-containing bioactive glasses," *Acta Biomaterialia*, vol. 7, no. 4, pp. 1827–1834, 2011.

[37] F. A. Shah, D. S. Brauer, R. M. Wilson, R. G. Hill, and K. A. Hing, "Influence of cell culture medium composition on in vitro dissolution behavior of a fluoride-containing bioactive glass," *Journal of Biomedical Materials Research Part A*, vol. 102, no. 3, pp. 647–654, 2014.

[38] M. Mneimne, R. G. Hill, R. Langford, D. Gillam, and J. Earl, "FIB-SEM depth profiling of dentine treated with novel bioactive glasses," in *Proceedings of the IADR General Session and Exhibition*, Cape Town, South Africa, September 2014.

26

Zirconia Implants in Esthetic Areas: 4-Year Follow-Up Evaluation Study

Andrea Enrico Borgonovo,[1] Rachele Censi,[2] Virna Vavassori,[1] Oscar Arnaboldi,[3] Carlo Maiorana,[3] and Dino Re[4]

[1] School of Oral Surgery, University of Milan, Department of Oral Rehabilitation, Istituto Stomatologico Italiano, 20122 Milan, Italy

[2] Department of Implantology and Periodontology, Istituto Stomatologico Italiano, 20122 Milan, Italy

[3] Department of Implantology, Dental Clinic, Fondazione IRCCS Cà Granda Ospedale Maggiore Policlinico, School of Oral surgery, University of Milan, 20122 Milan, Italy

[4] Head Department of Oral Rehabilitation, Istituto Stomatologico Italiano, 20122 Milan, Italy

Correspondence should be addressed to Virna Vavassori; virna.vavassori@hotmail.it

Academic Editor: Burak Demiralp

Objectives. The aim is to evaluate the survival and success rates, as well as the marginal bone loss (MBL) and periodontal indexes of zirconia implants positioned in the esthetic jaw areas. *Materials and Method*. 13 patients were selected and 20 one-piece zirconia implants were used for the rehabilitation of single tooth or partially edentulous ridge in the esthetic jaw areas. Six months after surgery and then once a year, a clinical-radiographic evaluation was performed in order to estimate peri-implant tissue health and marginal bone loss. *Results*. The survival and success rates were 100%. The average marginal bone loss from baseline to 48 months after surgery was +2.1 mm. Four years after surgery, the median and the mode for visible Plaque Index and Bleeding On Probing resulted 1 whereas Probing Pocket Depth amounted to 3 mm (SD = ±0.49 mm). *Conclusion*. One-piece zirconia dental implants are characterized by high biocompatibility, low plaque adhesion, and absence of microgap that can be related to the clinical success of these implants even in the esthetic areas.

1. Introduction

The original concept of implant surgery as described by Branemark [1] is that the fixture is placed in the bone and completely covered by mucoperiosteal flaps. After the healing period of at least 3 months in the mandible and up to 6 months in the maxilla, the implant is exposed and a healing abutment is connected.

Since the material composition and the surface topography of the implants play a fundamental role in osseointegration, various chemical and physical surface modifications have been developed in order to reduce the time of osseous healing, and it was observed that increased surface roughness of dental implants resulted in greater bone apposition [2] and reduced healing time [3]. However, even if the original protocol by Branemark was modified by modern works

of research, patients expect a rehabilitation to be finalized within the shortest time span possible especially if the edentulism involves the esthetic regions. Moreover, patients require implants that are esthetic as well as functional and, for this reason, more recently higher interest is directed towards the esthetic of the prosthetic rehabilitations.

The use of ceramic components based on alumina or yttrium-stabilized zirconium oxide in conjunction with all-ceramic restorations allows to achieve implant osseointegration, which was examined in several animal experiments [4–6], and to solve esthetic problems. In fact, even if several studies reported high success rates for titanium dental implants [7], it is important to consider that bone resorption of the vestibular cortical bone and recession of the peri-implant soft tissue can occur over time [8]. Consequently, the titanium components may be visible and cause discoloration of the gingiva, particularly in cases of thin biotype and high smile line [9]. The first ceramic material that was used in the past for dental implants was aluminium oxide. This material showed good osseointegration but it did not have sufficient mechanical properties for long-term loading [10]. More recently, new generation ceramic materials such as zirconia were introduced. Zirconia is characterized by more favorable mechanical properties (high flexural strength (900–1200 Mpa), hardness (1200 Vickers), and Weibull modulus (10–12)) than aluminium oxide. In addition, this biomaterial has a high biocompatibility and low plaque adhesion [11], and several animal studies showed bone-to-implant contact similar to titanium [5, 6, 12]

The aim of this study is to evaluate the survival and success rates, the marginal bone loss (MBL), radiographic measurements, and periodontal indexes (Plaque Index (PI), Bleeding On Probing (BOP), Probing Pocket Depth (PPD), and implant mobility) of zirconia dental implants positioned in the maxillary and mandibular esthetic areas.

2. Materials and Methods

At the Department of Implantology, Dental Clinic, Fondazione IRCCS Cà Granda Policlinico, University of Milan, the authors did a retrospective study of patients treated using monocomponent endosseous zirconia dental implants for the rehabilitation of esthetic areas.

22 one-piece endosseous dental implants made of sintered and yttrium-stabilized zirconium oxide were used for the rehabilitation of single tooth or partially edentulous ridge in the esthetic areas in the maxilla or the mandible. It was considered that the esthetic zone of the jaw includes the central and lateral incisors, the canines, and the first premolars.

The implants used in the clinical study are made of sintered and yttrium-stabilized zirconium oxide (WhiteSky, Bredent, Senden, Germany) and are featured by a conical implant body and a double, cylindrical thread. The endosteal portion has a sandblasted surface, whereas, transmucosally, the implant includes a machined neck with a height of 2 mm. The implant surface is treated with a sanding process. The microscopical surface characteristics of medium rugosity (Ra 0.9-1 m) are similar to the surface of last-generation machine-finished titanium implants.

The abutment surface is smooth and it has a length of 6.8 mm which can be modified by grinding after implant positioning.

For this study, 14 patients in need of a single or multiple teeth replacements in the maxillary esthetic areas were selected (Figures 1, 2, and 3). All sites should present adequate bone volume (minimum bone height and thickness, respectively, of 8 and 5.5 mm). Implants positioned in regenerated bone were excluded from this protocol because the regenerative procedures associated with implant rehabilitation can influence the results in terms of marginal bone loss. In fact, it has been demonstrated that the marginal bone loss is greater in the regenerated bone than in the native bone [13]. Moreover, patients with oral problems such as

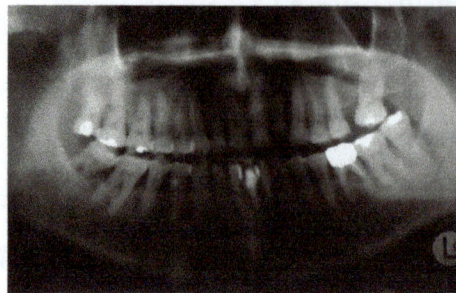

FIGURE 1: Preoperative orthopantomography.

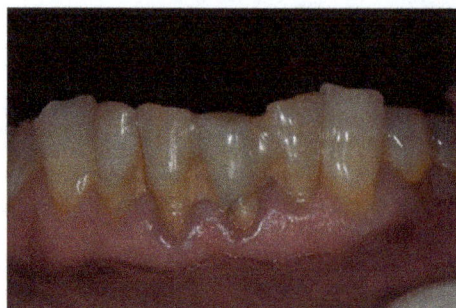

FIGURE 2: Preoperative clinical view.

active periodontal disease or parafunctions, bisphosphonates treatment, smoking more than 10 cigarettes per day, poor oral hygiene, and low compliance and patients with previous or concomitant systemic diseases such as immunodeficiency, head and neck radiotherapy, metabolic disorders, and hematological diseases, together with patients under 18 years of age were not included in this study.

All patients were previously informed about zirconia implants and possible alternatives and gave a written consent. Seven days before surgery, the patients underwent professional oral hygiene and they were instructed to start rinsing mouth twice a day with chlorhexidine 0.2% (Corsodyl, Glaxo, UK) until two weeks after surgery. Antibiotic prophylaxis with 2 gr of Amoxicillin and Clavulanic Acid (Laboratori Eurogenerici, Milan, Italy) was prescribed 1 hour prior to surgery.

The surgical procedure has involved the positioning of implants according to the protocol suggested by Bredent Medical, which is similar to the standard surgical protocol for titanium dental implants. All implants were inserted using a guide device prepared on a diagnostic wax-up (Figure 4). Mucoperiosteal flaps were elevated avoiding vertical releasing incisions in order to reduce the risk of blemishes. After preparing the implant sites, fixture insertion was performed by a surgical microengine. The fixtures were screwed until the rough surface of the implant body was positioned completely inside the bone, whereas implant abutment with smooth neck performed the function of the transmucosal element (Figure 5). All the implants were placed in the correct three-dimensional positioning according to esthetic protocol by Tarnow et al. [14]. Flaps were released through periosteal incisions to attain primary wound closure, and, at the end,

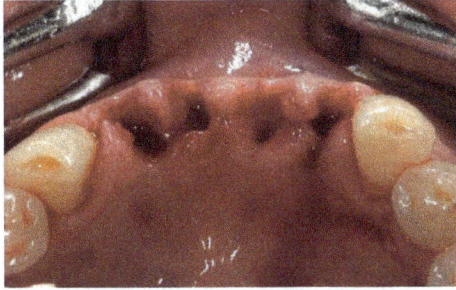

FIGURE 3: Dental extractions.

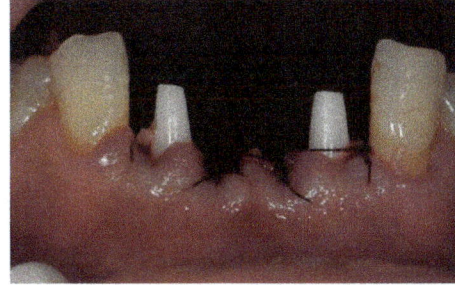

FIGURE 4: Surgical guide.

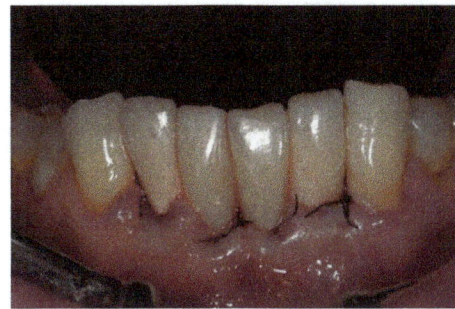

FIGURE 5: Two monocomponent zirconia implants are placed in the areas 3.2 and 4.2.

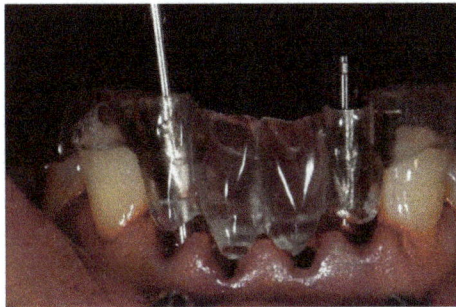

FIGURE 6: Immediate temporary restoration.

flaps were sutured with 4/0 monofilament suture (Premilene, Braun Melsungen, Germany).

After implant insertion, standardized periapical radiography using the Rinn alignment system (Dentsply, Constanz, Germany) with customized silicon bites (Orthogum Zermack, Badia Polesine, Rovigo, Italy) was obtained. The radiographic control was permitted to evaluate the correct positioning of implants.

Immediately after surgery, considering that zirconium oxide ceramics are bad thermal conductors, implant abutments were refined in order to correct their axis, length, or undercuts if present, using double diamond burs suited for zirconia (ETERNA Bredent, Senden, Germany) and water cooling. Temporary restorations obtained from diagnostic wax-up were relined with acrylic resin and luted with temporary cement (TEMPBOND, Kerr West Collins Orange, CA, USA). Single restorations were attached to the adjacent teeth by means of composite bonding, whereas multiple implants were connected together by provisional restoration in order to reduce the risk of implant mobility or extra occlusal load (in particular, tongue and lips movements) (Figure 6).

Patients were given oral hygiene suggestions and were instructed not to chew or eat on implant site until healing was completed. Antibiotic therapy (1 gr every 8 hours) and chlorhexidine mouth rinses were continued for 7 days, and Paracetamol 500 mg (Tachipirina, Angelini, Rome, Italy) was prescribed to use if necessity was felt. Sutures were removed 7 days after surgery and follow-up controls were programmed after 1 week, 2 weeks, and, subsequently, once a month for the following 6 months.

Six months after the surgery (Figures 7 and 8), definitive impressions (IMPREGUM, 3M, ESPE, St Paul, MN, USA)

were taken using a retraction cord (Ultrapak Cord, Ultradent, South Jordan, UT, USA) or an impression cap to register implant shoulder margins. The definitive restorations were made with CAD-CAM system (LAVA, 3M, ESPE, St Paul, MN, USA) (Figure 9) and cemented with glass ionomer cement (GC Fuji CEM, GC America, Alsip, IL, USA) (Figure 10).

One week after definitive restorations delivery and, subsequently, every year after implants placement, clinical-radiographic evaluation was performed. The periodontal evaluation was performed using a calibrated probe (Hu-Friedy, N. Rockwell Chicago, IL, USA) and the following periodontal indexes were investigated: Plaque Index (PI), Bleeding On Probing (BOP), Probing Pocket Depth (PPD), and implant mobility.

Moreover, the follow-up protocol included the radiographic control examination (Figures 10 and 11). The radiographs were taken using the customized silicon bite record prepared immediately after surgery. The radiographs were converted in digital images with a scanner (Epson 1680 Pro, Seiko Epson Cooperation, Nagano, Japan) and saved in JPG format. Each image was processed with a specific piece of software (CorelDraw 10.0; Corel Corp and Coral Ltd., Ottawa, Canada) and analyzed at ×20 magnification in order to calculate marginal bone loss. Mesial and distal marginal bone levels of all the implants were measured at baseline and on recall evaluations. The known length of the implant (measured from the implant shoulder to the implant apex) according to the manufacturer was used as a reference point. The distance from implant shoulder to crestal bone level was measured on the magnified images. To analyze the variability,

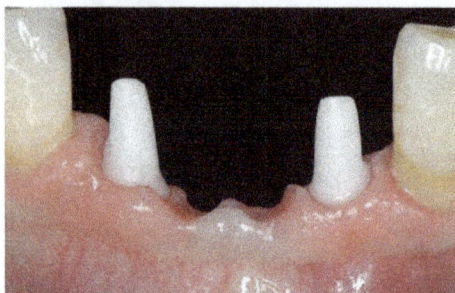

FIGURE 7: Soft tissue health 6 months after surgery.

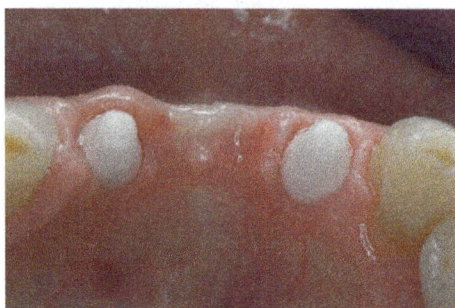

FIGURE 8: Occlusal view.

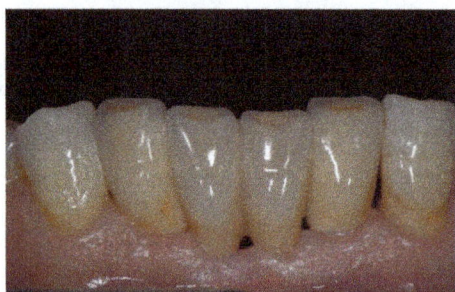

FIGURE 9: Definitive restoration.

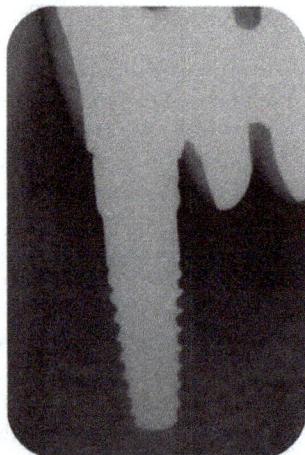

FIGURE 10: X-ray image of the zirconia implant placed in area 4.2, six months after surgery.

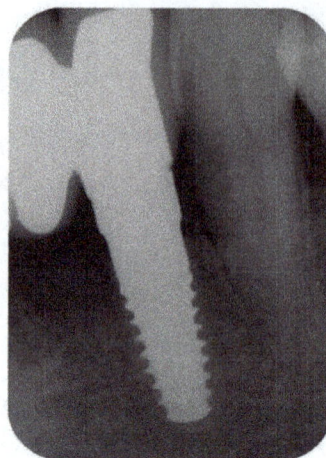

FIGURE 11: X-ray picture of the zirconia implant placed in area 3.2, six months after surgery.

the implant dimension (length) on the magnified X-ray was measured and compared to the real dimension, and ratios were calculated to adjust for distortion. Bone level changes were calculated at the distal and mesial surfaces of all implants by applying the distortion coefficient.

Data analysis was performed with descriptive statistics and the arithmetic mean; the median and the standard deviations were calculated. Clinical and radiographic control examination was repeated every year (Figures 12, 13, and 14).

At the end, success criteria and survival criteria were formulated in accordance with Albrektsson criteria for implants success [15]. Survival criteria were identified as the survival of loaded functionalized asymptomatic implants, whereas success criteria refer to four parameters, absence of implant mobility, absence of self-reported pain or paresthesia, absence of peri-implant radiolucency, and marginal bone loss inferior to 1.5 mm in the first year and to 0.2 mm in the following years.

3. Results

At the Department of Implantology, Dental Clinic, IRCCS Fondazione Cà Granda Ospedale Maggiore Policlinico, University of Milan, 14 patients were treated for the rehabilitation of the esthetic jaw areas. Average age was 60 years (ranging from 38 to 75 years), 13 male patients and one female. Starting from January 2007 and recruited in a period of one year, 14 patients were included in the study. The data were recorded to July 2012 when the implants had a minimal observation period of 4 years.

17 implants were placed in the maxilla, whereas 5 implants were placed in the mandible.

Considering the maxillary implants, 10 zirconia dental implants were used for the rehabilitation of single or multiple cases of edentulism in the incisor region; 3 implants replaced the canines, and the other 4 maxillary implants were placed in place of the missing first premolars. All mandibular implants were used for the rehabilitation of edentulism in the incisor

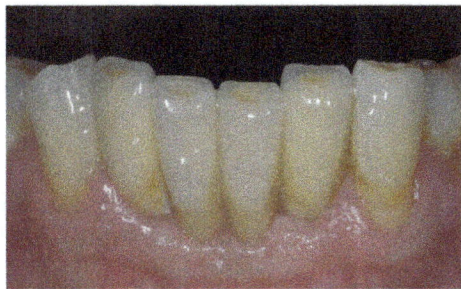

FIGURE 12: Clinical control 4 years after surgery.

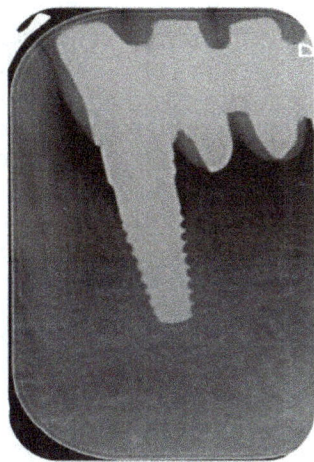

FIGURE 13: Radiographic control 4 years after implant insertions.

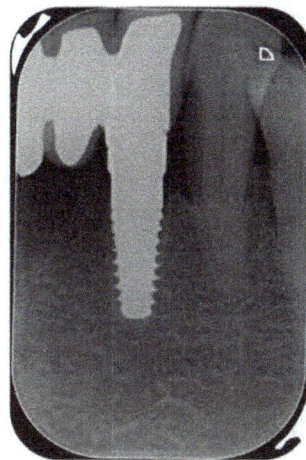

FIGURE 14: Radiographic control 4 years after implant insertions.

region, except 2 implants that were positioned in area of the missing right mandibular first premolar.

Considering patients' selection criteria, one patient with two implants placed in places of the upper right canine and the first premolar was excluded from this protocol because regenerative procedures were performed. For this reason, the data reported in this study refer exclusively to 20 implants. The follow-up period ranged from 6 to 48 months after implant insertion.

During the 48 months of follow-up, no implant failure was reported, with no pain or paresthesia, and, at the radiographic evaluation, peri-implant radiolucency was not detected. Thus, the cumulative survival rate was 100% after 4 years.

At follow-up controls, the median for PI and BOP was 1 and 0, respectively, and the mean values of PI and BOP were 0.54 and 0.23, respectively.

48 months after surgery, the median and the mode for visible Plaque Index (PI) and Bleeding On Probing (BOP) resulted 1. Overall Probing Pocket Depth (PPD) amounted to 3 mm (SD = ±0.49 mm). Mobility was not present at any site, and no pain (spontaneous or on percussion) or paresthesia was reported.

The mean marginal bone level after 4 years was +2,1045 mm, without a difference between mesial and distal sites. In particular, mean marginal bone loss was +1.50 mm

(SD = ±1.03) 6 months after implant insertion and +0.446 mm (SD = ±0.64) 6 months after prosthetic finalization.

From 1 year up to 2 years after implant positioning, an improvement of peri-implant bone level value was observed probably due to the formation of new bone trabeculae as a result of maturation of bone (-0.198 ± 0.50 mm).

A minimal bone remodeling with a further marginal bone loss of +0.18 mm (SD = ±0.28) and +0.17 mm (SD = ±0.11), respectively, was also observed at 3 and 4 years follow-up.

For implants placed in the maxilla, the average marginal bone loss from baseline to 6 months after surgery was $+1.50 \pm 1.03$ mm, from 6 months to 1 year was $+0.65 \pm 0.7$ mm, from 1 year to 2 years was -0.12 ± 0.57 mm, from 2 years to 3 years was $+0.12 \pm 0.25$ mm, and from 3 years to 4 years was -0.17 ± 0.11 mm.

Four patients were treated for multiple cases of edentulism with 8 zirconia dental implants, and, after surgery, all multiple implants were splinted together by provisional restoration. Considering the marginal bone loss adjacent to free-standing implants and multiple implants, it was observed that there is a statistically significant difference between the two groups ($P = 0.799$).

The success rate was 100%.

4. Discussion

The clinical success of the implant rehabilitation is in connection with the interface between bone tissue and implants surface. Several studies showed successful osseointegration of zirconia dental implants in different animal models [5–7, 12]. In the work by Thomsen et al. [16], the interface between the rabbit tibia bone tissue and the surfaces of gold, titanium, and zirconia implants was investigated, and the histological examination disclosed that the bone-implant contact ratio (BIC) is similar for zirconia and titanium implants, whereas gold implants had a lower degree of BIC. In the study by Scarano et al. [17], a great amount of newly formed bones was observed in close contact with the surfaces of zirconia implants positioned in rabbits, and the BIC ratio was 68%. Furthermore, the BIC ratio was better investigated by

Akagawa et al. [18] who demonstrated that the bone-implant contact ratio ranged from 54% to 69.8% at 12 months and from 66.2% to 67.7% at 24 months.

The bone-implant contact ratio is the result of bone formation, and it is related to the characteristics of implant surface. Sennerby et al. [19] evaluated the bone tissue reaction to titanium implants and zirconia dental implants with and without different surface modifications. The titanium implants and the zirconia implants with the surface modifications showed the highest surface roughness in comparison to the nonmodified zirconia implants, and, consequently, machined implants presented a lower degree of BIC than titanium and modified zirconia implants.

The reported studies demonstrate a bone-implant contact for zirconia dental implants, similar to those of titanium implants, and these findings suggest that zirconia dental implants can reach firm stability in bones.

More recently, the osseointegration of zirconia dental implants was histologically demonstrated in one human patient [20]. In this study, a two-piece zirconia implant was placed in the maxilla of a healthy woman and 6 months after surgery, the retrieval of the dental implant was performed. The surrounding soft and hard tissues were harvested and processed for histological evaluation. The processed sample of zirconia dental implant provided the histological evidence of osseointegration. Moreover, the scanning electron microscopic analyses showed a good maintenance of the crestal bone level; in fact, it was possible to evaluate that the first bone-to-implant contact was occlusal to the implant-abutment junction.

This finding can be related to the excellent characteristics of zirconia dental implants which present high biocompatibility and low plaque adhesion [17, 21]. In fact, it is important to note that a bacterial adhesion to implant surfaces is the first stage of peri-implant mucositis and peri-implantitis with the resulting loss of the supporting bone in the tissues surrounding the implants [22]. On the contrary, the reduction of bacterial adhesion on the surface of zirconia dental implants promotes early formation of the biological width and, therefore, the formation of a mucosal seal that stops early marginal bone resorption. As demonstrated by Scarano et al. [23], zirconium oxide surfaces showed a significant reduction of the presence of bacteria, and this fact is probably important for the health of the peri-implant soft tissues.

Moreover, the implant system adopted in our study is characterized by monocomponent dental implants. Several studies have shown that bone resorption around the implant neck is related to the presence of the microgap between implant and abutment [14, 24, 25]. This microgap leads to bacterial leakage and a microbial colonization of the gap at the bone level. Peri-implant soft tissues develop an inflammatory response which promotes osteoclast formation and activation to result in alveolar bone loss. According to the authors, the reduction of marginal bone loss is mainly due to the one-piece morphology of zirconia dental implants, through which there is no implant-abutment microgap and its microbial contamination; there are no micromovements of the prosthetic component and repeated screwing and unscrewing [26, 27].

For these reasons, it has been proposed that peri-implant marginal bone loss is more extended around two-piece implants than around one-piece implants as a result of the location of the microgap [28–30].

Another retrospective study suggests that zirconia endosseous implants can achieve a survival rate similar to that of titanium implants with healthy and stable soft and hard tissues. In the work by Brüll et al. [31] 121 zirconia implants (66 two-piece implants and 55 one-piece implants) were inserted in 74 patients. After a mean observation period of 18 months, the cumulative implant survival rate was of 96.5%. The clinical examination revealed that PPD and BOP were statistically significantly lower around implants than around teeth (mean PPD of 1.8 ± 0.4 mm – mean BOP scores of $4.1\% \pm 4.2\%$), whereas the radiographic evaluation demonstrated that peri-implant marginal bone levels were stable (mean bone loss of 0.1 ± 0.6 mm) after 3-year follow-up.

Even if the results regarding the rehabilitation of the esthetic areas with zirconia monocomponent implants are encouraging, further scientific information concerning the clinical use of zirconia dental implants is needed, as well as prospective long-term clinical studies in order to understand whether zirconia implants may represent a valid alternative to titanium implants.

5. Conclusion

In this study, it was evaluated that there is a preservation of the crestal bone adjacent to zirconia dental implants. In particular, the radiographic measurements of marginal bone loss showed values below 0.9–1.6 mm during the first year in function and not exceeding 0.2 mm 1 year up to 4 years after surgery in accordance with Albrektsson implant success criteria [15]. This finding can be related to some properties which characterize zirconia dental implants. These properties are the high biocompatibility of zirconia surfaces, the low plaque adhesion on zirconia dental implants, and the absence of microgap between fixture and abutment [32, 33].

Conflict of Interests

All the authors declare that they do not have any conflict of interests regarding the publication of the current work.

References

[1] P. I. Brånemark, B. O. Hansson, R. Adell et al., "Osseointegrated implants in the treatment of the edentulous jaw. Experience from a 10-year period," *Scandinavian Journal of Plastic and Reconstructive Surgery. Supplementum*, vol. 16, pp. 1–132, 1977.

[2] D. Buser, N. Broggini, M. Wieland et al., "Enhanced bone apposition to a chemically modified SLA titanium surface," *Journal of Dental Research*, vol. 83, no. 7, pp. 529–533, 2004.

[3] D. L. Cochran, D. Buser, C. M. Ten Bruggenkate et al., "The use of reduced healing times on ITI implants with a sandblasted and acid-etched (SLA) surface: early results from clinical trials on ITI SLA implants," *Clinical Oral Implants Research*, vol. 13, no. 2, pp. 144–153, 2002.

[4] R. J. Kohal, D. Weng, M. Bächle, and J. R. Strub, "Loaded custom-made zirconia and titanium implants show similar osseointegration: an animal experiment," *Journal of Periodontology*, vol. 75, no. 9, pp. 1262–1268, 2004.

[5] L. Sennerby, A. Dasmah, B. Larsson, and M. Iverhed, "Bone tissue responses to surface-modified zirconia implants: a histomorphometric and removal torque study in the rabbit," *Clinical Implant Dentistry and Related Research*, vol. 7, no. 1, pp. S13–S20, 2005.

[6] M. Gahlert, T. Gudehus, S. Eichhorn, E. Steinhauser, H. Kniha, and W. Erhardt, "Biomechanical and histomorphometric comparison between zirconia implants with varying surface textures and a titanium implant in the maxilla of miniature pigs," *Clinical Oral Implants Research*, vol. 18, no. 5, pp. 662–668, 2007.

[7] P. I. Brånemark, B. O. Hansson, R. Adell et al., "Osseointegrated implants in the treatment of the edentulous jaw. Experience from a 10-year period." *Scandinavian journal of plastic and reconstructive surgery. Supplementum*, vol. 16, pp. 1–132, 1977.

[8] G. Heydecke, R. Kohal, and R. Gläser, "Optimal esthetics in single-tooth replacement with the Re-Implant system: a case report," *International Journal of Prosthodontics*, vol. 12, no. 2, pp. 184–189, 1999.

[9] A. Wohlwend, S. Studer, and P. Schärer, "The zirconium oxide abutment—a new all-ceramic concept for esthetically improving suprastructures in implantology," *Quintessenz Zahntechnik*, vol. 22, pp. 364–381, 1996 (German).

[10] W. Schulte and B. d'Hoedt, "Thirteen years of the Tubigen implant system made by Frialit—additional results," *Zeitschrift für Zahnärztliche Implantologie*, vol. 3, pp. 167–172, 1988 (German).

[11] A. Scarano, F. Di Carlo, M. Quaranta, and A. Piattelli, "Bone response to zirconia ceramic implants: an experimental study in rabbits," *The Journal of Oral Implantology*, vol. 29, no. 1, pp. 8–12, 2003.

[12] R. Depprich, H. Zipprich, M. Ommerborn et al., "Osseointegration of zirconia implants: an SEM observation of the bone-implant interface," *Head and Face Medicine*, vol. 4, no. 1, article 25, 2008.

[13] N. U. Zitzmann, P. Schärer, and C. P. Marinello, "Long-term results of implants treated with guided bone regeneration: a 5-year prospective study," *International Journal of Oral and Maxillofacial Implants*, vol. 16, no. 3, pp. 355–366, 2001.

[14] D. P. Tarnow, S. C. Cho, and S. S. Wallace, "The effect of inter-implant distance on the height of inter-implant bone crest," *Journal of Periodontology*, vol. 71, no. 4, pp. 546–549, 2000.

[15] T. Albrektsson, G. Zarb, P. Worthington, and A. R. Eriksson, "The long-term efficacy of currently used dental implants: a review and proposed criteria of success," *The International Journal of Oral & Maxillofacial Implants*, vol. 1, no. 1, pp. 11–25, 1986.

[16] P. Thomsen, C. Larsson, L. E. Ericson, L. Sennerby, J. Lausmaa, and B. Kasemo, "Structure of the interface between rabbit cortical bone and implants of gold, zirconium and titanium," *Journal of Materials Science: Materials in Medicine*, vol. 8, no. 11, pp. 653–665, 1997.

[17] A. Scarano, F. Di Carlo, M. Quaranta, and A. Piattelli, "Bone response to zirconia ceramic implants: an experimental study in rabbits," *The Journal of oral implantology*, vol. 29, no. 1, pp. 8–12, 2003.

[18] Y. Akagawa, R. Hosokawa, Y. Sato, and K. Kamayama, "Comparison between freestanding and tooth-connected partially stabilized zirconia implants after two years' function in monkeys: a clinical and histologic study," *The Journal of Prosthetic Dentistry*, vol. 80, no. 5, pp. 551–558, 1998.

[19] L. Sennerby, A. Dasmah, B. Larsson, and M. Iverhed, "Bone tissue responses to surface-modified zirconia implants: a histomorphometric and removal torque study in the rabbit," *Clinical Implant Dentistry and Related Research*, vol. 7, supplement 1, pp. S13–S20, 2005.

[20] M. Nevins, M. Camelo, M. L. Nevins, P. Schupbach, and D. M. Kim, "Pilot clinical and histologic evaluations of a two-piece zirconia implant." *The International journal of periodontics & restorative dentistry*, vol. 31, no. 2, pp. 157–163, 2011.

[21] M. G. Doyle, C. J. Goodacre, C. A. Munoz, and C. J. Andres, "The effect of tooth preparation design on the breaking strength of Dicor crowns: 3," *The International Journal of Prosthodontics*, vol. 3, no. 4, pp. 327–340, 1990.

[22] L. W. Lindquist, G. E. Carlsson, and T. Jemt, "A prospective 15-year follow-up study of mandibular fixed prostheses supported by osseointegrated implants: clinical results and marginal bone loss," *Clinical Oral Implants Research*, vol. 7, no. 2, pp. 329–336, 1996.

[23] A. Scarano, M. Piattelli, S. Caputi, G. A. Favero, and A. Piattelli, "Bacterial adhesion on commercially pure titanium and zirconium oxide disks: an in vivo human study," *Journal of Periodontology*, vol. 75, no. 2, pp. 292–296, 2004.

[24] J. S. Hermann, D. L. Cochran, P. V. Nummikoski, and D. Buser, "Crestal bone changes around titanium implants. A radiographic evaluation of unloaded nonsubmerged and submerged implants in the canine mandible," *Journal of Periodontology*, vol. 68, no. 11, pp. 1117–1130, 1997.

[25] N. Broggini, L. M. McManus, J. S. Hermann et al., "Persistent acute inflammation at the implant-abutment interface," *Journal of Dental Research*, vol. 82, no. 3, pp. 232–237, 2003.

[26] G. Rasperini, M. Maglione, P. Cocconcelli, and M. Simion, "In vivo early plaque formation on pure titanium and ceramic abutments: a comparative microbiological and SEM analysis," *Clinical Oral Implants Research*, vol. 9, no. 6, pp. 357–364, 1998.

[27] T.-J. Oh, J. Yoon, C. E. Misch, and H.-L. Wang, "The causes of early implant bone loss: myth or science?" *Journal of Periodontology*, vol. 73, no. 3, pp. 322–333, 2002.

[28] A. E. Borgonovo, A. Fabbri, V. Vavassori, R. Censi, and C. Maiorana, "Multiple teeth replacement with endosseous one-piece yttrium-stabilized zirconia dental implants," *Medicina Oral, Patologia Oral y Cirugia Bucal*, vol. 17, no. 6, pp. 981–987, 2012.

[29] A. E. Borgonovo, V. Vavassori, R. Censi, J. L. Calvo, and D. Re, "Behavior of endosseous one-piece yttrium stabilized zirconia dental implants placed in posterior areas," *Minerva Stomatologica*, vol. 62, no. 7-8, pp. 247–257, 2013.

[30] A. Borgonovo, R. Censi, M. Dolci, V. Vavassori, A. Bianchi, and C. Maiorana, "Use of endosseous one-piece yttrium-stabilized zirconia dental implants in premolar region: a two-year clinical preliminary report," *Minerva Stomatologica*, vol. 60, no. 5, pp. 229–241, 2011.

[31] F. Brüll, A. J. van Winkelhoff, and M. S. Cune, "Zirconia dental implants: a clinical, radiographic and microbiologic evaluation up to 3 years," *The International Journal of Oral & Maxillofacial Implants*, vol. 29, no. 4, pp. 914–920, 2014.

[32] A. E. Borgonovo, O. Arnaboldi, R. Censi, M. Dolci, and G. Santoro, "Edentulous jaws rehabilitation with yttrium-stabilized zirconium dioxide implants: two years follow-up experience.," *Minerva stomatologica*, vol. 59, no. 7-8, pp. 381–392, 2010.

[33] A. E. Borgonovo, R. Censi, V. Vavassori et al., "Evaluation of the success criteria for zirconia dental implants: a four-year clinical and radiological study," *International Journal of Dentistry*, vol. 2013, Article ID 463073, 7 pages, 2013.

27

A Study of Success Rate of Miniscrew Implants as Temporary Anchorage Devices in Singapore

Song Yi Lin,[1] **Yow Mimi,**[1] **Chew Ming Tak,**[1]
Foong Kelvin Weng Chiong,[2] **and Wong Hung Chew**[3]

[1]National Dental Centre Singapore, 5 Second Hospital Avenue, Singapore 168938
[2]Faculty of Dentistry, National University of Singapore, 11 Lower Kent Ridge Road, Singapore 119083
[3]Yong Loo Lin School of Medicine, National University of Singapore, 1E Kent Ridge Road, NUHS Tower Block, Level 11, Singapore 119228

Correspondence should be addressed to Song Yi Lin; song.yi.lin@ndcs.com.sg

Academic Editor: Carla Evans

Objective. To find out the success rate of miniscrew implants in the National Dental Centre of Singapore (NDCS) and the impact of patient-related, location-related, and miniscrew implant-related factors. *Materials and Methods.* Two hundred and eighty-five orthodontic miniscrew implants were examined from NDCS patient records. Eleven variables were analysed to see if there is any association with success. Outcome was measured twice, immediately after surgery prior to orthodontic loading (T1) and 12 months after surgery (T2). The outcome at T2 was assessed 12 months after the miniscrew's insertion date or after its use as a temporary anchorage device has ceased. *Results.* Overall success rate was 94.7% at T1 and 83.3% at T2. Multivariate analysis revealed only the length of miniscrew implant to be significantly associated with success at both T1 ($P = 0.002$) and T2 ($P = 0.030$). Miniscrew implants with lengths of 10–12 mm had the highest success rate (98.0%) compared to other lengths, and this is statistically significant ($P = 0.035$). At T2, lengths of 10–12 mm had significantly ($P = 0.013$) higher success rates (93.5%) compared to 6-7 mm (76.7%) and 8 mm (82.1%) miniscrew implants. *Conclusion.* Multivariate statistical analyses of 11 variables demonstrate that length of miniscrew implant is significant in determining success.

1. Introduction

Anchorage has always been one of the most difficult aspects of orthodontic treatment. Traditional methods of anchorage preparation often rely on patients' cooperation and thus may be unpredictable. To ensure attainment of ideal treatment goals, temporary anchorage devices (TADs) are slowly gaining importance with their advantages over the traditional treatment modalities. TADs are devices temporarily fixed to bone for the purpose of enhancing orthodontic anchorage and which are subsequently removed after use. A commonly used TAD would be the miniscrew implant, which is a fixation device placed for anchorage control using mechanical stability without the intention of osseointegration [1]. Miniscrew implants are often chosen among other TADs due

to its ease of insertion and removal, relative affordability, and numerous applications in various anatomical locations [2].

In the National Dental Centre of Singapore (NDCS), miniscrew implants were first introduced in the year 2004 but there is currently no available datum on their success rate in NDCS. Success rates seem to vary amongst operators and its use is not widespread due to the purported high dislodgement rate and the need for surgical placement. In the orthodontic literature, there is also no clear information on whether patient-related, location-related, or miniscrew implant-related factors influence the success of miniscrews in NDCS. Meta-analyses [3, 4] conducted have shown that a myriad of factors seem to affect their failure rates, but most variables still need additional evidence to support any possible associations. This is due to the extensive types and

TABLE 1: Clinical variables examined.

Categories	Variables	
Patient-related	Age	<20/≥20 years old
	Gender	Male/Female
	Skeletal malocclusion (sagittal)	Class I/II/III
	Skeletal malocclusion (vertical)	High/average/low angle
	Dental malocclusion	Class I/II/III
Location-related	Side	Right/left/midline
	Jaw	Maxilla/mandible
	Position	(Anterior region/posterior region/retromolar/palate)
Miniscrew-related	Type	AbsoAnchor/VectorTAS
	Length	6-7/8/10–12 mm
	Diameter	1.3/1.4/2.0 mm

brands of miniscrew implants used and the heterogeneity of the included studies which may affect the success rates reported.

Thus, the aim of this retrospective study is to find out the success rate of miniscrew implants in NDCS pertaining to our local population, and whether they are a reliable form of TAD. Secondary objectives of this research will include finding out if patient-related factors, location-related factors, and miniscrew implant-related factors have any impact on success rates.

2. Materials and Methods

Records of patients who received miniscrew implants as part of their orthodontic treatment plan during the period of January 2010 to June 2012 were retrospectively examined. This amounted to 136 patients with a total of 285 miniscrew implants. Details of these patients were obtained from the surgical logbooks maintained in the Day Surgery Department in NDCS.

Patients with the following data on the electronic dental records of NDCS were included:

(i) comprehensive demographic information including dental and skeletal relationships,

(ii) dates of miniscrew placement, miniscrew loading, and miniscrew removal or dislodgement,

(iii) type, length, and diameter of miniscrew,

(iv) location of the miniscrew.

Smokers and patients with systemic medical conditions or those on long-term medications were excluded.

To see if there is any association with clinical success of miniscrew implants, 11 variables were collected for analysis. The 11 variables were divided into 3 categories: patient-related, miniscrew implant location-related, or miniscrew implant design-related factors as shown in Table 1.

Patient-related factors include the age and gender of the patient, the dental malocclusion according to the British Standards Institute incisor classification, and the skeletal (sagittal and vertical) relationship based on the orthodontist's clinical diagnosis and documentation.

Location-related factors of the miniscrew include the side of placement (right, left, or at the midline) and the jaw involved (maxilla or mandible). The miniscrew position in the oral cavity (anterior region, posterior region, retromolar, palate) was also examined. The anterior region refers to the labial dentoalveolus mesial to the canines. The posterior region refers to the buccal dentoalveolus distal to the canines, the tuberosity area and the infrazygomatic crest area.

Miniscrew implant-related factors include the type (VectorTAS or AbsoAnchor) of miniscrew, its length (6 mm, 7 mm, 8 mm, 10 mm, 12 mm), and its diameter (1.3 mm, 1.4 mm, 2.0 mm).

The miniscrew implant placement surgery was done by randomly assigned periodontists or oral and maxillofacial surgeons working in NDCS. Full consent was taken before the surgical procedure. The patients were also instructed on standard postoperative care instructions after the surgery. They were told to brush the surgical site gently to maintain good oral hygiene and a bottle of 0.2% chlorhexidine mouth rinse was prescribed to be used twice daily for a week.

This study examines early and late successes of the miniscrews at 2 time points: on the day of orthodontic loading and 12 months after insertion of the miniscrew implant. The outcome examined at the first time point (T1) will be the miniscrew implant's initial stability, prior to orthodontic loading. Success of the miniscrew implant at that juncture is defined by absence of infection of the surrounding soft tissues or any reason warranting its immediate removal or replacement prior to loading. Failure of the miniscrew implant is defined as dislodgement of the miniscrew implant prior to loading or a miniscrew that have become excessively mobile such that orthodontic anchorage objectives cannot be met. Likewise, if the miniscrew implant has caused irreversible biological damage to adjacent structures as recorded by the clinician and was thus unusable, it was also considered a failure.

The outcome at the second time point (T2) was assessed 12 months after the miniscrew's insertion date or after its use as skeletal anchorage has ceased, whichever came first. Success of the miniscrew implant at this juncture is defined by no dislodgement from the date of initial loading to the 12-month mark after the date of insertion or when intentional

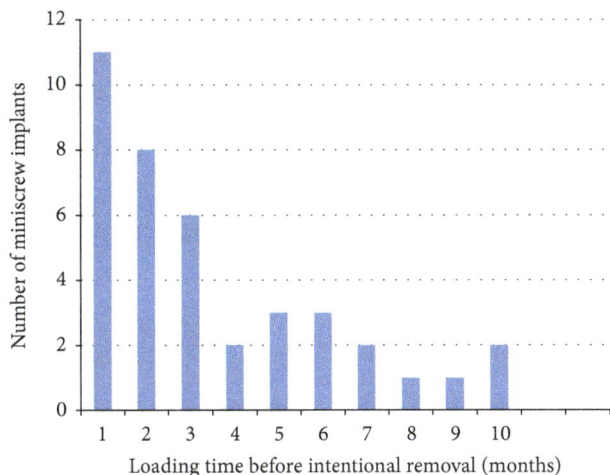

FIGURE 1: Loading time of successful miniscrew implants removed intentionally.

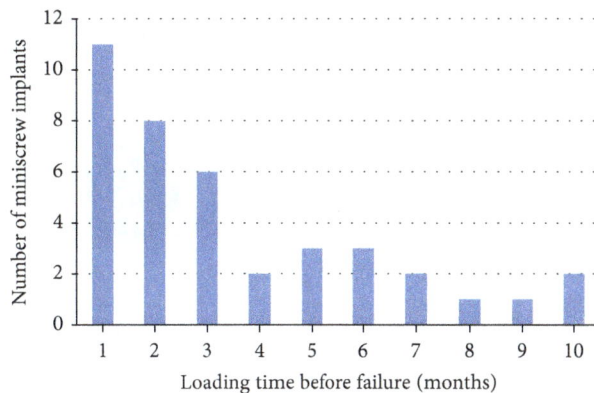

FIGURE 2: Loading time of failed miniscrew implants.

removal is carried out prior to the 12-month mark. It will mean that the miniscrew has sustained orthodontic loading forces throughout that time period and has served its skeletal anchorage function. Similarly, failure of the miniscrew will be defined as dislodgement from the surgical site after orthodontic loading, any time before the 12-month period.

The research protocol was approved by the SingHealth Institutional Review Board with CIRB reference 2012/1057/D.

Descriptive statistics were initially performed to calculate the overall success rate of the miniscrew implants, as well as their specific success rates with regard to the 11 variables studied. Multiple miniscrew implants in a patient were assumed to be independent entities. Logistic regression was used to evaluate factors associated with the success of miniscrew implant. The datum was analyzed using SAS version 9.2. Statistical significance was set at 5%. For any pairwise comparisons in the univariate analyses, the Bonferroni technique was applied. The Hosmer-Lemeshow test was used to test for goodness of fit for the logistic regression model and results showed a good fit (at T1, $P = 0.70$; at T2, $P = 0.11$).

3. Results

The overall success rate was 94.7% at T1 (95% CI 92.1%–97.3%) and 83.3% at T2 (95% CI 78.7%–87.9%). The detailed information on success rates at T1 and T2 is shown in Tables 2 and 3.

Out of the 214 successful miniscrew implants at T2, 37 of them were removed intentionally prior to the 12-month mark. These 37 miniscrews had a successful loading duration ranging from 2 to 12 months, and this is presented in Figure 1. Mean loading time for failed miniscrews at T2 was 3.5 months, ranging from 1 to 10 months and this is shown in Figure 2.

3.1. Success Rate at T1. In the univariate analyses, length of miniscrew was significantly associated with success at T1 ($P = 0.001$). In the multivariate analysis of success rate at T1, only length of miniscrew implant was still found to be significantly associated ($P = 0.002$) with miniscrew implant success after being adjusted for age, gender, vertical skeletal malocclusion, recipient jaw, and type of miniscrew implant. Due to multicollinearity, some variables in the univariate analyses were not included in the multivariate analysis.

3.2. Success Rate at T2. In the univariate analyses, sagittal skeletal malocclusion ($P = 0.025$) and vertical skeletal malocclusion ($P = 0.028$) were significantly associated with miniscrew implant success at T2. Multivariate analysis of the success of miniscrew implants at T2 found vertical skeletal malocclusion ($P = 0.043$) and length of miniscrew ($P = 0.030$) to be significantly associated with success rate.

3.3. Patient-Related Factors. Of the patient-related factors, there were no statistically significant differences between the variables at T1. But using univariate analyses at T2, there were associations between sagittal skeletal malocclusion and miniscrew implant success and also between vertical skeletal malocclusion and miniscrew implant success. Miniscrew implants placed in patients with class III malocclusion had a lower chance of success compared with those placed in patients with class I malocclusion ($P = 0.01$, OR = 0.26, 95% CI 0.08–0.79). Miniscrew implants in average angle patients had a higher chance of success compared with those placed in high angle patients ($P = 0.025$, OR = 3.18, 95% CI 1.13–8.98). After adjusting for age, gender, sagittal skeletal malocclusion, dental malocclusion, recipient jaw, type of miniscrew implant, and length of miniscrew, vertical skeletal malocclusion was still found to be significantly associated ($P = 0.043$) with miniscrew implant success. Miniscrew implants in average angle patients had a higher chance of success compared with those placed in high mandibular plane angle patients ($P = 0.013$, OR = 4.22, 95% CI 1.35–13.16).

3.4. Location-Related Factors. None of the location-related factors was significantly associated with success at T1 and T2. Although at T1, for side of placement, there seem to be higher success rates for miniscrew implants placed in the midline

TABLE 2: Success rate of miniscrew implants at T1.

	Success rate at T1 (%)	Number of 1st outcome successes/Total number	Unadjusted odds ratio (95% CI)	Unadjusted P value	Adjusted odds ratio (95% CI)	Adjusted P value
Overall success	94.7	270/285				
Age at surgery				0.877		0.251
<20 years	94.6	193/204	0.91 (0.28 to 2.95)		2.31 (0.55 to 9.62)	
≥20 years	95.1	77/81	1		1	
Gender				0.502		0.288
Female	93.8	120/128	1		2.01 (0.55 to 7.31)	
Male	95.5	150/157	1.43 (0.50 to 4.05)		1	
Sagittal skeletal malocclusion				0.421		
Class I	92.6	87/94	1			
Class II	94.7	126/133	1.45 (0.43 to 4.82)	1		
Class III	100	36/36	6.26 (0.22 to 177.92)	0.523		
Vertical skeletal malocclusion				0.918		0.524
High angle	93.8	106/113	1	1	1	
Average	95.1	97/102	1.28 (0.332 to 4.940)	1	2.12 (0.55 to 8.18)	0.276
Low angle	94.1	16/17	1.06 (0.09 to 12.50)		2.38 (0.19 to 29.38)	0.499
Dental malocclusion				0.361		
Class I	96.5	55/57	1	1		
Class II Div. I	93.4	155/166	0.61 (0.11 to 3.42)	0.554		
Class III	100	41/41	3.74 (0.09 to 164.50)	0.316		
Class II Div. 2	87.5	7/8	0.23 (0.01 to 3.55)			
Side of placement				0.928		
Left	94.9	129/136	1.07 (0.34 to 3.41)	1		
Midline	100	4/4	0.56 (0.01 to 25.32)	1		
Right	94.5	137/145	1			
Recipient jaw				0.290		0.286
Maxilla	94.1	222/236	1		1	
Mandible	98.0	48/49	3.03 (0.39 to 23.58)		3.40 (0.36 to 32.15)	
Site of placement				0.647		
Anterior region	93.3	14/15	0.36 (0.03 to 4.96)	1		
Posterior region	93.4	169/181	0.50 (0.09 to 2.76)	1		
Retromolar	100	20/20	1.52 (0.03 to 70.74)	1		
Palate	97.1	67/69	1			
Miniscrew implant type				0.606		0.887
AbsoAnchor	92.6	25/27	1		1	
Vector TAS	94.9	244/257	1.50 (0.32 to 7.04)		1.14 (0.19 to 6.85)	
Miniscrew length				0.001*		0.002*
6-7 mm	82.7	43/52	1		1	
8 mm	97.3	177/182	7.41 (2.01 to 27.38)	0.001*	11.88 (2.73 to 51.71)	0.001*
10-12 mm	98.0	50/51	10.47 (0.94 to 116.31)	0.058	10.50 (1.18 to 93.51)	0.035

TABLE 2: Continued.

	Success rate at T1 (%)	Number of 1st outcome successes/Total number	Unadjusted odds ratio (95% CI)	Unadjusted P value	Adjusted odds ratio (95% CI)	Adjusted P value
Miniscrew diameter						
1.3 mm	92.9	26/28	0.30 (0.02 to 4.86)	0.601		
1.4 mm	94.3	200/212	0.38 (0.04 to 4.02)	0.658		
2.0 mm	97.8	44/45	1	0.714		

* $P \leq 0.05$.

TABLE 3: Success rate of miniscrew implants at T2.

	Success rate at T2 (%)	Number of 2nd outcome successes/Total number	Unadjusted odds ratio (95% CI)	Unadjusted P value	Adjusted odds ratio (95% CI)	Adjusted P value
Overall success	83.3	214/257				
Age at surgery				0.082		0.270
<20 years	80.7	151/187	0.47 (0.20 to 1.10)		0.49 (0.14 to 1.73)	
≥20 years	90.0	63/70	1		1	
Gender				0.482		0.109
Female	81.4	92/113	1		1	
Male	84.7	122/144	1.27 (0.66 to 2.44)		2.12 (0.85 to 5.31)	
Sagittal skeletal malocclusion				0.025*		0.487
Class I	89.5	77/86	1		1	
Class II	83.5	101/121	0.59 (0.23 to 1.54)	0.438	0.88 (0.25 to 3.19)	0.852
Class III	68.6	24/35	0.26 (0.08 to 0.79)	0.014*	0.25 (0.02 to 2.56)	0.240
Vertical skeletal malocclusion				0.028*		0.043*
High angle	79.6	82/103	1		1	
Average	92.6	87/94	3.18 (1.13 to 8.98)	0.025*	4.22 (1.35 to 13.16)	0.013*
Low angle	75.0	12/16	0.77 (0.19 to 3.13)	1	2.20 (0.36 to 13.33)	0.391
Dental malocclusion				0.260		0.770
Class I	88.9	48/54	1		1	
Class II Div. I	84.0	126/150	0.69 (0.22 to 2.16)	1	0.81 (0.18 to 3.70)	0.787
Class III	75.0	30/40	0.39 (0.03 to 2.66)	1	1.25 (0.09 to 17.71)	0.339
Class II Div. 2	71.4	5/7	0.30 (0.10 to 1.47)		0.22 (0.01 to 5.02)	0.868
Side of placement				0.590		
Left	85.4	105/123	1.38 (0.65 to 2.93)	1		
Midline	100	4/4	2.18 (0.05 to 94.33)	1		
Right	80.8	105/130	1			
Recipient jaw				0.081		0.065
Maxilla	81.4	175/215	1		1	
Mandible	92.9	39/42	2.97 (0.87 to 10.10)		9.59 (0.87 to 105.86)	
Site of placement				0.404		
Anterior region	92.9	13/14	2.45 (0.18 to 33.59)	1		
Posterior region	80.9	131/162	0.80 (0.31 to 2.07)	1		
Retromolar	94.4	17/18	3.21 (0.24 to 43.06)	0.848		
Palate	84.1	53/63	1			
Miniscrew implant type				0.508		0.769
AbsoAnchor	78.3	18/23	1		1	
Vector TAS	83.7	195/233	1.43 (0.50 to 4.07)		1.22 (0.33 to 4.53)	
Miniscrew length				0.108		0.030*
6-7 mm	76.7	33/43	1		1	
8 mm	82.1	138/168	1.39 (0.55 to 3.52)	0.843	2.91 (0.93 to 9.13)	0.067
10-12 mm	93.5	43/46	4.34 (0.91 to 20.75)	0.071	17.95 (1.83 to 176.01)	0.013*

TABLE 3: Continued.

	Success rate at T2 (%)	Number of 2nd outcome successes/Total number	Unadjusted odds ratio (95% CI)	Unadjusted P value	Adjusted odds ratio (95% CI)	Adjusted P value
Miniscrew diameter				0.122		
1.3 mm	79.2	19/24	0.20 (0.03 to 1.41)	0.128		
1.4 mm	81.2	156/192	0.22 (0.04 to 1.19)	0.089		
2.0 mm	95.1	39/41	1			

* $P \leq 0.05$.

(100%) compared to the left (94.9%) or ride side (94.5%). This was also reflected at T2; midline miniscrew implants had a 100% success rate compared to the left (85.4%) or right (80.8%). For recipient jaw, success rate of miniscrew implants in the mandible is higher at both T1 and T2 compared to the maxilla. But this is also not significant. Similarly, the different sites of placement had no significant difference in success rates, although the retromolar area showed the highest success at T1 (100%) and T2 (94.4%).

3.5. Miniscrew Implant-Related Factors. Of the miniscrew implant-related factors, only length of miniscrew implant was significantly associated with success in the multivariate analyses at T1 ($P = 0.002$) and at T2 ($P = 0.030$). Those with length 8 mm and 10–12 mm had a higher chance of success at T1 compared to those with length 6-7 mm, respectively (8 mm: OR = 11.88, 95% CI 2.73–51.71, $P = 0.001$; 10–12 mm: OR = 10.50, 95% CI 1.18–93.51, $P = 0.035$). At T2, those with length 10–12 mm were found to have a higher chance of success compared with those with 6-7 mm (OR = 17.95, 95% CI 1.83–176.01, $P = 0.013$). Type of miniscrew implant and diameter had no significant association with miniscrew implant success.

4. Discussion

The success rate of miniscrew implants in our study was 94.7% at T1 and 83.3% at T2. Success rate at T1 is comparable to the success rate by Lim et al. [5] who reported a 93.1% success rate when they assessed initial stability of the miniscrews 1 week after placement. Similarly, success rate at T2 is comparable to the rates in other retrospective studies of Asian patients, (83.8%–89.9%) [6–9]. This is in spite of the various miniscrew implant systems used, the varying operators and surgical techniques, and diverse management protocols reported by the different centres.

The mean loading time for failed miniscrews in this study was 3.5 months, ranging from 1 to 10 months. Most of the failures (30 out of 39) occurred within the first 5 months after loading. This is in accord with the findings [10] which estimated that the highest failure rate occurred during the first 50–150 days following loading.

Although a success rate of 83.3% is reasonable, there is still a 1 in 5 chance of failure using miniscrew implants for orthodontic anchorage. Schätzle et al. [11] demonstrated that palatal implants and miniplates showed a better survival rate compared to miniscrews. It will be interesting to find out how the success rate of other skeletal anchorage systems is compared against miniscrew implants in NDCS, and whether they can provide an improved and significantly more reliable form of TAD for orthodontic use. This will be elucidated in a future study.

4.1. Limitations of Study. Due to the retrospective nature of this study, datum was sometimes lacking and not every variable mentioned in the literature was investigated and confounding factors may be present.

The miniscrew implant placement surgery was done by randomly assigned periodontists or oral and maxillofacial surgeons working in NDCS. Other than standard postoperative care instructions given to the patient, surgical techniques and surgical experience of the clinician may vary and affect the results of our study. Operator's surgical experience in miniscrew placement has been investigated in the literature [5], but this variable was excluded as we felt it was difficult to classify clinicians into groups according to years of experience or number of miniscrews inserted. This is because some clinicians do not work full time in NDCS, and it will be inaccurate to place a clinician in the "inexperienced" group who may have had prior experience in other centres before operating in NDCS.

Unlike a study in laboratory settings, insertion torque, loading forces, and direction of insertion were not recorded to numerical precision on a routine clinical basis. Thus, no data on the above variables could be obtained from the patient charts and treatment note records. Also, it is clinically hard to record accurately a constant magnitude of force due to the rapid force level decay of orthodontic elastomeric chains, which are most commonly used in NDCS for orthodontic loading.

The effect of delayed, early, or immediate loading on success rates was also not investigated as the individual patient's orthodontic appointment varies after insertion of the miniscrew implant and there are no standard loading protocols followed by the orthodontists.

Types of tooth movement involved were investigated by other studies [12] on success rates but this was not investigated as miniscrew implants are sometimes used for a combination of movements (e.g., both intrusion and distalization), thus making it difficult for any meaningful comparison of success rates to be made between any particular tooth movement.

4.2. Patient-Related Factors. Using univariate analysis at T2, sagittal skeletal malocclusion was associated with success rate. Miniscrew implants placed in patients with class III malocclusion had lower success compared with class I malocclusion. However, according to studies by Antoszewska et al. [12] and Miyawaki et al. [6], among groups with different skeletal patterns, there are no significant differences in success. There is no obvious physiological reason why dentoalveolar abnormality or malocclusion type should affect success rate. Hence, our initial finding may just be due to chance.

Using a multivariate analysis of success at T2, vertical skeletal malocclusion was significantly associated with success rate of miniscrew implants. This was agreed upon by Antoszewska et al. [12] who found that, out of all the patient-related factors, only the vertical dimension seemed to play a role in determining success rates. Our results showed that average mandibular plane angle patients had a significantly higher success rate compared to high mandibular plane angle patients. This corresponds with the study by Miyawaki et al. [6] who reported that the average mandibular plane angle group had significantly higher success rates compared to the high mandibular plane angle group. It was found that density of cortical bone was higher in subjects with small Frankfort-mandibular plane angles and gonial angles [13]. Accordingly, high mandibular angle patients may have less dense cortical bone and this might affect success rates of miniscrew implants placed. This is supported by results of a meta-analysis [14] which showed a positive association between the primary stability of miniscrew implants and cortical bone thickness of the surgical site.

4.3. Miniscrew Location-Related Factors. None of the location-related factors was significantly associated with success at both T1 and T2. For side of placement, at both T1 and T2, success rates for miniscrew implants placed in the midline were the highest, followed by the left then the right side but this did not reach statistical significance. Park et al. [15] and Wu et al. [9] reported that the left side had significantly higher success rates than the right side. In this study, placement of miniscrew implants on the left side does has a slightly higher success rate compared to the right side at both T1 and T2. This may be because most surgeons are right-handed, making it easier to insert miniscrews on the patient's left side. Also, there may be better hygiene maintenance on the left side in right-handed patients, who are most prevalent in the population. Miniscrews located in the midline had the highest success rate in our study and these were all located in the palate. This is similar to the results of a study by Lim et al. [5] which showed a 100% success rate in the mid-palatal area. Reasons for a high success rate in the mid-palatal region might be due to the abundance of compact bone and thin gingival tissue in the area, optimizing miniscrew implant insertion. The success rate of miniscrew implants in the mandible is higher compared to the maxilla at both T1 and T2 but this is not significant. This concurred with results from studies by Miyawaki et al. [6] and Lim et al. [5] who found no statistically significant association with success rates in the maxilla or mandible. The slightly higher success rate in the mandible may be attributed to thicker cortical bone in the mandible which is ideal for miniscrew implant stability [16].

The different sites of placement had no significant difference in success rates in our study, and this supports the results by Chen et al. [17] who showed that placement site (maxilla or mandible, left or right side, anterior or posterior) presented no statistically significant association with success rates. This is in contrast to the study by Tseng et al. [18] who found that the only statistically significant factor affecting miniscrew success rates was location. Success rates were the highest in the anterior tooth-bearing region of the maxilla, followed by the posterior tooth-bearing region of the maxilla, and success declines correspondingly in the anterior dentoalveolus of the mandible, posterior dentoalveolus of the mandible, and lastly the ramus. Chen et al. [7] also observed that the differences in success rates were significant in the different sites: success rate was best in maxillary anterior dentoalveolus followed by maxillary posterior dentoalveolus and then lastly in the mandibular posterior dentoalveolus.

In this study, the success rates of miniscrews were compared at the anterior or posterior dentoalveolus separately from those inserted in the maxillary or the mandibular basal bone. Since both maxillary and mandibular anterior miniscrews are grouped into one general category and vice versa for the posterior miniscrews, this may have decreased the statistical significance of the results.

4.4. Miniscrew Implant-Related Factors. Of the miniscrew implant-related factors, only length of miniscrew implant was significantly associated with success at both T1 and T2. Lengths of 10–12 mm had the highest success rate, followed by 8 mm and then the 6-7 mm lengths. This is probably due to the fact that longer miniscrews have the highest contact surface area for mechanical retention. This is in accord with the findings of Chen et al. [7] who found that length of microimplant is a significant risk factor. Success rate for the longer microimplant (8 mm) used in their study was significantly higher than the shorter microimplant (6 mm). Similarly, Tseng et al. [18] found that as success rate increases with length, it was the highest for miniscrews with lengths 12 mm and 14 mm.

Diameter of miniscrew implant had no statistically significant association with success in our study though it shows increasing success with increasing diameters.

Type of miniscrew implant showed no significant association with success although higher success rates were reported for the VectorTAS miniscrews compared to Absoanchor microimplant at both T1 and T2. This could be due to the larger diameter of VectorTAS miniscrews used in NDCS. In NDCS, the more popular AbsoAnchor microimplants used are the small head (SH1312) series, which has a diameter of 1.3 mm only and the lengths used in our study sample range from 6 to 10 mm, depending on the site of placement. In contrast, the VectorTAS miniscrews used in this study sample have a diameter of at least 1.4 mm or 2.0 mm, and lengths that range from 6–12 mm. Due to the larger diameter and longer length of the VectorTAS miniscrews, success rates may be similarly increased. However, since there are no prior studies evaluating the success rates of the two types of miniscrew implants, no comparisons can be made.

5. Conclusion

The overall success rate is 83.3% after 12 months. Patient-related factors like vertical skeletal malocclusion were found to influence success: average mandibular plane angle patients have a higher chance of success compared to high mandibular angle patients probably due to the less dense cortical bone of the latter. Miniscrew implant location-related factors have no significant effect on success but careful site selection must still be done to avoid encroaching on vital structures and to optimize orthodontic mechanics. Of the miniscrew implant-related factors, only length of miniscrew implant was significantly correlated with success. Thus, as long as surrounding anatomy permits, a longer miniscrew implant for better mechanical retention is recommended for higher success rate.

Conflict of Interests

The authors declare that there is no conflict of interests regarding the publication of this paper.

References

[1] J. B. Cope, "Temporary anchorage devices in orthodontics: a paradigm shift," *Seminars in Orthodontics*, vol. 11, no. 1, pp. 3–9, 2005.

[2] H. Wehrbein and P. Göllner, "Skeletal anchorage in orthodontics—basics and clinical application," *Journal of Orofacial Orthopedics*, vol. 68, no. 6, pp. 443–461, 2007.

[3] M. A. Papadopoulos, S. N. Papageorgiou, and I. P. Zogakis, "Clinical effectiveness of orthodontic miniscrew implants: a meta-analysis," *Journal of Dental Research*, vol. 90, no. 8, pp. 969–976, 2011.

[4] S. N. Papageorgiou, I. P. Zogakis, and M. A. Papadopoulos, "Failure rates and associated risk factors of orthodontic miniscrew implants: a meta-analysis," *The American Journal of Orthodontics and Dentofacial Orthopedics*, vol. 142, no. 5, pp. 577.e7–595.e7, 2012.

[5] H.-J. Lim, Y.-J. Choi, C. A. Evans, and H.-S. Hwang, "Predictors of initial stability of orthodontic miniscrew implants," *European Journal of Orthodontics*, vol. 33, no. 5, pp. 528–532, 2011.

[6] S. Miyawaki, I. Koyama, M. Inoue, K. Mishima, T. Sugahara, and T. Takano-Yamamoto, "Factors associated with the stability of titanium screws placed in the posterior region for orthodontic anchorage," *The American Journal of Orthodontics and Dentofacial Orthopedics*, vol. 124, no. 4, pp. 373–378, 2003.

[7] C.-H. Chen, C.-S. Chang, C.-H. Hsieh et al., "The use of microimplants in orthodontic anchorage," *Journal of Oral and Maxillofacial Surgery*, vol. 64, no. 8, pp. 1209–1213, 2006.

[8] C.-H. Moon, D.-G. Lee, H.-S. Lee, J.-S. Im, and S.-H. Baek, "Factors associated with the success rate of orthodontic miniscrews placed in the upper and lower posterior buccal region," *Angle Orthodontist*, vol. 78, no. 1, pp. 101–106, 2008.

[9] T.-Y. Wu, S.-H. Kuang, and C.-H. Wu, "Factors associated with the stability of mini-implants for orthodontic anchorage: a study of 414 samples in Taiwan," *Journal of Oral and Maxillofacial Surgery*, vol. 67, no. 8, pp. 1595–1599, 2009.

[10] D. Wiechmann, U. Meyer, and A. Büchter, "Success rate of mini- and micro-implants used for orthodontic anchorage: a prospective clinical study," *Clinical Oral Implants Research*, vol. 18, no. 2, pp. 263–267, 2007.

[11] M. Schätzle, R. Männchen, M. Zwahlen, and N. P. Lang, "Survival and failure rates of orthodontic temporary anchorage devices: a systematic review," *Clinical Oral Implants Research*, vol. 20, no. 12, pp. 1351–1359, 2009.

[12] J. Antoszewska, M. A. Papadopoulos, H.-S. Park, and B. Ludwig, "Five-year experience with orthodontic miniscrew implants: a retrospective investigation of factors influencing success rates," *American Journal of Orthodontics and Dentofacial Orthopedics*, vol. 136, no. 2, pp. 158.e1–158.e10, 2009.

[13] H. Sato, A. Kawamura, M. Yamaguchi, and K. Kasai, "Relationship between masticatory function and internal structure of the mandible based on computed tomography findings," *American Journal of Orthodontics & Dentofacial Orthopedics*, vol. 128, no. 6, pp. 766–773, 2005.

[14] M. Marquezan, C. T. Mattos, E. F. SantAnna, M. M. de Souza, and L. C. Maia, "Does cortical thickness influence the primary stability of miniscrews?: A systematic review and meta-analysis," *The Angle Orthodontist*, vol. 84, no. 6, pp. 1093–1103, 2014.

[15] H.-S. Park, S.-H. Jeong, and O.-W. Kwon, "Factors affecting the clinical success of screw implants used as orthodontic anchorage," *The American Journal of Orthodontics and Dentofacial Orthopedics*, vol. 130, no. 1, pp. 18–25, 2006.

[16] A. Ono, M. Motoyoshi, and N. Shimizu, "Cortical bone thickness in the buccal posterior region for orthodontic mini-implants," *International Journal of Oral and Maxillofacial Surgery*, vol. 37, no. 4, pp. 334–340, 2008.

[17] Y.-J. Chen, H.-H. Chang, H.-Y. Lin, E. H.-H. Lai, H.-C. Hung, and C.-C. J. Yao, "Stability of miniplates and miniscrews used for orthodontic anchorage: experience with 492 temporary anchorage devices," *Clinical Oral Implants Research*, vol. 19, no. 11, pp. 1188–1196, 2008.

[18] Y.-C. Tseng, C.-H. Hsieh, C.-H. Chen, Y.-S. Shen, I.-Y. Huang, and C.-M. Chen, "The application of mini-implants for orthodontic anchorage," *International Journal of Oral and Maxillofacial Surgery*, vol. 35, no. 8, pp. 704–707, 2006.

28

A Three-Dimensional Finite Element Study on the Biomechanical Simulation of Various Structured Dental Implants and Their Surrounding Bone Tissues

Gong Zhang,[1] Hai Yuan,[1] Xianshuai Chen,[1] Weijun Wang,[1] Jianyu Chen,[2] Jimin Liang,[1] and Peng Zhang[3]

[1]Guangzhou Institute of Advanced Technology, Chinese Academy of Sciences, Guangzhou 511458, China
[2]Hospital of Stomatology, Sun Yat-sen University Hospital, Guangzhou 510000, China
[3]Foshan Stomatology Hospital, Foshan 528000, China

Correspondence should be addressed to Gong Zhang; gong.zhang@giat.ac.cn

Academic Editor: Natasa N. Jakoba

Background/Purpose. This three-dimensional finite element study observed the stress distribution characteristics of 12 types of dental implants and their surrounding bone tissues with various structured abutments, implant threads, and healing methods under different amounts of concentrated loading. *Materials and Methods.* A three-dimensional geometrical model of a dental implant and its surrounding bone tissue was created; the model simulated a screw applied with a preload of 200 N or a torque of 0.2 N·m and a prosthetic crown applied with a vertical or an inclined force of 100 N. The Von Mises stress was evaluated on the 12 types of dental implants and their surrounding bone tissues. *Results.* Under the same loading force, the stress influence on the implant threads was not significant; however, the stress influence on the cancellous bone was obvious. The stress applied to the abutment, cortical bone, and cancellous bone by the inclined force applied to the crown was larger than the stress applied by the vertical force to the crown, and the abutment stress of the nonsubmerged healing implant system was higher than that of the submerged healing implant system. *Conclusion.* A dental implant system characterised by a straight abutment, rectangle tooth, and nonsubmerged healing may provide minimum value for the implant-bone interface.

1. Introduction

Since osseointegrated dental implants are introduced for the rehabilitation of the edentulous patient in the late 1960s, a tremendous awareness and subsequent demand have been arising in the field [1–3]. Recently, dental implants have been increasingly applied in oral rehabilitation and orthopedics used as replacements after the natural teeth are lost or partially damaged, which could restore human mastication functions [4]. Previous studies showed that dental implantation could have a high success rate: retention rate is in excess of 95% over a 5-year period if dental implants were correctly designed, manufactured, and inserted [5–7].

However, dental implant treatments are still failing frequently. One of the major causes of failure is that an artificial implant may never function as perfectly as the living tissues it replaces.

As a matter of fact, the success of dental implant is strongly affected by a number of biomechanical factors, including the type of loading, material properties of implant and prosthesis, implant geometry, surface structure, quality and quantity of surrounding bone, nature of implant-bone interface, and surgical procedures [8]. As far as implant shape is concerned, main design parameters affecting load transfer mechanisms include implant diameter and length of implant-bone interface [9], as well as thread pitch, shape, and depth in the case of threaded implants [10, 11]. In consideration of increasing surfaces appointed for osseous integration, threaded implants are generally preferred to smooth cylindrical ones [12].

The use of screw-type implants increases contact area and improves implant stability [13]. Other designs, such as the stepped implant and the tapered body of threaded implant, have also been proposed to mimic the root anatomy and to enhance the bony support in spongy bone, thereby creating a favorable load distribution [14, 15]. In addition, the thread size, thread profile, and surface roughness may affect the stress pattern in the surrounding bone [16–18].

Otherwise, occlusal loading may often be applied to an implant within 48 h after implant placement [19]. Nevertheless, the effectiveness of an immediately loaded implant is less predictable than that of the delay-loaded implant [20]. The main concern is the occurrence of fibrous encapsulation instead of osseointegration around implants [21].

The objective of this research is to compare the biomechanical effects of the immediately loaded dental implants and the surrounding bone tissue with various abutments (straight and angled), implant threads (trapezia tooth, rectangle tooth, and saw tooth), and healing methods (submerged and nonsubmerged) using a three-dimensional finite element analysis, accounting for the interaction between the dental implants and the supporting bone tissues. Three contact models and four types of loading conditions are used to simulate different integration qualities at the implant-bone interface during the osseointegration process. Extensive numerical simulation results show the influences of compositional profile, occlusal force orientations, and preload types on the static and dynamic behavior of the implant/bone system.

2. Materials and Methods

2.1. CAD Modeling. The three-dimensional geometrical model of the dental implant (Figure 1) and surrounding bone system (shown in Figure 2) was created using the CAD software Unigraphics NX 4.0 (Siemens PLM Software Inc., Germany). The geometry of the adult mandible took the shape created from CT database through image segmentation and spline reconstruction with STP format [24].

The dental implant/supporting bone system comprised abutment, an implant, an internal screw connecting the abutment and implant, and prosthetic crown duplicated from the molar, surrounding cortical bone and cancellous bone in the mandibular section (Figure 3).

As shown in Figure 4, the abutments were divided into straight abutment (shorted for "St") and angled abutment (shorted for "An"), respectively. The maximum diameter was 5.1 mm, wearing gingiva length was 5 mm, and the inclined angle of angled abutment was 15° (Straumann Product Catalog 2012, Straumann AG, Switzerland).

In dentistry, platform switching was a method used to preserve alveolar bone levels around dental implants. A narrower abutment diameter for a given implant platform diameter was used [25].

The diameter and length of the implant were 4.1 mm and 14 mm, respectively (Straumann Product Catalog 2012, Straumann AG, Switzerland). Figure 5 illustrated external thread of the implant comprising trapezia tooth shorted for "Tr" (pitch P was 0.6 mm, thread depth was 0.5P, and thread

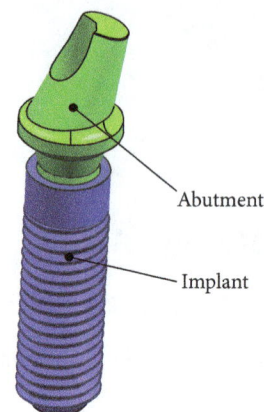

Figure 1: Dental implant system.

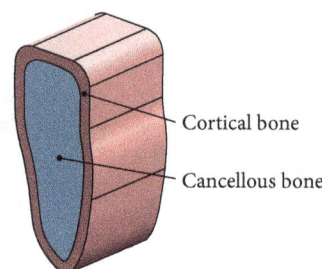

Figure 2: Surrounding bone tissues.

angle was 30°), rectangle tooth shorted for "Re" (pitch P was 0.6 mm, thread depth is 0.5P, and thread angle was 0°), and saw tooth shorted for "Sa" (pitch P is 0.6 mm, thread depth was 0.75P, face flank angle was 3°, and nonface flank angle was 30°).

In the connection of the implant and the abutment, we adopted internal hexagon and Morse taper. Figure 6 depicted two healing methods of submerged one shorted for "Su" (smooth neck height was 1.2 mm) and nonsubmerged one shorted for "Ns" (smooth neck height was 1.2 mm, the inclination angle was 15°, and total height was 2.0 mm) (Straumann Product Catalog 2012, Straumann AG, Switzerland).

According to the various structured abutments, implant threads, and healing methods, 12 combinations of the dental implant systems were exhibited (Figure 7 and Table 1).

2.2. Finite Element Modeling. All 12 models described above were combined using Boolean operations, and the parasolid format of the solid model was then imported into ANSYS Workbench 14.0 (ANSYS, Inc., USA) to generate the FE model (Figure 8) using 10-node tetrahedral h-elements (ANSYS SOLID187 elements).

The convergence of the FEM analysis depended largely on the mesh grid. A standard convergence study was conducted by FEM analysis for mesh grids with different mesh refinement levels. A refined mesh was used in the threaded areas and the surrounding bone. For mesh grid, the relative errors for the maximum Von Mises stress in the implant system and the surrounding bone were computed as the

TABLE 1: 12 combinations of the dental implant systems.

Category	Abutment	Implant	Healing	Nodes
1#	"St"	"Tr"	"Su"	124,128
2#	"St"	"Re"	"Su"	123,676
3#	"St"	"Sa"	"Su"	123,684
4#	"St"	"Tr"	"Ns"	123,060
5#	"St"	"Re"	"Ns"	123,294
6#	"St"	"Sa"	"Ns"	124,433
7#	"St"	"Tr"	"Su"	129,202
8#	"An"	"Re"	"Su"	128,994
9#	"An"	"Sa"	"Su"	129,578
10#	"An"	"Tr"	"Ns"	127,706
11#	"An"	"Re"	"Ns"	128,938
12#	"An"	"Sa"	"Ns"	128,721

St: straight; An: angled; Tr: trapezia; Re: rectangle; Sa: saw; Su: submerged; Ns: nonsubmerged.

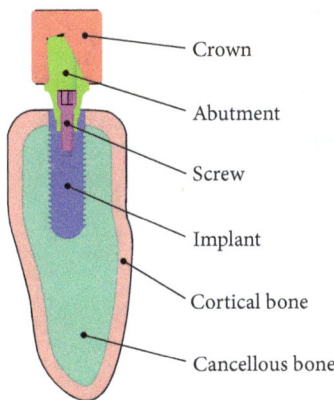

FIGURE 3: Dental implant/bone system.

percent differences between the current stress values and their counterparts predicted by the previous trial run. The calculation was considered to be convergent and the mesh grid was accepted when the relative errors were less than 1%. Number of total nodes is listed in Table 1, respectively.

2.3. Materials and Load Conditions. The abutment, implant, screw, cortical bone, and cancellous bone were treated as isotropic homogeneous linear elastic materials. Table 2 listed Young's modulus (E), Poisson's ratio (v), and Tensile Strength (Ts) of the materials used in the numerical examples. Because the elements were quite small, the material properties were assumed to be constant within each element.

The bottom of the mandible was treated as fixed boundaries, and both side planes were frictionless, which was normal constraint (Figure 9). Two different contact models ("bonded" and "frictional") are used to simulate different integration qualities at the implant and the supporting bone tissues during the osseointegration process. Using contact type of frictional to describe the integration quality among the abutment, implant, and screw interface and among implant, cortical bone, and cancellous bone interface

(Table 3), the friction coefficient was 0.5 and 0.4, respectively [26]. Frictional contact implied that a gap between the implant and the peri-implant part might exist under an occlusal force. The rest of the contact surfaces were Bonded contact (Table 3). The "bonded" type simulated perfect osseointegration in which the implant and the surrounding parts were fully integrated so that neither sliding nor separation in the implant-bone interface was possible.

Based on oral physiology, four types of loading conditions (Figure 6) were simulated:

(1) A vertical occlusal force of 100 N ($\theta = 0$) applied on the crown top surface [4], a preload of 200 N applied to the screw [27].

(2) A vertical occlusal force of 100 N ($\theta = 0$) applied on the crown top surface [4], a torque of 0.2 N·m applied to the screw [27].

(3) An inclined occlusal force of 100 N ($\theta = 15°$) applied on the crown top surface [4], a preload of 200 N applied to the screw [27].

(4) An inclined occlusal force of 100 N ($\theta = 15°$) applied on the crown top surface [4], a torque of 0.2 N·m applied to the screw [27].

3. Results

Figure 7 gave the Von Mises stress distributions of the typical dental implants and the surrounding bone tissues under loading condition (1), (2), (3), or (4), respectively.

As shown in Figure 10, the stress was mainly concentrated at the inner hexagon positioning junction because the force was just applied only on the contact surface. Application of the preload or torque applied to the screw resulted in the stress concentration on the screw, and fatigue failure would occur in the process of long-term use. The stresses in the cortical bone and cancellous bone, which were conjoint with implant, were relatively small due to the design concept of platform switching, which could reduce the stresses gradually at junction between the implant and the surrounding bone tissues, thus avoiding bone level being decreased in the long-term use.

Then we compared the maximum Von Mises stress distributions of 12 types of the dental implants and surrounding bone tissues (Figure 11).

Figure 11(a) exhibited the stress distribution of the abutment. When vertical force was applied on the crown, the abutment stress of the torque applied to the screw was larger than that of the preload condition while in the inclined force the abutment stress of the preload applied to the screw was larger than that of the torque condition. Both in the preload and in torque condition, the abutment stress of the inclined force was significantly higher than that in the vertical force of the crown. Taken together, the abutment maximum stresses of 1#, 2#, 3#, 7#, 8#, and 9# were rather small.

Figure 11(b) presented stress distribution of the implant. In the preloaded screw application, the stress difference was small in both the vertical force and the inclined force conditions. In the torque condition, the implant stress in

TABLE 2: Material properties used in this study.

Material	Region	E (MPa)	υ	Ts (MPa)	Reference
Titanium	Implant, abutment, screw	102,000	0.35	485	[22]
Porcelain	Crown	68,900	0.28	835	[22]
Cortical bone	Mandible	13,000	0.30	133.9	[23]
Cancellous bone	Mandible	690	0.30	56	[23]

TABLE 3: Contact methods.

	Abutment	Screw	Implant	Cortical bone	Cancellous bone
Crown	Bonded	—	—	—	—
Abutment	—	Frictional	Frictional	—	—
Screw	—	—	Frictional	—	—
Implant	—	—	—	Frictional	Frictional
Cortical bone	—	—	—	—	Bonded

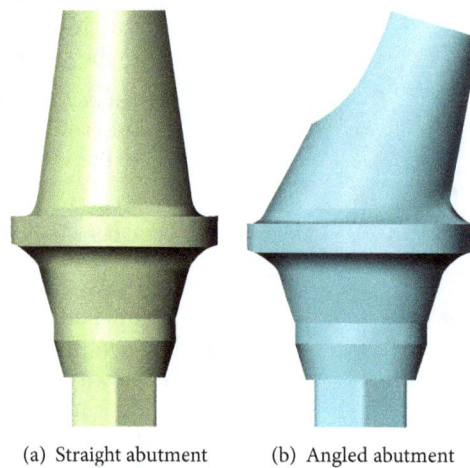

(a) Straight abutment   (b) Angled abutment

FIGURE 4: Abutment category.

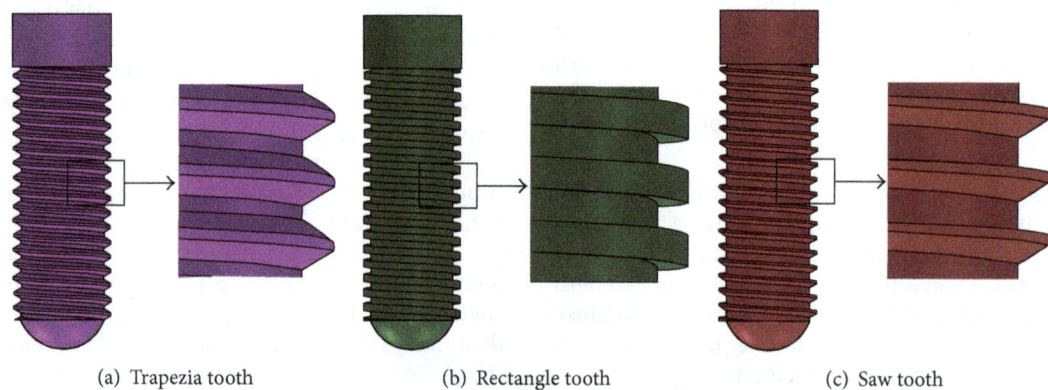

(a) Trapezia tooth   (b) Rectangle tooth   (c) Saw tooth

FIGURE 5: Thread category of the implant.

the inclined force was larger than that in the vertical force. Both in the vertical and the inclined force, the preloaded application had great effect on the implant stress. Taken together, the implant maximum stresses of 3#, 4#, 5#, 10#, and 11# were rather small.

Figure 11(c) depicted the stress distribution of the screw. Whether in the preloaded or in torque application, the vertical and inclined force of the crown application had little effect on screw stress. However, under same loading conditions, the screw stress of the preloaded screw had greater effect than the

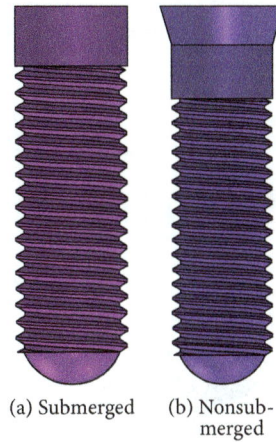

(a) Submerged   (b) Nonsub-
                          merged

FIGURE 6: Healing method.

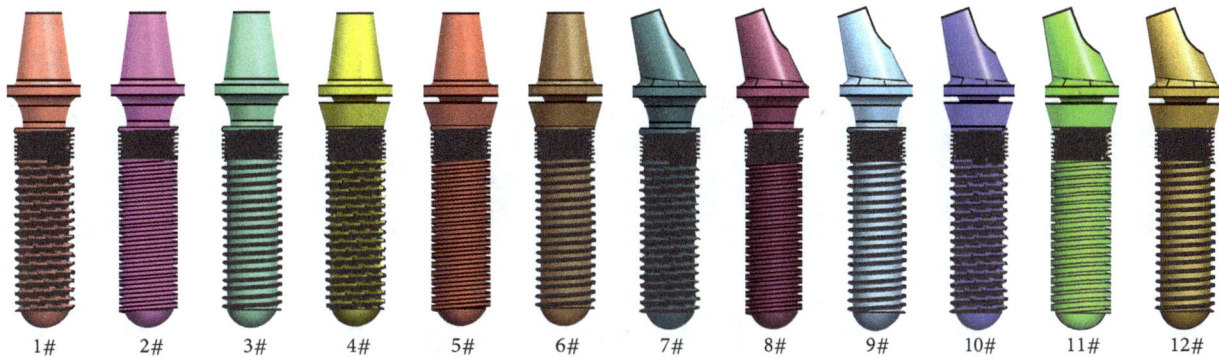

1#   2#   3#   4#   5#   6#   7#   8#   9#   10#   11#   12#

FIGURE 7: 3D model of 12 dental implant systems.

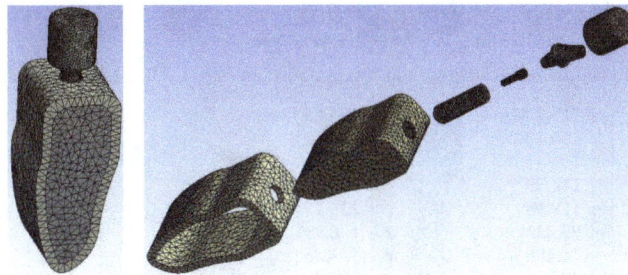

FIGURE 8: Finite element mesh view.

torque one. Taken together, the screw maximum stresses of 1#, 3#, 5#, 7#, 9#, and 11# were rather small.

Figure 11(d) represented the stress distribution of the cortical bone. The cortical bone stress was relatively small. Whether in the preload or in torque application of the screw, the cortical bone stress of the inclined force was larger than the vertical force while in the vertical force the torqued screw application had greater effect on screw stress than the preloaded one. However, in the inclined force application, the torqued screw had smaller effect on screw stress than the preload condition. Taken together, the cortical bone maximum stresses of 4#, 5#, 6#, 10#, 11#, and 12# were rather small.

Figure 11(e) showed the stress distribution of the cancellous bone. The cancellous bone stress was relatively small. Whether in the preload or in torque application of the screw, the cancellous bone stress of the inclined force was larger than that of the vertical force. However, under same load conditions, the preloaded screw had greater effect on screw stress than the torque condition. Taken together, the cancellous bone maximum stresses of 4#, 5#, 6#, 9#, 10#, and 11# were rather small.

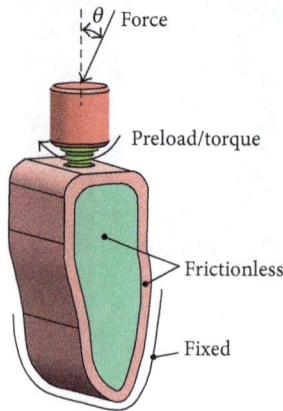

FIGURE 9: Load conditions of dental implant-bone tissue.

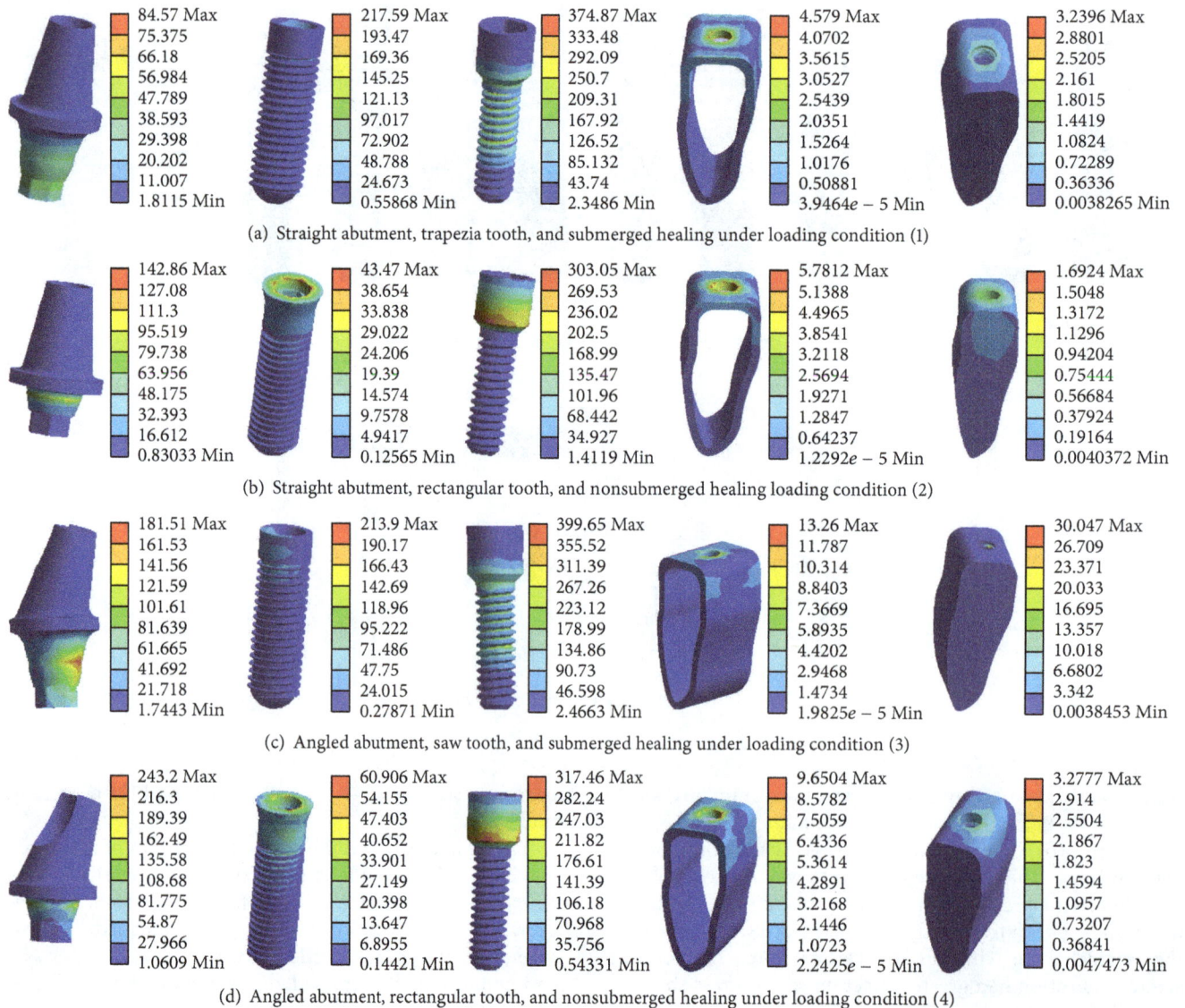

(a) Straight abutment, trapezia tooth, and submerged healing under loading condition (1)

(b) Straight abutment, rectangular tooth, and nonsubmerged healing loading condition (2)

(c) Angled abutment, saw tooth, and submerged healing under loading condition (3)

(d) Angled abutment, rectangular tooth, and nonsubmerged healing under loading condition (4)

FIGURE 10: Stress distributions in the typical dental implants and the surrounding bone tissues.

(a) Maximum stress of the abutment

(b) Maximum stress of the implant

(c) Maximum stress of the screw

(d) Maximum stress of the cortical bone

(e) Maximum stress of the cancellous bone

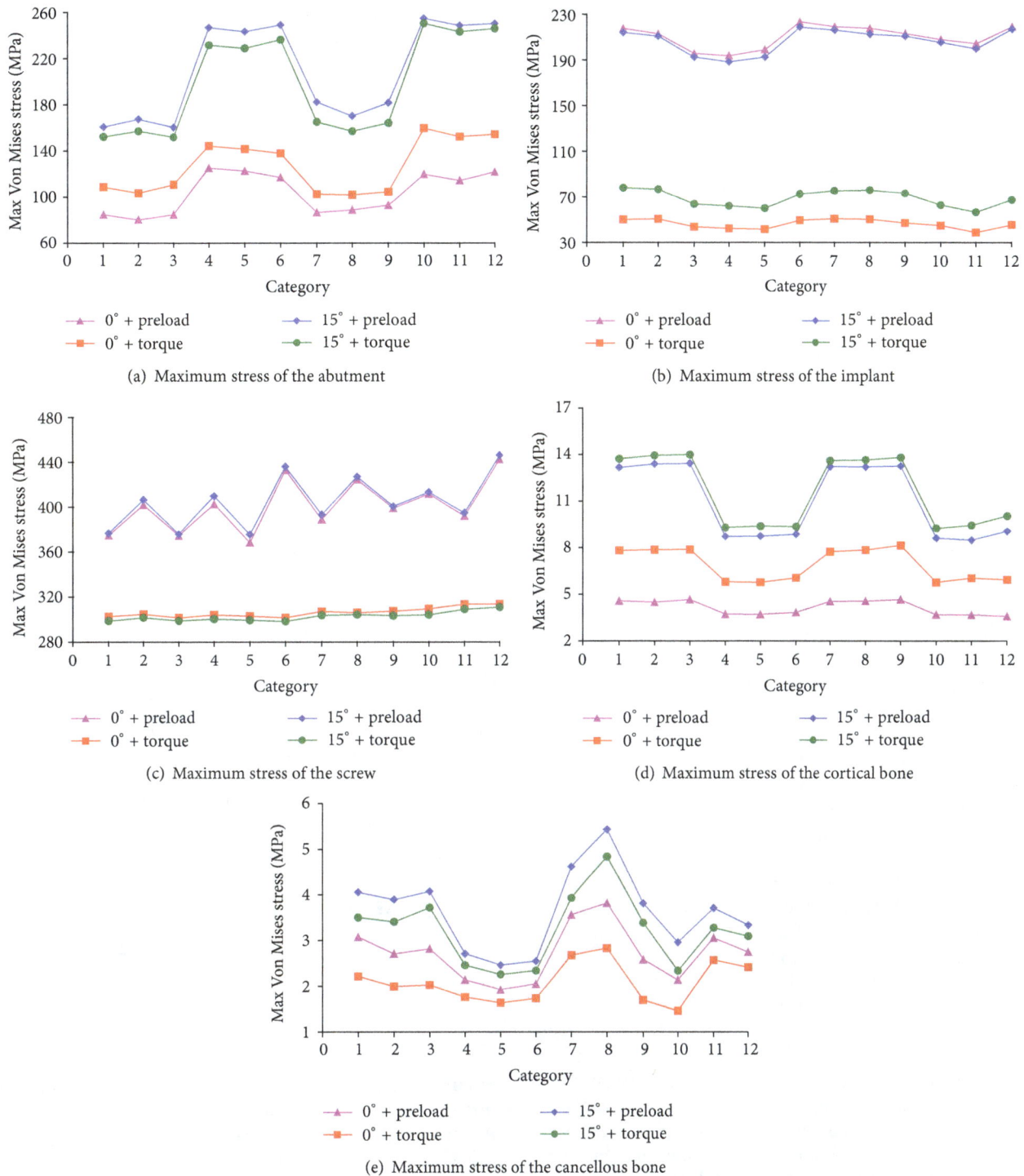

FIGURE 11: Maximum stress distributions of the dental implants and surrounding bone tissues.

4. Discussion

Stress fields around endosteal implants and the supporting bone tissues were closely related to the type of loading and implant geometry [4]. In order to realistically simulate the stress state of the implant/bone system, four types of loading conditions (Figure 9) were studied.

Our results showed that the stress was mainly concentrated at the inner hexagon positioning junction because of the force just applied on the contact surface. The application of the preloaded or torqued screw resulted in stress concentration on the screw. However, the stresses in the cortical bone and cancellous bone which were conjoint with implant were relatively small.

TABLE 4: Stress comparisons of 12 implants-bone tissues.

		Dental implant-bone system					
		Abutment	Implant	Screw	Cortical bone	Cancellous bone	Frequency
Implant combinations	1#	+		+			2
	2#	+					1
	3#	+	+	+			3
	4#		+		+	+	3
	5#		+	+	+	+	4
	6#				+	+	2
	7#	+		+			2
	8#	+					1
	9#	+		+			2
	10#				+	+	2
	11#		+	+	+		3
	12#				+	+	2

The symbol of "+" meant the unit with minimum stress of the implant-bone tissues.

Under same loading direction of the crown, the stress influence on the torqued screw was greater than that of the preload condition in the abutment and cortical bone while the stress influence of the preloaded screw was greater than that of the torqued condition for the implant, screw, and cancellous bone. The reason was mainly that the torque acted on the upper inner surface of the hexagonal hole of the screw while the preload was applied to the lower outer surface of the screw.

Meanwhile, under same loading mode of the screw, the stress distributions of the abutment, cortical bone, and cancellous bone in the inclined force on the crown were larger than those in the vertical force, up to 2 to 3 times. However, as for the implant and screw, the stress influence with different loading direction applied on the crown was not large. It was mainly due to the fact that the vertical force made stress distribution of the surrounding bone uniform through the cross section and the thread of implant. While the inclined force generated shear force and bending moment on the implant, thus the stress concentration at the implant's neck and bone contact area has taken place.

In addition, the abutment stress of nonsubmerged implant was larger than that of the submerged one under same load conditions. However, the implant, cortical bone, and cancellous bone stresses of nonsubmerged implant were smaller than those of submerged one indicating that if an overload condition occurred during chewing, the abutment of nonsubmerged system and the implant of submerged system would be susceptible to be broken, which could affect the long-term retention rate of the implant system. Therefore, doctors and patients need to take certain protective measures in use.

Table 4 listed stress distributions of 12 combinations of the dental implants and surrounding bone tissues (The symbol of "+" meant the unit with minimum stress of the implant-bone tissues). It was seen from Table 4 that 5# was the best option, which was the straight abutments, rectangular tooth, and nonsubmerged dental implant system. Meanwhile, 3#, 4#, and 11# were also provided with a certain application value.

5. Conclusion

Under same loading conditions, the thread had no significant effect on the implant stress but a greater impact on the cancellous bone stress. The stress distributions of the abutment, cortical bone, and cancellous bone in the inclined force of the crown were larger than that in the vertical force. The abutment stress of nonsubmerged healing implant system was larger than that of the submerged healing one. However, the implant, cortical bone, and cancellous bone stresses of nonsubmerged implant system were smaller than those of submerged one.

In conclusion, a dental implant system characterised by a straight abutment, rectangular tooth, and nonsubmerged healing method is the optimal design.

Conflict of Interests

The authors declare that there is no conflict of interests regarding the publication of this paper.

Acknowledgments

Financial support from the National Natural Science Foundation of China (51307170), the Cooperation Project of Chinese Academy of Sciences and Foshan City Government of China (2014HT10008), the Guangzhou City Key Laboratory project (15180003), and the Guangzhou Nansha District High-Tech Industrialization Project of China (201202005) is gratefully acknowledged.

References

[1] H. İplikçioğlu and K. Akça, "Comparative evaluation of the effect of diameter, length and number of implants supporting three-unit fixed partial prostheses on stress distribution in the bone," Journal of Dentistry, vol. 30, no. 1, pp. 41–46, 2002.

[2] R. Adell, B. Eriksson, U. Lekholm, P. I. Brånemark, and T. Jemt, "Long-term follow-up study of osseointegrated implants in the

treatment of totally edentulous jaws," *The International Journal of Oral & Maxillofacial Implants*, vol. 5, no. 4, pp. 347–359, 1990.

[3] R. Adell, U. Lekholm, B. Rockler, and P. I. Branemark, "A 15-year study of osseointegrated implants in the treatment of the edentulous jaw," *International Journal of Oral Surgery*, vol. 10, no. 6, pp. 387–416, 1981.

[4] J. Yang and H.-J. Xiang, "A three-dimensional finite element study on the biomechanical behavior of an FGBM dental implant in surrounding bone," *Journal of Biomechanics*, vol. 40, no. 11, pp. 2377–2385, 2007.

[5] R. Calandriello and M. Tomatis, "Immediate occlusal loading of single lower molars using br anemark system(R) wide platform TiUnite implants: a 5-year follow-up report of a prospective clinical multicenter study," *Clinical Implant Dentistry and Related Research*, vol. 19, pp. 381–396, 2009.

[6] G. O. Gallucci, C. B. Doughtie, J. W. Hwang, J. P. Fiorellini, and H.-P. Weber, "Five-year results of fixed implant-supported rehabilitations with distal cantilevers for the edentulous mandible," *Clinical Oral Implants Research*, vol. 20, no. 6, pp. 601–607, 2009.

[7] F. E. Lambert, H.-P. Weber, S. M. Susarla, U. C. Belserand, and G. O. Gallucci, "Descriptive analysis of implant and prosthodontic survival rates with fixed implant-supported rehabilitations in the edentulous maxilla," *Journal of Periodontology*, vol. 80, no. 8, pp. 1220–1230, 2009.

[8] J. B. Brunski, "Biomechanics of dental implants," in *Implants in Dentistry*, M. Block, J. N. Kent, and L. R. Guerra, Eds., no. 2, pp. 63–71, W.B. Saunders, Philadelphia, Pa, USA, 1997.

[9] T. Li, K. Hu, L. Cheng et al., "Optimum selection of the dental implant diameter and length in the posterior mandible with poor bone quality—A 3D finite element analysis," *Applied Mathematical Modelling*, vol. 35, no. 1, pp. 446–456, 2011.

[10] C.-C. Lee, S.-C. Lin, M.-J. Kang, S.-W. Wu, and P.-Y. Fu, "Effects of implant threads on the contact area and stress distribution of marginal bone," *Journal of Dental Sciences*, vol. 5, no. 3, pp. 156–165, 2010.

[11] H.-L. Huang, C.-H. Chang, J.-T. Hsu, A. M. Fallgatter, and C.-C. Ko, "Comparison of implant body designs and threaded designs of dental implants: a 3-dimensional finite element analysis," *International Journal of Oral and Maxillofacial Implants*, vol. 22, no. 4, pp. 551–562, 2007.

[12] C. E. Misch and M. W. Bidez, "A scientific rationale for dental implant design," in *Contemporary Implant Dentistry*, C. E. Misch, Ed., pp. 329–343, Mosby, St. Louis, Mo, USA, 2nd edition, 1999.

[13] N. Sykaras, A. M. Iacopino, V. A. Marker, R. G. Triplett, and R. D. Woody, "Implant materials, designs, and surface topographies: their effect on osseointegration. A literature review," *International Journal of Oral and Maxillofacial Implants*, vol. 15, no. 5, pp. 675–690, 2000.

[14] C. Maiorana and F. Santoro, "Maxillary and mandibular bone reconstruction with hip grafts and implants using Frialit-2 implants," *International Journal of Periodontics and Restorative Dentistry*, vol. 22, no. 3, pp. 221–229, 2002.

[15] G. H. Nentwig, "Ankylos implant system: concept and clinical application," *Journal of Oral Implantology*, vol. 30, no. 3, pp. 171–177, 2004.

[16] S. Hansson and M. Werke, "The implant thread as a retention element in cortical bone: the effect of thread size and thread profile: A finite element study," *Journal of Biomechanics*, vol. 36, no. 9, pp. 1247–1258, 2003.

[17] L. Kong, K. Hu, D. Li et al., "Evaluation of the cylinder implant thread height and width: a 3-dimensional finite element analysis," *International Journal of Oral and Maxillofacial Implants*, vol. 23, no. 1, pp. 65–74, 2008.

[18] H.-L. Huang, J.-T. Hsu, L.-J. Fuh, D.-J. Lin, and M. Y. C. Chen, "Biomechanical simulation of various surface roughnesses and geometric designs on an immediately loaded dental implant," *Computers in Biology and Medicine*, vol. 40, no. 5, pp. 525–532, 2010.

[19] D. L. Cochran, D. Morton, and H.-P. Weber, "Consensus statements and recommended clinical procedures regarding loading protocols for endosseous dental implants," *International Journal of Oral and Maxillofacial Implants*, vol. 19, no. 5, pp. 109–113, 2004.

[20] C. E. Misch, H.-L. Wang, C. M. Misch, M. Sharawy, J. Lemons, and K. W. M. Judy, "Rationale for the application of immediate load in implant dentistry: part I," *Implant Dentistry*, vol. 13, no. 3, pp. 207–217, 2004.

[21] R. Gapski, H.-L. Wang, P. Mascarenhas, and N. P. Lang, "Critical review of immediate implant loading," *Clinical Oral Implants Research*, vol. 14, no. 5, pp. 515–527, 2003.

[22] J. Chen, X. Lu, N. Paydar, H. U. Akay, and W. E. Roberts, "Mechanical simulation of the human mandible with and without an endosseous implant," *Medical Engineering and Physics*, vol. 16, no. 1, pp. 53–61, 1994.

[23] J. Y. Rho, R. B. Ashman, and H. Turner, "Young's modulus of trabecular and cortical bone material: ultrasonic and microtensile measurements," *Journal of Biomechanics*, vol. 26, no. 2, pp. 111–119, 1993.

[24] A. N. Natali, P. G. Pavan, and A. L. Ruggero, "Analysis of bone-implant interaction phenomena by using a numerical approach," *Clinical Oral Implants Research*, vol. 17, no. 1, pp. 67–74, 2006.

[25] Y. Maeda, J. Miura, I. Taki, and M. Sogo, "Biomechanical analysis on platform switching: is there any biomechanical rationale?" *Clinical Oral Implants Research*, vol. 18, no. 5, pp. 581–584, 2007.

[26] Z. Enwei and G. Fei, "Analysis of static force and fatigue between thread structure of dental implant and contact surface," *Journal of Clinical Rehabilitative Tissue Engineering*, vol. 14, no. 30, pp. 5531–5534, 2010.

[27] C. Luo, "Effects of different shape of occlusal screws on stability for single implant-supported crowns," *Chinese Journal of Oral Implantology*, vol. 14, no. 2, pp. 44–47, 2009.

29

Comparison of the Mechanical Properties of Early Leukocyte- and Platelet-Rich Fibrin versus PRGF/Endoret Membranes

Hooman Khorshidi,[1] Saeed Raoofi,[1] Rafat Bagheri,[2] and Hodasadat Banihashemi[3]

[1]Department of Periodontology, School of Dentistry, Shiraz University of Medical Sciences, Shiraz, Iran
[2]Department of Dental Materials, School of Dentistry, Shiraz University of Medical Sciences, Shiraz, Iran
[3]Periodontology Department, Faculty of Dentistry, Shahid Sadoughi University of Medical Sciences, Yazd, Iran

Correspondence should be addressed to Hodasadat Banihashemi; hoda.banihashemi@gmail.com

Academic Editor: Andrija Bosnjak

Objectives. The mechanical properties of membranes are important factors in the success of treatment and clinical handling. The goal of this study was to compare the mechanical properties of early leukocyte- and platelet-rich fibrin (L-PRF) versus PRGF/Endoret membrane. *Materials and Methods*. In this experimental study, membranes were obtained from 10 healthy male volunteers. After obtaining 20 cc venous blood from each volunteer, 10 cc was used to prepare early L-PRF (group 1) and the rest was used to get a membrane by PRGF-Endoret system (group 2). Tensile loads were applied to specimens using universal testing machine. Tensile strength, stiffness, and toughness of the two groups of membranes were calculated and compared by paired t-test. *Results*. The mean tensile strength and toughness were higher in group 1 with a significant difference ($P < 0.05$). The mean stiffness in group 1 was also higher but not statistically significant ($P > 0.05$). *Conclusions*. The results showed that early L-PRF membranes had stronger mechanical properties than membranes produced by PRGF-Endoret system. Early L-PRF membranes might have easier clinical handling and could be a more proper scaffold in periodontal regenerative procedures. The real results of the current L-PRF should be in fact much higher than what is reported here.

1. Introduction

Periodontal reconstruction is the ideal goal of periodontal treatment and since 1970, many researches led to developing various methods to achieve it. Among these methods, guided tissue regeneration (GTR) and guided bone regeneration (GBR) use barrier membranes to separate the periodontal ligament and bone from the epithelium and connective tissue which allow the former to regenerate the defects [1]. Recently, various growth factors have been studied in periodontal regeneration [2] and it is indicated that they might strongly alter the healing process [3]. A new method in this field is using concentrated platelet products which are the source of autologous platelet derived growth factors and transforming growth factors [4].

Among various concentrated platelet products, preparation rich in growth factor (PRGF) is an autologous platelet-rich plasma product which accelerates local release of growth factors and bioactive proteins following its activation. With various formulations, this product can be used in form of liquid or in form of clot as a membrane which is a biocompatible, dense, and elastic membrane [5]. The new form of concentrated platelet is platelet-rich fibrin (PRF) that can be used directly as a clot or as a strong membrane after compression [6, 7]. PRF as a membrane has shown slow release of growth factors such as vascular endothelial growth factor (VEGF), transforming growth factor (TGF-β), and platelet derived growth factor (PDGF) for at least 7 days in vitro [8]. Leukocyte- and platelet-rich fibrin (L-PRF) can be considered as a second-generation platelet concentrate. It forms a

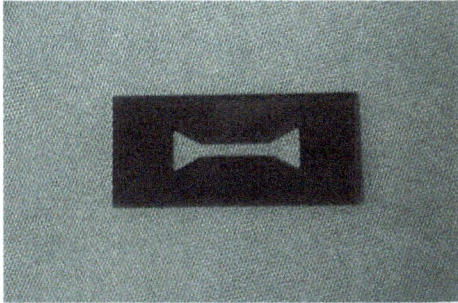

FIGURE 1: The dog-bone-shape plexiglass mold.

strong fibrin matrix with a complex three-dimensional architecture, in which most of the platelets and leucocytes from the harvested blood are concentrated [9]. Platelet-rich fibrin membranes can be used in various regenerative treatments [10, 11] to accelerate healing, to progress the regeneration process, and also as a scaffold in tissue engineering.

Besides scientific evidences about efficacy, for selection of an appropriate membrane, there are other important parameters including mechanical properties and clinical handling [12, 13]. Mechanical characteristics of the membrane may affect the final results of GBR [14]. Tensile strength of a material when sutured may affect the clinical result of following healing [15]. Moreover strong mechanical characteristics of a scaffold provide a more suitable support for regeneration [16].

It is reported that increasing fibrinogen concentrates and adding calcium chloride increase the adhesion and tensile strength of fibrin clot [17]. It is also indicated that increasing thrombin and fibrinogen may increase the stiffness of fibrin matrix [18].

To the best of authors' knowledge, a comparison of mechanical characteristics of PRF and PRGF membranes is missing in previous studies. The goal of this study was to compare the mechanical properties of early L-PRF and the PRGF membranes. The null hypothesis was that there is no difference between mechanical properties of early L-PRF and PRGF membranes.

2. Materials and Methods

In this experimental study, 20 cc venous blood was obtained from 10 healthy volunteer males with age range of 25 to 35 years. The exclusion criteria were suffering from a known systemic disease, history of taking any anticoagulant medication, smoking, and history of taking any medicine in the past 3 months.

2.1. Preparing a Mold. A specially designed plexiglass mold was fabricated to make the fibrin specimens identical in size, volume, and figure, following a modification of the dog-bone-shape mold in Alston's study [17]. The thickness of the mold was 2 mm and the width was 2 mm in the narrow middle part and 6 mm in the larger ends. The total volume of the mold was 104 mm^3. The narrow neck provided the weakest point where the specimen would break (Figure 1).

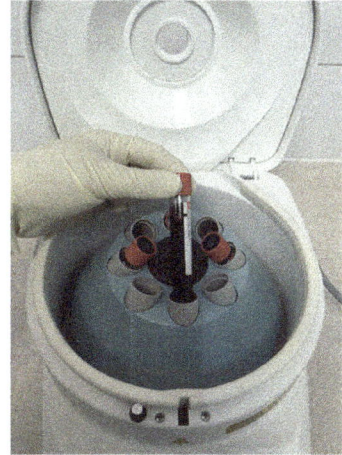

FIGURE 2: Tube containing blood in the centrifuge machine.

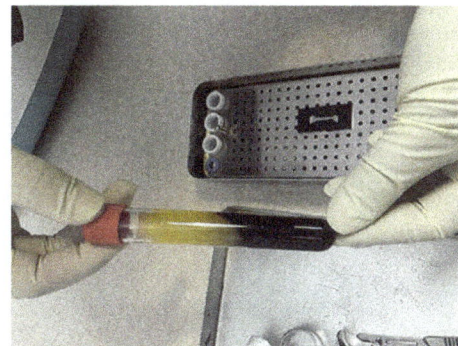

FIGURE 3: Tube containing early L-PRF after centrifuge.

2.2. Blood Collection. After obtaining informed consent approved by the ethical committee of Shiraz University of Medical Science (Grant number 92-01-03-6162) from all donors, 20 cc venous blood was collected by sterile syringe. 10 cc was placed in a dry sterile tube specific for PC-02 machine and the rest was divided into two 5 cc blood samples placed in two tubes containing 0.5 cc 3.8% concentrate of sodium citrate as anticoagulant specific for PRGF-Endoret system.

2.3. Preparing the Membranes. Platelet-rich membranes were obtained by two different protocols:

The first one was producing early L-PRF [7] by PC-02 machine (Process Ltd., Nice, France) in which the tube that contained blood was centrifuged immediately after blood collection in speed of 400 gr for 10 min [19] (Figure 2). The outcome was a fibrin clot containing platelets in the middle of the tube, between acellular plasma at the top and the red blood cell layer at the bottom (Figure 3). This clot was removed from the tube (Figure 4) and the attached red blood cells were scraped off and discarded. The early L-PRF clot was then placed in the mold (Figure 5) which was placed on the grid in the PRF Box [20] (Process

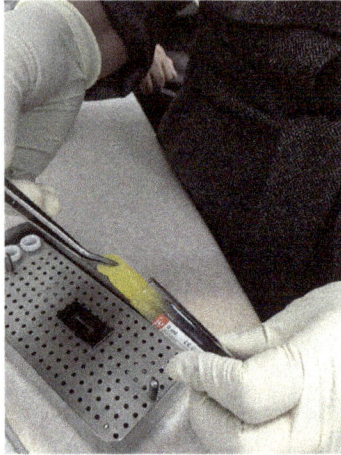

FIGURE 4: Removing the early L-PRF from the tube.

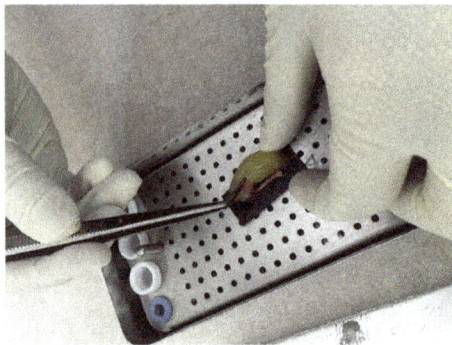

FIGURE 5: Placing the early L-PRF clot into the mold.

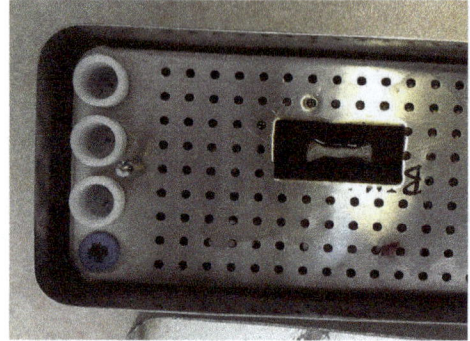

FIGURE 6: A fibrin specimen in the mold.

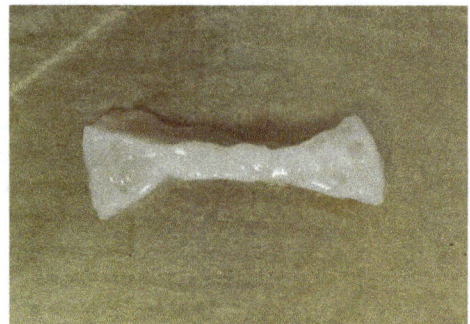

FIGURE 7: A formed specimen.

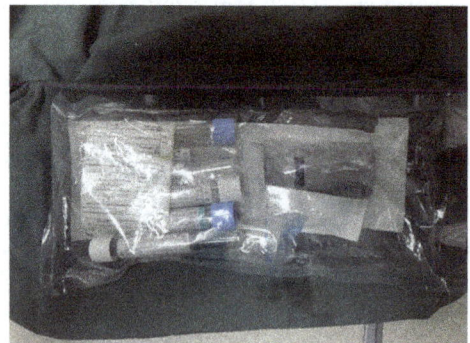

FIGURE 8: A BTI kit.

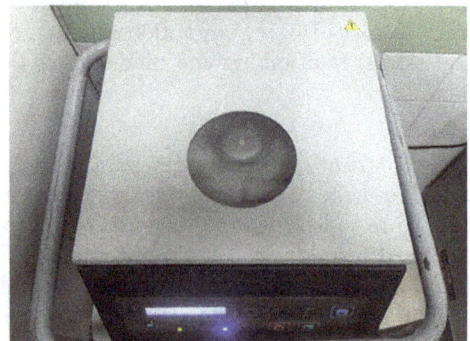

FIGURE 9: BTI centrifuging machine.

Ltd., Nice, France) (Figure 6) and covered with the compressor and lid. After 10 min the formed early L-PRF membrane was prepared (Figure 7).

The second protocol was performed using PRGF-Endoret system (BTI, Spain) (Figure 8). The two 5 cc tubes were centrifuged in speed of 400 gr for 8 min with BTI centrifuge machine (BTI, Spain) (Figure 9). Then each tube contained red blood cell at the bottom and plasma at the top with a thin layer of WBC in the middle (Figure 10). The inferior half of the plasma which was rich in platelets and growth factors was removed by plasma transfer device 2 (PTD2) (BTI, Spain) and placed in another tube. As the manufacturer instructions, 0.05 mL PRGF-Endoret activator per 1 mL plasma was added and then placed on incubator at 37°C for 30 min to obtain the clot (Figure 11). The clot was placed in the mold and after 10 min the formed membrane was obtained (Figure 12).

2.4. Tensile Test. Tensile test was performed using universal testing machine (Zwick/Roll Z020, Zwick GmbH & Co., Germany) (Figure 13). The larger ends of the dog-bone shape specimen were held with the clips of the machine without any

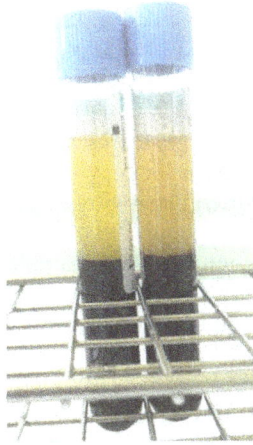

FIGURE 10: Tubes containing PRGF after centrifuge.

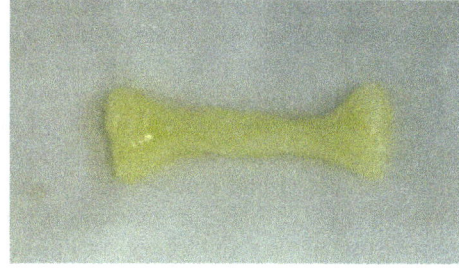

FIGURE 11: Mixture of the platelet-rich plasma and the activator on the incubator.

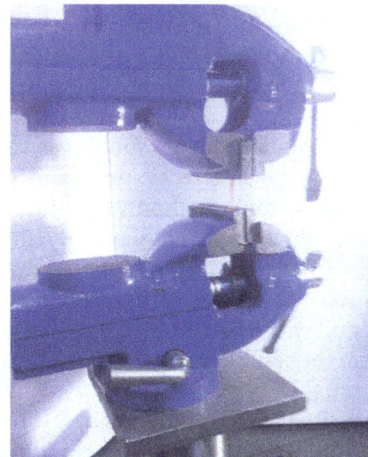

FIGURE 12: A formed specimen.

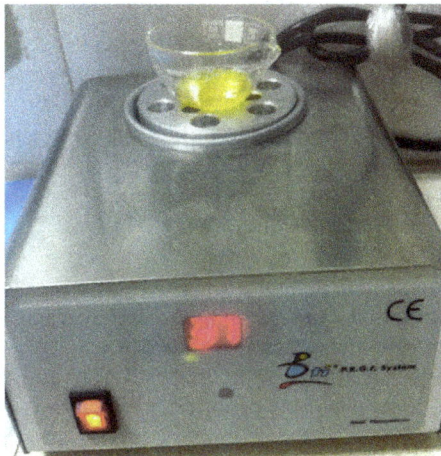

FIGURE 13: The universal testing machine.

tension. Tensile loading was applied at a cross head speed of 2 mm/min; the maximum load at specimen failure was recorded and tensile strength was calculated using following formula: $S = F/A$, where F is maximum force (N) and A is unit area (m^2).

Stress-strain curve was recorded with test Xpert II software simultaneously. Stiffness of the specimen (modulus of elasticity) was obtained by stress/strain and the total area under the curve designated as toughness of the specimens.

2.5. Data Analysis. Data were collected and analyzed using SPSS version 16; Student t-test was used to compare the groups: the early L-PRF as group 1 and the PRGF-Endoret system as group 2.

3. Results

The results of all tests for two groups are summarized in Table 1.

TABLE 1: Mean values and standard deviation (±SD) for all tested properties in the two groups.

Measured values	Group	Mean ± SD	P value
Tensile strength (MPa)	1	0.20 ± 0.06	0.049
	2	0.14 ± 0.07	
Modulus of elasticity (MPa)	1	0.13 ± 0.07	0.69
	2	0.11 ± 0.09	
Toughness (Joule/m^3)	1	1.87 ± 0.61	0.001
	2	0.81 ± 0.53	

Tensile strength of early L-PRF group with mean value of 0.20 ± 0.06 MPa was significantly higher than PRGF group with mean value of 0.14 ± 0.07 MPa ($P = 0.049$). Early L-PRF group was slightly stiffer than PRGF group but was not statistically significant ($P = 0.69$). Toughness of early L-PRF group was significantly higher than PRGF group ($P = 0.001$).

4. Discussion

This study experienced that the mechanical properties of early L-PRF membranes are stronger than the PRGF-Endoret membranes.

Platelet-rich fibrin membrane releases various growth factors such as PDGF, TGF-β, and VEGF slowly [21] and its supportive fibrin matrix plays an important role in its therapeutic effects [6]. The potential of platelet-rich membrane in accelerating regeneration has led to its application in various regenerative treatments like sinus floor elevation, ridge augmentation, socket preservation, root coverage, intrabony defects, and furcation defects [22–31]. It has been shown that fibrin membranes could be better scaffolds for proliferation of periosteal and osseous cells than collagen membranes in vitro [32, 33]. The membranes that are used in regenerative procedures should have strong mechanical properties to protect blood clot and healing process [13]. As a scaffold, they provide better support against forces from infiltrating cells and adjacent tissues [16, 34].

The specimens of this study were selected from healthy male individuals with the age range of 25–35 to prevent possible bias from varieties in blood components of different sexes, ages, and systemic conditions. These issues were not considered together in the previous studies on fibrin clots [17, 35, 36]. The dog-bone-shape mold was used to make the specimens identical in size, volume, and shape. It was a modification of Alston's method [17], since the volume of clot we could obtain and consequently the volume of our specimen were lesser than Alston's study. Mechanical measurements were performed by universal testing machine as some other studies [17, 35–38].

According to the results of our study, the tensile strength, stiffness, and toughness of early L-PRF membranes were higher than the PRGF-Endoret membranes though the stiffness difference was not significant. This result may be due to their structural differences which may be affected by some factors like their differences in polymerization. The mode of polymerization has significant effects on mechanical properties of fibrin matrix [39]. This is consistent with the studies that evaluated their polymerization and internal structure [9, 39]. The last stage of clotting, in which fibrinogen is converted to fibrin, can be accelerated by adding calcium chloride [40]. In PRGF-Endoret system, calcium chloride is used to initiate the last coagulation stage; then sudden fibrin polymerization occurs [39]. Therefore the fibrin matrix is immature and most of the fibrils are thin [9]. On the other hand, a slow and natural polymerization occurs during the centrifuge process in L-PRF producing method. The fibrin fibrillae can be assembled in 2 different biochemical architectures during gelling process: condensed tetramolecular or bilateral junctions and connected trimolecular or equilateral junctions [39]. PRGF mostly have the bilateral junctions which are weaker than the equilateral junctions [9] that are mostly found in L-PRF. This provides a flexible and elastic fibrin network [39]. L-PRF has thick fibers and strong matrix [9].

The density of the final fibrin matrix is another important factor that has an influence on the mechanical properties [41] and fibrinogen concentration affects this parameter. Fibrinogen mostly originates from the α-granules of the platelet in PRGF so the final fibrin has low density, while the circulating fibrinogen present in L-PRF strengthens the final fibrin matrix [9]. Alston et al. (2007) and Duong et al. (2009) indicated that increase in fibrinogen concentration makes the final fibrin matrix stronger [17, 18].

Another difference of these two membranes is the presence of large quantities of leukocytes in L-PRF and lack of them in PRGF. Some studies indicated that leukocytes have a key role in immune regulation, anti-infection properties [42–45], and angiogenesis [46] in platelet-rich concentrates. On the other hand, some authors claim that leukocytes may destroy the extracellular matrix of fibrin by the anti-inflammatory effects of proteases and hydrolase; therefore they suggest removing the leukocytes from platelet-rich concentrates to prevent their negative effects on autologous fibrin formation [5, 47]. The interaction of platelets and leukocytes in platelet-rich concentrates is not completely analyzed; they may also show synergistic effect [9]. Therefore the negative effects of leukocytes on fibrin matrix are controversial yet and our results suggest that these effects are not significant.

In producing the early L-PRF, no anticoagulant is employed but, in PRGF, sodium citrate is used. This difference of these two methods may affect the fibrin matrix. Kingston showed that high concentration of sodium citrate in blood samples decreases the ionized calcium of plasma leading to decrease in platelet accumulation and fibrinogen binding [48]. However, it is not obvious that 0.5 cc 3.8% concentration of sodium citrate can have such an effect on PRGF matrix and controlled studies are needed to confirm this issue.

The room temperature during the process and the speed of centrifuge were the same in both groups but the duration was less in PRGF. Perez et al. showed that longer duration of centrifuge increases the platelet recovery [49] so this may affect the plasma components and final fibrin matrix properties.

Parameters such as manufacturing property of the blood collecting tubes and the pressure applied during the process do not affect the biomaterial structure [8].

It should be noted that we used the early protocol (3000 rpm, 10 minutes) to produce L-PRF, while since years the 2700 rpm/12 minutes protocol is mostly used that gives much better polymerized L-PRF and therefore stronger membranes than the 3000 rpm/10 min protocol. The real results of the current L-PRF should be in fact much higher than what is reported here. However the material we used is adequate for the production of a good quality original L-PRF (early protocol). The original L-PRF system now exists only in one CE/FDA cleared form that is termed Intra-Spin L-PRF (Intra-lock, Boca Raton, FL, USA), and, legally, it is the only kit/system allowed in Western countries (CE/FDA).

5. Conclusion

Considering the limitations, this study showed that early L-PRF membranes have stronger mechanical properties than platelet-rich membranes obtained by PRGF-Endoret system. Probably, they have easier clinical application and handling, and they may also be stronger during suturing and provide more supportive scaffold in periodontal regeneration. The real results of the current L-PRF should be in fact much higher than what is reported here.

Conflict of Interests

The authors declare that there is no conflict of interests regarding the publication of this paper.

Acknowledgments

The authors thank the Vice-Chancellory of Research Shiraz University of Medical Science for supporting this research (Grant no. 92-01-03-6162). This paper is based on the thesis by Dr. Hodasadat Banihashemi. The authors also thank Dr. Mehrdad Vosooghi of the Dental Research Development Center, of the School of Dentistry, for the statistical analysis and Dr. Shahram Hamedani for his suggestions and editorial assistance in the paper.

References

[1] M. G. Newman, H. Takei, P. R. Klokkevold, and F. A. Carranza, *Carranza's Clinical Periodontology*, Elsevier Health Sciences, 2011.

[2] P. J. Boyne, R. E. Marx, M. Nevins et al., "A feasibility study evaluating rhBMP-2/absorbable collagen sponge for maxillary sinus floor augmentation," *The International Journal of Periodontics & Restorative Dentistry*, vol. 17, no. 1, pp. 11–25, 1997.

[3] Z. Schwartz, D. L. Carnes Jr., R. Pulliam et al., "Porcine fetal enamel matrix derivative stimulates proliferation but not differentiation of pre-osteoblastic 2T9 cells, inhibits proliferation and stimulates differentiation of osteoblast-like MG63 cells, and increases proliferation and differentiation of normal human osteoblast NHOst cells," *Journal of Periodontology*, vol. 71, no. 8, pp. 1287–1296, 2000.

[4] R. E. Marx, E. R. Carlson, R. M. Eichstaedt, S. R. Schimmele, J. E. Strauss, and K. R. Georgeff, "Platelet-rich plasma: growth factor enhancement for bone grafts," *Oral Surgery, Oral Medicine, Oral Pathology, Oral Radiology, and Endodontics*, vol. 85, no. 6, pp. 638–646, 1998.

[5] E. Anitua, M. Sánchez, G. Orive, and I. Andia, "Delivering growth factors for therapeutics," *Trends in Pharmacological Sciences*, vol. 29, no. 1, pp. 37–41, 2008.

[6] M. Toffler, N. Toscano, D. Holtzclaw, M. Corso, and D. D. Ehrenfest, "Introducing Choukroun's platelet rich fibrin (PRF) to the reconstructive surgery milieu," *The Journal of Implant & Advanced Clinical Dentistry*, vol. 1, no. 6, pp. 21–32, 2009.

[7] D. M. Dohan, J. Choukroun, A. Diss et al., "Platelet-rich fibrin (PRF): a second-generation platelet concentrate. Part I: technological concepts and evolution," *Oral Surgery, Oral Medicine, Oral Pathology, Oral Radiology and Endodontology*, vol. 101, no. 3, pp. E37–E44, 2006.

[8] D. M. Dohan Ehrenfest, G. M. de Peppo, P. Doglioli, and G. Sammartino, "Slow release of growth factors and thrombospondin-1 in Choukroun's platelet-rich fibrin (PRF): a gold standard to achieve for all surgical platelet concentrates technologies," *Growth Factors*, vol. 27, no. 1, pp. 63–69, 2009.

[9] D. M. D. Ehrenfest, L. Rasmusson, and T. Albrektsson, "Classification of platelet concentrates: from pure platelet-rich plasma (P-PRP) to leucocyte- and platelet-rich fibrin (L-PRF)," *Trends in Biotechnology*, vol. 27, no. 3, pp. 158–167, 2009.

[10] M. Del Corso, A. Vervelle, A. Simonpieri et al., "Current knowledge and perspectives for the use of Platelet-Rich Plasma (PRP) and Platelet-Rich Fibrin (PRF) in oral and maxillofacial surgery part 1: periodontal and dentoalveolar surgery," *Current Pharmaceutical Biotechnology*, vol. 13, no. 7, pp. 1207–1230, 2012.

[11] A. Simonpieri, M. Del Corso, A. Vervelle et al., "Current knowledge and perspectives for the use of platelet-rich plasma (PRP) and platelet-rich fibrin (PRF) in oral and maxillofacial surgery part 2: bone graft, implant and reconstructive surgery," *Current Pharmaceutical Biotechnology*, vol. 13, no. 7, pp. 1231–1256, 2012.

[12] J. Lindhe, T. Karring, and N. Lang, *Clinical Periodontology and Implant Dentistry*, Blackwell Munksgaard Blackwell Publishing, Oxford, UK, 5th edition, 2008.

[13] Y. Zhang, X. Zhang, B. Shi, and R. Miron, "Membranes for guided tissue and bone regeneration," *Annals of Oral & Maxillofacial Surgery*, vol. 1, no. 1, article 10, 2013.

[14] S.-B. Lee, J.-S. Kwon, Y.-K. Lee, K.-M. Kim, and K.-N. Kim, "Bioactivity and mechanical properties of collagen composite membranes reinforced by chitosan and β-tricalcium phosphate," *Journal of Biomedical Materials Research Part B: Applied Biomaterials*, vol. 100, no. 7, pp. 1935–1942, 2012.

[15] J. B. Herrmann, "Changes in tensile strength and knot security of surgical sutures in vivo," *Archives of Surgery*, vol. 106, no. 5, pp. 707–710, 1973.

[16] S. E. Lynch, *Tissue Engineering: Applications in Oral and Maxillofacial Surgery and Periodontics*, Quintessence Publishing Company, 2008.

[17] S. M. Alston, K. A. Solen, A. H. Broderick, S. Sukavaneshvar, and S. F. Mohammad, "New method to prepare autologous fibrin glue on demand," *Translational Research*, vol. 149, no. 4, pp. 187–195, 2007.

[18] H. Duong, B. Wu, and B. Tawil, "Modulation of 3D fibrin matrix stiffness by intrinsic fibrinogen-thrombin compositions and by extrinsic cellular activity," *Tissue Engineering—Part A*, vol. 15, no. 7, pp. 1865–1876, 2009.

[19] D. M. D. Ehrenfest, M. Del Corso, A. Diss, J. Mouhyi, and J.-B. Charrier, "Three-dimensional architecture and cell composition of a Choukroun's platelet-rich fibrin clot and membrane," *Journal of Periodontology*, vol. 81, no. 4, pp. 546–555, 2010.

[20] D. M. D. Ehrenfest, "How to optimize the preparation of leukocyte- and platelet-rich fibrin (L-PRF, Choukroun's technique) clots and membranes: introducing the PRF Box," *Oral Surgery, Oral Medicine, Oral Pathology, Oral Radiology and Endodontology*, vol. 110, no. 3, pp. 275–278, 2010.

[21] J. Gottlow, S. Nyman, T. Karring, and J. Lindhe, "New attachment formation as the result of controlled tissue regeneration," *Journal of Clinical Periodontology*, vol. 11, no. 8, pp. 494–503, 1984.

[22] J. Choukroun, A. Diss, A. Simonpieri et al., "Platelet-rich fibrin (PRF): a second-generation platelet concentrate. Part V: histologic evaluations of PRF effects on bone allograft maturation in sinus lift," *Oral Surgery, Oral Medicine, Oral Pathology, Oral Radiology and Endodontology*, vol. 101, no. 3, pp. 299–303, 2006.

[23] Z. Mazor, R. A. Horowitz, M. Del Corso, H. S. Prasad, M. D. Rohrer, and D. M. D. Ehrenfest, "Sinus floor augmentation with simultaneous implant placement using Choukroun's platelet-rich fibrin as the sole grafting material: a radiologic and histologic study at 6 months," *Journal of Periodontology*, vol. 80, no. 12, pp. 2056–2064, 2009.

[24] F. Inchingolo, M. Tatullo, M. Marrelli et al., "Trial with platelet-rich fibrin and Bio-Oss used as grafting materials in the treatment of the severe maxillar bone atrophy: clinical and radiological evaluations," *European Review for Medical and Pharmacological Sciences*, vol. 14, no. 12, pp. 1075–1084, 2010.

[25] M. Del Corso, M. Toffler, and D. Dohan Ehrenfest, "Use of an autologous leukocyte and platelet-rich fibrin (L-PRF) membrane in post-avulsion sites: an overview of Choukroun's PRF," *The Journal of Implant & Advanced Clinical Dentistry*, vol. 1, no. 9, pp. 27–35, 2010.

[26] J.-H. Zhao, C.-H. Tsai, and Y.-C. Chang, "Clinical and histologic evaluations of healing in an extraction socket filled with platelet-rich fibrin," *Journal of Dental Sciences*, vol. 6, no. 2, pp. 116–122, 2011.

[27] B. I. Simon, P. Gupta, and S. Tajbakhsh, "Quantitative evaluation of extraction socket healing following the use of autologous platelet-rich fibrin matrix in humans," *The International Journal of Periodontics & Restorative Dentistry*, vol. 31, no. 3, pp. 285–295, 2011.

[28] K. Anilkumar, A. Geetha, Umasudhakar, T. Ramakrishnan, R. Vijayalakshmi, and E. Pameela, "Platelet-rich-fibrin: a novel root coverage approach," *Journal of Indian Society of Periodontology*, vol. 13, no. 1, pp. 50–54, 2009.

[29] S. Aroca, T. Keglevich, B. Barbieri, I. Gera, and D. Etienne, "Clinical evaluation of a modified coronally advanced flap alone or in combination with a platelet-rich fibrin membrane for the treatment of adjacent multiple gingival recessions: a 6-month study," *Journal of Periodontology*, vol. 80, no. 2, pp. 244–252, 2009.

[30] Y.-C. Chang and J.-H. Zhao, "Effects of platelet-rich fibrin on human periodontal ligament fibroblasts and application for periodontal infrabony defects," *Australian Dental Journal*, vol. 56, no. 4, pp. 365–371, 2011.

[31] A. Sharma and A. R. Pradeep, "Autologous platelet-rich fibrin in the treatment of mandibular degree II furcation defects: a randomized clinical trial," *Journal of Periodontology*, vol. 82, no. 10, pp. 1396–1403, 2011.

[32] V. Gassling, T. Douglas, P. H. Warnke, Y. Açil, J. Wiltfang, and S. T. Becker, "Platelet-rich fibrin membranes as scaffolds for periosteal tissue engineering," *Clinical Oral Implants Research*, vol. 21, no. 5, pp. 543–549, 2010.

[33] V. Gassling, J. Hedderich, Y. Açil, N. Purcz, J. Wiltfang, and T. Douglas, "Comparison of platelet rich fibrin and collagen as osteoblast–seeded scaffolds for bone tissue engineering applications," *Clinical Oral Implants Research*, vol. 24, no. 3, pp. 320–328, 2013.

[34] T. E. Orr, P. A. Villars, S. L. Mitchell, H.-P. Hsu, and M. Spector, "Compressive properties of cancellous bone defects in a rabbit model treated with particles of natural bone mineral and synthetic hydroxyapatite," *Biomaterials*, vol. 22, no. 14, pp. 1953–1959, 2001.

[35] E. Lucarelli, R. Beretta, B. Dozza et al., "A recently developed bifacial platelet-rich fibrin matrix," *European Cells and Materials*, vol. 20, pp. 13–23, 2010.

[36] J. L. Velada, D. A. Hollingsbee, A. R. Menzies, R. Cornwell, and R. A. Dodd, "Reproducibility of the mechanical properties of Vivostat system patient-derived fibrin sealant," *Biomaterials*, vol. 23, no. 10, pp. 2249–2254, 2002.

[37] S. L. Rowe, S. Lee, and J. P. Stegemann, "Influence of thrombin concentration on the mechanical and morphological properties of cell-seeded fibrin hydrogels," *Acta Biomaterialia*, vol. 3, no. 1, pp. 59–67, 2007.

[38] B. Blombäck and N. Bark, "Fibrinopeptides and fibrin gel structure," *Biophysical Chemistry*, vol. 112, no. 2-3, pp. 147–151, 2004.

[39] R. V. Kumar and N. Shubhashini, "Platelet rich fibrin: a new paradigm in periodontal regeneration," *Cell and Tissue Banking*, vol. 14, no. 3, pp. 453–463, 2013.

[40] M. H. Boyer, J. R. Shainoff, and O. D. Ratnoff, "Acceleration of fibrin polymerization by calcium ions," *Blood*, vol. 39, no. 3, pp. 382–387, 1972.

[41] T. Kawase, K. Okuda, L. F. Wolff, and H. Yoshie, "Platelet-rich plasma-derived fibrin clot formation stimulates collagen synthesis in periodontal ligament and osteoblastic cells in vitro," *Journal of Periodontology*, vol. 74, no. 6, pp. 858–864, 2003.

[42] P. A. M. Everts, A. van Zundert, J. P. A. M. Schönberger, R. J. J. Devilee, and J. T. A. Knape, "What do we use: platelet-rich plasma or platelet-leukocyte gel?" *Journal of Biomedical Materials Research—Part A*, vol. 85, no. 4, pp. 1135–1136, 2008.

[43] A. Cieslik-Bielecka, T. S. Gazdzik, T. M. Bielecki, and T. Cieslik, "Why the platelet-rich gel has antimicrobial activity?" *Oral Surgery, Oral Medicine, Oral Pathology, Oral Radiology, and Endodontology*, vol. 103, no. 3, pp. 303–305, 2007.

[44] D. J. F. Moojen, P. A. Everts, R. M. Schure et al., "Antimicrobial activity of platelet-leukocyte gel against *Staphylococcus aureus*," *Journal of Orthopaedic Research*, vol. 26, no. 3, pp. 404–410, 2008.

[45] H. El-Sharkawy, A. Kantarci, J. Deady et al., "Platelet-rich plasma: growth factors and pro- and anti-inflammatory properties," *Journal of Periodontology*, vol. 78, no. 4, pp. 661–669, 2007.

[46] K. Werther, I. J. Christensen, and H. J. Nielsen, "Determination of Vascular Endothelial Growth Factor (VEGF) in circulating blood: significance of VEGF in various leucocytes and platelets," *Scandinavian Journal of Clinical & Laboratory Investigation*, vol. 62, no. 5, pp. 343–350, 2002.

[47] E. Anitua, M. Sánchez, G. Orive, and I. Andía, "The potential impact of the preparation rich in growth factors (PRGF) in different medical fields," *Biomaterials*, vol. 28, no. 31, pp. 4551–4560, 2007.

[48] J. K. Kingston, W. M. Bayly, D. C. Sellon, K. M. Meyers, and K. J. Wardrop, "Effects of sodium citrate, low molecular weight heparin, and prostaglandin E_1 on aggregation, fibrinogen binding, and enumeration of equine platelets," *American Journal of Veterinary Research*, vol. 62, no. 4, pp. 547–554, 2001.

[49] A. G. Perez, J. F. S. Lana, A. A. Rodrigues, A. C. M. Luzo, W. D. Belangero, and M. H. A. Santana, "Relevant aspects of centrifugation step in the preparation of platelet-rich plasma," *ISRN Hematology*, vol. 2014, Article ID 176060, 8 pages, 2014.

30

Pyogenic Granuloma/Peripheral Giant-Cell Granuloma Associated with Implants

Enric Jané-Salas,[1] Rui Albuquerque,[2] Aura Font-Muñoz,[1] Beatríz González-Navarro,[1] Albert Estrugo Devesa,[1] and Jose López-López[1]

[1] *School of Dentistry, University of Barcelona, Pabellón de Gobierno, University Campus of Bellvitge, C/Feixa Llarga s/n, L'Hospitalet de Llobregat, 08907 Barcelona, Spain*
[2] *School of Dentistry, University of Birmingham, St. Chads Queensway, Birmingham B4 6NN, UK*

Correspondence should be addressed to Jose López-López; 18575jll@gmail.com

Academic Editor: Manal Awad

Introduction. Pyogenic granuloma (PG) and peripheral giant-cell granuloma (PGCG) are two of the most common inflammatory lesions associated with implants; however, there is no established pathway for treatment of these conditions. This paper aims to illustrate the successful treatment of PG and PGCG and also report a systematic review of the literature regarding the various treatments proposed. *Methods*. To collect relevant information about previous treatments for PG and PGCG involving implants we carried out electronic searches of publications with the key words "granuloma", "oral", and "implants" from the last 15 years on the databases Pubmed, National Library of Medicine's Medline, Scielo, Scopus, and Cochrane Library. *Results*. From the electronic search 16 case reports were found showing excision and curettage as the main successful treatment. As no clinical trials or observational studies were identified the authors agreed to present results from a review perspective. *Conclusion*. This is the largest analysis of PG and PGCG associated with implants published to date. Our review would suggest that PGCG associated with implants appears to have a more aggressive nature; however the level of evidence is very limited. Further cohort studies with representative sample sizes and standard outcome measures are necessary for better understanding of these conditions.

1. Introduction

Reactive lesions are characterized as excessive proliferation of connective tissue as a response to chronic irritation [1]. Among these types of lesions, those seen in the oral cavity include pyogenic granuloma (PG), peripheral fibroma, fibroepithelial hyperplasia, peripheral ossifying fibroma, and peripheral giant-cell granuloma (PGCG). PG and PGCG appear to be the ones commonly associated with implants, as in the past few years multiple case reports have been published [1, 2].

PG is defined as an inflammatory hyperplasia that usually appears as a response to irritants, trauma, hormonal changes, or certain medications [3, 4]. Although classically it is called PG, a more correct name would be focal epithelial hyperplasia since the lesion is not strictly a granuloma or an infection [3, 4]. Peripheral giant-cell granuloma (PGCG) is considered

a reactive hyperplastic lesion, although its etiology is not entirely known. It is believed that its pathogenesis includes an excessive activation of osteoclasts, which is associated with a proliferation of macrophages, and possibly causes major bone resorption [2, 5].

PG is more frequent in women in their 20s, with a ratio of 3 : 2 [4]. In 75% of cases it occurs in keratinized gingiva, with location in order of frequency of tongue, lips, and then buccal mucosa [3, 4]. It is more common in the maxilla than in the mandible and in anterior as opposed to posterior areas [4]. In contrast, PGCG usually appears in patients who are between their 40s and 60s, and it is slightly more frequent in women and tends to appear more often in the mandible than in the maxilla (Table 1) [4, 5]. The treatment of these lesions generally involves eliminating the irritating factors as well as performing surgical removal [1, 2]. Commonly associated with periodontal disease, where calculus is the irritating

TABLE 1: Summarizing the differential diagnosis between pyogenic granuloma and peripheral giant-cell granuloma.

	Pyogenic granuloma	Peripheral giant-cell granuloma
Age	20s	40s–60s
Sex	Women	Women
Localization	Anterior maxilla	Posterior mandible
Symptomology	Asymptomatic	Asymptomatic
Color	Reddish	Reddish-purple
Sessile/with a pedicle	Both	Both
Bone involvement	No	Possible

factor, surgical removal along with nonsurgical debridement is well described in the literature [6].

Implant rehabilitation has become more common in the last decade and several factors have been studied which could interfere with osteointegration and longevity [7]. Factors such as smoking, diabetes, and periodontal disease have been studied [7–11]. However, with regard to reactive lesions such as PG and PGCG there is no clear pathway for intervention or treatment to manage these lesions and maintain healthy tissue around the implants [7].

The aim of this paper is to demonstrate the successful management of cases of PG and PGCG associated with implants and to review the literature for the various treatment options.

2. Materials and Methods

To collect all relevant information about previous published treatments for PG and PGCG involving implants, the authors carried out an electronic search from to January 2000 to June 2015 (Pubmed Central, National Library of Medicine's Medline, Scielo, Scopus, and Cochrane Library) for reactive lesions related to implants (key words: "granuloma", "oral", and "implants"). These articles were obtained, and a hand search of their bibliographies identified any pertinent secondary references. This process was repeated until no further new articles could be identified. The inclusion criteria included clinical trials, cohort studies, case-controlled studies, case series, and case reports, published in English, Portuguese, French, and Spanish, which included a clear description of the treatment employed. The search was limited to human studies and all articles which did not fit into the criteria were excluded. The full papers and abstracts identified through the search were independently reviewed by all authors (EJN, RA, AFM, BGM, AED, and JLL) for inclusion in this systematic review. If there was insufficient information provided in the abstract or if there was a disagreement between reviewers, the authors reviewed the full text before reaching consensus through discussion. Data extraction was then completed in duplicate by the same independent reviewers. The following data were collected: study year, gender, age, location of the implant/PG/PGCG, treatment used, relapse, follow-up, and histopathology (Table 2).

The author (JLL) prepared data extraction tables and all authors contributed to summary reports of the selected journal articles and review of the literature.

The case reports protocol was carried out with patient informed consent following guidelines according to the Helsinki Declaration of 1975, as revised in 2000.

3. Results

From the 55 articles initially selected, 39 studies were excluded as they were related to teeth or not directly related to implants. All 16 articles selected were case reports; these ranged from reports of a single case to articles describing up to a maximum of 3 cases, such that a total of 21 patients were reported. Of these there were 15 cases of PGCG [2, 5, 9–16, 21] and 6 of PG [4, 14, 17–20] (Table 2). As no experimental or observational studies were identified the authors agreed that it would not be reasonable to critically appraise the quality of the studies and consequently the results are presented from a review perspective.

The majority of patients with PGCG were women (3 : 1) while PG was seen more commonly in males (2 : 1) (Table 2). The average age of the population who suffered PGCG was 49.6 while for PG it was 50.3. The majority of published cases of PGCG associated with implants had suffered bone loss around the implant [2, 5, 11–15], as only 4 of the published cases of PGCG did not experience bone loss [9, 10, 12, 21] (26.7%). On the other hand bone loss did not occur in cases of PG [4, 14, 17–20].

The six cases of PG were treated with excision of the lesion and curettage, though one case involved excision with Er-YAG Laser [18].

The cases of PGCG were treated with a number of different strategies. In all of the cases the lesion was surgically removed, but in addition to this, in nine cases curettage was also performed [2, 4, 8, 9, 11, 14, 21], in two cases the prosthesis was replaced [10, 11], in one case the prostheses were temporarily removed [15], in another case a graft was performed [13], and in four cases the implant was explanted [2, 5, 12] (Table 2).

The 6 cases which suffered relapse all were PGCG. Three of these were treated with excision and curettage only [2, 9, 12], while the other 3 also underwent explantation [2, 8, 12] (Table 2). In fact, from the ones that underwent explantation, one had a PGCG with 8 times of recurrence [12] and the other case which had three times [2] was treated with curettage [2].

3.1. Case Report: Pyogenic Granuloma. A 52-year-old male came for consultation reporting two swellings intraorally

TABLE 2: Most highlighted characteristics from published cases of PG and PGCG associated with implants.

Author (year)	Sex	Age	Localization	Bone loss	Final treatment	Relapse	Follow-up (months)	PG/PGCG
Hanselaer et al. (2010) [9]	F	34	Posterior maxilla	No	Excision + curettage	1	8	PGCG
	M	31	Posterior mandible	Yes	Excision + curettage	1	—	PGCG
Hirshberg et al. (2003) [12]	F	69	Anterior maxilla	No	Excision + explantation	1	—	PGCG
	M	44	Posterior mandible	Yes	Excision + explantation	8	—	PGCG
Bischof et al. (2004) [10]	F	56	Posterior mandible	No	Excision + new prosthesis + control of plaque	No	36	PGCG
Scarano et al. (2008) [13]	F	48	Posterior maxilla	Yes	Excision + soft tissue graft	No	—	PGCG
Cloutier et al. (2007) [5]	M	21	Posterior mandible	Yes	Excision + explantation	No	12	PGCG
	F	62	Posterior mandible	Yes	Excision + curettage	No	2	PGCG
Hernández et al. (2009) [2]	F	45	Posterior mandible	Yes	Excision + curettage	5	108	PGCG
	F	36	Posterior maxilla	Yes	Excision + explantation	3	12	PGCG
Ozden et al. (2009) [11]	F	60	Posterior mandible	Yes	Excision + new prosthesis	No	12	PGCG
Olmedo et al. (2010) [14]	F	64	Anterior maxilla	Yes	Excision + curettage	No	24	PGCG
	F	75	Posterior mandible	No	Excision + curettage	No	48	PG
Dojcinovic et al. (2010) [4]	M	32	Posterior maxilla	No	Excision + curettage	No	18	PG
Peñarrocha-Diago et al. (2012) [15]	F	54	Posterior mandible	Yes	Excision + curettage + temporary removal of the prosthesis	No	12	PGCG
Galindo-Moreno et al. (2013) [16]	M	74	Anterior maxilla	No	Excision	No	6	PGCG
Etöz et al. (2013) [17]	M	55	Posterior mandible	No	Excision + curettage	No	8	PG
Kaya et al. (2013) [18]	M	39	Posterior mandible	No	Excision with an Er-YAG Laser	No	6	PG
Kang et al. (2014) [19]	M	68	Posterior maxilla	No	Excision + curettage	No	12	PG
Trento et al. (2014) [20]	F	33	Posterior mandible	No	Excision + curettage	No	6	PG
Brown et al. (2015) [21]	F	46	Posterior mandible	No	Excision + curettage	No	6	PGCG

M: male; F: female; PG: pyogenic granuloma; PGCG: peripheral giant-cell granuloma.

adjacent to implants that had been placed three years earlier. These lesions had developed over 6 months and were not painful but did bleed on brushing. With regard to his medical history, of interest, he was diagnosed with antiphospholipid syndrome in 2001 and suffered an acute myocardial infarction in August 2011. He also suffered from focal segmental glomerulosclerosis and chronic kidney failure since 2010 but did not require hemodialysis and could be linked to systemic lupus erythematosus. With respect to his dental history, he suffered from advanced chronic generalized periodontal disease and had plaque and calculus deposits both supra- and subgingivally. Due to his advanced periodontal disease the remaining upper and lower teeth had been splinted two years earlier.

The patient's regular medicines included 4 mg aceno-coumarol, 100 mg acetylsalicylic acid, pantoprazole 40 mg (proton pump inhibitors), atorvastatin 40 mg (HMG-CoA reductase inhibitors), amlodipine (calcium channel blockers), bisoprolol 5 mg (beta-blocker), and 360 mg mycophenolic acid. No habits of substance abuse were reported.

Oral examination revealed two nodular erythematous sessile lumps of 1.5 cm diameter, with elastic consistency and granulomatous appearance. They were associated with the gingiva, located on the buccal and palatal/lingual sides of implants 3.6, 1.6, and 1.7 (Figure 1). Radiographic investigation revealed 5 mm of peri-implant bone loss associated with both lesions. The presumptive diagnosis was that of pyogenic granuloma or peripheral giant-cell granuloma. An excisional biopsy was performed along with curettage and irrigation with chlorhexidine 0.5% of both the surgical site and the exposed implant threads. The microscopic description was that of ulcerated lesions covered by a fibrin and leukocyte

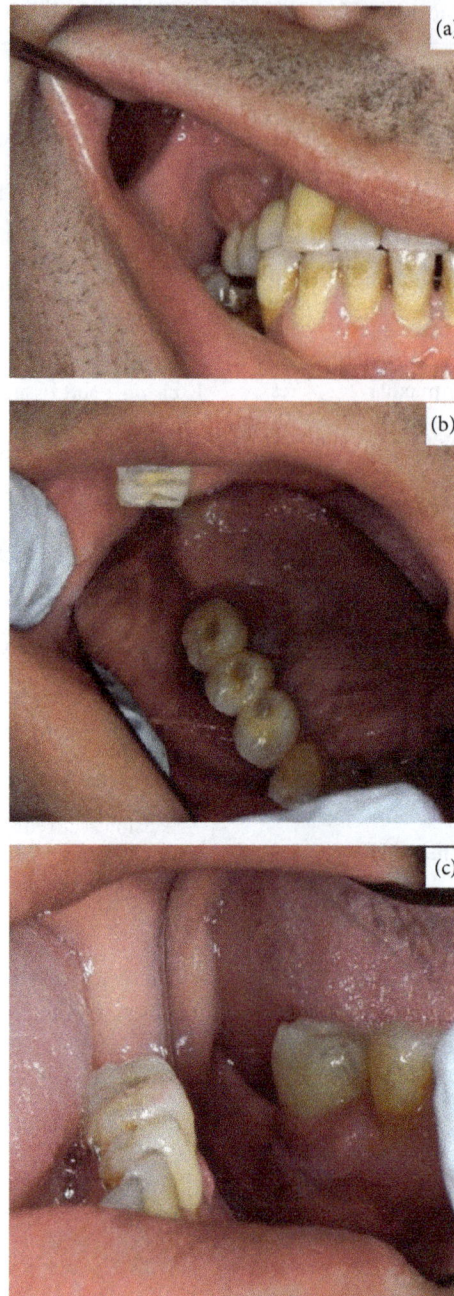

FIGURE 1: (a) Exophytic granulomatous lesion in 16 and 17 implants. (b) Palatal view of the granulomatous lesion in 16 and 17. (c) Granulomatous lesion in 36.

membrane and made up of granulation tissue with a mixed inflammatory infiltrate with polymorphonuclears, together with vascular proliferation (Figure 2). Squamous epithelium with parakeratosis, dyskeratosis, acanthosis, and elongation of the epithelial peaks was observed at the far extremes. The epithelial maturation was conserved and no dysplasia-like phenomenon was observed. The results were compatible with a diagnosis of pyogenic granuloma, without any suggestion of malignancy. Postoperatively there were no further issues and there was no evidence of relapse at 12-month follow-up (Figure 3).

3.2. Case Report: Peripheral Giant-Cell Granuloma. A 64-year-old male came for consultation regarding a 15-day history of an exophytic mass associated with the buccal marginal gingiva of an implant supported dental prosthesis in the lower right quadrant. This had been placed 8 years earlier. The lesion was asymptomatic, but the patient reported bleeding on brushing.

The patient's medical history revealed complete atrioventricular block, coronary atherothrombosis with acute myocardial infarction in 2006, left ventricular dysfunction, pericarditis, and diabetes mellitus type 2. The patient's

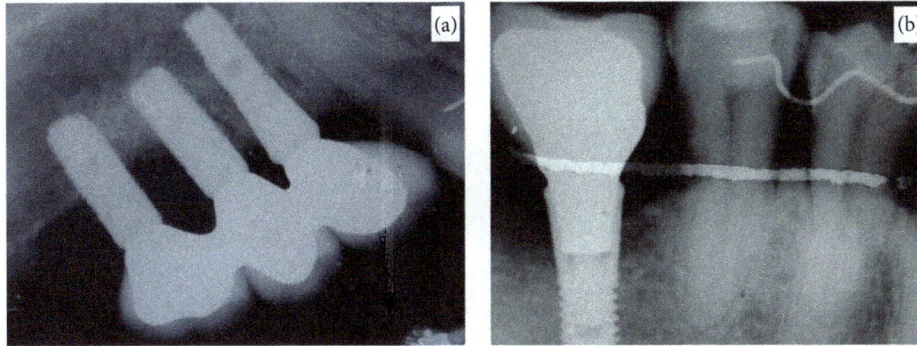

FIGURE 2: (a) Periapical radiograph that shows bone loss in implants 16 and 17. (b) Periapical radiograph that shows bone involvement in implant 36.

regular medicines included carvedilol 6.25 mg, 1/day (beta-blocker), enalapril 5 mg, 1/day (ACE inhibitor), furosemide 40 mg, 1/day (sulphonamide), Tromalyt 150 mg, 1/a day (acetylsalicylic acid), omeprazole 20 mg, 1/day (proton pump inhibitors), and variable dosage of insulin. No habits of substance abuse were reported. With respect to the patient's dental history, he was partially dentate in the mandible as a result of periodontal disease and had multiple implant supported fixed prostheses, with a total of 10 implants placed 8 years earlier.

On examination intraorally there was a swelling of 1 cm diameter on the buccal surface of implant 4.6. The lesion was reddish-purple in color and was well defined with an elastic consistency and an irregular texture. It was not mobile and was sessile. Periapical radiograph revealed bone loss of 4 mm affecting both the mesial and distal surfaces of the implant (Figure 4).

Histopathology confirmed that it was an ulcerated peripheral giant-cell granuloma, without suggestion of malignancy (Figure 5). Histologically it was described as a lesion covered by a parakeratinized stratified squamous epithelium, with areas of atrophy and ulceration in its thickness. A dense proliferation of multinucleated giant cells was dispersed on a stroma of the tissue, which was highly vascularized, with areas of hemorrhage, deposits of hemosiderin, and infiltrate due to accumulation of lymphoplasmacytic inflammatory cells. Laboratory tests showed no abnormalities with regard to calcium/phosphate metabolism or parathyroid gland function.

Treatment involved complete excision of the lesion, curettage of the exposed implant threads, and irrigation with chlorhexidine 0.5%. Postoperative healing was good and at 12-month follow-up there was no evidence of recurrence (Figure 6).

4. Discussion

Peri-implantitis with progressive bone loss is reported to be the most frequent complication associated with implants [2]. Its treatment is challenging and to do so correctly we must identify the pathology leading to peri-implantitis [2]. In our view recognition of the soft tissue pathology by biopsy should be the first step for potential successful treatment.

The etiology of these conditions when associated with implants is similar to that which is described when they are associated with teeth, where factors such as trauma, plaque deposits, or chronic infection have a major role [1]. In cases associated with implants, incorrect or inadequate prosthesis (implant cap or healing cap, poorly adjusted suprastructures, etc.) is also considered to be a possible causative factor [2, 9]. With regard to inadequate prosthesis, Bischof et al. [10], Ozden et al. [11], and Peñarrocha-Diago et al. [15] replaced the prosthesis or temporarily removed the prosthesis, allowing for better plaque control, and they reported no recurrence. Another suggested potential cause, although controversial, is that an inflammatory response to titanium may lead to development of granulomas [10, 12–15, 22].

The clinical presentation and age group of the PG and PGCG cases described appeared to be similar when associated with teeth [23–27]. Our data collection showed PGCG is more frequent in women and in the posterior mandible [2]. One could propose this may be due to greater plaque accumulation posteriorly due to difficult access for thorough oral hygiene. When associated with teeth, PG is also commonly seen in females [1, 2]. This is in contrast with our findings which suggest that when associated with implants it is more prevalent in men. Nonetheless this may be an inaccurate conclusion and due to the small number of cases reported.

In females, pregnancy can have a role in this condition. It has been suggested that the increase of estrogen and progesterone can influence gingival physiology, enhancing the tissue response to the local microbiota, with a predominance of more pathogenic microorganisms [20, 27, 28].

Data from the selected articles suggests that bone loss from the implant site is more commonly associated with PGCG [2, 5, 11–15] than PG. Hernández et al. [2], Cloutier et al. [5], and Bischof et al. [10] support the hypothesis that bone loss occurs first, exposing the implant collar, which then contributes to irritating factors that lead to PGCG. This is also more prevalent when lesions present posteriorly. Again this could be related to difficult access for thorough oral hygiene though this may also be due to the greater occlusal load experienced posteriorly, as opposed to that experienced by the anterior teeth [2, 5, 10].

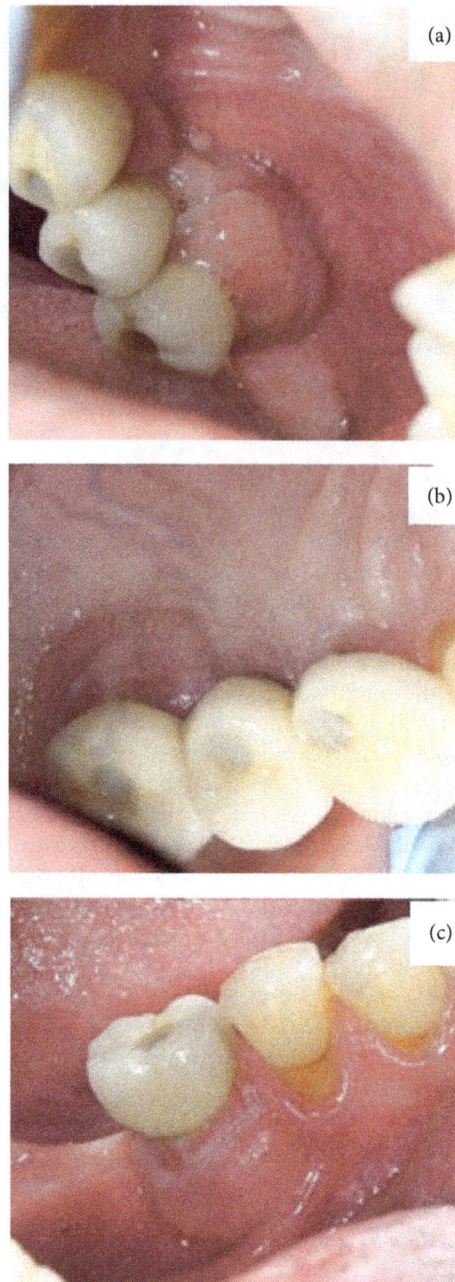

FIGURE 3: (a) 12-month postexcision follow-up of the lesion in 16 and 17 area. (b) Palatal view of the 12-month postexcision follow-up of the lesion in 16 and 17. (c) 12 month postexcision follow-up of the lesion in 36.

The prevalence of recurrence in cases of PG and PGCG is estimated to be 2.9–8.2% and 5–11%, respectively, but in cases associated with implants these figures increase [2, 9, 16, 17, 21]. Recurrence has been reported in 6 of the 15 published cases of PGCG associated with implants (Table 2). Lester et al. [23], in a review of 279 cases, noted a total of 10 recurrences on 5 implant cases; 1 implant case had 2 recurrences, and another case with multiple implants had 8 recurrences. It was noted that while 2 of the 5 implant cases (40%) had multiple recurrences, 6 of 237 non-implant-related cases (2.5%) presented with multiple recurrences too. Several possible explanations are considered, such as incomplete excision, but in addition these lesions may have been caused by combination of irritating factors, which therefore makes it challenging to eradicate all possible causes [2, 5, 8].

Several treatments have been described when treating PG/PGCG when associated with implants, with excision and curettage being the most common. This is consistent with normal convention when these lesions are associated with teeth (being a relatively simple technique and with satisfactory results [1, 2, 9, 10, 12, 25, 26, 29]).

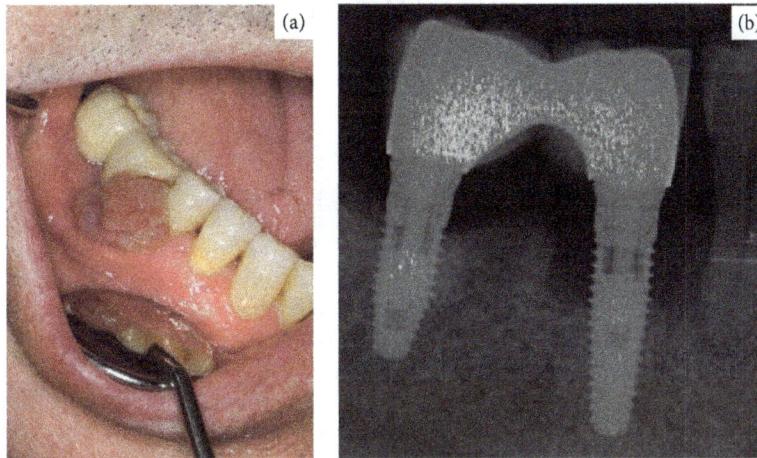

FIGURE 4: (a) Exophytic granulomatous lesion in 4.6. (b) Periapical radiograph that shows bone involvement in implant 46.

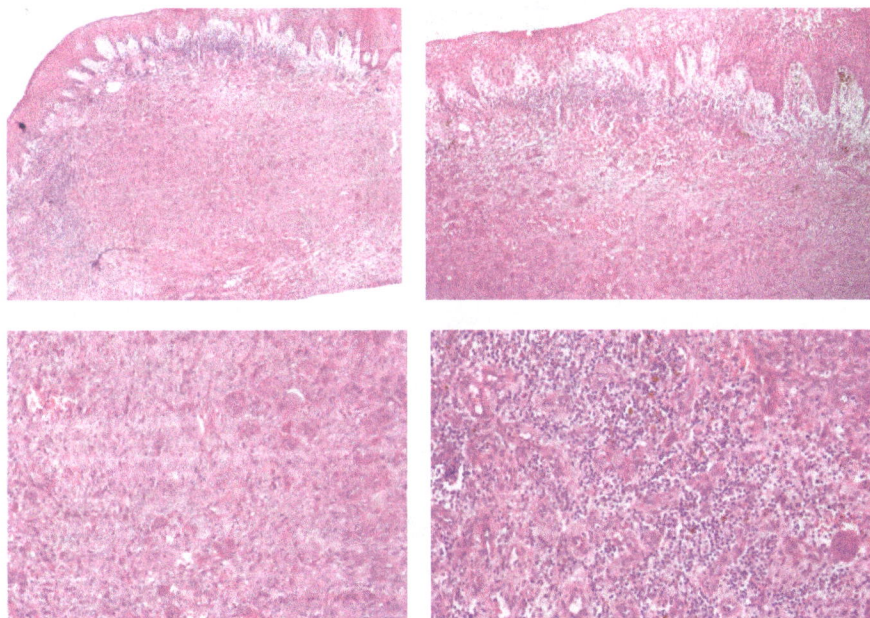

FIGURE 5: Histopathology of peripheral giant-cell granuloma.

Other options have been described such as the use of Er-YAG Laser [18] or explantation of the implant and the provision of a new prosthesis [10, 11] or indeed temporary removal [15]. It is suggested that use of the Er-YAG Laser for granuloma excision offers advantages in comparison to conventional surgery techniques, especially by reducing the risk of bleeding, pain, and postoperative edema and also eliminating the need for sutures at the end of the procedure [18].

Given the small number of cases published, it is difficult to evaluate if explantation of the implant affects the number of recurrences or the amount of bone loss. Recurrences of PG and PGCG have been described when associated with bad plaque control but also due to hormonal imbalance during pregnancy, especially in PG cases [30]. The authors believe that more aggressive treatments such as explanation

can be used as a secondary technique, only after excision and curettage have failed as explantation could be beneficial in improving plaque control and consequently reduce the number of relapses and amount of bone loss. However the data available about its use in implants is still limited. The use of antimicrobials such as chlorhexidine, as described in our cases, is reported to offer improved plaque control in the treatment of peri-implantitis [29].

5. Conclusion

In conclusion, we believe the primary approach to manage these two soft tissue conditions should be excisional biopsy and subsequent histopathology. The authors believe oral hygiene instruction should be one of the first steps in management as good plaque control could help reduce number

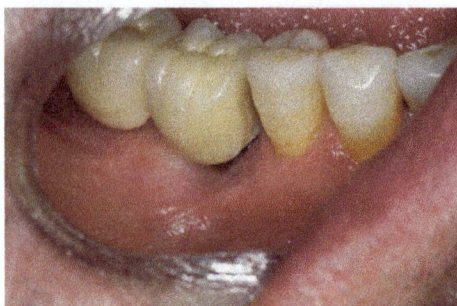

FIGURE 6: 12-month postexcision follow-up of the lesion located in 46.

of recurrences. This review of the literature highlights that histopathological diagnosis is important, as if PGCG is diagnosed histologically, then the clinician will be aware of a higher risk of bone loss and higher rate of recurrence. This would highlight the need of close monitoring and regular review. However, we recognize the limitations of this analysis due to the limited number of case reports published and consequently these conclusions should be interpreted with caution. Further cohort studies with representative sample sizes, control group, and standard outcome measures are necessary.

Conflict of Interests

The authors declare that there is no conflict of interests regarding the publication of this paper.

References

[1] P. K. Verma, R. Srivastava, H. C. Baranwal, T. P. Chaturvedi, A. Gautam, and A. Singh, "'Pyogenic granuloma—hyperplastic lesion of the gingiva: case reports," *Open Dentistry Journal*, vol. 6, no. 1, pp. 153–156, 2012.

[2] G. Hernández, R. M. López-Pintor, J. Torres, and J. C. de Vicente, "Clinical outcomes of peri-implant peripheral giant cell granuloma: a report of three cases," *Journal of Periodontology*, vol. 80, no. 7, pp. 1184–1191, 2009.

[3] N. Mahabob, S. Kumar, and S. Raja, "Palatal pyogenic granulomaa," *Journal of Pharmacy and Bioallied Sciences*, vol. 5, no. 2, pp. 179–181, 2013.

[4] I. Dojcinovic, M. Richter, and T. Lombardi, "Occurrence of a pyogenic granuloma in relation to a dental implant," *Journal of Oral and Maxillofacial Surgery*, vol. 68, no. 8, pp. 1874–1876, 2010.

[5] M. Cloutier, M. Charles, R. P. Carmichael, and G. K. B. Sándor, "An analysis of peripheral giant cell granuloma associated with dental implant treatment," *Oral Surgery, Oral Medicine, Oral Pathology, Oral Radiology and Endodontology*, vol. 103, no. 5, pp. 618–622, 2007.

[6] J. Mailoa, G.-H. Lin, V. Khoshkam, M. MacEachern, H.-L. Chan, and H.-L. Wang, "Long-term effect of four surgical periodontal therapies and one non-surgical therapy: a systematic review and meta-analysis," *Journal of Periodontology*, vol. 86, no. 10, pp. 1150–1158, 2015.

[7] H.-J. Han, S. Kim, and D.-H. Han, "Multifactorial evaluation of implant failure: a 19-year retrospective study," *The International Journal of oral & Maxillofacial Implants*, vol. 29, no. 2, pp. 303–310, 2014.

[8] N. Ramer, C. Wadhwani, A. Kim, and D. Hershman, "Histologic findings within peri-implant soft tissue in failed implants secondary to excess cement: report of two cases and review of literature," *The New York State Dental Journal*, vol. 80, no. 2, pp. 43–46, 2014.

[9] L. Hanselaer, J. Cosyn, H. Browaeys, and H. De Bruyn, "Giant cell peripheral granuloma surrounding a dental implant: case report," *Revue Belge de Médecine Dentaire (1984)*, vol. 65, no. 4, pp. 152–158, 2010.

[10] M. Bischof, R. Nedir, and T. Lombardi, "Peripheral giant cell granuloma associated with a dental implant," *International Journal of Oral and Maxillofacial Implants*, vol. 19, no. 2, pp. 295–299, 2004.

[11] F. O. Ozden, B. Ozden, M. Kurt, K. Gündüz, and O. Günhan, "Peripheral giant cell granuloma associated with dental implants: a rare case report," *International Journal of Oral & Maxillofacial Implants*, vol. 24, no. 6, pp. 1153–1156, 2009.

[12] A. Hirshberg, A. Kozlovsky, D. Schwartz-Arad, O. Mardinger, and I. Kaplan, "Peripheral giant cell granuloma associated with dental implants," *Journal of Periodontology*, vol. 74, no. 9, pp. 1381–1384, 2003.

[13] A. Scarano, G. Iezzi, L. Artese, E. Cimorelli, and A. Piattelli, "Peripheral giant cell granuloma associated with a dental implant. A case report," *Minerva Stomatologica*, vol. 57, no. 10, pp. 529–534, 2008.

[14] D. G. Olmedo, M. L. Paparella, D. Brandizzi, and R. L. Cabrini, "Reactive lesions of peri-implant mucosa associated with titanium dental implants: a report of 2 cases," *International Journal of Oral and Maxillofacial Surgery*, vol. 39, no. 5, pp. 503–507, 2010.

[15] M. A. Peñarrocha-Diago, J. Cervera-Ballester, L. Maestre-Ferrin, and D. Penarrocha-Oltra, "Peripheral giant cell granuloma associated with dental implants: clinical case and literature review," *Journal of Oral Implantology*, vol. 38, no. 1, pp. 527–532, 2012.

[16] P. Galindo-Moreno, P. Hernández-Cortes, R. Rios, E. Sanchez-Fernández, M. Camara, and F. O'Valle, "Immunophenotype of dental implant-associated peripheral giant cell reparative granuloma in a representative case report," *Journal of Oral Implantology*, 2013.

[17] O. A. Etöz, E. Soylu, K. Kiliçl, Ö. Günhan, H. Akcay, and A. Alkan, "A reactive lesion (pyogenic granuloma) associated with dental implant: a case report," *Journal of Oral Implantology*, vol. 39, no. 6, pp. 733–736, 2013.

[18] A. Kaya, F. Ugurlu, B. Basel, and C. B. Sener, "Oral pyogenic granuloma associated with a dental implant treated with an Er:YAG laser: a case report," *Journal of Oral Implantology*, 2013.

[19] Y.-H. Kang, J.-H. Byun, M.-J. Choi et al., "Co-development of pyogenic granuloma and capillary hemangioma on the alveolar ridge associated with a dental implant: a case report," *Journal of Medical Case Reports*, vol. 8, no. 1, article 192, 2014.

[20] G. L. Trento, V. C. Veltrini, R. N. M. dos Santos, and V. T. de Gois Santos, "Granuloma gravídico associado a implante osseointegrado: relato de caso," *Revista de Odontologia da UNESP*, vol. 43, no. 2, pp. 148–152, 2014.

[21] A. L. Brown, P. Camargo de Moraes, M. Sperandio, A. Borges Soares, V. C. Araújo, and F. Passador-Santos, "Peripheral giant

cell granuloma associated with a dental implant: a case report and review of the literature," *Case Reports in Dentistry*, vol. 2015, Article ID 697673, 6 pages, 2015.

[22] H. M. Al-Shamiri, N. A. Alaizari, S. A. Al-Maweri, and B. Tarakji, "Development of pyogenic granuloma and hemangioma after placement of dental implants: a review of literature," *Journal of International Society of Preventive and Community Dentistry*, vol. 5, no. 2, pp. 77–80, 2015.

[23] S. R. Lester, K. G. Cordell, M. S. Rosebush, A. A. Palaiologou, and P. Maney, "Peripheral giant cell granulomas: a series of 279 cases," *Oral Surgery, Oral Medicine, Oral Pathology and Oral Radiology*, vol. 118, no. 4, pp. 475–482, 2014.

[24] O. A. Effiom, W. L. Adeyemo, and O. O. Soyele, "Focal reactive lesions of the Gingiva: an analysis of 314 cases at a tertiary Health Institution in Nigeria," *Nigerian Medical Journal*, vol. 52, pp. 35–40, 2011.

[25] M. A. Gordón-Núñez, M. De Vasconcelos Carvalho, T. G. Benevenuto, M. F. F. Lopes, L. M. M. Silva, and H. C. Galvão, "Oral pyogenic granuloma: a retrospective analysis of 293 cases in a Brazilian population," *Journal of Oral and Maxillofacial Surgery*, vol. 68, no. 9, pp. 2185–2188, 2010.

[26] T. Al-Khateeb and K. Ababneh, "Oral pyogenic granuloma in Jordanians: a retrospective analysis of 108 cases," *Journal of Oral and Maxillofacial Surgery*, vol. 61, no. 11, pp. 1285–1288, 2003.

[27] E. S. Sills, D. J. Zegarelli, M. M. Hoschander, and W. E. Strider, "Clinical diagnosis and management of hormonally responsive oral pregnancy tumor (pyogenic granuloma)," *Journal of Reproductive Medicine*, vol. 41, no. 7, pp. 467–470, 1996.

[28] A. O. Ojanotko-Harri, M. P. Harri, H. M. Hurttia, and L. A. Sewón, "Altered tissue metabolism of progesterone in pregnancy gingivitis and granuloma," *Journal of Clinical Periodontology*, vol. 18, no. 4, pp. 262–266, 1991.

[29] A. Mombelli and N. P. Lang, "Antimicrobial treatment of peri-implant infections," *Clinical Oral Implants Research*, vol. 3, no. 4, pp. 162–168, 1992.

[30] H. Jafarzadeh, M. Sanatkhani, and N. Mohtasham, "Oral pyogenic granuloma: a review," *Journal of Oral Science*, vol. 48, no. 4, pp. 167–175, 2006.

31

Impact of Orthodontic Treatment on Periodontal Tissues: A Narrative Review of Multidisciplinary Literature

Angelina Gorbunkova,[1,2] **Giorgio Pagni,**[1,2] **Anna Brizhak,**[1,2] **Giampietro Farronato,**[1,2] **and Giulio Rasperini**[1,2]

[1]*Department of Biomedical, Surgical and Dental Sciences, University of Milan, Milan, Italy*
[2]*UOC Maxillofacial and Dental Surgery, Foundation IRCCS Ca' Granda Polyclinic, 20142 Milan, Italy*

Correspondence should be addressed to Giulio Rasperini; giulio.rasperini@unimi.it

Academic Editor: Andreas Stavropoulos

The aim of this review is to describe the most commonly observed changes in periodontium caused by orthodontic treatment in order to facilitate specialists' collaboration and communication. An electronic database search was carried out using PubMed abstract and citation database and bibliographic material was then used in order to find other appropriate sources. Soft and hard periodontal tissues changes during orthodontic treatment and maintenance of the patients are discussed in order to provide an exhaustive picture of the possible interactions between these two interwoven disciplines.

1. Introduction

Thanks to the increasing demand in appearance, orthodontic treatment is being more and more adopted in the adult population. As adult orthodontic patients may also have restorative and periodontal needs, the interaction between different specialties becomes even more important. Many periodontal patients may present with pathological tooth migration or other deformities where orthodontics may represent an important part of their treatment. Both periodontists and orthodontists should understand the results of one's work on the other's and cooperate in clinical practice to deliver the best possible treatment to their patients.

The number of publications evaluating orthodontics and periodontal interactions keeps increasing (Figure 1). The number of papers published in the last 5 years equals that of those published in the previous 10 years (2000–2010), which, in turn, almost equals the one of the previous 60 years (1940–2000).

The aim of this review is to explore this vast body of literature, select specific critical concepts and multidisciplinary connections, and highlight the importance of specialties cooperation.

An electronic database search was carried out using PubMed abstract and citation database with the keywords: "periodontology" AND "orthodontics" published in English. Reviews, clinical trials, animal studies, comparative studies, evaluation studies, and case reports were selected. Two authors, Angelina Gorbunkova and Anna Brizhak, selected the papers. Bibliographic material from the papers was then used in order to find other appropriate sources.

Observations of soft and hard periodontal tissues' changes during the orthodontic tooth movement (OTM) in orthodontic and periodontal literature will be described.

2. Soft Tissue Changes

Orthodontic treatment can be implemented to improve dental aesthetics not only by correcting position of the jaws and deformities of dentition, but also by creating the conditions for improved gingival health. Adult patients previously affected by periodontal disease often present with "black triangles" due to missed interdental papillae height. By means of orthodontics, it is possible to correct teeth position and to improve soft tissue aesthetics. It was suggested that orthodontic teeth approximation might change the topography of

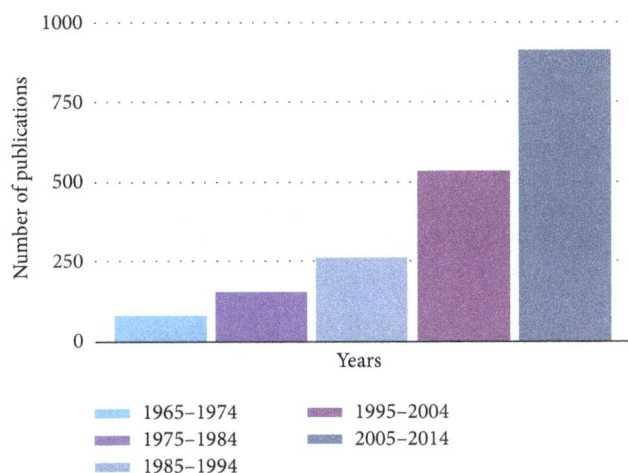

FIGURE 1: Increasing number of data observing orthodontics with periodontology reflects the increasing interest in multidisciplinary approach with time.

the interproximal alveolar crest level and enhance the position of the interdental papilla [1] although black triangles may also appear as a consequence of teeth alignment when resolving crowding. Tarnow et al. in 1992 [2] and Wu et al. in 2003 [3] suggested that the filling of the interdental space with the papilla could be determined by the position of the contact point with respect to the bone crest position. Tooth reshaping may help moving the contact point more apically during orthodontic teeth approximation which might help to achieve good aesthetic results in the interdental area [4].

It should however be taken into consideration that during OTM some adverse effects on the soft periodontal tissue may be observed. The most frequently occurring changes in soft tissues are gingival overgrowth (GO), gingival recessions (GR), and gingival invaginations (GIs), which commonly occur in orthodontic extraction cases.

Gingival overgrowth is a very common condition in the orthodontic population that is characterized by gingival enlargement possibly resulting in pseudo-pocketing with or without attachment loss. When involving the anterior region, it may have an impact on oral health-related quality of life [5]. Traditionally, GO was considered as an inflammatory reaction consecutive to bacterial plaque accumulation [6]. Other factors as chemical irritation produced by materials used for banding, mechanical irritation by bands, and food impaction have been suggested to explain the pathogenesis of GO [7]. In 1972, S. Zachrisson and B. U. Zachrisson [8] had reported gingival enlargement in patients maintaining excellent oral hygiene. More recently, Şurlin et al. [9] evaluated orthodontic patients with good dental hygiene exhibiting GO without any clinical signs of gingival inflammation. These patients exhibited elevated matrix metalloproteinase-8 (MMP-8) and matrix metalloproteinase-9 (MMP-9) levels in gingival crevicular fluid (GCF). It was considered that, during orthodontic treatment, the mechanical stress appeared to be one of the key factors determining the increase of MMP-9 production and the onset of GO. Some authors also evaluated the possible role of an allergic reaction to nickel, releasing

from the orthodontic appliances made of stainless steel. In vitro and in vivo studies suggest that released nickel ions may cause an exposure time dependent allergic reaction characterized by an upregulated proliferation of keratinocytes and increased epithelial cell proliferation [10, 11]. It may be therefore important to treat patients with nickel-free appliances and to adopt questionnaires to evaluate previous history of allergies to metals as they have been linked to an increased frequency of GO [12–14].

Enlargement of interdental papillae and accumulation of gingival tissue may appear due to the application of compressive or retraction forces at the site of extraction space closure. In orthodontic treatment, the extraction of teeth, most commonly, first or second premolars, may be required. Orthodontic space closure of extraction sites may result in gingival invagination or accumulation of gingival tissue [15].

Gingival ingrowth was defined by Robertson et al. [16] as a linear invagination of the interproximal tissue with mesial and distal orientation and an intragingival probing depth of at least 1 mm. The frequency of GI is reported to be high and may be observed more often in the lower jaw [16–18]. Due to its location, GI may render adequate plaque control complicated, possibly contributing to gingival and periodontal disease occurrence [16, 19]. There is a correlation between gingival cleft and timing of OTM. Significantly more GIs were reported when there was a delay in space closure and orthodontic treatment was initiated late after tooth extraction [17, 20]; therefore, proper communication between specialists is particularly important. Gingival ingrowth may exhibit a high degree of variability, ranging from a minor superficial crease in the gingiva to severe defects with complete penetration of the alveolar ridge (25% of all clefts) [17]. According to the GI severity, treatment strategies may vary. When GI is located in soft tissues only, it may be treated using a cold blade or the electric cautery with no significant difference between the two gingivectomy techniques [21]. Soft tissue diode laser in the management of mucogingival problems may present some advantages because of the minimal postoperative pain reposted with the use of these devices [22]. To prevent GI formation during OTM in the postextraction area, guided bone regeneration (GBR) can be applied; however, the best timing for tooth approximation to be initiated after surgery is still under discussion [23–25].

Both orthodontic and periodontal literature have thoroughly discussed gingival recession that may lead to unsatisfactory aesthetics, root sensitivity, increased susceptibility to caries, tooth abrasion, and following difficulties in maintenance of oral hygiene. OTM may either promote GR formation or improve soft tissue conditions [26–32]. Among orthodontic patients, up to 10–12% exhibited gingival recessions [26, 33]. One of the main reasons for GR development is believed to be a continuous mechanical trauma by toothbrush [34, 35], but Matthews [36] and Rajapakse et al. [37] suggested that there is no good evidence of direct link between toothbrushing and appearance of noninflammatory GR. Several anatomical and morphological characteristics were suggested to play a role in GR formation. During OTM, alveolar bone dehiscences may occur when tooth roots move through the alveolar cortical bone [38–40]. More often, this type of movement is carried out in patients with a small alveolar process, thin buccal or lingual bone plates, eccentric position of teeth, basally extended maxillary sinus, and progressive alveolar bone loss [41]. It should be noted that if the tooth is moved within the envelope of the alveolar bone, the risk of harmful side effect on the marginal soft tissue is minimal [40, 41]. The direction of applied orthodontic forces may also have an impact on soft tissues. Some studies suggested that controlled proclination of mandibular incisors could be carried out in orthodontic patients with no risk of periodontal breakdown if good level of dental hygiene is provided [27, 33, 42, 43]. Recent studies suggested that [44, 45] proinclination orthodontic movement may be significantly associated with a reduction of the keratinized tissue width. These findings are supported by other previous studies suggesting that labial tooth movement may result in decreased buccolingual tissue thickness and reduce the height of the free gingiva facilitating GR. On the other hand, lingual tooth movement may have the opposite effect [29, 38, 44]. Periodontal biotype also has been suggested to be an important factor in GR development. A strong correlation was found between thin biotype and proinclination orthodontic movement in terms of GR depth and keratinized tissue width. In contrast to patients who performed a thick gingival biotype, those with a thin-scalloped biotype are considered at risk [44, 45]. Thin periodontal biotype and amount of attached gingiva were found to be significantly related to labial plate thickness and alveolar crest position. Thin periodontium demonstrates decreased resistance to mechanical stress or inflammation and may correlate with development of GR [28, 42, 45, 46]. In light of this, an accurate evaluation of gingival thickness before starting OTM is definitely recommended [44, 45].

As for any condition with multifactorial etiology, it is important to weight the importance of any contributing factor to evaluate patient predisposition prior to initiating therapy. Because of this, we recommend critically evaluating each specific case before coming to a definitive treatment plan. Patient-related factors may also play an important role in the decision making process.

While awaiting more evidence-based information on how to proceed in different case scenarios, we would like to provide our personal opinion in order to highlight areas of interest for possible future research.

Mucogingival surgery during orthodontic treatment aims to change soft tissue characteristics in order to create more favourable conditions for the mechanical stress resistance. Nevertheless, improved gingival characteristics may not guarantee the absence of gingival recession after OT especially when significant dental arch expansion or labial proclination is performed and a second surgery may be needed after the end of orthodontics.

Our insight when evaluating orthodontic cases at risk for possible GR is that patients with a thin biotype should receive soft tissue grafting prior to OTM in order to reduce the risk and the extent of the possible GR. Thus far, it is not clear which gingival and movement characteristics may predispose to GR and what would be the incidence of GR in each specific scenario. The efficacy of preventive surgeries should also be further analysed: in example, we would like to

know the number of preventive surgeries in correspondence with the number of patients that would actually develop GR. We would also like to know how many patients receiving a preventive surgery will also require a second corrective surgical procedure.

A different scenario can be found, should GR occur during OTM. In these cases, soft tissue grafting is indicated and should be performed as soon as possible given that all other parameters (gingival inflammation, trauma, etc.) are controlled. The aim is to treat the recession once it is still minimal and improve treatment prognosis. Orthodontic therapy should be carefully evaluated in this period of time in order to determine whether to stop or to slow down OTM until wound healing is complete. Clearly, the timing of appearing of the GR is important and we should better understand the implications of a GR occurring in the initial third of orthodontic treatment versus close to the end of OTM.

When preexisting GRs are found before orthodontic treatment, the impact of orthodontic treatment should be carefully evaluated. Should the tooth be planned for lingual tooth movement, mucogingival surgery may not even be required and OTM alone may end up treating or at least not aggravating the recession. When necessary, the prognosis of mucogingival surgery may be improved after the tooth is moved lingually. Should the tooth be moved labially instead, a corrective mucogingival procedure aiming to avoid disease progression should be taken into consideration. OTM may be initiated once wound healing is complete (3-4 months). At the end of orthodontic therapy, the site should be reevaluated and a second intervention may be needed in limited cases.

Every clinical case may include a combination of different predisposing and precipitating factors that can affect the treatment outcome; therefore, it is important to evaluate risk factors while planning orthodontic treatment in order to avoid undesired consequences of the delivered therapy. Risk management is possibly the most important factor when treatment planning these patients. We encourage researchers to further evaluate unclear aspects such as patient/tooth/site predisposition to gingival recession and ideal type and timing of treatment and to generate incremental systems for hierarchical clustering, which would be able to put together different probabilistic nodes in the determination of specific clinical solutions.

3. Bone Changes

Mechanical force during OTM results in bone resorption and bone apposition widely discussed in both orthodontic and periodontal literature. In health, during OTM, all components of periodontal attachment apparatus, including the osseous structure, periodontal ligament, and the soft tissue components, move together with the tooth. The same applies to patients with reduced but healthy periodontal tissues [32, 47, 48]. After periodontal treatment, light orthodontic forces combined with good dental hygiene control may be enough to result in teeth alignment when periodontal support is reduced.

OTM in presence of intrabony pockets presents a different challenge for clinicians. Several studies suggested that OTM after surgical periodontal treatment may have an impact on the morphology of bone defects, decrease pocket depth, and enhance connective tissue healing. All the positive changes in supporting apparatus were achieved only when a good dental hygiene control had been implemented. Some authors applied intrusive orthodontic forces and reported clinical and radiological improvements [49, 50]. Also, it was reported in histological study by Melsen et al. [51] that new cementum formation and new collagen attachment may be obtained by orthodontic intrusion in presence of good dental hygiene. da Silva et al. [52] in their study on dogs intruded teeth with furcation defects and suggested that class-III defects may be clinically eliminated or reduced resulting in clinical attachment level gain. Another study investigated the influence of tilting movements in presence of intrabony pockets and reinforced the conclusion that OTM may be performed in teeth with bone defects without damage to the periodontal attachment level [53]. Polson et al. [47] further evaluated the attachment apparatus on such teeth and reported the presence of long junctional epithelium between the bone and the root surface after teeth movement into and through the defect, suggesting no regeneration from the supporting apparatus. Therefore, it was recommended to apply GTR techniques in the treatment of intrabony defects before orthodontic therapy in order to achieve regeneration instead of repair.

Effectiveness of periodontal regeneration in the treatment of intrabony defects is well documented and supported by histological studies. All the benefits of guided tissue regeneration (GTR) may be maintained over a long period of time (over 10 years) [54, 55]. It is commonly believed that bony pocket topography is important for the prognosis of the regenerative treatment; however, a recent systematic review claimed clinical outcomes of periodontal regeneration to be influenced by patient behaviors and surgical approach more than by tooth and defect characteristics [56]. The combined adoption of orthodontic therapy and periodontal regeneration of teeth with infrabony defects may be suggested in multiple situations. Orthodontic extrusion, intrusion, and sagittal tooth movements with different timing of OTM after GTR were described in the literature. Evaluating apical downgrowth of junctional epithelium, Nemcovsky et al. [57] suggested that periodontal regeneration might be indicated prior to OTM. In 2003, Diedrich et al. [58] performed a study on orthodontic intrusion and translation of teeth with 3-wall bony defects previously treated with open flap debridement combined with enamel matrix protein. In the intrusion group, a slight epithelial downgrowth, extensive cementogenesis, and bone apposition were documented leading to results comparable to those noted on the tension site of translation group. Defects on the pressure side were additionally covered with resorbable membrane and after OTM showed markedly reduced bone apposition. These results may indicate the possible influence of biomaterial degradation on regenerative outcomes, which was also suggested in other studies [52, 59]. Araújo et al. [60] suggested that it was possible to move teeth into areas previously augmented with biomaterial.

Orthodontic forces were applied 3 months after grafting and no impediment in OTM was observed. Some authors suggested that the optimal timing to begin OTM after GTR is 4 weeks after surgery when mitotic activity of periodontal cells is increased and OTM occurs in immature bone [52, 61]. Attia et al. [62, 63], evaluating the effectiveness of different timing for initiating active orthodontic treatment after GTR, suggested that significant improvements of periodontal regeneration may be observed in defects treated with the immediate application of orthodontic forces after surgery. Others demonstrated that orthodontic treatment provided 1 year after GTR, when both hard and soft tissues are mature, caused no detrimental effect on periodontal regeneration outcomes [4]. Taking into account the results of these different studies, it may be concluded that several factors such as direction of tooth movement and timing and choice of biomaterials should be taken into consideration during treatment planning, although more well-designed clinical trials are needed to further clarify the mechanisms involved with wound healing when orthodontic forces are applied [64].

4. Maintenance

Our initial search included a large amount of studies evaluating the effects of different levels of oral hygiene in patients undergoing OTM. This highlights the importance of maintenance in dental practice especially in cases where orthodontics is combined with periodontal treatment. For all patients undergoing orthodontic treatment on fixed appliances or wearing fixed retainers, it is difficult to maintain a good level of oral hygiene, because orthodontic constructions and accessories may hinder conventional brushing and flossing. Meanwhile, deficient oral hygiene in orthodontic patients appears to be a key factor in the development of white spot lesions, dental caries, and gingival inflammation due to the presence of dental plaque accumulation [65, 66]. In the presence of insufficient dental hygiene, orthodontic treatment may lead to the transposition of the supragingival dental plaque subgingivally resulting in infrabony pocket formation [67].

The type of appliance (fixed or removable), bracket material, bonding technique (lingual or buccal bonding), and type of retainer selected for orthodontic therapy may all influence the patient ability to maintain a good level of plaque control. During OTM oral malodor, plaque index and gingival index increase and first changes may be observed immediately after bonding [66, 68].

Some authors suggested dental plaque accumulation in patients wearing fixed appliances to be greater than that in patients wearing removable appliances [69]. While the evidence supporting this sentence is not that strong and more well-designed clinical trials should be carried out in order to investigate clinical parameters of periodontal status in two different treatment modalities, clinicians may want to consider this piece of information when treatment planning periodontal patients for orthodontic therapy. Lingual orthodontic appliances showed higher plaque retention compared to labial orthodontic appliances due to more difficult access for daily maintenance [70]. Despite the fact that there was no significant difference in plaque accumulation with regard to the type of ligation [71, 72], bracket material also seems to influence quantity and location of plaque accumulation. Stainless steel brackets appeared to harvest significantly bigger amount of plaque when compared to ceramic, sapphire, and polycarbonate brackets. When using ceramic brackets, the greatest amount of plaque was shown to accumulate on occlusal and gingival surfaces, while mesial and distal surfaces were shown to accumulate more plaque when adopting stainless steel brackets [73–75]. In addition, stainless steel surfaces were suggested to attract less biofilm than gold [76–78]. The presence of fixed retainers may be associated with a risk of higher level of plaque accumulation, gingival recession, and bleeding on probing. Patients with multistrand wire retainers exhibited more plaque accumulation on the distal surfaces of the lower anterior teeth in comparison with a single span, round wire retainers [79, 80].

In order to reduce risks of periodontal breakdown during and after OTM, more attention should be paid to the orthodontic devices' characteristics while planning. Periodontal status in orthodontically treated patients might be assessed not only during therapy and after debonding, but likely also during follow-ups in retention period. In periodontal patients undergoing orthodontic therapy, plaque control has to be closely monitored.

Numerous articles extensively discussed advantages and disadvantages of different types of toothbrushes: manual toothbrushes, sonic, orthodontic, powered, oscillating-rotating, ultrasonic, and ionic [81–84]. According to the recent update of a Cochrane review [85] based on 51 articles with a total of 4624 participants, it was suggested that powered toothbrushes may provide a significant benefit when compared with manual toothbrushes. Several studies in orthodontic patients also supported these findings and demonstrated higher effectiveness of oscillating-rotating toothbrushes in dental plaque removal and gingivitis reduction when compared to manual brushes [86, 87]. It should be taken into consideration that patients' motivation and repeated oral hygiene instructions may be a crucial factor for patients undergoing OTM with fixed appliances [88, 89]. Motivation of orthodontic patients may include different educational techniques: oral hygiene instructions, showing images of possible complications, the use of plaque-disclosing tablets, demonstrations of brushing techniques on models, and even showing patients phase contrast microscopy of their plaque samples [90, 91].

Orthodontic patients who are not able to establish satisfactory oral hygiene levels are recommended to receive some additional aids such as dental varnishes, gels, mouth washes, or dentifrices. Chlorhexidine (CHX) which may be included in different kinds of vehicles shows antibacterial effectiveness against gingival inflammation and cariogenic bacteria and may also reduce the severity of traumatic ulcers during OTM [92–96]. The discussion on the side effects related to long-term use of CHX such as tooth staining is commonly debated and is considered to be related to its concentration. By using

mouthrinses and dentifrices with lower concentrations of CHX, it is possible to reduce tooth decoloration without significant difference in reduction plaque formation and gingival inflammation [96, 97]. The inclusion of fluoride in CHX dentifrices may help in providing better prophylaxis of white spot lesion formation while simultaneously reducing gingival inflammation [98].

Patient's compliance, motivation, and oral hygiene maintenance are universally recognized as important factors when evaluating the impact of OTM on their periodontal status. These parameters are important for maintaining the periodontal condition after nonsurgical and surgical periodontal therapy and should be continued afterwards. Taking into account additional difficulties in daily dental hygiene for orthodontic patients during treatment with fixed appliances, regular monitoring of adults with predisposition for periodontal breakdown during OTM is mandatory. Orthodontists should pay great attention to the dental health education, emphasizing oral hygiene instructions and regular periodontal care. Periodontal check-ups and good quality professional hygiene maintenance appointments are essential even after the completion of orthodontic treatment. In other words, periodontal maintenance should be provided from the beginning of periodontal therapy, through all the steps of periodontal treatment, it should be even more closely monitored during orthodontic treatment, and it should be continued throughout the lifetime of the patient.

5. Conclusions

Well-coordinated multidisciplinary dental treatment aims to provide satisfactory aesthetics, function, and long-term prognosis for patients. An effective cooperation makes it possible to observe clinical problems from different perspectives and to better understand the interactions between different specialties. Periodontal health is essential for any form of dental treatment. In order to avoid undesirable consequences during and after OTM, a thorough assessment of periodontal health should be provided. Attention should be paid to dental hygiene parameters especially in patients wearing fixed appliances and in periodontally susceptible individuals.

In this review, we elected some clinical aspects where periodontal and orthodontic knowledge come together to provide a more exhaustive picture of the orthodontic treatments impact on periodontium. We discussed possible effects of OTM on soft and hard periodontal tissues accompanied by fixed orthodontic appliances wearing. Finally, the importance of maintenance on patients' health, function, and aesthetics following active therapy was stressed as a priority in the management of both specialties' populations.

Other interesting fields where the interaction between orthodontics and periodontology is very important have not been adequately explored yet. The timing of orthodontic treatment of patient that underwent active periodontal therapy is one area where very little evidence has yet been produced. While most clinicians may agree that orthodontic movement should start after the end of active therapy, there is still no universal protocol that can be applied to patients with periodontally compromised dentition undergoing combined ortho-perio treatment. The influence of the adopted surgical protocol may also have an impact on the timing and regenerative therapies may require longer periods of time compared to traditional periodontal treatments when a translatorily movement direction is required.

Despite the high number of published articles, we realized there is a lack of good evidence about many of the treatments including both orthodontics and periodontal therapy. Well-designed clinical trials evaluating the interaction between these only apparently distant specialties must be encouraged in the dental community. Evaluating patient care from just one specialty eye may limit the possibilities of treatment when compared to a coordinated view of each particular condition. A good perspective can only exist with two points of view.

Conflict of Interests

The authors declare that there is no conflict of interests regarding the publication of this paper.

References

[1] Y. Kim, E. Kwon, Y. Cho, J. Lee, S. Kim, and J. Choi, "Changes in the vertical position of interdental papillae and interseptal bone following the approximation of anterior teeth," *The International Journal of Periodontics & Restorative Dentistry*, vol. 34, no. 2, pp. 219–224, 2014.

[2] D. P. Tarnow, A. W. Magner, and P. Fletcher, "The effect of the distance from the contact point to the crest of bone on the presence or absence of the interproximal dental papilla," *Journal of Periodontology*, vol. 63, no. 12, pp. 995–996, 1992.

[3] Y.-J. Wu, Y.-K. Tu, S.-M. Huang, and C.-P. Chan, "The influence of the distance from the contact point to the crest of bone on the presence of the interproximal dental papilla," *Chang Gung Medical Journal*, vol. 26, no. 11, pp. 822–828, 2003.

[4] C. Ghezzi, S. Masiero, M. Silvesth, G. Zanotti, and G. Rasperini, "Orthodontic treatment of periodontally involved teeth after tissue regeneration," *International Journal of Periodontics & Restorative Dentistry*, vol. 28, no. 6, pp. 559–567, 2008.

[5] F. B. Zanatta, T. M. Ardenghi, R. P. Antoniazzi, T. M. P. Pinto, and C. K. Rösing, "Association between gingival bleeding and gingival enlargement and oral health-related quality of life (OHRQoL) of subjects under fixed orthodontic treatment: a cross-sectional study," *BMC Oral Health*, vol. 12, no. 1, article 53, 2012.

[6] H. A. Eid, H. A. M. Assiri, R. Kandyala, R. A. Togoo, and V. S. Turakhia, "Gingival enlargement in different age groups during fixed orthodontic treatment," *Journal of International Oral Health*, vol. 6, no. 1, pp. 1–4, 2014.

[7] J. S. Kloehn and J. S. Pfeifer, "The effect of orthodontic treatment on the periodontium," *Angle Orthodontist*, vol. 44, no. 2, pp. 127–134, 1974.

[8] S. Zachrisson and B. U. Zachrisson, "Gingival condition associated with orthodontic treatment," *The Angle Orthodontist*, vol. 42, no. 1, pp. 26–34, 1972.

[9] P. Şurlin, A.-M. Rauten, D. Pirici, B. Oprea, L. Mogoantă, and A. Camen, "Collagen IV and MMP-9 expression in hypertrophic gingiva during orthodontic treatment," *Romanian Journal of Morphology and Embryology*, vol. 53, no. 1, pp. 161–165, 2012.

[10] U. K. Gursoy, O. Sokucu, V.-J. Uitto et al., "The role of nickel accumulation and epithelial cell proliferation in orthodontic treatment-induced gingival overgrowth," *European Journal of Orthodontics*, vol. 29, no. 6, pp. 555–558, 2007.

[11] C. Marchese, V. Visco, L. Aimati et al., "Nickel-induced keratinocyte proliferation and up-modulation of the keratinocyte growth factor receptor expression," *Experimental Dermatology*, vol. 12, no. 4, pp. 497–505, 2003.

[12] C. A. Pazzini, L. S. Marques, M. L. Marques, G. O. J. Nior, L. J. Pereira, and S. M. Paiva, "Longitudinal assessment of periodontal status in patients with nickel allergy treated with conventional and nickel-free braces," *The Angle Orthodontist*, vol. 82, no. 4, pp. 653–657, 2012.

[13] C. Maspero, L. Giannini, G. Galbiati, F. Nolet, L. Esposito, and G. Farronato, "Titanium orthodontic appliances for allergic patients," *Minerva Stomatologica*, vol. 63, no. 11-12, pp. 403–410, 2014.

[14] M. C. G. Pantuzo, E. G. Zenóbio, H. D. A. Marigo, and M. A. F. Zenóbio, "Hypersensitivity to conventional and to nickel-free orthodontic brackets," *Brazilian Oral Research*, vol. 21, no. 4, pp. 298–302, 2007.

[15] J. Kurol, A. Ronnerman, and G. Heyden, "Long-term gingival conditions after orthodontic closure of extraction sites. Histological and histochemical studies," *European Journal of Orthodontics*, vol. 4, no. 2, pp. 87–92, 1982.

[16] P. B. Robertson, L. D. Schultz, and B. M. Levy, "Occurrence and distribution of interdental gingival clefts following orthodontic movement into bicuspid extraction sites," *Journal of Periodontology*, vol. 48, no. 4, pp. 232–235, 1977.

[17] C. Reichert, L. Gölz, C. Dirk, and A. Jäger, "Retrospective investigation of gingival invaginations: Part I: clinical findings and presentation of a coding system," *Journal of Orofacial Orthopedics*, vol. 73, no. 4, pp. 307–316, 2012.

[18] A. L. R. Circuns and J. F. C. Tulloch, "Gingival invagination in extraction sites of orthodontic patients: their incidence, effects on periodontal health, and orthodontic treatment," *American Journal of Orthodontics*, vol. 83, no. 6, pp. 469–476, 1983.

[19] L. Gölz, C. Reichert, C. Dirk, and A. Jäger, "Retrospective investigation of gingival invaginations: part II: microbiological findings and genetic risk profile," *Journal of Orofacial Orthopedics*, vol. 73, no. 5, pp. 387–396, 2012.

[20] P. Diedrich and H. Wehrbein, "Orthodontic retraction into recent and healed extraction sites. A histologic study," *Journal of Orofacial Orthopedics*, vol. 58, no. 2, pp. 90–99, 1997.

[21] S. Malkoc, T. Buyukyilmaz, I. Gelgor, and M. Gursel, "Comparison of two different gingivectomy techniques for gingival cleft treatment," *The Angle Orthodontist*, vol. 74, no. 3, pp. 375–380, 2004.

[22] I. N. Ize-Iyamu, B. D. Saheeb, and B. E. Edetanlen, "Comparing the 810 nm diode laser with conventional surgery in orthodontic soft tissue procedures," *Ghana Medical Journal*, vol. 47, no. 3, pp. 107–111, 2013.

[23] M. L. B. Pinheiro, T. C. Moreira, and E. J. Feres-Filho, "Guided bone regeneration of a pronounced gingivo-alveolar cleft due to orthodontic space closure," *Journal of Periodontology*, vol. 77, no. 6, pp. 1091–1095, 2006.

[24] J. Tiefengraber, P. Diedrich, U. Fritz, and P. Lantos, "Orthodontic space closure in combination with membrane supported healing of extraction sockets (MHE). A pilot study," *Journal of Orofacial Orthopedics*, vol. 63, no. 5, pp. 422–428, 2002.

[25] C. Reichert, M. Wenghöfer, W. Götz, and A. Jäger, "Pilot study on orthodontic space closure after guided bone regeneration," *Journal of Orofacial Orthopedics*, vol. 72, no. 1, pp. 45–50, 2011.

[26] A. M. Renkema, P. S. Fudalej, A. A. P. Renkema, F. Abbas, E. Bronkhorst, and C. Katsaros, "Gingival labial recessions in orthodontically treated and untreated individuals: a case—control study," *Journal of Clinical Periodontology*, vol. 40, no. 6, pp. 631–637, 2013.

[27] D. Allais and B. Melsen, "Does labial movement of lower incisors influence the level of the gingival margin? A case-control study of adult orthodontic patients," *European Journal of Orthodontics*, vol. 25, no. 4, pp. 343–352, 2003.

[28] G. W. Coatoam, R. G. Behrents, and N. Bissada, "The width of keratinized gingiva during orthodontic treatment: its significance and impact on periodontal status," *Journal of Periodontology*, vol. 52, no. 6, pp. 307–313, 1981.

[29] A. Andlin-Sobocki and L. Bodin, "Dimensional alterations of the gingiva related to changes of facial/lingual tooth position in permanent anterior teeth of children. A 2-year longitudinal study," *Journal of Clinical Periodontology*, vol. 20, no. 3, pp. 219–224, 1993.

[30] H. S. Dorfman, "Mucogingival changes resulting from mandibular incisor tooth movement," *American Journal of Orthodontics*, vol. 74, no. 3, pp. 286–297, 1978.

[31] S. Re, D. Cardaropoli, R. Abundo, and G. Corrente, "Reduction of gingival recession following orthodontic intrusion in periodontally compromised patients," *Orthodontics & Craniofacial Research*, vol. 7, no. 1, pp. 35–39, 2004.

[32] S. Re, G. Corrente, R. Abundo, and D. Cardaropoli, "Orthodontic treatment in periodontally compromised patients: 12-year report," *International Journal of Periodontics & Restorative Dentistry*, vol. 20, no. 1, pp. 31–39, 2000.

[33] G. Djeu, C. Hayes, and S. Zawaideh, "Correlation between mandibular central incisor proclination and gingival recession during fixed appliance therapy," *The Angle Orthodontist*, vol. 72, no. 3, pp. 238–245, 2002.

[34] M. Vehkalahti, "Occurrence of gingival recession in adults," *Journal of Periodontology*, vol. 60, no. 11, pp. 599–603, 1989.

[35] L. Checchi, G. Daprile, M. R. A. Gatto, and G. A. Pelliccioni, "Gingival recession and toothbrushing in an Italian School of Dentistry: a pilot study," *Journal of Clinical Periodontology*, vol. 26, no. 5, pp. 276–280, 1999.

[36] D. C. Matthews, "No good evidence to link toothbrushing trauma to gingival recession," *Journal of Evidence-Based Dental Practice*, vol. 9, no. 2, article 49, 2008.

[37] P. S. Rajapakse, G. I. McCracken, E. Gwynnett, N. D. Steen, A. Guentsch, and P. A. Heasman, "Does tooth brushing influence the development and progression of non-inflammatory gingival recession? A systematic review," *Journal of Clinical Periodontology*, vol. 34, no. 12, pp. 1046–1061, 2007.

[38] J. L. Wennström, "Mucogingival considerations in orthodontic treatment," *Seminars in Orthodontics*, vol. 2, no. 1, pp. 46–54, 1996.

[39] C. Richman, "Is gingival recession a consequence of an orthodontic tooth size and/or tooth position discrepancy? A paradigm shift," *Compendium of Continuing Education in Dentistry*, vol. 32, no. 4, pp. e73–e79, 2011.

[40] Y. A. Mostafa, F. A. El Sharaby, and A. R. El Beialy, "Do alveolar bone defects merit orthodontists' respect?" *World Journal of Orthodontics*, vol. 10, no. 1, pp. 16–20, 2009.

[41] R. Fuhrmann, "Three-dimensional interpretation of periodontal lesions and remodeling during orthodontic treatment. Part III," *Journal of Orofacial Orthopedics*, vol. 57, no. 4, pp. 224–237, 1996.

[42] B. Melsen and D. Allais, "Factors of importance for the development of dehiscences during labial movement of mandibular incisors: a retrospective study of adult orthodontic patients," *American Journal of Orthodontics and Dentofacial Orthopedics*, vol. 127, no. 5, pp. 552–561, 2005.

[43] S. Ruf, K. Hansen, and H. Pancherz, "Does orthodontic proclination of lower incisors in children and adolescents cause gingival recession?" *American Journal of Orthodontics and Dentofacial Orthopedics*, vol. 114, no. 1, pp. 100–106, 1998.

[44] R. Acunzo, G. Rasperini, P. Cannalire, and G. Farronato, "Influence of periodontal biotype on root surface exposure during orthodontic treatment: a preliminary study," *International Journal of Periodontology and Restaurative Dentistry*, vol. 35, no. 5, pp. 665–675, 2015.

[45] K. H. Zawawi and M. S. Al-Zahrani, "Gingival biotype in relation to incisors' inclination and position," *Saudi Medical Journal*, vol. 35, no. 11, pp. 1378–1383, 2014.

[46] D. R. Cook, B. L. Mealey, R. G. Verrett et al., "Relationship between clinical periodontal biotype and labial plate thickness: an in vivo study," *The International Journal of Periodontics & Restorative Dentistry*, vol. 31, no. 4, pp. 345–354, 2011.

[47] A. Polson, J. Caton, A. P. Polson, S. Nyman, J. Novak, and B. Reed, "Periodontal response after tooth movement into intrabony defects," *Journal of Periodontology*, vol. 55, no. 4, pp. 197–202, 1984.

[48] C. C. Cirelli, J. A. Cirelli, J. C. D. R. Martins et al., "Orthodontic movement of teeth with intraosseous defects: histologic and histometric study in dogs," *American Journal of Orthodontics and Dentofacial Orthopedics*, vol. 123, no. 6, pp. 666–675, 2003.

[49] G. Corrente, R. Abundo, S. Re, D. Cardaropoli, and G. Cardaropoli, "Orthodontic movement into infrabony defects in patients with advanced periodontal disease: a clinical and radiological study," *Journal of Periodontology*, vol. 74, no. 8, pp. 1104–1109, 2003.

[50] D. Cardaropoli, S. Re, G. Corrente, and R. Abundo, "Intrusion of migrated incisors with infrabony defects in adult periodontal patients," *American Journal of Orthodontics and Dentofacial Orthopedics*, vol. 120, no. 6, pp. 671–677, 2001.

[51] B. Melsen, N. Agerbæk, J. Erikson, and S. Terp, "New attachment through periodontal treatment and orthodontic intrusion," *American Journal of Orthodontics and Dentofacial Orthopedics*, vol. 94, no. 2, pp. 104–116, 1988.

[52] V. C. da Silva, C. C. Cirelli, F. S. Ribeiro et al., "Intrusion of teeth with class III furcation: a clinical, histologic and histometric study in dogs," *Journal of Clinical Periodontology*, vol. 35, no. 9, pp. 807–816, 2008.

[53] C. C. Cirelli, J. A. Cirelli, J. C. da Rosa Martins et al., "Orthodontic movement of teeth with intraosseous defects: histologic and histometric study in dogs," *American Journal of Orthodontics and Dentofacial Orthopedics*, vol. 123, no. 6, pp. 666–675, 2003.

[54] M. Silvestri, G. Rasperini, and S. Milani, "120 Infrabony defects treated with regenerative therapy: long-term results," *Journal of Periodontology*, vol. 82, no. 5, pp. 668–675, 2011.

[55] M. A. Reynolds, R. T. Kao, P. M. Camargo et al., "Periodontal regeneration—intrabony defects: a consensus report from the AAP regeneration workshop," *Journal of Periodontology*, vol. 86, supplement 2, pp. S105–S107, 2015.

[56] R. T. Kao, S. Nares, and M. A. Reynolds, "Periodontal regeneration—intrabony defects: a systematic review from the AAP regeneration workshop," *Journal of Periodontology*, vol. 86, no. 2, supplement, pp. S77–S104, 2015.

[57] C. E. Nemcovsky, M. Sasson, L. Beny, M. Weinreb, and A. D. Vardimon, "Periodontal healing following orthodontic movement of rat molars with intact versus damaged periodontia towards a bony defect," *European Journal of Orthodontics*, vol. 29, no. 4, pp. 338–344, 2007.

[58] P. Diedrich, U. Fritz, G. Kinzinger, and J. Angelakis, "Movement of periodontally affected teeth after guided tissue regeneration (GTR)—an experimental pilot study in animals," *Journal of Orofacial Orthopedics*, vol. 64, no. 3, pp. 214–227, 2003.

[59] V. C. da Silva, C. C. Cirelli, F. S. Ribeiro, M. R. Costa, R. C. Comelli Lia, and J. A. Cirelli, "Orthodontic movement after periodontal regeneration of class II furcation: a pilot study in dogs," *Journal of Clinical Periodontology*, vol. 33, no. 6, pp. 440–448, 2006.

[60] M. G. Araújo, D. Carmagnola, T. Berglundh, B. Thilander, and J. Lindhe, "Orthodontic movement in bone defects augmented with Bio-Oss. An experimental study in dogs," *Journal of Clinical Periodontology*, vol. 28, no. 1, pp. 73–80, 2001.

[61] S. Ogihara and H.-L. Wang, "Periodontal regeneration with or without limited orthodontics for the treatment of 2- or 3-wall infrabony defects," *Journal of Periodontology*, vol. 81, no. 12, pp. 1734–1742, 2010.

[62] M. S. Attia, E. A. Shoreibah, S. A. Ibrahim, and H. A. Nassar, "Histological evaluation of osseous defects combined with orthodontic tooth movement," *Journal of the International Academy of Periodontology*, vol. 14, no. 1, pp. 7–16, 2012.

[63] M. S. Attia, E. A. Shoreibah, S. A. Ibrahim, and H. A. Nassar, "Regenerative therapy of osseous defects combined with orthodontic tooth movement," *Journal of the International Academy of Periodontology*, vol. 14, no. 1, pp. 17–25, 2012.

[64] R. Rotundo, T. Bassarelli, E. Pace, G. Iachetti, J. Mervelt, and G. P. Prato, "Orthodontic treatment of periodontal defects. Part II: a systematic review on human and animal studies," *Progress in Orthodontics*, vol. 12, no. 1, pp. 45–52, 2011.

[65] K. C. Julien, P. H. Buschang, and P. M. Campbell, "Prevalence of white spot lesion formation during orthodontic treatment," *The Angle Orthodontist*, vol. 83, no. 4, pp. 641–647, 2013.

[66] M. M. C. de Melo, M. G. Cardoso, J. Faber, and A. Sobral, "Risk factors for periodontal changes in adult patients with banded second molars during orthodontic treatment," *The Angle Orthodontist*, vol. 82, no. 2, pp. 224–228, 2012.

[67] I. Ericsson, B. Thilander, J. Lindhe, and H. Okamoto, "The effect of orthodontic tilting movements on the periodontal tissues of infected and non-infected dentitions in dogs," *Journal of Clinical Periodontology*, vol. 4, no. 4, pp. 278–293, 1977.

[68] H. Babacan, O. Sokucu, I. Marakoglu, H. Ozdemir, and R. Nalcaci, "Effect of fixed appliances on oral malodor," *American Journal of Orthodontics and Dentofacial Orthopedics*, vol. 139, no. 3, pp. 351–355, 2011.

[69] R.-R. Miethke and S. Vogt, "A comparison of the periodontal health of patients during treatment with the Invisalign system and with fixed orthodontic appliances," *Journal of Orofacial Orthopedics*, vol. 66, no. 3, pp. 219–229, 2005.

[70] L. Lombardo, Y. Ö. Ortan, Ö. Gorgun, C. Panza, G. Scuzzo, and G. Siciliani, "Changes in the oral environment after placement of lingual and labial orthodontic appliances," *Progress in orthodontics*, vol. 14, article 28, 2013.

[71] A. J. Ireland, V. Soro, S. V. Sprague et al., "The effects of different orthodontic appliances upon microbial communities," *Orthodontics and Craniofacial Research*, vol. 17, no. 2, pp. 115–123, 2014.

[72] W. Sukontapatipark, M. A. El-Agroudi, N. J. Selliseth, K. Thunold, and K. A. Selvig, "Bacterial colonization associated with fixed orthodontic appliances. A scanning electron microscopy study," *European Journal of Orthodontics*, vol. 23, no. 5, pp. 475–484, 2001.

[73] I. D. Lindel, C. Elter, W. Heuer et al., "Comparative analysis of long-term biofilm formation on metal and ceramic brackets," *The Angle Orthodontist*, vol. 81, no. 5, pp. 907–914, 2011.

[74] T. Eliades, G. Eliades, and W. A. Brantley, "Microbial attachment on orthodontic appliances: I. Wettability and early pellicle formation on bracket materials," *American Journal of Orthodontics and Dentofacial Orthopedics*, vol. 108, no. 4, pp. 351–360, 1995.

[75] H. F. Saloom, H. S. Mohammed-Salih, and S. F. Rasheed, "The influence of different types of fixed orthodontic appliance on the growth and adherence of microorganisms (in vitro study)," *Journal of Clinical and Experimental Dentistry*, vol. 5, no. 1, pp. e36–e41, 2013.

[76] M. P. Dittmer, C. F. Hellemann, S. Grade et al., "Comparative three-dimensional analysis of initial biofilm formation on three orthodontic bracket materials," *Head & Face Medicine*, vol. 11, article 110, 2015.

[77] M. A. Jongsma, F. D. H. Pelser, H. C. van der Mei et al., "Biofilm formation on stainless steel and gold wires for bonded retainers in vitro and in vivo and their susceptibility to oral antimicrobials," *Clinical Oral Investigations*, vol. 17, no. 4, pp. 1209–1218, 2013.

[78] M. A. Jongsma, H. C. van der Mei, J. Atema-Smit, H. J. Busscher, and Y. Ren, "*In vivo* biofilm formation on stainless steel bonded retainers during different oral health-care regimens," *International Journal of Oral Science*, vol. 7, no. 1, pp. 42–48, 2015.

[79] L. Levin, G. R. Samorodnitzky-Naveh, and E. E. Machtei, "The association of orthodontic treatment and fixed retainers with gingival health," *Journal of Periodontology*, vol. 79, no. 11, pp. 2087–2092, 2008.

[80] K. Al-Nimri, R. Al Habashneh, and M. Obeidat, "Gingival health and relapse tendency: a prospective study of two types of lower fixed retainers," *Australian Orthodontic Journal*, vol. 25, no. 2, pp. 142–146, 2009.

[81] A. Silvestrini Biavati, L. Gastaldo, M. Dessì, F. Silvestrini Biavati, and M. Migliorati, "Manual orthodontic vs. Oscillating-rotating electric toothbrush in orthodontic patients: a randomised clinical trial," *European Journal of Paediatric Dentistry*, vol. 11, no. 1, pp. 200–202, 2010.

[82] M. R. Costa, V. C. Silva, M. N. Miqui, T. Sakima, D. M. P. Spolidorio, and J. A. Cirelli, "Efficacy of ultrasonic, electric and manual toothbrushes in patients with fixed orthodontic appliances," *The Angle Orthodontist*, vol. 77, no. 2, pp. 361–366, 2007.

[83] A. Borutta, E. Pala, and T. Fischer, "Effectiveness of a powered toothbrush compared with a manual toothbrush for orthodontic patients with fixed appliances," *Journal of Clinical Dentistry*, vol. 13, no. 4, pp. 131–137, 2002.

[84] J. Hickman, D. T. Millett, L. Sander, E. Brown, and J. Love, "Powered vs manual tooth brushing in fixed appliance patients: a short term randomized clinical trial," *The Angle Orthodontist*, vol. 72, no. 2, pp. 135–140, 2002.

[85] M. Yaacob, H. V. Worthington, S. A. Deacon et al., "Powered versus manual toothbrushing for oral health," *Cochrane Database of Systematic Reviews*, no. 6, Article ID CD002281, 2014.

[86] C. Erbe, M. Klukowska, I. Tsaknaki, H. Timm, J. Grender, and H. Wehrbein, "Efficacy of 3 toothbrush treatments on plaque removal in orthodontic patients assessed with digital plaque imaging: a randomized controlled trial," *American Journal of Orthodontics and Dentofacial Orthopedics*, vol. 143, no. 6, pp. 760–766, 2013.

[87] A. Silvestrini Biavati, L. Gastaldo, M. Dessì, F. Silvestrini Biavati, and M. Migliorati, "Manual orthodontic vs. oscillating-rotating electric toothbrush in orthodontic patients: a randomised clinical trial," *European Journal of Paediatric Dentistry*, vol. 11, no. 1, pp. 200–202, 2010.

[88] C. Kossack and P.-G. Jost-Brinkmann, "Plaque and gingivitis reduction in patients undergoing orthodontic treatment with fixed appliances-comparison of toothbrushes and interdental cleaning aids. A 6-month clinical single-blind trial," *Journal of Orofacial Orthopedics*, vol. 66, no. 1, pp. 20–38, 2005.

[89] I. Marini, F. Bortolotti, S. Incerti Parenti, M. R. Gatto, and G. Alessandri Bonetti, "Combined effects of repeated oral hygiene motivation and type of toothbrush on orthodontic patients: a blind randomized clinical trial," *The Angle Orthodontist*, vol. 84, no. 5, pp. 896–901, 2014.

[90] S. Acharya, A. Goyal, A. K. Utreja, and U. Mohanty, "Effect of three different motivational techniques on oral hygiene and gingival health of patients undergoing multibracketed orthodontics," *The Angle Orthodontist*, vol. 81, no. 5, pp. 884–888, 2011.

[91] Y. Peng, R. Wu, W. Qu et al., "Effect of visual method vs plaque disclosure in enhancing oral hygiene in adolescents and young adults: a single-blind randomized controlled trial," *American Journal of Orthodontics and Dentofacial Orthopedics*, vol. 145, no. 3, pp. 280–286, 2014.

[92] G. B. Anderson, J. Bowden, E. C. Morrison, and R. G. Caffesse, "Clinical effects of chlorhexidine mouthwashes on patients undergoing orthodontic treatment," *American Journal of Orthodontics and Dentofacial Orthopedics*, vol. 111, no. 6, pp. 606–612, 1997.

[93] K. W. Albertsson, A. Persson, and J. W. V. van Dijken, "Effect of essential oils containing and alcohol-free chlorhexidine mouthrinses on cariogenic micro-organisms in human saliva," *Acta Odontologica Scandinavica*, vol. 71, no. 3-4, pp. 883–891, 2013.

[94] R. Attin, E. Yetkiner, A. Aykut-Yetkiner, M. Knösel, and T. Attin, "Effect of chlorhexidine varnish application on *Streptoococcus mutans* colonisation in adolescents with fixed orthodontic appliances," *Australian Orthodontic Journal*, vol. 29, no. 1, pp. 52–57, 2013.

[95] O. Baygin, T. Tuzuner, M.-B. Ozel, and O. Bostanoglu, "Comparison of combined application treatment with one-visit varnish treatments in an orthodontic population," *Medicina Oral, Patologia Oral y Cirugia Bucal*, vol. 18, no. 2, pp. e362–e370, 2013.

[96] P. V. P. Oltramari-Navarro, J. M. Titarelli, J. A. Marsicano et al., "Effectiveness of 0.50% and 0.75% chlorhexidine dentifrices in orthodontic patients: a double-blind and randomized controlled trial," *American Journal of Orthodontics and Dentofacial Orthopedics*, vol. 136, no. 5, pp. 651–656, 2009.

[97] C.-P. Ernst, K. Prockl, and B. Willershausen, "The effectiveness and side effects of 0.1% and 0.2% chlorhexidine mouthrinses: a clinical study," *Quintessence International*, vol. 29, no. 7, pp. 443–448, 1998.

[98] K. P. K. Olympio, P. A. P. Bardal, J. R. D. M. Bastos, and M. A. R. Buzalaf, "Effectiveness of a chlorhexidine dentifrice in orthodontic patients: a randomized-controlled trial," *Journal of Clinical Periodontology*, vol. 33, no. 6, pp. 421–426, 2006.

Permissions

All chapters in this book were first published in IJD, by Hindawi Publishing Corporation; hereby published with permission under the Creative Commons Attribution License or equivalent. Every chapter published in this book has been scrutinized by our experts. Their significance has been extensively debated. The topics covered herein carry significant findings which will fuel the growth of the discipline. They may even be implemented as practical applications or may be referred to as a beginning point for another development.

The contributors of this book come from diverse backgrounds, making this book a truly international effort. This book will bring forth new frontiers with its revolutionizing research information and detailed analysis of the nascent developments around the world.

We would like to thank all the contributing authors for lending their expertise to make the book truly unique. They have played a crucial role in the development of this book. Without their invaluable contributions this book wouldn't have been possible. They have made vital efforts to compile up to date information on the varied aspects of this subject to make this book a valuable addition to the collection of many professionals and students.

This book was conceptualized with the vision of imparting up-to-date information and advanced data in this field. To ensure the same, a matchless editorial board was set up. Every individual on the board went through rigorous rounds of assessment to prove their worth. After which they invested a large part of their time researching and compiling the most relevant data for our readers.

The editorial board has been involved in producing this book since its inception. They have spent rigorous hours researching and exploring the diverse topics which have resulted in the successful publishing of this book. They have passed on their knowledge of decades through this book. To expedite this challenging task, the publisher supported the team at every step. A small team of assistant editors was also appointed to further simplify the editing procedure and attain best results for the readers.

Apart from the editorial board, the designing team has also invested a significant amount of their time in understanding the subject and creating the most relevant covers. They scrutinized every image to scout for the most suitable representation of the subject and create an appropriate cover for the book.

The publishing team has been an ardent support to the editorial, designing and production team. Their endless efforts to recruit the best for this project, has resulted in the accomplishment of this book. They are a veteran in the field of academics and their pool of knowledge is as vast as their experience in printing. Their expertise and guidance has proved useful at every step. Their uncompromising quality standards have made this book an exceptional effort. Their encouragement from time to time has been an inspiration for everyone.

The publisher and the editorial board hope that this book will prove to be a valuable piece of knowledge for researchers, students, practitioners and scholars across the globe.

List of Contributors

Ochiba Mohammed Lukandu and Lionel Sang Koech
Department of Maxillofacial Surgery, Oral Medicine, Pathology and Radiology, School of Dentistry, Moi University, P.O. Box 4606, Eldoret 30100, Kenya

Paul Ngugi Kiarie
Department of Oral Biology, Anatomy, Physiology and Biochemistry, School of Dentistry, Moi University, P.O. Box 4606, Eldoret 30100, Kenya

Shipra Singh, Rajni Nagpal and Shashi Prabha Tyagi
Department of Conservative Dentistry and Endodontics, Kothiwal Dental College and Research Centre, Moradabad 244001, India

Naveen Manuja
Department of Pediatric Dentistry, Kothiwal Dental College and Research Centre, Moradabad 244001, India

G. Lo Giudice, G. Iannello, A. Terranova, R. Lo Giudice and G. Pantaleo
Medical Sciences and Stomatology Department, School of Dentistry, University of Messina, Via Consolare Valeria, 98100 Messina, Italy

M. Cicciù
Human Pathology Department, School of Dentistry, University of Messina, Via Consolare Valeria, 98100 Messina, Italy

Ranya F. Elemam
Department of Restorative Dentistry and Periodontology, School of Dentistry, Libyan International Medical University (LIMU), Benghazi, Libya
University of Porto, Porto, Portugal

Ziad Salim AbdulMajid
Department of Restorative Dentistry and Periodontology, School of Dentistry, Libyan International Medical University (LIMU), Benghazi, Libya

Matt Groesbeck
Salt Lake City, UT, USA

Álvaro F. Azevedo
Faculty of Dentistry, EPIUNIT-ISPUP, University of Porto, Porto, Portugal

Shariq Najeeb
Restorative Dental Sciences, Al-Farabi Colleges, King Abdullah Road, P.O. Box 85184, Riyadh 11891, Saudi Arabia

Zohaib Khurshid
School of Metallurgy and Materials, University of Birmingham, Edgbaston, Birmingham B15 2TT, UK

Jukka Pekka Matinlinna
Dental Materials Science, Faculty of Dentistry,The University of Hong Kong, 4/F,The Prince Philip Dental Hospital, 34 Hospital Road, Sai Ying Pun, Hong Kong

Fahad Siddiqui
Division of Oral Health & Society, 2001 McGill College, Suite 500, Montreal, QC, Canada H3A 1G1

Mohammad Zakaria Nassani
Restorative Dental Sciences, Al-Farabi Colleges, King Abdullah Road, P.O. Box 85184, Riyadh 11891, Saudi Arabia

Kusai Baroudi
Preventive Dental Sciences, Al-Farabi Colleges, King Abdullah Road, P.O. Box 85184, Riyadh 11891, Saudi Arabia

P. Santiago-Medina and N. Diffoot-Carlo
Department of Biology, University of Puerto Rico, Mayaguez, PR 00680, USA

P. A. Sundaram
Department of Mechanical Engineering, University of Puerto Rico, Mayaguez, PR 00680, USA

T. Malarkodi and S. Sathasivasubramanian
Department of Oral Medicine & Radiology, Faculty of Dental Sciences, Sri Ramachandra University, Porur, Chennai 600116, India

P. Diogo, P. Palma and J.M. Santos
Faculty of Medicine, University of Coimbra (FMUC), Avenida Bissaya Barreto, 3000-075 Coimbra, Portugal

T. Gonçalves
Faculty of Medicine, University of Coimbra (FMUC), Avenida Bissaya Barreto, 3000-075 Coimbra, Portugal

Centre for Neuroscience and Cell Biology (CNC), University of Coimbra, Coimbra, Portugal

Joao Carames
Faculty of Dental Medicine at the University of Lisbon, Lisbon, Portugal

Loana Tovar Suinaga, Yung Cheng Paul Yu, Alejandro Pérez and Mary Kang
Ashman Department of Periodontology and Implant Dentistry, New York University College of Dentistry, 345 East 24th Street, Suite 3W, New York, NY 10010, USA

Zahra Heidari, Hamidreza Mahmoudzadeh-Sagheb and Bita Moudi
Infectious Diseases and Tropical Medicine Research Center, Zahedan University of Medical Sciences, Zahedan 98167-43175, Iran
Department of Histology, School of Medicine, Zahedan University of Medical Sciences, Zahedan 98167-43175, Iran

Mohammad Hashemi
Cellular and Molecular Research Center, Zahedan University of Medical Sciences, Zahedan 98167-43175, Iran
Department of Clinical Biochemistry, School of Medicine, Zahedan University of Medical Sciences and Health Services, Zahedan 98167-43175, Iran

Somayeh Ansarimoghaddam
Department of Periodontology, School of Dentistry, Zahedan University of Medical Sciences, Zahedan 98167-43175, Iran

Nadia Sheibak
Department of Histology, School of Medicine, Zahedan University of Medical Sciences, Zahedan 98167-43175, Iran

Andreas S. Gkogkos, Ioannis K. Karoussis, Ioannis D. Prevezanos, Kleopatra E.Marcopoulou, Kyriaki Kyriakidou, and Ioannis A. Vrotsos
Department of Periodontology, School of Dentistry, University of Athens, 2Thivon Street, Goudi, 115 27 Athens, Greece

M. Daas
Department of Prosthodontics, Ren´e Descartes University, Paris, France
Private Practice, 62 Boulevard de la Tour Maubourg, 75007 Paris, France

A. Assaf
Department of Prosthodontics, Beirut Arab University, Beirut, Lebanon
Department of Prosthodontics, Lebanese University, Beirut, Lebanon

K. Dada
Private Practice, 62 Boulevard de la Tour Maubourg, 75007 Paris, France
Former Clinical Associate, Louis Mournier Hospital, Colombes, France

J.Makzoumé
Department of Removable Prosthodontics, Saint-Joseph University, Beirut, Lebanon

Andreas L. Ioannou, Georgios A. Kotsakis, James E. Hinrichs and Michelle G. McHale
Advanced Education Program in Periodontology, University of Minnesota, 515 Delaware Street SE, Minneapolis, MN 55455, USA

Donald E. Lareau
Advanced Education Program in Periodontology, University of Minnesota, 515 Delaware Street SE, Minneapolis, MN 55455, USA
Private Practice, Edina, MN 55435, USA

Georgios E. Romanos
Department of Periodontology, School of Dental Medicine, Stony Brook, NY 11794, USA

Peter Fairbairn
Department of Periodontology and Implant Dentistry, School of Dentistry, University of Detroit Mercy, 2700 Martin Luther King Jr. Boulevard, Detroit, MI 48208, USA

Minas Leventis
Department of Oral and Maxillofacial Surgery, Dental School, University of Athens, 2Thivon Street, Goudi, 115 27 Athens, Greece

Valiollah Arash, Saeed Javanmard, Zeinab Eftekhari and Manouchehr Rahmati-Kamel
Department of Orthodontics, Faculty of Dentistry, Babol University of Medical Sciences, Babol, Iran
Dental Materials Research Center, Babol University of Medical Sciences, Babol, Iran

Mohammad Bahadoram
Medical Student Research Committee & Social Determinant of Health Research Center, Ahvaz Jundishapur University of Medical Sciences, Ahvaz, Iran

Ahmed Elkhaweldi, Takanori Suzuki and Zev Kaufman
Department of Periodontology and Implant Dentistry, New York University College of Dentistry, 345 East 24th Street, New York City, NY 10010, USA

Carmen Rincon Soler and Rodrigo Cayarga
Universidad Francisco Marroqu´ın, 01010 Guatemala City, Guatemala

Robert G. Hill
Dental Physical Sciences, Barts and The London School of Medicine and Dentistry, Queen Mary University of London (QMUL), London E1 4NS, UK

Xiaohui Chen
School of Dentistry, The University of Manchester, Manchester M13 9PL, UK

David G. Gillam
Centre for AdultOralHealth, Barts andThe London School of Medicine andDentistry,QueenMary University of London (QMUL), London E1 2AD, UK

Akshaya Srikanth Bhagavathula
Department of Clinical Pharmacy, University of Gondar, College of Medicine and Health Sciences, School of Pharmacy, Gondar, Ethiopia

Nazrin Bin Zakaria and Shazia Qasim Jamshed
Department of Pharmacy Practice, Kulliyyah of Pharmacy, International Islamic University Malaysia, Kuantan, Pahang, Malaysia

Maryam Paknahad
Oral Radiology Department, Dental School, Shiraz University of Medical Sciences, Shiraz 7145613466, Iran
Prevention of Oral and Dental Disease Research Center, Dental School, Shiraz University of Medical Sciences, Shiraz 7145613466, Iran

Shoaleh Shahidi, Shiva Iranpour and SabahMirhadi
Oral Radiology Department, Dental School, Shiraz University of Medical Sciences, Shiraz 7145613466, Iran

Majid Paknahad
Radiology Department, Medical School, Shiraz University of Medical Sciences, Shiraz 7145613466, Iran

Tamanna Tiwari, Judith Albino and Terrence S. Batliner
Centers for American Indian and Alaska Native Health, Colorado School of Public Health, University of Colorado Anschutz Medical Campus, Aurora, CO 80045, USA

Mohammad E. Rokaya
Department of Endodontics, Faculty of Dentistry, Al-Azhar University, Assiut, Egypt

Khaled Beshr and Samah Samir Pedir
Department of Restorative Dental Sciences, Al-Farabi Colleges, Riyadh, Saudi Arabia

Abeer HashemMahram
Department of Restorative Dental Sciences, Al-Farabi Colleges, Riyadh, Saudi Arabia
Department of Endodontics, Faculty of Dentistry, Ain Shams University, Cairo, Egypt

Kusai Baroudi
Department of Preventive Dental Sciences, Al-Farabi Colleges, Riyadh, Saudi Arabia

Amanpreet Singh Natt, Amandeep Kaur Sekhon, SudhirMunjal, Rohit Duggal, Anup Holla, Prahlad Gupta, Piyush Gandhi and Sahil Sarin
Dasmesh Institute of Research and Dental Sciences, Faridkot, Punjab, India

Antoine Hanna and Joseph G. Ghafari
Division of Orthodontics and Dentofacial Orthopedics, Department of Otolaryngology/Head and Neck Surgery, American University of Beirut Medical Center, Beirut, Lebanon

Monique Chaaya, Khalil El Asmar and Miran Jaffa
Department of Epidemiology and Population Health, Faculty of Health Sciences, American University of Beirut, Beirut, Lebanon

Celine Moukarzel
Private Practice, Beirut, Lebanon

Atsushi Kameyama
Department of Endodontics and Clinical Cariology, Tokyo Dental College, Tokyo, Japan
Division of General Dentistry, Tokyo Dental College Chiba Hospital, Chiba, Japan

Kurumi Ishii and Chihiro Tatsuta
Tokyo Dental College School of Dental Hygiene, Chiba, Japan

Sachiyo Tomita
Department of Periodontology, Tokyo Dental College, Tokyo, Japan

Toshiko Sugiyama, Toshiyuki Takahashi and Masatake Tsunoda
Division of General Dentistry, Tokyo Dental College Chiba Hospital, Chiba, Japan

Yoichi Ishizuka
Department of Epidemiology and Public Health, Tokyo Dental College, Tokyo, Japan

Melissa H. X. Tan, Robert G. Hill and Paul Anderson
Centre for Oral Growth and Development, Barts and The London School of Medicine and Dentistry, Unit of Dental Physical Sciences, Queen Mary University of London, Mile End Road, London E1 4NS, UK

Andrea Enrico Borgonovo
School of Oral Surgery, University of Milan, Department of Oral Rehabilitation, Istituto Stomatologico Italiano, 20122 Milan, Italy

Rachele Censi
Department of Implantology and Periodontology, Istituto Stomatologico Italiano, 20122 Milan, Italy

Virna Vavassori
School of Oral Surgery, University of Milan, Department of Oral Rehabilitation, Istituto Stomatologico Italiano, 20122 Milan, Italy

Oscar Arnaboldi and CarloMaiorana
Department of Implantology, Dental Clinic, Fondazione IRCCS C`a Granda Ospedale Maggiore Policlinico, School of Oral surgery, University of Milan, 20122 Milan, Italy

Dino Re
Head Department of Oral Rehabilitation, Istituto Stomatologico Italiano, 20122 Milan, Italy

Song Yi Lin, YowMimi and Chew Ming Tak
National Dental Centre Singapore, 5 Second Hospital Avenue, Singapore 168938

Foong KelvinWeng Chiong
Faculty of Dentistry, National University of Singapore, 11 Lower Kent Ridge Road, Singapore 119083

WongHung Chew
Yong Loo Lin School of Medicine, National University of Singapore, 1E Kent Ridge Road, NUHS Tower Block, Level 11, Singapore 119228

Gong Zhang, Hai Yuan, Xianshuai Chen, Weijun Wang and Jimin Liang
Guangzhou Institute of Advanced Technology, Chinese Academy of Sciences, Guangzhou 511458, China

Jianyu Chen
Hospital of Stomatology, Sun Yat-sen University Hospital, Guangzhou 510000, China

Peng Zhang
Foshan Stomatology Hospital, Foshan 528000, China

Hooman Khorshidi and Saeed Raoofi
Department of Periodontology, School of Dentistry, Shiraz University of Medical Sciences, Shiraz, Iran

Rafat Bagheri
Department of Dental Materials, School of Dentistry, Shiraz University of Medical Sciences, Shiraz, Iran

Hodasadat Banihashemi
Periodontology Department, Faculty of Dentistry, Shahid Sadoughi University of Medical Sciences, Yazd, Iran

Enric Jané-Salas, Beatríz González-Navarro, Aura Font-Muñoz Albert, Estrugo Devesa and Jose López-López
School of Dentistry, University of Barcelona, Pabell´on de Gobierno, University Campus of Bellvitge, C/Feixa Llarga s/n, L'Hospitalet de Llobregat, 08907 Barcelona, Spain

Rui Albuquerque
School of Dentistry, University of Birmingham, St. Chads Queensway, Birmingham B4 6NN, UK

Angelina Gorbunkova, Giorgio Pagni, Anna Brizhak, Giampietro Farronato and Giulio Rasperini
Department of Biomedical, Surgical and Dental Sciences, University of Milan, Milan, Italy
UOC Maxillofacial and Dental Surgery, Foundation IRCCS Ca' Granda Polyclinic, 20142 Milan, Italy

www.ingramcontent.com/pod-product-compliance
Lightning Source LLC
Chambersburg PA
CBHW080459200326
41458CB00012B/4031